Attachment and Bonding

Report of the 92nd Dahlem Workshop on
Attachment and Bonding
Berlin, September 28 to October 3, 2003

Held and published on behalf of the President, Freie Universität Berlin

Scientific Advisory Board: H. Keupp and R. Tauber, Chairpersons
                                  N. S. Baer, G. Braun, P. J. Crutzen,
                                  E. Fischer-Lichte, F. Hucho, K. Labitzke,
                                  R. Menzel, J. Renn, H.-H. Ropers,
                                  E. Sandschneider, M. Schäfer-Korting,
                                  L. Wöste

Executive Director: W. de Vivanco

Program Director, Series Editor: J. Lupp

Assistant Editors: C. Rued-Engel, G. Custance

Goals for this Dahlem Workshop
To explore the integrative nature of attachment and bonding from different
scientific perspectives, with a focus on human behavior and mental health.

Attachment and Bonding
A New Synthesis

edited by

C. S. Carter, L. Ahnert, K. E. Grossmann, S. B. Hrdy,
M. E. Lamb, S. W. Porges, and N. Sachser

Program Advisory Committee:

C. S. Carter, and L. Ahnert, Chairpersons
K. E. Grossmann, S. B. Hrdy,
M. E. Lamb, S. W. Porges, and N. Sachser

The MIT Press
Cambridge, Massachusetts
London, England

in cooperation with Dahlem University Press

This book was set in Times New Roman by BerlinScienceWorks.

Dahlem Workshop on Attachment and Bonding: A New Synthesis (92nd : 2003 : Berlin, Germany)

Library of Congress Cataloging-in-Publication Data
Attachment and bonding : a new synthesis / edited by C.S. Carter ... [et al.] ; program advisory committee, C.S. Carter ... [et al.].
   p. cm. — (Dahlem workshop reports)
Includes bibliographical references and indexes.
ISBN: 978-0-262-03348-0 (hc. alk. paper)—978-0-262-52854-2 (pb.)
   1. Attachment behavior—Congresses. I. Carter, Carol Sue, 1944– II. Series.

BF575.A86A775 2005
155.42′28—dc22

                                               2005047190

The MIT Press is pleased to keep this title available in print by manufacturing single copies, on demand, via digital printing technology.

Contents

The Dahlem Workshops

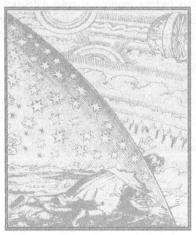

History

During the last half of the twentieth century, specialization in science greatly increased in response to advances achieved in technology and methodology. This trend, although positive in many respects, created barriers between disciplines and could have inhibited progress if left unchecked. Understanding the concepts and methodologies of related disciplines became a necessity. Reuniting the disciplines to obtain a broader view of an issue became imperative, for problems rarely fall conveniently into the purview of a single scientific area. Interdisciplinary communication and innovative problem solving within a conducive environment were perceived as integral yet lacking to this process.

In 1971, an initiative to create such an environment began within Germany's scientific community. In discussions between the *Deutsche Forschungsgemeinschaft* (German Science Foundation) and the *Stifterverband für die Deutsche Wissenschaft* (Association for the Promotion of Science Research in Germany), researchers were consulted to compare the needs of the scientific community with existing approaches. It became apparent that something new was required: an approach that began with state-of-the-art knowledge and proceeded onward to challenge the boundaries of current understanding; a form truly interdisciplinary in its problem-solving approach.

As a result, the *Stifterverband* established *Dahlem Konferenzen* (the Dahlem Workshops) in cooperation with the *Deutsche Forschungsgemeinschaft* in 1974. Silke Bernhard, formerly associated with the Schering Symposia, was

Figure adapted from *L'Atmosphère: Météorologie Populaire*, Camille Flammarion. Paris: Librairie Hachette et Cie., 1888.

engaged to lead the conference team and was instrumental in implementing this unique approach.

The Dahlem Workshops take their name from a district of Berlin known for its strong historic connections to science. In the early 1900s, Dahlem was the seat of the Kaiser Wilhelm Institutes where, for example, Albert Einstein, Lise Meitner, Fritz Haber, and Otto Hahn conducted their research. Today the district is home to several Max Planck Institutes, the *Freie Universität Berlin*, the *Wissenschaftskolleg*, and the Konrad Zuse Center.

In its formative years, the Dahlem Workshops evolved in response to the needs of science. They soon became firmly embedded within the international scientific community and were recognized as an indispensable tool for advancement in research. To secure its long-term institutional stability, *Dahlem Konferenzen* was integrated into the *Freie Universität Berlin* in 1990.

Aim

The aim of the Dahlem Workshops is to promote an international, interdisciplinary exchange of scientific information and ideas, to stimulate international cooperation in research, and to develop and test new models conducive to more effective communication between scientists.

Concept

The Dahlem Workshops were conceived to be more than just another a conference venue. Anchored within the philosophy of scientific enquiry, the Dahlem Workshops represent an independently driven quest for knowledge: one created, nurtured, and carefully guided by representatives of the scientific community itself. Each Dahlem Workshop is an interdisciplinary communication process aimed at expanding the boundaries of current knowledge. This dynamic process, which spans more than two years, gives researchers the opportunity to address problems that are of high-priority interest, in an effort to identify gaps in knowledge, to pose questions aimed at directing future inquiry, and to suggest innovative ways of approaching controversial issues. The overall goal is not necessarily to exact consensus but to search for new perspectives, for these will help direct the international research agenda.

Governance

The Dahlem Workshops are guided by the Scientific Advisory Board, composed of representatives from the international scientific community. The board is responsible for the scientific content and future directions of the Dahlem Workshops and meets biannually to review and approve all workshop proposals.

Workshop Topics

Workshop topics are problem-oriented, interdisciplinary by nature, of high-priority interest to the disciplines involved, and timely to the advancement of science. Scientists who submit workshop proposals, and chair the workshops, are internationally recognized experts active in their field.

Program Advisory Committee

Once a proposal has been approved, a Program Advisory Committee is formed for each workshop. Composed of 6–7 scientists representing the various scientific disciplines involved, the committee meets approximately one year before the Dahlem Workshop to develop the scientific program of the meeting. The committee selects the invitees, determines the topics that will be covered by the pre-workshop papers, and assigns each participant a specific role. Participants are invited on the basis of their international scientific reputation alone. The integration of young German scientists is promoted through special invitations.

Dahlem Workshop Model

A Dahlem Workshop can best be envisioned as a week-long intellectual retreat. Participation is strictly limited to forty participants to optimize the interaction and communication process.

Participants work in four interdisciplinary discussion groups, each organized around one of four key questions. There are no lectures or formal presentations at a Dahlem Workshop. Instead, concentrated discussion — within and between groups — is the means by which maximum communication is achieved.

To enable such an exchange, participants must come prepared to the workshop. This is facilitated through a carefully coordinated pre-workshop dialog: Discussion themes are presented through "background papers," which review a particular aspect of the group's topic and introduce controversies as well as unresolved problem areas for discussion. These papers are circulated in advance, and everyone is requested to submit comments and questions, which are then compiled and distributed. By the time everyone arrives in Berlin, issues have been presented, questions have been raised, and the Dahlem Workshop is ready to start.

Discussion takes place in moderated sessions as well as through informal interactions. Cross-fertilization between groups is both stressed and encouraged. By the end of the week, through a collective effort directed by a rapporteur, each group has prepared a draft report of the ideas, opinions, and contentious issues raised by the group. Directions for future research are highlighted, as are problem areas still in need of resolution. On the final day, the results of the draft reports are discussed in a plenary session, to which colleagues from the Berlin–Brandenburg area are invited.

Dahlem Workshop Reports

After the workshop, attention is directed toward the necessity of communicating the results of the workshop to a wider audience. A two-tier review process guides the revision of the background papers, and discussion continues to finalize the group reports. The chapters are carefully edited to highlight the perspectives, controversies, gaps in knowledge, and proposed research directions.

The publication of the workshop results in book form completes the process of a Dahlem Workshop, as it turns over the insights gained to the broad scientific community for consideration and implementation. Each volume in the Dahlem Workshop Report series contains the revised background papers and group reports as well as an introduction to the workshop themes. The series is published in partnership with The MIT Press.

Julia Lupp, Program Director and Series Editor
Dahlem Konferenzen der Freien Universität Berlin
Thielallee 50, 14195 Berlin, Germany

List of Participants

Lieselotte Ahnert Fachbereich Erziehungswissenschaft und Psychologie, Freie Universität Berlin, 14195 Berlin, Germany
Early social and emotional development in humans in different contexts, including homes and child care centers

Gustl Anzenberger Department of Anthropology, University of Zurich, Winterthurerstr. 190, 8057 Zurich, Switzerland
Monogamy in nonhuman primates; proximate causes of behavior, especially motivation and hormones

Jay Belsky Institute for the Study of Children, Families and Social Issues, Birkbeck, University of London, 7 Bedford Square, London WC1B 3RA, U.K.
Child development; infant–parent attachment; parenting; evolutionary psychology

Katharina Braun Department of Zoology and Developmental Neurobiology, Faculty for Natural Sciences, Otto-von-Guericke-University of Magdeburg, Brenneckestr. 6, 39118 Magdeburg, Germany
Identification and characterization of cellular principles, including their neurochemical and molecular mechanisms, which underlie learning- and experience-driven development of the limbic brain circuits

C. Sue Carter Brain–Body Center, Department of Psychiatry, University of Illinois at Chicago, 1601 W. Taylor St., Chicago, IL 60612, U.S.A.
Behavioral endocrinology; biological basis of social support

Patricia Draper Department of Anthropology and Geography, University of Nebraska, 126 Bessy Hall, Lincoln, NE 68588, U.S.A.
Cross-cultural childhood; adult development and aging; evolutionary ecology; intergenerational relations

Alison S. Fleming Department of Psychology, University of Toronto at Mississauga, 3359 Mississauga Road North, Mississauga, Ontario L5L 1C6, Canada
Psychobiology of maternal behavior, psychneuroendocrinology, developmental neurobiology

Karin Grossmann Institut für Psychologie, Universität Regensburg, Universitätsstr. 31, 93040 Regensburg, Germany
Attachment development across the lifespan; father–child attachment relationship; cross-cultural universalities of attachment development; applied attachment theory

Klaus E. Grossmann Institut für Psychologie, Universität Regensburg, Universitätsstr. 31, 93040 Regensburg, Germany
Attachment; development; comparative psychology

Megan R. Gunnar Institute of Child Development, University of Minnesota, 51 East River Road, Minneapolis, MN 55455, U.S.A.
Neuroendocrinology, stress, relationships, temperament

Markus Heinrichs   Department of Clinical Psychology, University of Zurich, Zürichsbergstr. 43, 8044 Zurich, Switzerland
Psychoneuroendocrinology of social interaction; psychoneuroendocrinology of stress protection; oxytocin and behavior

Kate Hennighausen   Family Pathways Project, Harvard Medical School, 120 Beacon St., Somerville, MA 02143, U.S.A.
Identification of early predictors of childhood psychopathology

Michael B. Hennessy   Department of Psychology, 335 Fawcett Hall, Wright State University, Dayton, OH 45435, U.S.A.
Developmental psychology; early stress; attachment

Sarah B. Hrdy   Citrona Farms, 21440 Road 87, Winters, CA 95694, U.S.A.
Primatology, anthropology, sociobiology

Heidi Keller   Entwicklung und Kultur, Universität Osnabrück, Seminarstr. 20, 49069 Osnabrück, Germany
Evolutionary psychology; cultural psychology; interplay between culture, biology, and development

E. Barry Keverne   Animal Behaviour Department, University of Cambridge, Madingley, Cambridge CB3 8AA, U.K.
Brain and behavior

Gisela Klann-Delius   Institut für Deutsche Philologie, Freie Universität Berlin, Habelschwerdter Allee 45, 14195 Berlin, Germany
Language acquisition in securely and insecurely attached children; internal state language and theory of mind in Japanese, Turkish, and German toddlers; socio-emotional aspects of lexical acquisition and their neurophysiological correlates

Gary W. Kraemer   Department of Psychology, University of Toronto at Mississauga, 3359 Mississauga Road North, Mississauga ON L5L 1C6, Canada
Developmental psychobiology; attachment; neural plasticity

Michael E. Lamb   Department of Social and Developmental Psychology, Faculty of Social and Political Sciences, Cambridge University, Free School Lane, Cambridge CB2 3RQ, U.K.
The development and significance of relationships with parents and other care providers; effects of diverse patterns of care; cultural variation in child care and rearing; implications of attachment theory for forensic contexts; forensic interviewing

James F. Leckman   I-267 Sterling Hall of Medicine, Child Study Center, Yale University School of Medicine, 230 South Frontage Road, New Haven, CT 06520–7900, U.S.A.
Genes and environment; evolutionary perspectives on human psychopathology; early parental preoccupations and harm avoidant behavior and its relationship to obsessive-compulsive disorder

Giovanni A. Liotti Associazione Psicologia Cognitiva, Viale Castro Pretorio 116, 00185 Rome, Italy
Disorganized attachment as risk factor for borderline and dissociative disorders: implications for etiology and therapy; interactions between attachment and other inborn behavioral systems in the regulation of interpersonal behavior: implications for the therapeutic relationship

Karlen Lyons-Ruth Department of Psychiatry, Harvard Medical School, Cambridge Hospital, 1493 Cambridge Street, Cambridge, MA 02139, U.S.A.
Identification of early predictors of childhood psychopathology, including genetic factors, parent–child interactive processes, and disorganized attachment strategies; exploration of efficacy of early intervention

Gunther Meinlschmidt Department of Psychobiology, Division of Clinical and Theoretical Psychobiology, University of Trier, Johanniter Ufer 15, 54290 Trier, Germany
Long-term psychological consequences of early life experiences; stress protection and stress-related illnesses; clinical psychology and psychotherapy

Thomas G. O'Connor Department of Psychiatry, University of Rochester Medical Center, 300 Crittenden Blvd., Rochester, NY 14642, U.S.A.
Attachment, behavioral genetics, early experience and long-term development

Cort A. Pedersen Department of Psychiatry, CB #7160, University of North Carolina, Chapel Hill, NC 27599–7160, U.S.A.
Behavioral neuroendocrinology; biological psychiatry

Stephen W. Porges Brain–Body Center, Department of Psychiatry, University of Illinois at Chicago, 1601 W. Taylor St., Chicago, IL 60612, U.S.A.
Human neurobiology and development; neural regulation of the autonomic nervous system; developmental psychophysiology

Norbert Sachser Department of Behavioural Biology, University of Münster, Badestr. 9, 48149 Münster, Germany
Behavioral biology, stress and welfare, behavioral endocrinology, mammalian social systems

Axel Schölmerich Fakultät für Psychologie, Entwicklungspsychologie, Ruhr-Universität Bochum, 44780 Bochum, Germany
Emotional regulation and reactivity; cultural factors in human development

Carsten Schradin Eco-physiological Studies Research Group, School of Animal, Plant and Environmental Sciences, University of the Witwatersrand, Private Bag 3, Wits 2050, Johannesburg, South Africa
Integrative approach to paternal care with the striped mouse as a model species; social flexibility; ulitmate and proximate causes of group living

Simone Sommer Zoologisches Institut und Zoologisches Museum, Universität Hamburg, Martin-Luther-King Platz 3, 20146 Hamburg, Germany
Ecological basis for the evolution and maintenance of monogamous social and mating systems; the role of major histocompatibility complex genes in mate choice, inbreeding avoidance and parasite resistance; effects of mating systems on the genetic variability of mammals

Gottfried Spangler Institut für Psychologie, Universität Erlangen-Nürnberg, Bismarckstr. 6/11, 91054 Erlangen, Germany
Attachment development, psychobiology of attachment; the role of individual disposition, normative development of the inner working model of attachment

Miriam Steele Anna Freud Centre, 21 Maresfield Gardens, London NW3 53D, U.K. and Department of Psychology, New School for Social Research, 65 Fifth Ave., New York, NY 10003, U.S.A.
Intergenerational patterns of attachment; clinical applications of attachment theory and research; adoption and foster care

Ross A. Thompson Department of Psychology, University of California, One Shields Ave., 279 Young Hall, Davis, CA 95616, U.S.A.
Early emotional, moral, and sociopersonality development; parent–child relationships; developmental science and public policy

Dietrich P. Tietze Institut für Kleinkindpädagogik, Freie Universität Berlin, Takustr. 4, 14195 Berlin, Germany
Early childhood education and care: quality and long-term effects

Dietrich Todt Institut für Biologie, Verhaltensbiologie, Freie Universität Berlin, Haderslebener Str. 9, 12163 Berlin, Germany
Early socialization; bonding in birds; vocal communication; social intelligence; behavioral processes; development of signal repertoires; social model learning

Colwyn Trevarthen Department of Psychology, University of Edinburgh, 7 George Square, Edinburgh, EH8 9JZ, Scotland, U.K.
Development of mutual awareness between child and others by sympathetic communication; the psychobiology of companionship in shared experience — the adaptive goal of attachment; rhythms and expressive forms of body movement; "communicative musicality" and the acoustic analysis of rhythmic and melodic patterns in teachers' talk and in music therapy; moral emotions and the acquisition of cultural skills, including language

Eckart Voland Zentrum für Philosophie und Grundlagen der Wissenschaft der Justus-Liebig-Universität, Otto-Behaghel-Str. 10/C1 II. OG, 35394 Giessen, Germany
Differential parental investment; reproductive strategies; behavioral ecology; sociobiology; evolutionary anthropology

Dietrich von Holst Lehrstuhl für Tierphysiologie, Universität Bayreuth, Gebäude, NW I, 95440 Bayreuth, Germany
Ethoendocrinology; psychoimmunology; social stress; pair bonding; population biology: behavior of mammals

Sheila Wang The Judith Nan Miller Integrative Medicine Initiative, Children's Memorial Hospital, 2300 Children's Plaza, Box 73, Chicago, IL 60614, U.S.A.
Psychoendocrinology, attachment behavior, hormonal and autonomic regulation of emotions

Larry J. Young Yerkes Research Center, Emory University, 954 Gatewood Rd., Atlanta, GA 30322, U.S.A.
Molecular, cellular, and neurobiological mechanisms underlying social attachment

1

Introduction

C. S. CARTER and L. AHNERT, Chairpersons

K. E. GROSSMANN, S. B. HRDY, M. E. LAMB, S. W. PORGES,

and N. SACHSER, Program Advisory Committee

Snow is rare in Berlin in late March, and it was an unexpected six inches of snow that stranded Sue Carter (on her way to an international conference) at the Ahnert home. Briefly housebound, they began a discussion that ran late into the night. Both Ahnert and Carter studied something they called "attachment," yet as they talked, it was obvious that their perception of this construct had little in common except for the word. Furthermore, it became apparent that the differences in the way developmental psychologists (such as Ahnert) and behavioral biologists (such as Carter) viewed and studied attachment went well beyond semantics.

This chance occurrence was the first stage of a proposal for a Dahlem Workshop. With the support of Dahlem's Scientific Advisory Board, a program advisory committee (PAC), consisting of Ahnert, Carter, Klaus Grossmann, Stephen Porges, and Norbert Sachser, was convened in 2002 to select the participants for the workshop and refine the scientific scope of the discussion themes. Although unable to attend the PAC, Sarah Hrdy and Michael Lamb contributed to this meeting and helped, as did the other members of the PAC, in the editing of this volume. We are especially grateful to Julia Lupp and the other members of the Dahlem Konferenzen staff (Caroline Rued-Engel, Gloria Custance, Angela Daberkow), who worked tirelessly to make this workshop and volume possible.

The goals of the 92nd Dahlem Workshop (held in Berlin, September 28 to October 3, 2003) were to explore the concepts of attachment and bonding from different scientific perspectives. To our knowledge, this workshop represents the first systematic attempt to bring together scientists with very diverse perspectives on this topic. At the workshop, we sought to initiate a dialog, question assumptions, reveal new directions for research, and to suggest the foundations of a synthesis or consilience[1] (Wilson 1998).

---

[1] As described by E.O. Wilson (1998, p. 8), the term "consilience" was coined by William Whewell in 1840, as a " 'jumping together' of knowledge by the linking of facts and fact-based theory across disciplines to create a common groundwork of explanation."

Attachment, bonding, and related concepts have intrigued and inspired scientists and nonscientists alike and have been at the center of an intellectual maelstrom for several decades. These words — attachment and bonding — and the concepts that they represent have attracted scientists from many disciplines, including anthropology, psychology, psychiatry, pediatrics, neurobiology, endocrinology, and even molecular biology.

It is important at the onset to recognize that both attachment and bonding are hypothetical constructs. No one has ever seen an attachment or a social bond or directly measured their qualities or strengths. As the authors of this volume write about these constructs, we are still struggling to give words to processes that emerged long before modern human cognition. In addition, "attachment" and "bonding" have acquired colloquial meanings within different disciplines. Common to definitions of these words are selective social behaviors or feelings toward another individual. Beyond attempts to define attachment and bonding, most studies, including those summarized here, seek to understand either the causes or the consequences of attachment and bonding, in general, and their different qualities in individual development, in particular.

COMMON THEMES

There was general acceptance at this workshop that attachment and bonding are evolved processes which were once, and in many situations still are, adaptive. The mechanisms that permit the development of selective social bonds are assumed to be very ancient, based on neural circuitry and endocrine processes rooted deep in mammalian evolution (Hrdy; Keverne; Sachser; all this volume), although the nature and timing of these processes, along with their ultimate (evolutionary) and proximate (ontogenetic, epigenetic, and physiological) causes, are only in the earliest stages of being understood. The proximate processes necessary for social bonding tend to be species-typical, shaped by phylogeny and the history of local populations. These same processes, however, can be quite plastic. Within the lifespan of a single individual, ontogenetic and epigenetic processes, including learning and different forms of cognitive and affective experience, can result in much variation between individuals belonging to the same species (Trevarthen, this volume). In particular, physical states of the body involving the status of the central and autonomic nervous system can alter the readiness of an individual to form attachments, and the environment can foster and hinder attachment processes (Porges, this volume).

Humans are highly social creatures, capable of exhibiting and eliciting social interactions as early as the first day of life. From birth onwards, social involvement is essential for normal development (Trevarthen, this volume). In all humans, we can find mechanisms for transmitting social experiences from one generation to the next. The physiological substrates for social bonds are shared with other processes, including those responsible for reproduction and the management of "stress" responses. The shared physiological substrates and shared experiences in turn allow social bonds to influence perceived safety or "psychological security," individual survival, and eventually genetic fitness.

Selective social relationships are not limited to humans and can be found in other highly social species, particularly those that are socially monogamous or which rear offspring cooperatively, so that survival or reproduction depend heavily on social bonds. This fact has facilitated experimental analysis of some proximate mechanisms underlying social bonds using animal models.

A BRIEF HISTORY

Contemporary theories regarding attachment and bonding are generally traced to the twentieth century. John Bowlby, a British psychiatrist trained in Freudian psychoanalysis, did much to delineate the concept of attachment. Strongly influenced by Konrad Lorenz, Niko Tinbergen, and Robert Hinde, Bowlby laid the groundwork for an evolutionary theory of human development. All of Bowlby's mentors were acutely sensitive to the role of early experience in the formation of social systems and social bonds. Bowlby wrote several volumes in which he defined and elaborated the concepts of attachment (1969), separation (1973), and grief at the loss of attachments (1980) and a secure base (1988). He saw attachment in the context of human evolution, and what he called the "environment of evolutionary adaptedness." Bowlby was galvanized by observations of children separated from their mothers, based on his own clinical work, as well as Rene Spitz's earlier studies of children in orphanages (Spitz 1945). Upon separation from their mother (or other consistent caretaker), toddlers tended to show protest, followed by despair and then apparent detachment.

Based on the science of his time, Bowlby created a theoretical framework to explain the dynamic interaction between human infants and their caretakers. Bowlby conceptualized human attachment in complex, multidimensional terms ranging from a cybernetic process to an individual trait (Thompson et al., this volume). Attachment theory specified a hypothetical "attachment system" in the young child. Attachment behaviors were the observable interactions between a child and its caretaker. The attachment relationship was seen as a "bond" shaped by interactions between a child and its primary caretaker. Also influential in the development of attachment theory were the experiments of Harry Harlow (1961), who reared young rhesus monkeys in various conditions of separation, in artificial family situations, on inanimate surrogates as well as in total isolation in "pits of despair." The atypical behaviors of surrogate-reared monkeys and motherless children were more than just strong support for the notion that early experience played a critical role in later social behaviors. When Harlow tried experimentally to see if rejection induces psychopathic behavior, it was John

Bowlby who told him that he had already seen more psychopathy in the single cages than anywhere else on the face of the earth (Blum 2002, p. 214).

ATTACHMENT

Developmental psychologists, working within the context of attachment theory (for details and references, see chapters by Grossmann and Grossmann; Belsky; Ahnert; Thompson et al.; and Kraemer et al.; all this volume), have defined attachment as a "phylogenetically programmed propensity" of one person (usually a child) to bond to another who is viewed as "stronger and wiser." Explicit in attachment theory is the notion that the attachment figure and the affectional bond cannot be replaced by another. In the absence of the security figure and especially as the child grows older, attachment theory posits another hypothetical construct termed the "internal working models" (IWMs). IWMs incorporate both cognitive and affective representations and expections regarding attachment figures. In the terminology of attachment theory, bonds are relatively long-lived ties to unique individuals. However, across the lifespan of the individual, multiple bonds may be formed, broken, and reformed. Also, according to the convention of attachment theory, a child forms one primary attachment to a caretaker (usually the mother) but may have many affectional bonds, including bonds formed by a parent (or other caretakers) for their child, or between two adults (Ahnert, this volume).

Over time, Bowlby's followers, especially Mary Ainsworth, Mary Main, Klaus and Karin Grossmann, and their students, have developed a subfield within developmental psychology — now commonly known as Attachment Theory. Standardized paradigms, with an emphasis on the response of a child to the presence or absence of its primary caretaker, were used to identify individual differences.

Ainsworth (1978) developed the Strange Situation tests, which categorized children based on how they responded to separation and reunion with caretakers, as well as their reactions to strangers. Children were identified as (a) avoidant insecurely-attached, (b) securely-attached, or (c) ambivalent insecurely-attached. Later, Mary Main and colleagues (Main and Solomon 1990) added a fourth category: (d) disorganized, which was used for previously hard to categorize children who displayed contradictory traits that did not fit the other categories or that resulted in a breakdown of organized secure or insecure strategies. They also devised an Adult Attachment Interview (AAI), which is increasingly used to examine the coherence between early measures of attachment and related adult behaviors (Thompson et al., this volume).

The usefulness of attachment classifications to predict social or cognitive response generations is discussed elsewhere in this volume. It has become common to search for relationships between measures of attachment (usually taken in early life) and other behavioral, physiological, or genetic processes (see

Belsky; Grossmann and Grossmann; Hennighausen and Lyons-Ruth; Kraemer et al.; all this volume).

BONDING

Whereas attachment theory focused on the child's response to its mother, another point of view, championed by Marshall Klaus and John Kennell (1982, 1995), emphasized the notion that human mothers were programmed to develop strong bonds with their own infants. Based on observations of the mother–infant dyad, Klaus and Kennell, suggested that the immediate postpartum period was a time of unique emotional sensitivity on the part of the mother to her newborn. Klaus and Kennell's emphasis on the novel capacity of a mother who had recently given birth to "bond" to her offspring was widely accepted and increased the attention on maternal–infant interactions in obstetrics and pediatrics. This theory, however, drew criticism from psychologists, who argued that other caretakers, including fathers and nonrelatives, could also form intense relationships with the newborn and that the social bonds could continue to form well beyond the time of birth (Pedersen et al., this volume).

Of particular value to an understanding of the substrates of social bonding has been the analysis of the selective responses of a mother toward her newborn infant (Fleming; Keverne; Leckman et al.; Pedersen et al.; all this volume). Neuroendocrine processes associated with birth and lactation have also been implicated in maternal behavior and more specifically in filial bonding. Studies of maternal bonding in turn provided clues regarding the neuroendocrine mechanisms necessary for the formation or expression of social bonds between adult animals (Pedersen et al., this volume). Animal research suggests that specific hormones and neurotransmitters, acting on definable (if at present incompletely understood) pathways, play a role in the formation of social bonds. Among the neuropeptide hormones that have been implicated in social bond formation are oxytocin, vasopressin, and corticotropin-releasing factor, all potentially capable of influencing social fear; under optimal conditions, these peptides may facilitate social engagement and other positive social interactions (Carter; Keverne; Porges; Pedersen et al.; all this volume). In addition, the salience of a relationship may be reinforced by neural mechanisms that are shared with reward and pleasure. At the core of the capacity to form selective social bonds are interactions among the above neuropeptides and other systems that rely on dopamine and the endogenous opioids (Fleming; Keverne; Leckman et al.; Pedersen et al., all this volume).

ATTACHMENT AND BONDING: THE SYNTHESIS

Because biologists often work with animal models, they have tended to use the terms *attachment* and *bonding* interchangeably. Positive social behaviors, such as selective approaches or physical contacts, were commonly used to measure attachment or a social bond. Responses to separation and reunion, such as distress vocalizations or attempts to reunite with a partner after separation, were used to determine the presence or absence of a social bond or an attachment. However, it can be difficult to demonstrate that these responses are specific to attachment or bonding. It is important to understand the evolutionary and ecological context in which these responses ordinarily occur. Such background is essential for understanding the neural and endocrine substrates underlying social bonds (Belsky; Carter; Gunnar; Keverne; Sachser; all this volume).

Semantic issues not withstanding, this workshop affirms the notion that social bonds and attachments do exist, although considerable differences between individuals are expected. Some of this variation will be adaptive, and some of it harmful to the individual and thus maladaptive (Kraemer et al., this volume). Under certain circumstances, the capacity or opportunity to engage socially and form social bonds may remain unexpressed or be defectively expressed (Porges; Trevarthen; this volume). The absence of close relationships and social bonds is associated throughout life with various kinds of maladaptive/atypical behaviors or "disorders" (Hennighausen and Lyons-Ruth; Kraemer et al.; Pedersen et al.; Thompson et al.; all this volume). Evidence is mounting that the absence of secure or sensitive infant–caregiver relationships will have impairing consequences for subsequent social behavior and for the capacity to regulate physical and emotional reactions to stressors (Gunnar, this volume). Due to ethical and logistical constraints, however, controlled experiments to test these theories in humans are rare.

So far, attempts to examine the relative contributions of early attachment experiences to emotional reactivity or later patterns of behavior have focused on children exposed to different patterns of childrearing. For example, atypical behavioral responses in some children who have experienced inadequate care or multiple caregivers offer support for the importance of caretaker consistency (Ahnert; Grossmann and Grossmann; Gunnar; Belsky; all this volume). Children raised under conditions of severe emotional deprivation in orphanages where they lacked opportunities to form selective social bonds during early development have provided some of the most extreme examples (O'Connor; Gunnar; this volume). Aberrant or atypical responses in such children have been categorized, but not explained, by the Diagnostic and Statistical Manuel (DSM-IV) of the American Psychiatric Association as "Reactive Attachment Disorder." It has been noted that some, but not all, institutionally reared children, especially those who experienced a pattern of inconsistent caretakers, may show indiscriminate social behaviors, without normal degrees of wariness — a pattern that has been termed "disinhibited disturbance." An alternative, but less common pattern, involves the failure to respond to social interactions and apparently fearful "inhibited" behaviors. Children with either response pattern are also at risk for a variety of other behavioral disorders. Children who have experienced foster care, insensitive parenting, and even maltreatment are also at risk for later psychopathology, but do not typically show disinhibited social behaviors.

These and many other examples leave little doubt that social bonds have consequences for virtually all aspects of behavior. Perceived social bonds may be protective in the face of both emotional and physical challenges. When positive social relationships are not present, either because attachments were not formed or because bonds are broken, the results may include changes in behavior and physiology that are considered "maladaptive" or pathological. The absence of normal social relationships and attachments may increase the risk for mental and physical illness. It is hypothesized that inconsistent early social experiences lead to disturbed relationships in later life. A variety of mental illnesses, such as autism, attention disorders, and depression, are conditions characterized by atypical attachment and bonding. Epidemiological studies suggest that the presence or absence of social bonds are important predictors of speed of recovery and subsequent longevity following illnesses as diverse as cancer and cardiovascular disease.

This volume, which grew out of the 92nd Dahlem Workshop, provides a snapshot of contemporary scientific theories and findings, presented in the form of background papers and the reports of the four discussion groups. Of course one workshop or book cannot unite diverse disciplines, especially in fields with such limited prior interaction. Our larger goal of a "synthesis" among various points of view must be viewed as a work still in progress. However, this volume is an already advanced progress report — one that we hope will encourage readers to engage in the interdisciplinary dialog and enrich the ongoing complex development of our understanding of attachment and bonding.

REFERENCES

Ainsworth, M.D.S., M.C. Blehar, E. Waters, and S. Wall. 1978. Patterns of Attachment: A Psychological Study of the Strange Situation. Hillsdale, NJ: Erlbaum.
Blum, D. 2002. Love at Goon Park: Harry Harlow and the Science of Affection. Cambridge, MA: Perseus.
Bowlby, J. 1969. Attachment. Attachment and Loss, vol. I. New York: Basic.
Bowlby, J. 1973. Separation: Anxiety and Anger. Attachment and Loss, vol. II. New York: Basic.
Bowlby, J. 1980. Loss. Attachment and Loss, vol. III. New York: Basic.
Bowlby, J. 1988. A Secure Base: Parent-Child Attachment and Healthy Human Development. New York: Basic.
Harlow, H.F. 1961. The development of affectional patterns in infant monkeys. In: Determinants of Infant Behavior, ed. B.M. Foss, vol. 1, pp. 75–97. New York: Wiley.
Klaus, M.H., and J.H. Kennell. 1982. Parent–Infant Bonding. St. Louis: Mosby.
Klaus, M.H., J.H. Kennell, and P.H. Klaus. 1995. Bonding. Reading, MA: Addison-Wesley.

Main, M., and J. Solomon. 1990. Procedures for identifying infants as disorganized/disoriented during the Ainsworth Strange Situation. In: Attachment in the Preschool Years: Theory, Research and Intervention, ed. M.T. Greenberg; D. Cicchetti, and E.M. Cummings, pp. 121–160. Chicago: Univ. of Chicago Press.

Spitz, R. 1945. Hospitalism: An inquiry into the genesis of psychiatric conditions in early childhood. *Psychoan. Stud. Child* **1**:53–75.

Wilson, E.O. 1998. Consilience: The Unity of Knowledge. New York: Knopf.

2

Evolutionary Context of Human Development

The Cooperative Breeding Model

S. B. HRDY

Department of Anthropology, University of California,
Davis, CA 95616–8522, U.S.A.

ABSTRACT

According to the Cooperative Breeding Hypothesis, allomaternal assistance was essential for child survival during the Pleistocene. This breeding system — quite novel for an ape — permitted hominid females to produce costly offspring without increasing interbirth intervals, and allowed humans to move into new habitats, eventually expanding out of Africa. Reliance on allomaternal assistance would make maternal commitment more dependent on the mother's perception of probable support from others than is the case in most other primates. One artifact of such conditional maternal investment would be newborns who needed to monitor and engage mothers, as well as older infants and juveniles who needed to elicit care from a range of caretakers across the prolonged period of dependence characteristic of young among cooperative breeders. Implications of this evolutionary context for the sociocognitive and emotional development of infants are explored.

INTRODUCTION: MOVING BEYOND BOWLBY

John Bowlby was the first evolutionary psychologist to explore how selection pressures encountered by our Pleistocene ancestors (what he termed "the environment of evolutionary adaptedness," or EEA) shaped the development of human infants. In a now classic book on attachment, Bowlby (1969) drew on personal and clinical experience with Western childrearing, on such evidence as was then available for hunter–gatherer childrearing as well as for maternal care in other primates — mostly macaques, baboons, and chimps. Based on these sources of information, Bowlby assumed that the mother was the primary, typically exclusive, caretaker in the EEA. In later versions of his book, Bowlby (influenced by Ainsworth and others) mentioned the possibility of multiple caretakers, but he nevertheless continued to center his model on a Victorian division of labor within a pair bond where a sexually monandrous mother nurtured off-spring provisioned by their father. The last quarter century has, however, pro-duced new evidence from primate sociobiology and from the behavioral ecol-ogy of foraging peoples that challenges this exclusive "sex contract" between mother and father as the fundamental economic unit for childrearing among our ancestors. Attention began to focus on assistance from group members other than the genetic parents. In the course of an ongoing — still controversial — par-adigm shift within anthropology, the long-standing ideal of an EEA character-ized by mother–father childrearing units is being replaced with a model based on cooperative breeding (Hrdy 1999).

WHAT IS MEANT BY "COOPERATIVE BREEDING"?

The Study of Cooperative Breeding

From wild dogs to elephants, meerkats, marmosets, acorn woodpeckers, and scrub jays, roughly 3% of mammals, and between 8% and 17% of bird species (Heinsohn and Double 2004) breed cooperatively. The literature on cooperative breeding in vertebrates is divided between studies of birds, of mammals other than primates, and primates except for humans. Although sometimes appropri-ate, this taxonomic compartmentalization has hindered synthetic analyses and led to a confusing array of taxonomically specific definitions for cooperative breeding. Here, I use a broad and simple definition: a breeding system in which group members, other than the genetic parents (alloparents), help one or both parents rear their offspring. Because we rarely know the genetic identity of fa-thers, it is often more accurate to confine the discussion to allomothers, individ-uals of either sex who are not the mother. Note that an allomother can be a male, or even the genetic father. Paternal assistance can be complicated in cases like marmosets or wild dogs where not only does more than one possible "father" help, but several males may actually father young in "multiple paternity" litters. More typically, males with different probabilities of paternity adjust their level of care in line with their past mating history with the mother. For example, male dunnocks calibrate food delivery to nestlings in line with how frequently these birds copulated with the mother during the period when she was last fertile (Davies 1992). Male baboons, whose partners have mated polyandrously with multiple males, intervene preferentially on behalf of older infants and juveniles likely to be their own (Buchan et al. 2003).

Theoretical Explanations

At a general level, the altruism of alloparents is explained by Hamilton's rule: The cost of helping should be less than benefits to offspring calibrated in line with the alloparent's degree of relatedness to his or her charge. Hence alloparents enhance their inclusive fitness by helping kin. Almost certainly, the neural and physiological underpinnings of helpful motivations first evolved in groups of closely related animals. Tendencies that led individuals to invest in unrelated infants at the expense of closely related infants would be selected against. However, there is continuing debate about how important kinship is in maintaining dispositions to help once they have evolved. In particular, complex patterns of migration often mean that male and female helpers are not that closely related, yet with varying levels of commitment, they continue to help.

Cooperative breeding was first studied in social insects and birds, animals without lactation where nonmothers are just as equipped to feed young as mothers are. Struck by how much allomothers were helping in hymenopteran social insects, Hamilton (1964) emphasized the unusually high degree of relatedness between mothers and helpers. His ideas about kin selection have received strong support. For example, cooperatively breeding carrion crows leave their natal groups and then seek out related individuals, preferring to help kin over nonkin. Today most theorists acknowledge that kinship facilitates the evolution of cooperative breeding, even if it is not necessarily essential to maintain helping behaviors in all contexts. Emlen (1997) has played a major role, emphasizing ecological constraints (such as saturated habitats or predation) that discourage relatives from dispersing. Cooperative breeding is especially likely to evolve where inherited resources are critical for reproduction since maturing animals must queue up. Others emphasize the benefits of philopatry (or remaining in the natal territory). Cockburn (1998) provides the most comprehensive, if aviocentric, review of how helpers might benefit from (a) enhanced production of nondescendant kin; (b) payment of "rent" allowing access to the territory or other group benefits in exchange for being allowed to stay; (c) opportunistic access to mating opportunities; (d) building up the territory or group in ways that enhance future breeding opportunities; (e) social advancement or better opportunities to signal quality to prospective mates; (f) buying time to mature or acquire skills within the security of a group.

Hence, even unrelated allomothers may sometimes benefit from caring for infants. For examples, consider the case of help from prereproductives whose own current breeding opportunities are limited. Furthermore, as animals age, and especially as female mammals approach the end of their reproductive careers at menopause, their threshold for helping may decline, while their "donative intent" increases (for langurs, see Hrdy 1977). In contrast, when physical reserves are at a low point, or when risks rise high, alloparents with prospects of breeding in the future may become less altruistic (for meerkats, see Russell et al. 2003). Still, even helpers with energy to spare or post-reproductives with little to lose should prioritize their service depending on the degree of relatedness and especially level of need. The "ideal" allomother's internalized version of Hamilton's rule reads: find infants appealing and help them if you can, so long as cost is not prohibitive and so long as it does not interfere with your own future reproductive career or caring for your own off-spring when you have them.

Ecological and Life-History Outcomes

Cooperative breeding systems tend to be flexible and dynamic. There are often one or more mated pairs, but depending on circumstances, which fluctuate from one habitat to another, and over the course of lifetimes, a breeding female may mate monogamously, polyandrously (i.e., with several males), or polygynously (sharing her mate with other females). Important features of such systems include delayed dispersal by maturing family members or migration into the group by nonreproducing (or only occasionally reproducing) adults who are neverthe-less responsive to maternal and offspring needs. At a physiological level there has to be sufficient phenotypic flexibility so individuals can shift between nonreproductive and reproductive roles. At a cognitive and emotional level, there has to be some prior predisposition among alloparents to respond to signs of infant need. That is, the underlying neural circuitry has to be there in both sexes and in virgin and parous females (see Fleming, this volume).

As a result of such help, usual quantity versus quality life-history tradeoffs constraining maternal decision making no longer pertain. This ecological re-lease permits mothers to produce more, larger, or more closely spaced offspring since the total cost of rearing each offspring to independence can go up without jeopardizing either her own survival or that of her offspring. Furthermore, re-duced opportunity costs from childrearing, along with benefits of group mem-bership, may mean higher rates of maternal survival (e.g., Rowley and Russell 1990). Humans exhibit the broadest range of mating permutations ever reported, produce some of the costliest infants, and have all the characteristics of a coop-erative breeder. Compared to other apes, humans take the longest to mature yet human infants are born after shorter intervals. (It was such observations that led anthropologists to devise the "sex contract" hypothesis in the first place.) Since provisioning by alloparents buffers immatures from starvation, it allows popu-lations to move into and spread throughout new habitats where mothers other-wise would not manage to rear surviving young. *Homo erectus*, which evolved in Africa prior to 1.8 million years ago and quickly spread into Eurasia and the Near East, exemplifies this pattern.

As early as 1966, Hamilton hypothesized that cooperative breeding would permit slower maturation. A strong correlation between cooperative breeding and prolonged dependence has since been documented in birds. In a sample of 261 species of passerines, 217 never bred cooperatively, 10 did so occasionally, while 34 species were frequent cooperative breeders. Average duration of post-fledging nutritional dependence was significantly longer in cooperative species, and up to twice as long in the obligately cooperative (Langen 2000). Langen attributed these extended periods of nutritional dependence to (a) the reduced cost of parenting produced by a division of labor between helpers who continued to feed youngsters and mothers who were able to resume breeding, and (b) the fact that provisioned offspring had less incentive to become independent. Logically, these same factors should also pertain in cooperatively breeding mammals. That is, slow maturation combined with short birth intervals would be feasible in cooperatively breeding species such as marmosets and tamarins, because allomothers (typically adult males) do so much of the heavy lifting and also help provision infants around the time of weaning. This may explain why, when the much smaller size of babies at birth is taken into account, Callitrichids mature at rates almost as slow as those found in humans. Nutritional independence is similarly delayed in other cooperatively breeding mammals, where immatures rely on special "baby foods" provided by allomothers. These include regurgitated meat provided to wolf and wild dog pups. In the case of lions and wild dogs, adults allow weaned but still inexperienced young access at pre-butchered kills, subsidizing long apprenticeships.

Primate Preadaptions for Cooperative Breeding and the Case of Male Primability

Thus far, members of the subfamily Callitrichidae provide the only "textbook" cases of cooperative breeding among primates, where allomothers provision and carry charges as in cooperatively breeding birds. By two weeks after birth, male *Calithrix jacchus* — typically former sexual partners of the mother — carry infants (typically twins) up to 60% of the time. By three weeks, other group members supplement mother's milk by providing small prey, even though the infant will not be weaned until around three months. The more allomaternal assistance available (especially from males), the higher the mother's reproductive success. *Saquinus oedipus* mothers are so dependent on such help that when kept in naturalistic social groups in captivity, mothers abandoned their newborns if allomaternal assistance was not forthcoming (Bardi et al. 2001). Humans are the only other primates so dependent on alloparental asssistance, characterized by situation-dependent levels of maternal commitment and comparably high rates of maternal abandonment (Hrdy 1999).

Even though members of the subfamily Callitrichidae, and perhaps (if I am right) humans, are the only primates classifiable as full-fledged "cooperative breeders," over all, the Order primates is composed of intensely social species. Many primate attributes predispose them to evolve some degree of shared caretaking. Relevant preadaptations for cooperative breeding range from a primate-wide tendency to be attracted to infants, and to protect infants in the group, to strong urges to hold or carry babies. Benefits of remaining in their natal group can be documented in all primates. These include practical advantages such as enhanced knowledge of local resources and protection from predation, as well as social advantages like support from kin. Not surprisingly, the rule of thumb among primates is that those who can remain in their natal troop, do so, thereby enjoying the benefits of social support. Typically it is those who cannot afford to stay who migrate. A main incentive for leaving is female reluctance to breed with males likely to be close kin, the relevant cue being familiarity from an early age. Males denied sexual access, decamp to find groups of unfamiliar females. Where males resist migrating and stay put, females are pressured to leave rather than breed with kin.

For many primates, especially mothers, remaining among matrilineal kin in multigenerational groups offers special benefits. Enhanced social support brings with it improved vigilance, stress reduction, health, and fitness benefits (e.g., von Holst 1986; Heinrichs et al. 2003; Silk et al. 2003; Sachser, this volume), which probably increase maternal survival rates. Kin support is especially important for primiparas around the time of first births, an especially vulnerable time for primates with universally higher rates of infant loss. Not only does the proximity of matrilineal kin enhance social support, but a mother's greater willingness to allow nulliparous daughters access to their younger siblings provides inexperienced daughters who remain nearby greater opportunities to practice and prepare for motherhood (Hrdy 1999, pp. 155–164; Fleming, this volume).

Females in all Old World monkeys and apes, as well as in New World monkeys of both sexes, exhibit a "lust" to touch, inspect, or carry newborns. The limiting factor is the mother's willingness to allow access. In infant-sharing species like langurs (where in both captivity and the wild, females other than the mother carry infants for up to 50% of daylight hours), mothers freely give up infants to group members (typically close kin). Even though shared care is species-typical, infant langurs prefer their mothers (with whom they always spend the night) and complain vociferously at being taken away. By contrast to langurs, mothers in other species, like rhesus macaques or chimps, deny access (Hrdy 1977). (It is interesting to speculate that if Bowlby had selected langurs as his "model primate" rather than rhesus macaques, attachment theory might have unfolded differently.)

Over half of all 175 or so species of primates exhibit some (often rudimentary) form of either biparental care (both mother and father protecting and caring) or shared protection involving allomothers. Such shared care varies from nonexclusive, occasional care (e.g., a male baboon sitting close to an offspring he might have sired, intervening if protection is needed) to care so costly that those providing it temporarily forego opportunities to forage or breed. Among infant-sharing species, shared care frees mothers to forage with the result that they breed at a faster pace (Mitani and Watts 1997).

The level of shared care varies, but underlying neural circuitry for responding to infants (especially signals of vulnerability and need) seems to be universally present. All simian females are attentive to sights and sounds of newborns, and many (especially young females) find newborns magnetically attractive regardless of whether they are related to them. By contrast, many male primates (e.g., chimps or langurs) tend to remain aloof from infants and, even in infant-sharing species, exhibit little interest in holding babies (Hrdy 1977). In species like titi monkeys or marmosets, holding and carrying newborns is a top male priority, and males are predisposed to caretake. Surprisingly, though, even in species of primates which do not normally caretake, males can be primed by experiences to do so, although the threshold for responding to infants is set higher (Hrdy 1999, pp. 211–214). Male primability provides an informative case study.

The most interesting findings involve prolactin-mediated systems (Schradin and Anzenberger 1999; Storey et al. 2000). The first hint that there was a correlation between prolactin levels and male care came from marmosets. This report was initially met with skepticism, partly because prolactin was viewed as a maternal hormone and also because prolactin is involved in stress responses. However the discovery was subsequently replicated using noninvasive techniques. Later still, researchers learned that the rise in prolactin levels was more pronounced among males who had prior caretaking experience (Snowdon 1996).

These were impressive findings, yet it took two decades along with a paradigm shift in the conceptualization of sex roles before researchers asked the same questions about humans. Only then did we learn that men cohabiting with pregnant women and new mothers experience hormonal changes similar to those in cooperatively breeding marmosets (Storey et al. 2000; Fleming et al. 2002; Fleming, this volume). Over the course of a woman's pregnancy, the man's prolactin levels gradually rise. In addition, men exposed to pregnant women and new babies experience a drop in testosterone after birth.

There is little doubt that hormonal changes during pregnancy and lactation are more pronounced in women than men. Except for species with obligate male care, like titi monkeys, female primates are more sensitive to infant appeals and signals than are males. No one is suggesting that fathers are equivalent to mothers, male caretakers the same as female ones. Physiological and sensory thresholds of the two sexes are so different that experimenters use different scales to measure them. The point is: even in animals with low levels of joint caretaking, both sexes can be primed to care. Neither birth, nor even the prospect of giving birth, are prerequisites for nurturing. Virgin females, or males, can be primed to nurture merely by prolonged exposure to infants or pregnant mothers. One possible interpretation is that in our evolutionary past, infants short on care could look to males as well as females to act as a substitute.

WHY HUMANS MUST HAVE EVOLVED AS COOPERATIVE BREEDERS

Humans are costly to produce, mature slowly, and rarely reach nutritional independence before age 18 or older. Even with four-year or longer birth intervals, a hunter–gatherer mother would have a new offspring before her last one became entirely self-sufficient (Kaplan et al. 2000). Assuming roughly 13 million calories to rear a child from infancy to nutritional independence, such outlays exceed what a mother could provide by herself. Among extant foragers, hunting and/or fishing are important sources of protein, but also risky pursuits. Even when men manage to kill a large animal, meat is typically shared with the group at large rather than channeled to a man's own mate and her offspring. For this reason, mothers who exclusively relied on "husbands" took a chance. When fathers die, or defect, have little luck hunting, or when they decide to share what they bring back with the group at large, what kept children from starvation? Part of the answer is that many early humans did starve. But which ones survived?

Availability of Allomothers in Pleistocene Societies

Recently, Hawkes et al. (1998) have focused attention on the role of older matrilineal kin, especially "hardworking" grandmothers studied among Hadza hunter–gatherers in Tanzania. In times of food shortage, children with older matrilineal kin on hand grew better. However, as critical as a grandmother (or great-aunt) might be, how likely were they to be present? The answer is not knowable. At best, such paleontological and archeological evidence as is available can be used in combination with demographic assumptions derived from extant hunter–gatherers, to estimate reasonable demographic profiles for groups under a range of circumstances. Using this methodology, Jeff Kurland and Corey Sparks (pers. comm.) estimate that under conditions of low mortality, a twenty-year-old primipara would have about a 50% chance of having a forty-year-old mother alive to help her. If higher mortality rates are used, this probability drops to 25%. Under both mortality conditions, the chance of a new mother having a five-year older sibling around would be about twice as high as the chance of having a grandmother. The chances of having one or more cousins would be higher still. Mothers would typically be coping with incomplete kinship sets, although deficits in allomaternal assistance could be offset by compensatory behavior on the part of opportunistic strategists (e.g., a grandmother might move to join the daughter who needed her most). The need to expand the number of available "kin" may help explain why classificatory kinship systems are so common, as well as why foragers place so much stock in trade networks and other reciprocal relationships (Wiessner 2002). Wiessner argues that one reason, besides prestige, that a talented hunter would expend effort hunting large game and sharing out the meat (which after all is not the most efficient way to provision his children) is that he thereby influenced the demographic composition and political dispositions of his group. By recruiting group members likely to be both efficient providers and/or generous allomothers, a hunter could thus enhance the survival chances of kin.

The Debate over Residence Patterns

Demographic reconstructions of Pleistocene family life rely on assumptions about residence patterns. Based on a two-pronged set of assumptions, it was long taken for granted that early humans lived patrilocally. First, it was taken as gospel that early humans lived in "male philopatric" associations because, unlike most mammals, the nonhuman Great Apes were assumed to do so. Sons remained near father, brothers, and cousins to form alliances of related males who cooperated to protect their access to resources (including breeding females) in their local area. Second, Murdock's cross-cultural analyses (1967) indicated that 67% of the world's cultures lived patrilocally, so it was assumed that Pleistocene humans did so as well. Fairly obviously, if women were moving away to live among their husband's kin, this severely constrained the availability of matrilineal relatives.

New data, however, suggest that ape females do not necessarily migrate. Based on molecular data, wild chimp "brotherhoods" may be no more closely related than females are. Furthermore, longitudinal observations from Gombe reveal that some females manage to remain in their natal territories (Pusey et al. 1997). In particular, the oldest daughter of a dominant female, who finds herself in a good situation, may remain to inherit her mother's territory along with her social position, backed up by high-ranking male kin in the area. Females thus privileged reach menarche earlier, breed at shorter intervals, and produce offspring more likely to survive. The new rule of thumb for female chimps is best summarized as "those who can, stay; those who can't, leave" (Hrdy 1999). Furthermore, Alvarez (2004) has painstakenly re-examined the original ethnographies used by Murdock (1967) to classify so many foragers as patrilocal. Murdock's criteria were undeniably precise. For example, a society classified as "ambilocal" (or bilocal) had to be one where "residence is optionally established with or near the parents of either the husband or the wife...where neither alternative exceeds the other in actual frequency by a ratio greater than two to one." Still, nowhere in the ethnographies could Alvarez locate the information needed to make such precise determinations. The majority of Murdock's assignments appear to have been based on hunches. Confining her analysis to those foraging societies with sufficient evidence to assign residence patterns confidently, only one-quarter (12 of 48) were patrilocal. Most were bilocal. Because of bride service (where the new husband hunted on behalf of his wife's family for a time), a daughter was likely to remain near her kin until after her first birth. Various strategic maneuvers could increase the availability of kin, even as harsh demographic realities worked to reduce it.

ALLOMOTHERS WERE NOT JUST HELPFUL BUT ESSENTIAL FOR SURVIVAL IN THE PLEISTOCENE

According to family historians, early European mothers with supportive matrilineal kin were less likely to abandon their babies, whereas for contemporary mothers and children, a vast sociological literature attests to the manifold benefits of extended families. Ethnographers, too, have long stressed the usefulness of child minders in non-Western societies (Levine et al. 1996; Tronick et al. 1987; Weisner and Gallimore 1977). It scarcely comes as news that supportive kin are helpful. What is new is the proposition that in societies with high rates of mortality, children without allomothers might be significantly less likely to survive. This is the basis for hypothesizing that alloparental assistance represents an ancient way of life integral to human adaptations in the EEA. Nomadic hunter–gatherer mothers would have confronted dilemmas like those that working mothers face today, except that given high rates of child mortality in the Pleistocene, few mothers without alloparental assistance managed to rear offspring successfully.

Early humans are presumed to have lived at low densities, and the remarkable lack of genetic variation among humans compared to chimps may be due to population crashes and population bottlenecks (although this is not the only interpretation). If early human groups were prone to local extinctions, the most plausible cause would be recurring periods of food shortage. Alternative explanations rely on sources of mortality (warfare or disease) that probably only increased after our numbers did, post-Neolithic. Diseases like malaria, cholera, diarrhea, and tuberculosis did not become big killers until after people adopted sedentary lifestyles and lived at higher densities. Based on what we know about primate mortality from food shortage, immatures — especially those just past weaning — are most susceptible. This would be the age group that benefits most from alloparental assistance. Indeed, data coming in from traditional societies now show that wherever child mortality rates are high, alloparents significantly affect their survival.

The Sibling Factor

One reason why the critical role of allomothers was overlooked was that sociologists studied Western populations with low rates of child mortality. By the end of the 1980s, however, anthropologists influenced by sociobiological studies of animals began to ask if allomaternal assistance mattered for human reproductive success. In a pioneering study, Turke (1988) found a correlation between the availability of allomaternal assistance and increased maternal reproductive success in a matrilineal, matrilocal population living on Ifaluk atoll. On this Pacific island, parents with a daughter to help rear subsequent children had higher reproductive success than parents whose first two children were sons. About the same time, another sociobiologist, Mark Flinn (1989), reported that Trinidadian mothers in households with nonreproductive helpers — usually daughters — had significantly higher reproductive success than mothers without such help. Neither study involved nomadic foragers, and both suffered from small sample sizes. Furthermore, if mothers with helpers had higher reproductive success, how can we be sure that this was due to their help? Perhaps some other factor (e.g., household resources) encouraged nonreproductive helpers to remain and also enhanced child well-being? Nevertheless, this was the beginning.

Accustomed to stratified, patriarchal societies, many of us took for granted that older siblings were a liability who received more parental investment and inherited the bulk of family resources, while younger siblings received less attention. Indeed, in many Asian societies, a daughter with several older siblings — especially if her family already had older daughters — risked being killed by her parents at birth. In doing so, we tended to overlook the fact that in less stratified traditional societies, older siblings can be an asset. For example, among horticulturalists living in the Gambia of West Africa, children with older sisters had significantly higher survival chances than did same-age children without older sisters (Sear et al. 2002, p. 58). In cases like Ifaluk, the beneficial effects of siblings depended on a precise configuration with daughters born first. Elsewhere, though, benefits of older siblings did not show up until later in life, when younger sibs themselves reproduced (for !Kung hunter–gatherers in Botswana, see Draper and Hames 2000). Mechanisms behind this correlation remain unknown. Possibly, adult siblings provide shelter or food in times of crisis, contributing to the survival of nieces and nephews. The point is, collateral kin have the potential to help at various times across the life cycle.

Although the lactating mother would typically be the primary caretaker in the first months, the prospect of allomaternal assistance promotes maternal commitment. Having child minders within easy reach, even inexperienced ones, frees the mother to forage more efficiently. With the approach of weaning, allomothers can offer soft foods to the infant. Experienced grandmothers and great-aunts seem to be especially important for the survival of just-weaned infants. For those whose mother is in poor shape or less than fully committed, allomothers can be critical at any age.

Grandmothers as a Special Class of Allomother

Ever since Hawkes et al. (1998) called attention to how hard and efficiently post-reproductive women foraged among the Hadza of Tanzania, data have been accumulating for a broad range of societies documenting increased survival for children with older matrilineal kin nearby. Such data are all the more remarkable because the correlation is found over such a broad spectrum of subsistence conditions. Well-documented cases come from African hunter–gatherers, West African horticulturalists (Sear et al. 2002), eighteenth-century German peasants (Voland and Beise 2002), and rice-growing peasants in nineteenth-century Tokugawa Japan (Jamison et al. 2002). Among patrilocal Bengalis, swidden agriculturalists in northeastern India, grandmothers contribute to shorter birth intervals, whereas among nearby matrilineal Khasi groups, their presence was correlated with increased child survival (for an overview, see Leonetti et al. 2005; Voland et al. 2004).

For German peasants (Voland and Beise 2002) and Gambian horticulturists (Sear et al. 2002), survival advantages from a nearby maternal grandmother

showed up around the age of weaning — an especially vulnerable life phase involving emotional stress and the introduction of new foods. The cause is unknown, but timing points to the provisioning by grandmothers. The Gambia
population is primarily Muslim, with mothers living patrilocally in their husband's home. At first glance, it seems odd that the maternal grandmother's presence mattered so much. Noting how common it is for West African mothers to
foster babies out at the time of weaning so babies "forget the breast," Sear et al.
(2002) suggest that the most solicitous caretaker not already living in the household would be — were she still alive and near-by — the maternal grandmother.

Once allomothers became essential for childrearing, selection would have
acted on life-history traits that made allomothers more available (e.g., delayed
dispersal, delayed maturity, longer lifespans). In particular, Hawkes et al. (1998)
argued that women's long postmenopausal lifespans evolved because post-reproductive women helped provision matrilineal kin, favoring the survival of
children whose great-aunts and grandmothers were genetically prone to
longevity.

How Much Do Fathers Help?

Perhaps the biggest surprise from the Gambia study was how little difference the
presence of either the father or older brothers made (see also Sugiyama and
Chacon 2004). Elsewhere, among Aché foragers in South America (Hill and
Hurtado 1996), death of the father undermines an infant's survival prospects. In
this and other traditional populations in South America, women line up alternative sources of support by identifying "back-up" fathers, relying on a convenient
biological fiction known as "partible paternity" to downplay jealousy and increase shared provisioning of young. Not only does the extent to which fathers
help vary, but whether or not their help even matters varies.

The Importance of Real and Perceived Allomaternal Support

Across mammals, the best single predictor of infant survival is maternal commitment. In humans, however, this commitment is influenced, at least initially,
by the mother's own perception of pre- and postpartum social support. The
ethnographic and historical record for societies in which child survival is far less
certain than in our own provides ample evidence that mothers short on
allomaternal support are more likely to abandon infants at birth (Hrdy 1999).
Even small increases in social support for the mother enhance how responsive
she is to her infant (Thompson et al., this volume). Adolescent U.S. mothers
(even those where the father remains with them) are more sensitive to their infants' needs and have more securely attached infants if a supportive grandmother is also present. Even "as if" kin in the persons of visiting nurses can increase maternal responsiveness and lower the incidence of child abuse in the

first two years, with benefits from these early interventions still detectable 15 years later (Olds et al. 1986, 2002). Social workers and medical personnel have long been aware that both mothers and their children derive emotional and material support from extended, multigenerational families. Even when socio-economic conditions are held steady, rates of child morbidity and mortality rise in single-parent homes (Weitoft et al. 2003). When times are tough, presence of allomaternal support may matter even more, e.g., if maternal competence is compromised by immaturity, inexperience, father absence, or resource scarcity. Beneficial effects also extend to sociocognitive skills. Prospects for children at risk can be improved through the presence of a supportive allomother, whether related (like a grandmother) or an unrelated teacher or mentor (Werner 1984). Furstenberg (1976), for example, found that babies born to unmarried, low-income U.S. teenagers test better on cognitive development if a grandmother is present. It is time to consider what prompts such individuals to help.

HAMILTON'S RULE AND THE PROXIMATE CAUSES OF HELPING

Allomaternal Responsiveness

For cooperative breeding to evolve in the first place, group members must be predisposed to respond to signals of infant need. Most primates are. Females in particular are attracted to babies and seek to touch, hold, or carry them. Across primates, prior caretaking experience matters for competent parenting. Presumably, such baby "lust" evolved to help insure that pre-reproductives are prepared for parenthood, neurologically primed as well as practiced (Fleming, this volume). In infant-sharing primates where females live in matrilineal kin groups, allomaternal assistance keeps the baby safe while the mother is free to forage, contributing to both her fitness and to the inclusive fitness of kin. Males may be attracted to babies as well, and in some species (like titi monkeys) have an even lower threshold for responding to them than mothers. To be convinced, one need only watch a male *Callithrix argentata* hovering near his mate at birth, grabbing at the emerging baby, even vying with the mother to eat the placenta. Males primed by prior experience with babies appear especially eager.

In humans, both sexes respond to infantile behaviors like smiling or babbling and, as first noted by Konrad Lorenz, both sexes are attracted by "cuteness" (round heads, small face, big eyes, immature body form, and obvious vulnerability), but there are significant differences in how the sexes respond (Alley 1983). Although both sexes respond to cuteness, and having a younger sibling increased this responsiveness, on average, women were more protective.

Strategic Calibration of Altruism

In many cooperatively breeding mammals, allomothers schedule assistance in ways that reduce costs to their fitness. They are most likely to help when they are

too young or too old to breed themselves, or when for social or ecological reasons, breeding would not be practical. Allomothers may be most eager to help
when in good condition, but when resources are scarce or when helping would
interfere with their own reproduction, their offer to help may decline. Simply
pretending to help is also an option. Among white-winged choughs, young helpers ostentatiously carry food to nestlings, only to swallow it themselves when
parents are not watching (Cockburn 1998, p. 161). There may also be penalties
for not helping, including reduced parental tolerance for shirking allomothers.
Such generalizations apply especially to humans where social sanctions operate
in many subtle, and not so subtle, ways and among whom pay-offs from generosity and kindness come in many currencies.

IMPLICATIONS OF THE COOPERATIVE BREEDING HYPOTHESIS FOR HUMAN DEVELOPMENT

A heritage of cooperative breeding has profound implications for psychological
adaptations across a broad range of life phases. This topic has only begun to be
explored. For example, even though human mothers, like other apes, produce
singleton young after a long period of gestation, if human mothers evolved as
cooperative breeders, women and their infants should theoretically have been
selected to seek and elicit support from a range of individuals. This has repercussions for the psychobiological underpinnings of male–female, female–female,
infant–mother, and infant–allomother relationships. Here I focus on the implications for the emotional and cognitive development of infants.

Primates produce costly singleton births. Quality control is built into the process at many levels. Only adequately nourished mothers ovulate, only selected
ovulations are fertile, only a single successful sperm is selected, only viable conceptions persist, and so forth. Once they give birth, nonhuman primates are predisposed to carry and care for any infant vigorous enough to catch hold of the
mother's fur, reach her nipples, and initiate lactation. Once born, even blind or
seriously deformed neonates are carried so long as they can cling. Even a stillborn infant may be carried at least for a few hours. In hundreds of thousands of
hours of observations, abandonment of full-term infants by their mothers has
rarely been observed in wild primates, and mothers in the wild have almost
never been observed to hurt their own infants deliberately. (Exceptions involve
inexperienced primiparae, anxious mothers trying to restrain infants, or mothers
who punish offspring they are trying to wean, and with the exception of incom-
petence such behaviors never result in injury.) Apart from inexperienced
primiparae, abandonment only occurs under extreme duress (e.g., mother in
very poor condition; infant threatened by infanticidal males). There are, however, two groups of primates to which these generalizations do not apply: cooperatively breeding Callitrichids and humans. In both, maternal commitment is
unusually contingent on social circumstances. Like tamarins, human females

respond to lack of support by failing to commit in the period right after birth, reducing or terminating investment in a newborn by abandoning it, or outright infanticide. Furthermore, human mothers are the only primates who have become discriminating about which infants they invest in, using criteria like sex, birth order, and viability (including birth weight and whether the baby appears full term; for review of vast ethnographic, historical, and ethological literatures on maternal abandonment and infanticide in humans, see Hrdy 1999).

Selection Pressures on Neonates Produced by Contingent Maternal Commitment

If human mothers are more discriminating about which babies to invest in, neonates that conform to maternal preferences would have been more likely to survive. Maternal preferences for babies that look plump and full term may explain why human infants are born fatter at birth than other primates. (The main alternative hypothesis has to do with the demands of brain growth, but this does not explain why fat is stockpiled prior to the difficult birth process.) Infants who engage their mothers right from birth would have an advantage over those who do not. Contingent maternal commitment meant that, compared to other apes, human infants had a greater need to monitor and interpret the moods and intentions of others, and if a caretaker seems likely to disengage, to work harder at engaging her.

Beyond clinging and the cries that baby apes emit when uncomfortable or separated, newborn humans seek out human-like faces and initiate contact with others. Soon after birth, human apes imitate faces, smile, and laugh in ways that have never been observed among the wild ape. Human babies are born with white sclera (not seen in other apes), which highlights the direction of their gaze. The extraordinary eagerness of human newborns to seek out faces and connect with eyes, well described by Baron-Cohen (1995/2001), may reflect their need to monitor, attract, and engage mothers. (In a remarkable set of experiments, increased eye contact, mutual face gazing, and more smiling was elicited in baby chimps by inserting a human allomother into the mother–infant dyad [Matsuzawa 2001; Bard 2004].) At the same time, sociocognitive skills thereby developed can also serve to attract allomothers later on, opening further possibilities.

THE NEED TO ATTRACT ALLOMOTHERS AND SELECTION PRESSURES ON OLDER INFANTS

A baby's primary source of information about the world would be the mother and her reactions to her world. However, if humans evolved as cooperative breeders, infants also needed to be sensitive to social support cues in their immediate community. Such cues would inform internal working models (see Kraemer et al., this volume), but also physiological "decisions," such as how

fast to grow. When infants feel confident of continued succor, they should invest
in rapid growth. Alternatively, indifference or neglect might signal that this was
a time for the child to shut down growth, conserving resources and increasing
the chances of surviving future neglect, one explanation for why children with
adequate food nevertheless "fail to thrive."

Human babies are born "connoisseurs" of solicitude. Even with the onset of
weaning, early learning biases persist, developing with age and experience. As a
baby becomes more discriminating about which caretakers to trust, his ability to
predict the behavior of others is further refined and reinforced (Tomasello
1999). Good mind readers become better mind readers (Baron-Cohen
1995/2001). Human infants seek out, fixate on, engage with eyes, and preferentially respond to a direct gaze. By three to four months, human infants smile less
at adults who avert their gaze, but resume smiling when the adult looks straight
at them (Farroni et al. 2002). Such propensities and sociocognitive tools for
monitoring others and reading their intentions by seeking out their eyes, following their gaze, etc., are not so well developed in other apes (Baron-Cohen 1995/
2001; pers. obs.). Evidence from field and lab studies (summarized by Whiten et
al. 2003) suggests that chimps are capable of reading intentions and learning
through observation and imitation, but by three to four years, humans are more
adept and eager at doing so. Children freely imagine what it is like to be someone
altogether different, even someone they have never seen, enjoy doing so, and de-
light in drawing others into this game (Harris 2000; Trevarthen, this volume).
This greater interest in "inter-subjectivity," in understanding what and why
someone else is trying to do something (Hennighausen and Lyons-Ruth, this
volume), coupled with an eagerness to share goals with others, improves our
ability to learn through observation. It makes humans especially prone to accumulate and transmit new knowledge (Tomasello 1999). Both Baron-Cohen and
Chisholm (2003) propose that such mental aptitudes for mind reading would be
valuable for predicting and interpreting the intentions of others, and hence in
affecting their behavior. But why should humans have been selected to be so
much better at this than chimps are?

WHY HUMANS ARE SO COOPERATIVE
AND "HYPER-SOCIAL"

According to proponents of the "Machiavellian intelligence" hypothesis (Byrne
and Whiten 1985), reading minds provides a strategic advantage in competitive
worlds characterized by shifting alliances. Given that many primates, and all
other apes, also live in complexly competitive societies, the need for Machiavellian intelligence fails to explain why humans should be so much better at imagining the intentions of others and moving into their conceptual worlds than other
apes are. Chimps, after all, are at least as dominance-oriented and competitive as
humans are, probably more so. Why should capacities for shared engagement be

so much better developed in humans; why should humans be (following Tomasello 1999) so "hyper-social"? Why are they hyper-altruistic (e.g., Fehr and Fischbacher 2003)? What distinguishes humans most from other apes is not so much our competitive heritage as our more cooperative one.

Infants born into cooperative breeding systems depend on a range of caretakers, and maternal commitment itself is contingent on the mother's perception of how much support she is likely to have from allomothers. To prosper in such a system, infants have to be adept at monitoring caretakers, reading their moods and intentions, and eliciting their solicitude. Chisholm (2003) argues that "theory of mind" reduces the uncertainties youngsters face, helping them to predict how others (both mothers and allomothers) are likely to respond. Through practice and conditional rewards, infants get incrementally better at reading intentions and learning to engage caretakers. This explains why infants with older siblings are better able to interpret the feelings and intentions of others (Ruffman et al. 1998).[1]

In the case of creatures as intelligent and manipulative as all apes are, precociously expressed abilities to read and interpret the intentions of others continue to develop through the first years of life. There is a racheting effect as early efforts develop into sophisticated mind reading (Tomasello 1999, p. 67; Baron-Cohen 1995/2001). Being able to intuit and care about what others are thinking, to put oneself cognitively and emotionally in someone else's place and think about what they are thinking, to play with them, learn from them, and share their goals (Trevarthen, this volume) has, in turn, had spectacular repercussions in the evolution of our peculiarly "hyper-social," information-sharing, and culture-transmitting species (Tomasello 1999). That is, neural underpinnings for mind reading are laid down in early and later infancy and provide the necessary underpinnings first for empathy and then for development of full-fledged theory of mind a few years later, usually between ages four to six. Once such traits were expressed in the phenotype, natural selection would have had an opportunity to favor any small changes in genes or gene expression that predispose the organism to develop them (West-Eberhard 2003).

Continuing in this speculative vein, I am struck by other unusual traits that humans share with cooperative breeders. Against all phylogenetic predictions, dogs can be better at extracting information from human social signals than are chimps (with the exception of chimps reared in close contact with humans). In an ingenious set of experiments, Hare et al. (2003) demonstrated that dogs (and even puppies not yet exposed to humans) were more skillful than chimps at using human social cues (e.g., direction of gaze, finger pointing, and finger

---

[1] It is noteworthy that cooperatively breeding tamarins gauge another individual's intentions in deciding on whether or not to share food (Hauser et al. 2003). Unfortunately, this pioneering study stands by itself, so we do not yet have any comparative information about which other primates, besides humans and tamarins, do and do not share such abilities.

tapping) to locate containers with hidden food. (Experimenters controlled for smell.) How could this be? Not only do dogs descend from cooperatively breeding wolves — and so are presumably neurologically equipped to read intentions — but domestic dogs also have a fifteen-thousand-year history of coevolving with humans. In this sense, the social environments of dogs were evolutionarily comparable to those of children: both depended on tolerance and handouts from larger, food-possessing human allomothers.

Babbling, the repetitive, rhythmical vocalizations long assumed to be uniquely human, represents the strangest of all such convergences. Babbling spontaneously emerges around seven months, about the same time that babies begin to grow "milk" teeth, beginning with two tiny incisors at the bottom, then four more on top. This is about the time that babies begin to distinguish familiar people from strangers and to accept pre-weaning foods. By age three or so there will be twenty sharp little teeth to help babies chew their first solids, mostly soft or mashed foods, or food premasticated by someone else. Babbling, as it turns out, is not unique to humans. Something like babbling crops up in Callitrichids, (the only primates besides humans, if I am right) with full-fledged cooperative breeding. In pygmy marmosets, babbling emerges between the first and third weeks, just about the time allomothers take over most of the care (Snowdon 2001). It seems likely that babbling in human babies, like smiling, originated for the same reason that babbling developed in Callitrichids: babbling (and the rhythmic movements of hands and feet that accompany it in humans) attracts the attention of caregivers and elicits interest, solicitude, and edible tidbits. Even as adults, Callitrichids continue to use vocalization as a means of locating and staying in contact with other group members. They engage in far more contact vocalizations than do chimps or other apes — with the exception of humans (Snowdon 2001).

It has long been assumed that infants babble because the practice helps them learn to talk. No doubt it does. However, I suspect that babbling evolved before language and for a different reason. Our ancestors were born clever apes who because they needed to engage caretakers babbled at them. Best babblers were best fed, and also learned to talk, thus entering into a world of new possibilities. Of course long childhoods are critical for such skills to develop, but longer periods of nutritional dependency are predictable corollaries of alloparental provisioning. According to this scenario, opportunities provided by slow development were in place before the evolution of sapient brains. Cooperative breeding in a species so clever as an ape was the novel feature of this experiment.

Dependence on allomaternal assistance produced more contingent maternal commitment and with it the need for babies born scanning and monitoring signals of commitment from those around them, equipped from birth and through childhood to engage and elicit investment from mothers and others. Present such a talented ape with a long, well-buffered phase in which to develop, and novel coevolutionary processes are likely to be unleashed.

Long Childhoods

To the extent that anthropologists thought about childhood, most viewed it as a unique stage in the life history of human beings which evolved some two million years ago to provide extra time for developing large brains and for learning. According to this view, the evolution of childhood and adolescence, the human capacity for symbolic language, and culture are the result of the inclusion of new life stages in human development. From a comparative sociobiological perspective, however, prolonged post-weaning or post-fledging dependence is a predictable corollary of allomaternal provisioning. Regardless of how big and costly their brains were, and even without the need to acquire special cognitive skills for complex tool use, language, and symbolic culture (all the uniquely human traits that long childhoods supposedly evolved to facilitate), early humans would be expected to take their time maturing. Other cooperative breeders far less brainy than we are (e.g., crested magpie jays and wolves) also have long "childhoods." I do not think it is a coincidence that animals like the Caledonian crow, which amaze us with their problem-solving and tool use (Chappell and Kacelnik 2002), are found in taxa with long histories of cooperative breeding.

Conventional explanations for the evolution of sapient brains emphasize the (undeniable) subsistence benefits of tools (Kaplan et al. 2000) or else the social and reproductive benefits of Machiavellian intelligence. However, other group-living apes stand to benefit from tools. After all, chimps use tools to obtain massive amounts of calories from nuts that they have laboriously learned to crack open. They too would benefit from enhanced learning. Yet chimps never evolved human-sized brains — why not? Because brains are energetically extremely costly and any delay in maturation is risky (Aiello and Wheeler 1995). How could a chimp just a little better at nut-cracking gain sufficient reproductive rewards to make delayed maturation and a little bit bigger brain worth it? The slightly dumber nutcracker would still be likely to outbreed him.

It is difficult to explain why such skills evolved only in the line leading to humans without knowing just what distinguished prehominids from other apes. The proposal made here is that the distinguishing condition was a reliance on allomaternal assistance, and with it (a) contingent maternal commitment (along with the sociocognitive capacities infants need to engage caretakers), and (b) the slow maturation that comes as a corollary of cooperative breeding. If the time until nutritional independence was already delayed, metabolically costly big brains would evolve at a discount. Using this logic, long periods of dependency preceded the coevolutionary processes that selected for increasingly larger brains and other trademarks of our "hyper-social" species. Among prehominid creatures who already possessed rudimentary theories of mind, and among whom greater intelligence did not have to compensate its possessors for the entire cost of delayed maturation, even small reproductive payoffs from being smarter would be sufficient to favor bigger brains.

OUTSTANDING QUESTIONS ABOUT INFANT NEEDS

The cooperative breeding hypothesis relies on a number of assumptions. Is social support really as important for human maternal commitment as assumed here? Are humans really different from other apes in this respect? Will the paleontological record confirm the prediction that long childhoods and delayed maturation precede expansion to sapient-sized brains, elaborate tool kits, and expansion out of Africa? Questions of particular relevance to this Dahlem Workshop, however, have to do with infant development.

We know from classic studies of hunter–gatherer childcare by Konner, Hewlett, Lamb, Ivey, Tronick, and others that !Kung and Aché babies are primarily held by mothers, whereas Aka and Efé babies are frequently held by allomothers (see Hewlett and Lamb 2004). It is impossible to know which pattern was more typical of Pleistocene families, although I think we can know how easily infants learn to prefer one specific caretaker. Usually, this is the mother. However, to reconstruct Pleistocene family lives, we need more. For example, right from birth newborn langurs are carried by a range of allomothers. Babies cling like glue to whichever female has them even, although they unabashedly prefer their mothers. Without the field observations (which we also lack for the Pleistocene), using infant predilections to reconstruct langurs' caretaking system would, by themselves, lead to the wrong conclusion about who cared for babies in these animals.

Accepting Bowlby's central premise about the importance of "a secure base," what options exist for providing a sufficiently secure base for adequate (?), optimal (?), particularly desired (?) outcomes (which one is a whole other issue). To date, most attachment research has relied on assumptions about the naturalness of more or less exclusive maternal care (cf. Sagi et al. 1995; Ahnert et al. 2000; Grossmann and Grossmann, this volume; Ahnert, this volume). To date, most studies compared mother-care with institutionalized daycare. Yet, the cooperative breeding hypothesis suggests that we should assume an EEA peopled by an array of potential caretakers. Assuming that Pleistocene babies developed in a world surrounded by familiar allomothers and rarely encountered strangers, how did (and how do) babies differentiate? I would like future research in developmental psychology to explore cues infants use for designating someone as "kin" (or at least, as-if kin). How familiar does an allomother have to be? As in other mammals, infants are monitoring smells and facial expressions. What role do other processes, like phenotype matching or dialect monitoring, play in distinguishing "allomothers" from strangers? I want to know more about infant comfort levels with different allomaternal regimens at different developmental ages. According to this new theoretical perspective, we should be asking about the different effects of a range of allomothers entering the lives of infants and children at various ages. But how many allomothers? At which ages? For how long? It is a theoretical framework that takes "other care" for granted and focuses on making "other" care better.

ACKNOWLEDGMENTS

I am indebted to Jim Chisholm, Barry Hewlett, Kristen Hawkes, Mel Konner, and Michael Lamb for discussion over many years about ideas presented here. Specific suggestions from Jim Leckman and Karin Grossmann were gratefully included in the final version.

REFERENCES

Ahnert, L., M. Lamb, and K. Seltenheim. 2000. Infant-care provider attachments in contrasting child care settings. I. Group-oriented care before German reunification. *Infant Behav. Dev.* **23**:197–209.

Aiello, L., and P. Wheeler. 1995. The expensive tissue hypothesis. *Curr. Anthro.* **36**: 199–221.

Alley, T. 1983. Growth-produced changes in body shape and size as determinants of perceived age and adult caregiving. *Child Dev.* **54**:241–248.

Alvarez, H. 2004. Residence groups among hunter-gatherers: A view of the claims and evidence for patrilocal bands. In: Kinship and Behavior in Primates, ed. B. Chapais and C. Berman, pp. 400–442. Oxford: Oxford Univ. Press.

Baron-Cohen, S., ed. 1995/2001. Mindblindness: An Essay on Autism and Theory of Mind. Cambridge, MA: MIT Press.

Bard, K. 2004. Emotions in young chimpanzees: The value of a comparative developmental approach to understand the evolutionary bases of emotions. In: Emotional Development: Recent Research Advances, ed. J. Nadel and D. Muir. Oxford: Oxford Univ. Press.

Bardi, M., A. Petto, and D. Lee-Parritz. 2001. Parental failure in captive cotton-top tamarins\(*Saguinus oedipus*). *Am. J. Primatol.* **54**:150–169.

Bowlby, J. 1969. Attachment. Attachment and Loss, vol. 1. New York: Basic.

Bowlby, J. 1982. Attachment. 2nd ed. Attachment and Loss, vol. 1. New York: Basic/Harper Collins.

Buchan, J.C., S.A. Alberts, J.B. Silk, and J. Altmann. 2003. True paternal care in a multi-male primate society. *Nature* **425**:179–181.

Byrne, R.W., and A. Whiten. 1985. Machiavellian Intelligence: Social Expertise and the Evolution of Intellect in Monkeys, Apes and Humans. Oxford: Clarendon.

Chappell, J., and A. Kacelnik. 2002. Selectivity of tool length by New Caledonian crows. *Anim. Cogn.* **5**:71–78.

Chisholm, J. 2003. Uncertainty, contingency and attachment: A life history theory of theory of mind. In: From Mating to Mentality: Evaluating Evolutionary Psychology, ed. K. Sterelny and J. Fitness, pp. 125–154. Hove: Psychology Press.

Cockburn, A. 1998. Evolution of helping behavior in cooperatively breeding birds. *Ann. Rev. Ecol. System.* **29**:141–177.

Davies, N. 1992. Dunnock Beahviour and Social Evolution. Oxford: Oxford Univ. Press.

Draper, P., and R. Hames. 2000. Birth order, sibling investment and fertility among the Ju/'hoansi (!Kung). *Hum. Nat.* **11**:117–156.

Emlen, S.T. 1997. Predicting family dynamics in social vertebrates. In: Behavioural Ecology: An Evolutionary Approach, ed. J.R. Krebs and N.B. Davies, pp. 228–253. 4th ed. Oxford: Blackwell.

Farroni, T., G. Csibra, F. Simion, and M. Johnson. 2002. Eye contact detection in humans from birth. *PNAS* **99**:9602–0605.

Fehr, E., and U. Fischbacher. 2003. The nature of human altruism. *Nature* **425**:785–791.

Fleming, A.S., C. Corter, J. Stallings, and M. Steiner. 2002. Testosterone and prolactin are associated with emotional responses to infant cries in new fathers. *Horm. Behav.* **42**:399–413.

Flinn, M.V. 1989. Household composition and female reproductive strategies in a Trinidadian village. In: The Sociobiology of Sexual and Reproductive Strategies, ed. A.E. Rasa, C. Vogel, and E. Voland, pp. 206–233. London: Chapman and Hall.

Furstenberg, F.F. 1976. Unplanned Parenthood: The Social Consequences of Unplanned Parenthood. New York: Free Press.

Hamilton, W.D. 1964. The genetical evolution of social behaviour. 1. *J. Theor. Biol.* **7**:1–18.

Hamilton, W.D. 1966. The moulding of senescence by natural selection. *J. Theor. Biol.* **12**:12–45.

Hare, B., M. Brown, C. Williamson, and M. Tomasello. 2003. The domestication of social cognition in dogs. *Science* **298**:1634–1636.

Harris, P. 2000. The Work of the Imagination. Oxford: Blackwell.

Hauser, M.D., M.K. Chen, F. Chen, and E. Chuang. 2003. Give unto others: Genetically unrelated cotton-top tamarins preferentially give food to those who altruistically give food back. *Proc. Roy. Soc. Lond. B* **270**:2363–2370.

Hawkes, K., J.F. O'Connell, N.G. Blurton Jones, E.L. Charnov, and H. Alvarez. 1998. Grandmothering, menopause, and the evolution of human life histories. *PNAS* **95**:1336–1339.

Heinrichs, M.T., T. Baumgartner, C. Kirschbaum, and U. Ehlert. 2003. Social support and oxytocin interact to suppress cortisol and subjective responses to psychosocial stress. *Biol. Psych.* **54**:1389–1398.

Heinsohn, R., and M.C. Double. 2004. Cooperate or speciate: New theory for the distribution of passerine birds. *Trends Ecol. Evol.* **19**:55–60.

Hewlett, B., and M. Lamb, eds. 2004. Hunter–Gatherer Childhood. Hawthorne, NY: Aldine.

Hill, K., and A. Hurtado. 1996. Ache Life History: The Ecology and Demography of a Foraging People. Hawthorne, NY: Aldine de Gruyter.

Hrdy, S.B. 1977. The Langurs of Abu: Female and Male Strategies of Reproduction. Cambridge: Harvard Univ. Press.

Hrdy, S.B. 1999. Mother Nature: A History of Mothers, Infants and Natural Selection. New York: Pantheon.

Ivey, P.K. 2000. Cooperative reproduction in Ituri forest hunter-gatherers: Who cares for Efe infants? *Curr. Anthro.* **41**:856–866.

Jamison, C.S., L.L. Cornell, P.L. Jamison, and H. Nakazato. 2002. Are all grandmothers equal? A review and a preliminary test of the "grandmother hypothesis" in Tokugawa, Japan. *Am. J. Phys. Anthro.* **119**:67–76.

Kaplan, H., K. Hill, J. Lancaster, and A.M. Hurtado. 2000. A theory of human life history evolution: Diet, intelligence and longevity. *Evol. Anthro.* **9**:156–185.

Langen, T.A. 2000. Prolonged offspring dependence and cooperative breeding in birds. *Behav. Ecol.* **11**:367–377.

Leonetti, D., D.C. Nath, N.S. Hemam, and D.B. Neill. 2005. Kinship organization and grandmother's impact on reproductive success among the matrilineal Khasi and patrilineal Bengali of N.E. India. In: Grandmotherhood: The Evolutionary Significance of the Second Half of Female Life, ed. E. Voland, A. Chasiotis, and W. Schiefenhoevel. Piscataway: Rutgers Univ. Press, in press.

Levine, R., S. Dixon, S. LeVine et al. 1996. Child Care and Culture: Lessons from Africa. Cambridge: Cambridge Univ. Press.

Matsuzawa, T. 2001. The Baby and Ai. Film made by Primate Research Institute, Kyoto, Japan. Distributed by Mico.

Mitani, J.C., and D. Watts. 1997. The evolution of nonmaternal caretaking among anthropoid primates: Do helpers help? *Behav. Ecol. Sociobiol.* **40**:213–240.

Murdock, G.P. 1967. Ethnographic Atlas. Pittsburgh: Univ. of Pittsburgh Press.

Olds, D., C.R. Henderson, R. Chaberlin, and R. Tatelbaum. 1986. Preventing child abuse and neglect: A randomized trial of nurse home visitiation. *Pediatrics* **78**:65–78.

Olds, D., J. Robinson, R. O'Brien et al. 2002. Home visiting by paraprofessionals and by nurses: A randomized controlled trial. *Pediatrics* **110**:486–496.

Pusey, A., J. Williams, and J. Goodall. 1997. The influence of dominance rank on the reproductive success of female chimpanzees. *Science* **277**:828–831.

Rowley, I., and E. Russell. 1990. Splendid fairy wrens: Demonstrating the importance of longevity. In: Cooperative Breeding in Birds, ed. P. Stacey and W. Koenig, pp. 3–30. Cambridge: Cambridge Univ. Press.

Ruffman, T., J. Perner, M. Naito, L. Parkin, and W. Clements. 1998. Older (but not younger) siblings facilitate false belief understanding. *Dev. Psychol.* **34**:161–174.

Russell, A.F., L.Sharp, P. Brotherton, and T.H. Clutton-Brock. 2003. Cost minimization by helpers in cooperative vertebrates. *PNAS* **100**:3333–3338.

Sagi, A., M. van IJzendooorn, O. Aviezer et al. 1995. Attachments in a multiple-caregiver and multiple-infant environment: The case of the Israeli kibbutzim. *Mono. Soc. Res. Child Dev.* **60**:71–91.

Sear, R., F. Steel, I. McGregor, and R. Mace. 2002. The effects of kin on child mortality in rural Gambia. *Demography* **39**:43–63.

Schradin, C., and G. Anzenberger. 1999. Prolactin, the hormone of paternity. *News Physiol. Sci.* **14**:221–331.

Silk, J.B., S.C. Alberts, and J. Altmann. 2003. Social bonds of female baboons enhance infant survival. *Science* **302**:1231–1234.

Snowdon, C. 1996. Infant care in cooperatively breeding species. *Adv. Stud. Behav.* **25**:643–689.

Snowdon, C.T. 2001. From primate communication to human language. In: Tree of Origin, ed. F. de Waal, pp. 195–227. Cambridge, MA: Harvard Univ. Press.

Storey, A., C.J. Walsh, R.L. Quinton, and K.E. Wynne-Edwards. 2000. Hormonal correlates of paternal responsiveness in new and expectant fathers. *Evol. Hum. Behav.* **21**:79–95.

Sugiyama, L., and R. Chacon. 2004. Juvenile responses to household ecology among the Yora of Peruvian Amazonia. In: Hunter–Gatherer Childhood, ed. B. Hewlett and M. Lamb. Hawthorne, NY: Aldine.

Tomasello, M. 1999. The Cultural Origins of Human Cognition. Cambridge, MA: Harvard Univ. Press.

Tronick, E.Z., G.A. Morelli, and S.A. Winn. 1987. Multiple caretaking of Efé (pygmy) infants. *Am. Anthropologist* **89**:96–106.

Turke, P. 1988. "Helpers at the nest": Childcare networks on Ifaluk. In: Human Reproductive Behaviour: A Darwinian Perspective, ed. L. Betzig, M. Borgherhoff Mulder, and P. Turke, pp.173–188. Cambridge: Cambridge Univ. Press.

Voland, E., and J. Beise. 2002. Opposite effects of maternal and paternal grandmothers on infant survival in historical Krummhoern. *Behav. Ecol. Sociobiol.* **52**:435–443.

Voland, E., A. Chasiotis, and W. Schiefenhoevel, eds. 2004. Grandmotherhood: The Evolutionary Significance of the Second Half of Female Life. Piscataway: Rutgers Univ. Press.

von Holst, D. 1986. Psychosocial stress and its pathophysiological effects in tree shrews (*Tupaia belangeri*). In: Biological and Psychological Factors in Cardiovascular Disease, ed. T.H. Schmidt, T.M. Dembroski, and G. Blumchen, pp. 476–489. Heidelberg: Springer.

Weisner, T., and R. Gallimore. 1977. My brother's keeper: Child and sibling caretaking. *Curr. Anthro.* **18**:169–170.

Weitoft, G.R., A. Hjern, B. Haglund, and M. Rosén. 2003. Mortality, severe morbidity, and injury in children living with single parents in Sweden: A population-based study. *Lancet* **361**:289–295.

Werner, E.E. 1984. Child Care: Kith, Kin and Hired Hands. Baltimore: Univ. Park Press.

West-Eberhard, M.J. 2003. Developmental Plasticity and Evolution. Oxford: Oxford Univ. Press.

Wiessner, P. 2002. Hunting, healing and hxaro exchange: A long-term perspective on !Kung (Ju/'hoansi) large-game hunting. *Evol. Hum. Behav.* **23**:407–436.

Whiten, A., V. Horner, and S. Marshall-Pescini. 2003. Cultural anthropology. *Evol. Anthro.* **2**:92–105.

3

The Role of Social Engagement in Attachment and Bonding

A Phylogenetic Perspective

S. W. PORGES

Brain–Body Center, Department of Psychiatry, University of Illinois at Chicago, Chicago, IL 60612, U.S.A.

ABSTRACT

This chapter focuses on the importance of social engagement as a mechanism that fosters the establishment of social attachment and social bonds. A model of social engagement derived from the Polyvagal Theory is presented. The model emphasizes phylogeny as an organizing principle and includes the following points: (1) there are well-defined neural circuits to support social engagement behaviors and the defensive strategies of fight, flight, and freeze, (2) these neural circuits form a phylogenetically organized hierarchy, (3) without being dependent on conscious awareness the nervous system evaluates risk in the environment (i.e., neuroception) and regulates visceral state to support the expression of adaptive behavior to match a neuroception of safety, danger, or life threat, (4) social engagement behaviors and the benefits of the physiological states associated with social support require a neuroception of safety, (5) social behaviors associated with nursing, reproduction, and the formation of strong pair bonds require a unique biobehavioral state characterized by immobilization without fear, and (6) immobilization without fear is mediated by a co-opting of the neural circuit regulating defensive freezing behaviors through the involvement of oxytocin, a neuropeptide involved in the formation of social bonds. The model provides a phylogenetic interpretation of the neural mechanisms mediating the behavioral and physiological features associated with stress and several psychiatric disorders.

DEFINING SOCIAL BEHAVIOR: THE GREAT CONCEPTUAL DIVIDE

An objective of this workshop was to build bridges among researchers who study the development of attachment and bonding from both animal model and clinical population perspectives. As a primary premise of organizing this workshop, it was assumed that both cohorts share similar constructs and interests in generating knowledge related to the mechanisms of normal and atypical social behavior into clinical practice. The contrasts between the research strategies and methods of the two cohorts are forcing a re-evaluation of this assumption.

Animal models often emphasize the role of a specific neural system, neurotransmitter, neuropeptide, hormone, or brain structure as a regulator of social behavior. In contrast, clinical research often focuses on studying aberrant psychological processes in clinical populations. When neurophysiological systems are studied with clinical populations, research designs focus on establishing correlations with the disorders and, in general, preclude the possibility of distinguishing whether physiological correlates are causes or effects of the disorder.

Although the two research strategies often use similar terms, the terms may reflect different domains of social behavior. Animal models tend to focus on the establishment of pair bonds and generate paradigms to evaluate the strength of these bonds. In contrast, research on human attachment is conducted primarily with young children and investigates normal and atypical reactions to strangers. Moreover, the terminology associated with measuring and defining social behavior differs when contrasting the compromised social engagement strategies expressed by an institutionalized child with the ability to establish pair bonds by a vole.

A final perplexing part of the conceptual divide relates to the translation of neuroscience principles and research findings into clinical practice. The clinician is the third limb of this triad. Paradoxically, although the link between social behavior and mental illness in children emerged directly from clinical observations, the features and dimensions of social behavior studied in both animal models and in laboratory studies of normal and atypical children often deviates from the features that clinicians use to define the pathology. Clinical researchers, who conduct studies of social behavior, are interested in either how outlier behaviors overlap with features of clinical diagnoses or how behavioral, psychological, and physiological parameters differentiate the clinical population from normal subjects. Often the parameters of interest or, at least, those that distinguish the clinical group from normal subjects, focus on processes that do not have an obvious relation to the behaviors observed in clinical settings or used to define the pathology (e.g., cortisol, heart rate variability).

Most research in psychopathology accepts the validity of clinical assessment and diagnostic systems (e.g., DSM-IV) as inclusion criteria and then attempts to demonstrate that deficits in psychological processes and/or atypical neurophysiological response patterns underlie the disorder. The research on processes and mechanisms, whether obtained from clinical populations or by studying animal models assumed to express behaviors similar to the clinical populations, does not easily enter the clinical realm and inform clinical assessment. Similarly, other than global diagnoses and quantitative information from standardized assessment instruments, little information from clinical observations regarding the specific features of behavior that have triggered the clinician's concern easily enters the research environment. Thus, constructs of social behavior and engagement are treated differently by researchers testing animal models, researchers studying normal social behavior, researchers studying the psychological and neurophysiological mechanisms and processes underlying a clinical diagnosis, and clinicians who diagnose and treat children with social behavior problems. Missing in this mix of metaphors, worldviews, paradigms, and diagnostic models, is a shared agenda to translate research findings into practice (i.e., assessment and treatment) and to use clinical information to inform the theoretical models being tested.

SOCIAL BEHAVIOR AND ATTACHMENT

Several researchers who study the development of social behavior in children have focused on the construct of attachment. Several of these researchers conduct studies derived from the observations of Bowlby (1982) and the paradigm-building research of Ainsworth (1978). Much of the current research on human attachment is based on the Ainsworth typology, which applies a paradigm assessing infant responses to separation. Clinicians and researchers in developmental psychopathology assume that the Ainsworth classification system and recent derivatives (Cassidy and Shaver 1999) will provide insights into the psychological mechanisms of specific disorders. In fact, diagnostic categories now include disorders such as "Reactive Attachment Disorder" (RAD).

The traditional attachment schema derived from the Bowlby theory constitutes only a small part of social behavior. Moreover, traditional attachment theory, by focusing on mother–infant relations, does not include other putative attachment behaviors that are observed in the enduring bonds between peers, siblings, and mates. Missing from the traditional attachment theories is an articulation of the mechanisms mediating engagement between the individuals bonding or forming attachments.

SOCIAL ENGAGEMENT: THE PREAMBLE
OF A SOCIAL BOND

To develop a social bond, individuals have to be in close proximity. This is true for the models focusing on both mother–infant attachment and the strong bonds associated with social monogamy. Both models test the strength and features of the relationship through separation paradigms. There are, of course, major differences between the contexts in which mother–infant attachment and the social bonds of reproductive partners are established and tested. One specific difference is the contrast in mobility between the mother–infant and reproductive partner dyads. In the mother–infant dyad there is an imbalance with the infant having limited abilities to move toward or away from the mother. However, in

the reproductive partner dyad, there is a balance between the behavioral repertoires of the two adults.

Although proximity is critical to the establishment of social bonds, proximity
is totally due to the ability to navigate across physical distance via voluntary behavior. If social bonds were dependent upon voluntary motor behaviors, then
the newborn infant would be greatly disadvantaged because the neural regulation of the spinal motor pathways are immature at birth and take several years to
fully develop. However, in mammals not all muscles are driven by corticospinal
pathways. Unlike the striated muscles controlling the trunk and limbs, in primates and especially humans, corticobulbar pathways regulate the striated muscles of the face and head. In humans, myelination of corticobulbar pathways
begins between 24 and 28 weeks gestation (Sarnat 2003) and is sufficiently developed at birth to be available to the full-term infant to signal a caregiver (e.g.,
vocalizations, grimace) and to engage the social (e.g., gaze, smile) and nutrient
(e.g., sucking) aspects of the world. Thus, the neural regulation of muscles that
provide important elements of social cueing are available to facilitate the social
interaction with the caregiver and function collectively as an integrated social
engagement system (Porges 2001).

The muscles of the face and head influence both the expression and receptivity of social cues and can effectively reduce or increase social distance. Neural
regulation of these muscles can reduce social distance by making eye contact,
expressing prosody in voice, displaying contingent facial expressions, and modulating the middle ear muscles to improve the extraction of human voice from
background sounds. Alternatively, by reducing the muscle tone to these muscles, the eyelids droop, prosody is lost, positive and contingent facial expressions are diminished, the ability to extract human voice from background
sounds is compromised, and the awareness of the social engagement behaviors
of others may be lost. Thus, the neural regulation of the striated muscles of the
face and head function both as an active social engagement system that reduces
psychological distance and as a filter that can influence the perception of the
engagement behaviors of others.

Special visceral efferent pathways mediate the neural regulation of the striated muscles of the face and head. Special visceral efferent pathways emerge
from three nuclei in the brainstem (nucleus of the trigeminal nerve, nucleus of
the facial nerve, and nucleus ambiguus) and provide motor pathways that are
contained within five cranial nerves (i.e., trigeminal, facial, hypoglossal, vagus,
accessory). These pathways regulate structures that evolved from the ancient
gill arches. From both clinical and research perspectives, the striated muscles of
the face and head provide potent information regarding the behavioral dimensions used to express as well as to evaluate the strength of attachment or the
stress to the social bond. For example, facial expressivity and prosody of vocalizations have been used as clinical indicators as well as quantifiable responses of
separation distress (Newman 1988).

THE SOCIAL ENGAGEMENT SYSTEM: PHYLOGENETIC ORIGINS OF BEHAVIORAL AND AUTONOMIC COMPONENTS

The phylogenetic origin of the behaviors associated with the social engagement system is intertwined with the phylogeny of the autonomic nervous system. As the striated muscles, via special visceral efferent pathways, evolved into a behavioral system that regulated social engagement behaviors, there was a profound shift in neural regulation of the autonomic nervous system. Phylogenetically, these changes in both somatomotor and visceromotor regulation are observed in the transition from reptiles to mammals. As the muscles of the face and head evolved into an ingestion (i.e., nursing) and social engagement system, a new component of the autonomic nervous system (i.e., a myelinated vagus) evolved that was regulated by a brainstem nucleus, which was also involved in the regulation of the striated muscles of the face and head (i.e., nucleus ambiguus). This convergence of neural mechanisms resulted in an integrated social engagement system with a synergism between behavioral and visceral features of social engagement. Thus, activation of the somatomotor component would trigger visceral changes that would support social engagement, while modulation of visceral state would either promote or impede social engagement behaviors. For example, stimulation of visceral states that would promote mobilization (i.e., fight or flight behaviors) would impede the ability to express social engagement behaviors, while increased activity through the myelinated vagus would promote the social engagement behaviors associated with a calm visceral state. Thus, we can infer the specific neural mechanisms related to the effectiveness that feeding and rocking have on promoting calm behavioral and visceral states. Specifically, both the ingestive behaviors associated with feeding and the passive rocking of an infant promote calmness by influencing the myelinated vagus. Feeding activates the muscles of mastication via trigeminal efferent pathways, which in turn provide afferent feedback input to the nucleus ambiguus (i.e., the source nucleus of the myelinated vagus). Rocking provides an efficient and direct influence on the vagus by stimulating vagal afferent pathways via the baroreceptors. Moreover, activation of the social engagement system dampens the neural circuits including the limbic structures that support fight, flight, or freeze behaviors.

THE POLYVAGAL THEORY: THREE NEURAL CIRCUITS REGULATING REACTIVITY

To survive, mammals must determine friend from foe, evaluate whether the environment is safe, and communicate with their social unit. These survival-related behaviors are associated with specific neurobehavioral states that limit the extent to which a mammal can be physically approached and whether the mammal can communicate or establish new coalitions. Through stages of phylogeny mammals, and especially primates, have evolved a functional neural organization that regulates visceral state to support social behavior. The Polyvagal Theory (Porges 1995, 1997, 1998, 2001) proposes that the evolution of the mammalian autonomic nervous system provides the neurophysiological substrates for the emotional experiences and affective processes that are major components of social behavior. The theory proposes that physiological state limits the range of behavior and psychological experience. In this context, the evolution of the nervous system determines the range of emotional expression, quality of communication, and the ability to regulate bodily and behavioral state. The Polyvagal Theory links the evolution of the autonomic nervous system to affective experience, emotional expression, facial gestures, vocal communication, and contingent social behavior. Thus, the theory provides a plausible explanation of several social, emotional, and communication behaviors and disorders.

The polyvagal construct emphasizes the neurophysiological and neuroanatomical distinction between two branches of the vagus and proposes that each branch supports different adaptive behavioral strategies. The Polyvagal Theory articulates three phylogenetic stages of the development of the mammalian autonomic nervous system. Each state is associated with a distinct autonomic subsystem that is retained in mammals. These autonomic subsystems are phylogenetically ordered and behaviorally linked to social communication (e.g., facial expression, vocalization, listening), mobilization (e.g., fight–flight behaviors), and immobilization (e.g., feigning death, vaso–vagal syncope, and behavioral shutdown). The social communication system (i.e., social engagement system, see below) is dependent upon the myelinated vagus, which serves to foster calm behavioral states by inhibiting the sympathetic influences to the heart and dampening the hypothalamic–pituitary–adrenal (HPA) axis (e.g., Bueno et al. 1989). The mobilization system is dependent on the functioning of the sympathetic nervous system. The most phylogenetically primitive component, the immobilization system, is dependent on the unmyelinated or "vegetative" vagus, which is shared with most vertebrates. With increased neural complexity due to phylogenetic development, the organism's behavioral and affective repertoire is enriched. The theory emphasizes the functional aspect of neural control of both the striated muscles of the face and the smooth muscles of the viscera, since their functions rely on common brainstem structures.

By investigating the phylogeny of the regulation of the vertebrate heart (Morris and Nilsson 1994), three principles can be extracted. First, there is a phylogenetic shift in the regulation of the heart from endocrine communication, to unmyelinated nerves, and finally to myelinated nerves. Second, there is a development of opposing neural mechanisms of excitation and inhibition to provide rapid regulation of graded metabolic output. Third, with increased cortical development, the cortex exhibits greater control over the brainstem via direct (e.g., corticobulbar) and indirect (e.g., corticoreticular) neural pathways originating in motor cortex and terminating in the source nuclei of the myelinated motor nerves emerging from the brainstem (e.g., specific neural pathways embedded within cranial nerves V, VII, IX, X, XI), controlling visceromotor structures (i.e., heart, bronchi, thymus) and somatomotor structures (muscles of the face and head). These phylogenetic principles provide a basis for speculations regarding the neural mechanisms underlying social engagement as well as fight–flight and freeze behaviors.

In general, phylogenetic development results in increased neural control of the heart via the myelinated mammalian vagal system, which can promote transitory mobilization and the expression of sympathetic tone without requiring sympathetic or adrenal activation. With this new vagal system, transitory incursions into the environment or withdrawals from a potential predator can be initiated without the severe biological cost of the metabolic excitation associated with sympathetic–adrenal activation. Paralleling this change in neural control of the heart is an enhanced neural control of the face, larynx, and pharynx that enables complex facial gestures and vocalizations associated with social communication. This phylogenetic course results in greater central nervous system regulation of behavior, especially behaviors needed to engage and disengage with environmental challenges. Is it possible that psychiatric disorders, such as autism or RAD, in which compromised social behavior is a diagnostic feature, are associated with neurobiological states that foster defensive and not social behaviors?

The Vagal Brake

Due to the tonic vagal influences to the sinoatrial node (i.e., the heart's pacemaker), resting heart rate is substantially lower than the intrinsic rate of the pacemaker. When the vagal tone to the pacemaker is high, the vagus acts as a brake on the rate the heart is beating. When vagal tone to the pacemaker is low, there is little or no inhibition of the pacemaker. Thus, the vagal brake may be used as a construct to describe the functional modulation of heart rate by the myelinated vagal efferent pathways. The vagal brake provides a neural mechanism to rapidly change visceral state by slowing or speeding heart rate. Consistent with the assumptions of the Polyvagal Theory, the vagal brake contributes to the modulation of cardiac output by decreasing the inhibitory vagal control of the heart to speed heart rate and by increasing the inhibitory vagal control of the heart to slow heart rate. Thus, neurophysiologically the vagal brake provides a mechanism to support the metabolic requirements for mobilization and communication behaviors. Functionally, the vagal brake, by modulating visceral state, enables the individual to rapidly engage and disengage with objects and other individuals and to promote self-soothing behaviors and calm behavioral states. Developmentally, the number of myelinated vagal fibers increases linearly from 24–28 weeks gestation (Sarnat 2003) until term, when the number of fibers is comparable to those observed in adolescence (Sachis et al. 1982). In term infants, the myelination process is active during the first year of life, particularly during the first three months (Pereyra et al. 1992). Thus, deficits in the regulation of the vagal brake may be causal in problems in social communication observed early in development. Basically, the expression of social engagement behaviors is dependent upon the regulation of visceral state by the vagal brake. If visceral homeostasis is challenged and the vagal brake is unable to regulate visceral homeostasis, then social engagement behaviors will be minimized. This may be part of the deficit observed in autism and in RAD, in which social engagement behaviors are obviously compromised.

The Social Engagement System

The Polyvagal Theory provides an explicit neurobiological model of how difficulties in spontaneous social behavior are linked to both facial expressivity and the regulation of visceral state, and, alternatively how social behavior may serve as a regulator of physiological activity. The theory proposes a possible mechanism to explain how these difficulties might form a core domain of several psychiatric profiles. Relevant to this focus on psychiatric disorders are the specific deficits associated with several diagnoses in both the somatomotor (e.g., poor gaze, low facial affect, lack of prosody, difficulties in mastication) and visceromotor (difficulties in autonomic regulation resulting in cardiopulmonary and digestive problems) components of the social engagement system. For example, clinicians and researchers have documented these deficits in individuals with autistic spectrum disorders. Deficits in the social engagement system would compromise spontaneous social behavior, social awareness, affect expressivity, prosody, and language development. In contrast, interventions that improve the neural regulation of the social engagement system would hypothetically enhance spontaneous social behavior, state and affect regulation, reduce stereotypical behaviors, and improve language skills.

Embryologically, components of several cranial nerves known as special visceral efferent pathways develop together to form the neural substrate of a social engagement system (see Porges 1998). This system, as illustrated in Figure 3.1, provides the neural structures involved in social and emotional behaviors. The social engagement system has a control component in the cortex (i.e., upper motor neurons) that regulates brainstem nuclei (i.e., lower motor neurons) to control eyelid opening (e.g., looking), facial muscles (e.g., emotional expression), middle ear muscles (e.g., extracting human voice from background noise), muscle of mastication (e.g., ingestion), laryngeal and pharyngeal muscles (e.g., prosody), and head tilting and turning muscles (e.g., social gesture and orientation). Collectively, these muscles function not only as determinants of engagement with the social environment, but also as filters that limit social stimuli (e.g., observing facial features and listening to human voice). In addition, the source

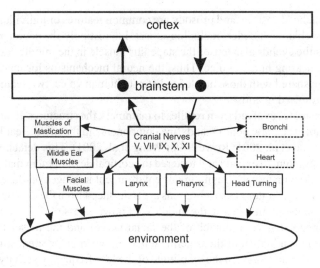

Figure 3.1 The social engagement system: Social communication is determined by the cortical regulation of medullary nuclei via corticobulbar pathways. The social engagement system consists of a somatomotor component (i.e., special visceral efferent pathways that regulate the muscles of the head and face) and a visceromotor component (i.e., the myelinated vagus that regulates the heart and bronchi). Solid blocks indicate the somatomotor component. Dashed blocks indicate the visceromotor component.

nuclei (i.e., lower motor neurons) of these nerves, which are located in the brainstem, communicate directly with an inhibitory neural system that slows heart rate, lowers blood pressure, and actively reduces arousal to promote calm states consistent with the metabolic demands of growth and restoration of our neurophysiological systems.

Direct corticobulbar pathways reflect the influence of frontal areas of the cortex (i.e., upper motor neurons) on the regulation of this system. Moreover, afferent feedback through the vagus to medullary areas (e.g., nucleus of the solitary tract) influences forebrain areas that are assumed to be involved in several psychiatric disorders. In addition, the anatomical structures involved in the social engagement system have neurophysiological interactions with the HPA axis, the neuropeptides of oxytocin and vasopressin, and the immune system (for an overview, see Porges 2001).

The study of comparative anatomy, evolutionary biology, and embryology may provide important hints regarding the functional relation between the neural control of the muscles of the face and head and emergent psychological experiences and behavior. Collectively, the neural pathways that regulate the muscles of the face and head are labeled as special visceral efferent. Special visceral efferent nerves innervate striated muscles, which regulate the structures derived during embryology from the ancient gill arches (Truex and Carpenter 1969). As a cluster, the difficulties in gaze, extraction of human voice, facial expression, head gesture, and prosody are common features of individuals with several psychiatric disorders including autism. Interestingly, the neural pathway that raises the eyelids also tenses the stapedius muscle in the middle ear, which facilitates hearing human voice. Thus, the neural mechanisms for making eye contact are shared with those needed to listen to human voice, two features that are compromised in autism.

As vertebrates evolved from reptiles to mammals, the structures at the end of the mandible (i.e., jaw bone) that define components in the middle ear became detached (Luo et al. 2001; Rowe 1996; Wang et al. 2001). This detachment allowed the cranium to expand and fostered the cortical development that characterizes modern mammals. Sound in our environment impinges on the eardrum and causes it to vibrate. These vibrations are transduced from the eardrum to the inner ear via the small bones in the middle ear known as ossicles. The stapedius muscle (innervated via a branch of the facial nerve) and the tensor tympani (innervated via a branch of the trigeminal nerve), when innervated, stiffen the ossicular chain and dampen the amplitude of the low-frequency activity reaching the inner ear. The functional impact of these muscles on the perceived acoustic environment is to markedly attenuate low-frequency sounds and to facilitate the extraction of high-frequency sounds associated with human voice. For example, our acoustic environment is often dominated by loud low-frequency sounds that have the functional effect of masking the soft high-frequency sounds associated with human voice. In humans, the ossicular chain is regulated primarily by the stapedius muscle and tensing the stapedius prevents this masking effect (see Borg and Counter 1989). In fact, individuals who can voluntarily contract middle ear muscles exhibit an attenuation of approximately 30 db at frequencies below 500 Hz, while there is no or minimal attenuation at frequencies above 1000 Hz (see Kryter 1985).

The evolution of the mammalian middle ear enabled low-amplitude, relatively high-frequency airborne sounds (i.e., sounds in the frequency of human voice) to be heard, even when the acoustic environment was dominated by low-frequency sounds. This phylogenetic innovation enables mammals to communicate in a frequency band that cannot be detected by reptiles, which were only able to hear lower frequencies due to their dependence on bone conduction to "hear." This ability to hear low-amplitude, high-frequency airborne sounds in an acoustic environment dominated by loud low-frequency sounds can only be accomplished when the middle ear muscles are tensed to increase the rigidity of the ossicular chain. Tensing the middle ear muscles prevents the low-frequency sounds from being transduced through the ossicular chain connecting the eardrum to the cochlear and, thus, facilitates the extraction of the high-frequency sounds associated with human voice.

Studies have demonstrated that the neural regulation of middle ear muscles, a necessary mechanism to extract the soft sounds of human voice from the loud sounds of low-frequency background noise, is defective in individuals with language delays, learning disabilities, and autistic spectrum disorders (Smith et al. 1988; Thomas et al. 1985). Middle ear infection (i.e., otitis media) may result in a total inability to elicit the "reflexive" contraction of the stapedius muscles (Yagi and Nakatani 1987). Disorders that influence the neural function of the facial nerve (i.e., Bell's Palsy), not only influence the stapedius reflex (Ardic et al. 1997), but also affect the patient's ability to discriminate speech (Wormald et al. 1995). Thus, the observed difficulties that many autistic individuals have in extracting human voice from background sounds may be dependent on the same neural system that regulates facial expression (i.e., the nerves that regulate the muscles of the face). Consistent with this speculation, there has been a report of an association between chronic otitis media and degenerative changes (e.g., demyelination) in the facial nerve (Djeric 1990).

Disorders of the Social Engagement System: Maladaptive or Adaptive Behavioral Strategies?

Individuals with several psychiatric and behavioral disorders have difficulties in establishing and maintaining relations. Several clinical diagnostic categories include features associated with difficulties both in expressing social behavior and in reading social cues (i.e., social awareness). These features are observed in individuals with a variety of primary psychiatric diagnoses including autism, social anxiety, posttraumatic stress disorder, and RAD.

Although a compromised social engagement system results in "maladaptive" social behavior, do these asocial behavioral strategies have "adaptive" features? The phylogeny of the vertebrate autonomic nervous system provides a guide (i.e., the Polyvagal Theory) to understand these adaptive features. Phylogenetically, the vertebrate autonomic nervous system follows three general stages of development. Each stage supports a different category of behavior with only the phylogenetically most recent innovation (i.e., the myelinated vagus) supporting social engagement behaviors. Since the neural regulation of the myelinated vagus is integrated into the social engagement system, when the social engagement system is compromised the effects are both behavioral and autonomic. The resultant changes in autonomic state support a range of adaptive defensive behaviors. Specifically, the compromised social engagement system is associated, neurophysiologically, with a change in autonomic regulation characterized by a reduction in the influence of the myelinated vagus (i.e., ventral vagal complex including nucleus ambiguus) on the heart. The removal of the regulatory influence of the ventral vagal complex on the heart potentiates the expression of the two phylogenetically older neural systems (i.e., sympathetic nervous system, dorsal vagal complex including dorsal nucleus of the vagus). These two older neural systems foster mobilization behaviors of fight and flight via the sympathetic nervous system or immobilization behaviors of death feigning, freezing, and behavioral shutdown via the dorsal vagal complex.

NEUROCEPTION: A NERVOUS SYSTEM
EVALUATION OF RISK

When individuals meet, what determines the biobehavioral sequence and consequence of their initial interactions? What contextual features and neural mechanisms trigger whether an individual expresses prosocial engagement or the specific defensive behaviors of fight, flight, or freeze? Regardless of the model of
attachment or its dependence on cognitive, affective, behavioral, or biological
constructs, the critical features that determine the valence of the interaction are
related to perceived safety. Thus, the perception of safety is the turning point in
the development of relationships for most mammals. The perception of safety
determines whether the behavior will be prosocial (i.e., social engagement) or
defensive. If the context and the other individual are perceived as safe, then the
candidates for the social bond may inhibit the adaptive primitive neurobiological reactions of defense to allow the expression of social engagement. The
three stages of the Polyvagal Theory articulate the neural systems that are available for social engagement and the defensive behaviors of fight, flight, and
freeze. However, how are the adaptive neurobiological systems for defense
functionally subdued to insure that attachment and the formation of social bonds
will be the products of appropriate social engagement?

Before a social bond can occur, both individuals have to perceive each other
as safe. What mediates the individual's ability to engage? Why would an infant
look and coo at a caregiver, while gaze avert and cry as a stranger approached?
Why would a gentle embrace be experienced as pleasurable when expressed by
a lover and be experienced as assault when expressed by a stranger? Mammals
have adaptive neurobehavioral systems for both defensive and social engagement behaviors. However, what enables engagement behaviors to occur, while
disenabling the mechanisms of defense? The Polyvagal Theory, with its focus
on the phylogeny of the vertebrate autonomic nervous system, provides a perspective to identify and to understand the plausible mechanisms that enable
mammals to functionally switch between positive social engagement and defensive behavioral strategies. To switch effectively from defensive to social engagement strategies, the mammalian nervous system needs to perform two
important processes: (a) to assess risk, and (b) if the environment is perceived as
safe, to inhibit the more primitive limbic structures that control fight, flight, or
freeze behaviors.

The nervous system, through the processing of sensory information from the
environment, continuously evaluates risk. Since the neural evaluation of risk
does not require conscious awareness, the term *neuroception* is introduced to
emphasize the neural circuits that function as a safety–threat detection system
capable of distinguishing among situations that are safe, dangerous, or life
threatening. Due to the phylogenetic heritage of mammals, neuroception can
operate without cognitive awareness via relatively primitive mechanisms that

are dependent upon subcortical structures (e.g., limbic). As a product of evolution, new neural systems evolved in mammals that involved cortical regulation of subcortical structures and, in many instances, co-opted the defense functions of the primitive structures to support other functions including those related to reproductive behavior and pair bonding (see Porges 1998).

Based on the relative risk of the environment, both social engagement and defense behaviors may be interpreted as either adaptive or maladaptive. For example, the inhibition of defense systems by the social engagement system would be adaptive and appropriate only in a safe environment. From a clinical perspective it would be the inability to inhibit defense systems in safe environments (e.g., anxiety disorders, RAD) or the inability to activate defense systems in risk environments (e.g., Williams Syndrome) that might contribute to the behavioral features that define specific psychopathologies. For example, an invalid neuroception of danger might contribute to maladaptive physiological reactivity and the expression of the defensive behaviors associated with specific psychiatric disorders. However, in most individuals neuroception accurately reflects risk and there is a consistency between the cognitive awareness of risk and the visceral response to risk.

There is a common feature between the invalid neuroception that identifies risk when no risk is there and McEwen's concept of "allostatic load" (McEwen and Wingfield 2003). The physiological reaction to a valid risk, although metabolically costly, is adaptive. Thus, the increased metabolic activity necessary to support the mobilization behaviors of fight and flight are adaptive in the short term, but costly to the organism if maintained. The duration of the response is an important feature that distinguishes between adaptive and maladaptive reactions. The complex mammalian nervous system evolved with a great dependence on oxygen and, unlike the reptile, can survive only for short periods without oxygen. Thus, breath holding for mammals is adaptive only for short periods. In contrast, apnea is adaptive for reptiles, who due to their limited needs for oxygen can inhibit breathing for long periods, while apnea is potentially lethal for mammals (Porges et al. 2003). Similarly, temporal features, in part, determine the construct of allostatic load. McEwen describes chronic stress or allostatic state as a physiological response that, although having adaptive functions in the short term, can be damaging if employed for long periods when it is no longer needed (i.e., invalid neuroception). This cost of adaptation or "maladaptation," McEwen refers to as "allostatic load."

SAFETY TRUMPS FEAR

In safe environments, autonomic state is adaptively regulated to dampen sympathetic activation and to protect the oxygen-dependent central nervous system from the metabolically conservative reactions via the dorsal vagal complex, a neural circuit shared with the vertebrates that preceded mammals. However, how does the nervous system know when the environment is safe, dangerous, or life threatening, and what neural mechanisms evaluate risk in the environment?

New technologies, such as fMRI, have identified specific neural structures that are involved in detecting risk. The temporal lobe is of particular interest in expanding the construct of neuroception and in identifying neural mechanisms that modulate the expression of adaptive defensive behaviors and autonomic states. Functional imaging techniques document that areas of the temporal cortex, fusiform gyrus (FG) and superior temporal sulcus (STS), are involved in detecting features such as movements, vocalizations, and faces, which contribute to an individual being perceived as safe or trustworthy (Adolphs 2002; Winston et al. 2002). Slight changes in these stimuli can pose threat or signal endearment. Connectivity between these areas of the temporal cortex and the amygdala suggests a top-down control in the processing of facial features that could actively inhibit activity of the structures involved in the expression of defensive strategies (Pessoa et al. 2002).

Neuroanatomical and neurophysiological research with animals provides additional information regarding the modulation and inhibition of defensive behaviors via well-defined connections between the amygdala and the periacqueductal gray (PAG). The PAG is a heterogeneous midbrain structure consisting of gray matter surrounding the cerebral aqueduct that connects the third and fourth ventricles. Studies have identified areas of the PAG that are organized to regulate flight, fight, or freeze behaviors and the autonomic states that support these behaviors (Keay and Bandler 2001). Stimulating rostrally within the lateral and dorsolateral PAG produces confrontational defensive behaviors (i.e., fight), whereas stimulating caudally within the lateral PAG and dorsolateral PAG produces escape behaviors (i.e., flight). Autonomic shifts such as increases in heart rate and blood pressure parallel these behaviors. In contrast, stimulation in the region of the PAG ventrolateral to the aqueduct (vlPAG) evokes a passive reaction of immobility, a drop in blood pressure, and a slowing of heart rate. Interestingly, excitation of the vlPAG evokes an opioid-mediated analgesia that might adaptively raise pain thresholds. In addition, there is evidence of a functional connection between the central nucleus of the amygdala and the vlPAG that modulates both antinociception and immobilization (Leite-Panissi et al. 2003). Consistent with the Polyvagal Theory, the vlPAG communicates with dorsal vagal complex, while the lPAG and dlPAG communicate with the sympathetic nervous system.

In the absence of threat, inhibitory projections from the FG and STS to the amygdala would be available to actively inhibit the limbic defense systems. This inhibition would provide an opportunity for social behavior to occur. Thus, the appearance of a friend or mate would subdue the limbic activation with the biobehavioral consequences of allowing proximity, physical contact, and other social engagement behaviors. In contrast, during situations in which the appraisal of risk is high, the amygdala and various areas of the PAG are activated.

Only the central nucleus of the amygdala shares connections with the PAG (Rizvi et al. 1991).

The detection of safety subdues the adaptive defensive systems dependent on limbic structures. Thus, providing a plausible model of how a *neural* detection of environmental risk (i.e., *neuroception*) would modulate behavior and physiological state to support adaptive behaviors in response to safe, dangerous, and life threatening environments. Conceptually, the process of detecting safety is inclusive of the detection of risk. Thus, the neural circuits that mediate the more primitive defense systems have, through the processes of evolution, been co-opted to support the social behavior necessary for mammalian survival. These behaviors include social engagement and the behaviors associated with social bonding (e.g., reproductive behaviors and nursing). With development, other neural circuits associated with learning and language may also be involved in inhibiting or triggering the primitive defense system systems.

CO-OPTING THE IMMOBILIZATION DEFENSE SYSTEM FOR REPRODUCTIVE BEHAVIORS, NURSING, AND THE FORMATION OF SOCIAL BONDS

Immobilization as a defense system is phylogenetically old and is associated with reduced metabolic demands and increased pain threshold. In reptiles, due to their limited need for oxygen, immobilization is a very effective defense strategy. In contrast, since mammals have a great need for oxygen, the inhibition of movement coupled with a shift in autonomic state to support the immobilization behavior (i.e., apnea and bradycardia) can be lethal (Hofer 1970; Richter 1957). However, several aspects of mammalian social behavior require immobilization, but immobilization without fear. Immobilization without fear is accomplished by co-opting the structures that regulate immobilization and pain thresholds to serve a broad range of social needs including reproduction, nursing, and pair bonding. By focusing on the area of the PAG that coordinates freezing behavior we can see how a primitive immobilization defense system has been modified through evolution to serve the intimate social needs of mammals. In addition, when we study the vlPAG we find that it is rich in receptors for oxytocin, a neuropeptide associated with partuition, nursing, and the establishment of pair bonds (Carter 1998; Insel and Young 2001).

Overlapping with the area of the PAG that organizes immobility (i.e., vlPAG) are areas that when stimulated produce lordosis and kyphosis. The lordosis reflex is a hormone-dependent behavior displayed by female rodents and other mammalian species during mating. In most mammals lordosis involves the female immobilizing in a crouching posture with her hind end available to the male for copulation. Neural tracing studies have demonstrated that the vlPAG is part of the neural circuit involved in regulating lordosis (Daniels et al. 1999). Kyphosis is an upright crouching posture that is accompanied by inhibition of limb movements. This posture is stimulated by nipple attachment and provides an opportunity for the dam to feed simultaneously a large litter. When dams initiate a nursing bout, behavioral state shifts immediately from high activity to immobility (Stern 1997). When the caudal portion of the vlPAG is lesioned there are important consequences: (a) kyphotic nursing decreases, (b) litter weight gains decrease, and (c) the lesioned rats are more aggressive and more frequently attack strange males (Lonstein and Stern 1998).

TEST OF THE MODEL

The processes of attachment and the formation of social bonds require appropriate social engagement strategies. In the sections above, elements of a preliminary model are presented that link social engagement to attachment and the formation of social bonds. The model is expanded from the Polyvagal Theory and emphasizes the following points: (a) there are well-defined neural circuits to support social engagement behaviors and the defensive strategies of fight, flight, and freeze, (b) without being dependent on conscious awareness, the nervous system evaluates risk in the environment and regulates the expression of adaptive behavior to match the neuroception of a safe, dangerous, or life-threatening environment, (c) social engagement behaviors and the benefits of the physiological states associated with social support require a neuroception of safety, (4) social behaviors associated with nursing, reproduction, and the formation of strong pair bonds require immobilization without fear, and (5) immobilization without fear is mediated by a co-opting of the neural circuit regulating defensive freezing behaviors through the involvement of oxytocin, a neuropeptide involved in the formation of social bonds (Carter and Keverne 2002; Winslow and Insel 2002).

Figures 3.2–3.4 illustrate the role that neuroception plays in determining the neural circuits recruited to regulate social engagement, fight, flight, and freeze behaviors. Each figure illustrates a different environment context (i.e., safe, dangerous, life threat). Figure 3.2 illustrates the assumed neural circuits involved in promoting social engagement behaviors in a safe context. The detection of safe or trustworthy features derived from face, voice, and movement activate a neural circuit that projects from the temporal cortex (i.e., FG, STS) to the central nucleus of the amygdala to inhibit defensive limbic functions (see Figures 3.3 and 3.4). This circuit disenables the limbic defense systems that organize and regulate fight, flight, and freeze behaviors and enables the corticobulbar pathways that regulate the social engagement behaviors (see Figure 3.1). Figure 3.3 illustrates the neural circuits involved in a response to a neuroception of danger. In response to danger, the limbic defense circuits function to adaptively protect the individual. The specificity of the defense strategy, whether confrontational or avoidant (i.e., fight or flight), is regulated by the

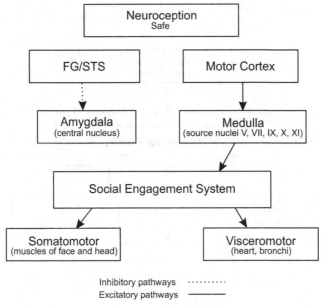

Figure 3.2 Neural structures and pathways involved in a neuroception of safety.

PAG. To support these mobilization behaviors, the sympathetic nervous system is activated and dominates autonomic state. Figure 3.4 illustrates the neural circuits involved in response to life threat. In response to life threat the mammalian nervous system promotes immobilization or freezing behavior. Freezing, as a defense strategy, is coordinated by the PAG. To inhibit metabolic activity during immobilization, autonomic state is under the control of the dorsal vagal complex. As proposed by the Polyvagal Theory, the autonomic reactions, during each adaptive behavioral strategy, are hierarchically organized following the phylogeny of both the changes in the vertebrate autonomic nervous system and changes in the behavioral repertoire from immobilization to mobilization to social engagement.

The ability to evaluate whether the environment is safe or if a person is trustworthy is difficult for individuals with a variety of psychiatric diagnoses. Current research suggests that the areas in the temporal cortex (i.e., FG, STS), which are assumed to inhibit limbic defense reactions, are not activated in clinical populations that have difficulties with social engagement behaviors (e.g., autism, schizophrenia). Moreover, individuals diagnosed with other psychiatric disorders such as anxiety disorders and depression, which have as diagnostic features compromised social behavior, have difficulties in regulating visceral state (e.g., lower vagal regulation of the heart) and supporting social engagement behaviors (e.g., reduced facial expressiveness and motor control of the striated

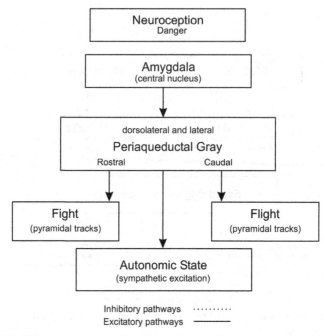

Figure 3.3 Neural structures and pathways involved in a neuroception of danger.

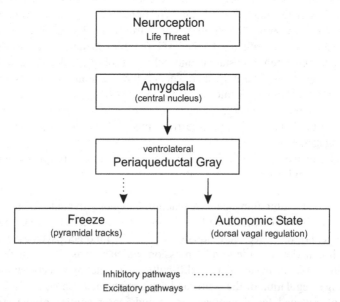

Figure 3.4 Neural structures and pathways involved in a neuroception of life threat.

muscles of the face and head). Thus, from a theoretical perspective, a potential root of several psychiatric disorders might be linked to an inability to detect safety in the environment and trustworthiness from interactions and, thus, the inability to express appropriate social engagement behaviors.

The study of attachment disorders, such as RAD, provides an intriguing test of the critical role of neuroception in mediating appropriate attachment and social behavior. RAD is described in both the DSM-IV (American Psychiatric Association 1994) and the ICD-10 (World Health Organization 1992) psychiatric diagnostic manuals. RAD comprises two clinical patterns (i.e., inhibited and uninhibited subtypes). The inhibited subtype is characterized by an emotionally withdrawn, unresponsive pattern in which there is an absence of attachment behaviors. The disinhibited subtype is characterized by indiscriminate attachment, which is often directed at strangers. These patterns have been described in institutionalized and maltreated children (Zeanah 2000). From a neuroception perspective, in both subtypes, the evaluation of the risk in the environment is not accurate.

Recent research on the outcomes of children raised in institutions in Romania has stimulated interest in RAD and in developing intervention strategies to remediate these devastating disturbances in social development. If an accurate neuroception of the environment is necessary for normal social behavior, then what features in the environment might potentiate normal social development? A recent study of Romanian toddlers (Smyke et al. 2002) provides insight into the process. In this study indices of RAD were evaluated in children as a function of the number of different caregivers. Two groups of institutionalized children were evaluated and contrasted to children who were never institutionalized. One group consisted of the standard institution unit in which 20 different caregivers worked rotating shifts with approximately three caregivers for 30 children on each shift. A second group consisted of a pilot unit in which the number of children was reduced to about ten and the pool of caregivers was reduced to four. If neuroception of safety is necessary to promote appropriate social behavior, then familiarity of caregiver would be critical. By having familiar caregivers, the child's detection of the caregiver's face, voice, and movements (the features that define a safe and trustworthy person) should trigger the inhibitory pathways to disenable the limbic defense system and foster the behaviors expressed by the social engagement system. In support of this model, the study demonstrated a monotonic relation between the number of different caregivers that a child had contact with and the indices of RAD. On all measures the standard unit children were more likely to have higher indices of RAD and on some measures the pilot group did not differ from the children who were never institutionalized. Thus, once we understand the contextual and social features that inhibit the neural circuits that mediate defensive behavioral strategies, we can optimize the developmental consequences of the neural circuits that promote social engagement behaviors.

CONCLUSIONS

The Polyvagal Theory forces us to interpret compromised social behavior and attachment from a different perspective. The theory emphasizes that the range of social behavior is limited by physiological state. The theory emphasizes that mobilization and immobilization behaviors may be adaptive strategies to a challenged (e.g., frightened) individual. Thus, it may be possible that creating states of calmness and exercising the neural regulation of brainstem structures may potentiate positive social behavior by stimulating the neural regulation of the social engagement system. This perspective forms the basis for our intervention research program. In our research we focus on biologically based behaviors, which trigger the neural substrate required for social engagement behaviors, in contrast to the more commonly administered behavioral and biochemical (i.e., pharmacological) intervention strategies.

ACKNOWLEDGMENTS

The preparation of this manuscript was supported in part by a grant from the National Institutes of Health (MH 60625). Several of the ideas presented in this manuscript are the products of discussions with C. Sue Carter.

REFERENCES

Adolphs, R. 2002. Trust in the brain. _Nature Neurosci._ **5**:192–193.
Ainsworth, M., M. Blehar, E. Waters, and S. Walls. 1978. Patterns of Attachment: A Psychological Study of the Strange Situation. Hillsdale, NJ: Erlbaum.
American Psychiatric Association. 1994. Diagnostic and Statistical Manual of Mental Disorders. 4th ed. Washington, D.C.: Am. Psychiatric Assn.
Ardic, F.N., I. Topaloglu, S. Oncel, F. Ardic, and M.Z. Uguz. 1997. Does the stapes reflex remain the same after Bell's Palsy? _Am. J. Otology_ **18**:761–765.
Borg, E., and S.A. Counter. 1989. The middle-ear muscles. _Sci. Am._ **26**:74–80.
Bowlby, J. 1982. Attachment. 2nd ed. Attachment and Loss, vol. 1. New York: Basic.
Bueno, L., M. Gue, M.J. Fargeas et al. 1989. Vagally mediated inhibition of acoustic stress-induced cortisol release by orally administered kappa-opioid substances in dogs. _Endocrinology_ **124**:1788–1703.
Carter, C.S. 1998. Neuroendocrine perspectives on social attachment and love. _Psychoneuroendocrin._ **23**:779–818.
Carter, C.S., and E.B. Keverne. 2002. The neurobiology of social affiliation and pair bonding. In: Hormones, Brain, and Behavior, ed. D.W. Pfaff et al., pp. 299–337. San Diego: Academic.
Cassidy, J., and P.R. Shaver, eds. 1999. Handbook of Attachment: Theory, Research, and Clinical Application. New York: Guilford.
Daniels, D., R.R. Miselis, and L.M. Flanagan-Cato. 1999. Central neuronal circuit innervating the lordosis-producing muscles defined by transneuronal transport of pseudorabies virus. _J. Neurosci._ **19**:2823–2833.

Djeric, D. 1990. Neuropathy of the facial nerve in chronic otitis media without associated facial paralysis: A human temporal bone study. *Eur. Arch. Otorhinolaryngology* **247**:232–236.

Hofer, M.A. 1970. Cardiac respiratory function during sudden prolonged immobility in wild rodents. *Psychosom. Med.* **32**:633–647.

Insel, T.R., and L.J. Young. 2001. The neurobiology of attachment. *Nat. Rev. Neurosci.* **2**:129–136.

Keay, K.A., and R. Bandler. 2001. Parallel circuits mediating distinct emotional coping reactions to different types of stress. *Neurosci. Biobehav. Rev.* **25**:669–678.

Kryter, K.D. 1985. The Effects of Noise on Man. New York: Academic.

Leite-Panissi, C.R., N.C. Coimbra, and L. Menescal-de-Oliveira. 2003. The cholinergic stimulation of the central amygdala modifying the tonic immobility response and antinociception in guinea pigs depends on the ventrolateral periaqueductal gray. *Brain Res. Bull.* **60**:167–178.

Lonstein, J.S., and J.M. Stern. 1998. Site and behavioral specificity of periaqueductal gray lesions on postpartum sexual, maternal, and aggressive behaviors in rats. *Brain Res.* **804**:21–35.

Luo, Z.X., A.W. Crompton, and A.L. Sun. 2001. A new mammaliaform from the early Jurassic and evolution of mammalian characteristics. *Science* **292**:1535–1540.

McEwen, B.S., and J.C. Wingfield. 2003. The concept of allostasis in biology and biomedicine. *Horm. Behav.* **43**:2–15.

Morris, J.L., and S. Nilsson. 1994. The circulatory system. In: Comparative Physiology and Evolution of the Autonomic Nervous System, ed. S. Nilsson and S. Holmgren, pp. 193–246. Chur: Harwood.

Newman, J.D. 1988. The Physiological Control of Mammalian Vocalizations. New York: Plenum.

Pereyra, P.M., W. Zhang, M. Schmidt, and L.E. Becker. 1992. Development of myelinated and unmyelinated fibers of human vagus nerve during the first year. *J. Neurol. Sci.* **110**:107–113.

Pessoa, L., M. McKenna, E. Gutierrez, and L.G. Ungerleider. 2002. Neuroprocessing of emotional faces requires attention. *PNAS* **99**:11,458–11,463.

Porges, S.W. 1995. Orienting in a defensive world: Mammalian modifications of our evolutionary heritage: A Polyvagal Theory. *Psychophysiology* **32**:301–318.

Porges, S.W. 1997. Emotion: An evolutionary by-product of the neural regulation of the autonomic nervous system. *Ann. NY Acad. Sci.* **807**:62–77.

Porges, S.W. 1998. Love: An emergent property of the mammalian autonomic nervous system. *Psychoneuroendocrin.* **23**:837–861.

Porges, S.W. 2001. The Polyvagal Theory: Phylogenetic substrates of a social nervous system. *Intl. J. Psychophysiol.* **42**:123–146.

Porges, S.W., T.C. Riniolo, T. McBride, and B. Campbell. 2003. Heart rate and respiration in reptiles: Contrasts between a sit-and-wait predator and an intensive forager. *Brain Cogn.* **52**:88–96.

Richter, C.P. 1957. On the phenomenon of sudden death in animals and man. *Psychosom. Med.* **19**:191–198.

Rizvi, T.A., M. Ennis, M.M. Behbehani, and M.T. Shipley. 1991. Connections between the central nucleus of the amygdala and the midbrain periaqueductal gray: Topography and reciprocity. *J. Comp. Neurol.* **303**:121–131.

Rowe, T. 1996. Coevolution of the mammalian middle ear and neocortex. *Science* **273**:651–654.

Sachis, P.N., D.L. Armstrong, L.E. Becker, and A.C. Bryan. 1982. Myelination of the human vagus from 24 weeks postconceptional age to adolescence. *J. Neuropath. Exp. Neurol.* **41**:466–472.

Sarnat, H.B. 2003. Functions of the corticospinal and corticobulbar tracts in the human newborn. *J. Pediatric Neurol.* **1**:3–8.

Smith, D.E.P., S.D. Miller, M. Stewart, T.L. Walter, and J.V. McConnell. 1988. Conductive hearing loss in autistic, learning-disabled, and normal children. *J. Autism Dev. Disorders* **18**:53–65.

Smyke, A.T., A. Dumitrescu, and C.H. Zeanah. 2002. Attachment disturbances in young children. I. The continuum of caretaking casuality. *J. Am. Acad. Child Adoles. Psych.* **41**:972–982.

Stern, J.M. 1997. Offspring-induced nurturance: Animal-human parallels. *Dev. Psychobiol.* **31**:19–37.

Thomas, W.G., G. McMurry, and H.C. Pillsbury. 1985. Acoustic reflex abnormalities in behaviorally disturbed and language delayed children. *Laryngoscope* **95**:811–817.

Truex, R.C., and M.B. Carpenter. 1969. Human Neuroanatomy. 6th ed. Baltimore: Williams and Wilkins.

Wang, Y., Y. Hu, J. Meng, and C. Li. 2001. An ossified Mechel's cartilage in two cretaceous mammals and origin of the mammalian middle ear. *Science* **294**:357–361.

Winslow, J.T., and T.R. Insel. 2002. The social deficits of the oxytocin knockout mouse. *Neuropeptides* **36**:221–229.

Winston, J.S., B.A. Strange, J. O'Doherty, and R.J. Dolan. 2002. Automatic and intentional brain responses during evaluation of trustworthiness of faces. *Nature Neurosci.* **5**:277–283.

World Health Organization. 1992. The ICD-10 Classification of Mental and Behavioural Disorders: Clinical Descriptions and Diagnostic Guidelines. Geneva: WHO.

Wormald, P.J., C. Rogers, and S. Gatehouse. 1995. Speech discrimination in patients with Bell's Palsy and paralysed stapedius muscle. *Clin. Otolaryngology* **20**:59–62.

Yagi, N., and H. Nakatani. 1987. Stapedial muscle electromyography in various diseases. *Arch. Otolarynogology: Head Neck Surg.* **113**:392–396.

Zeanah, C.H. 2000. Disturbances of attachment in young children adopted from institutions. *J. Dev. Behav. Pediat.* **21**:230–236.

4

"Stepping Away from the Mirror: Pride and Shame in Adventures of Companionship"

Reflections on the Nature and Emotional Needs of Infant Intersubjectivity

C. TREVARTHEN

Department of Psychology, The University of Edinburgh, Edinburgh, Scotland, U.K.

ABSTRACT

This chapter contends that classical attachment theory, and the contemporary transformation of it into a theory of maternal external regulation of the neonates physiology and emotional processes, fail to grasp the importance of motives for relationships between offspring and their parents that serve shared discovery of new ways of behaving. A good human mother is more than a protector of the human infant from fear, and more than a known and secure "base" from which the infant may explore and gain experience. She, like others whom the infant may know and like, is a friend and playmate.

Infants take initiative in their learning and have rich intersubjective powers. Descriptive studies of infant communication with any persons who offer sympathetic human response show that, from the moment of birth, other processes are active besides those that seek protection and regulation of vital state. There is a mental engagement between interests and purposes and an emotional evaluation of the quality of concordant activity to discover and use experiences. Developments before language show that meaning is discovered in playful collaborative friendships, and that its discovery is motivated by pleasure in dynamically responsive company. The young child seeks a place in a community of "common sense," not just security in attachments.

Investigation of core brain mechanisms — which coordinate and guide intentional and investigative movements, that infuse actions with emotion, that evaluate goals and discoveries aesthetically in the regulation of learning, and that signal all these motivating events to others — indicates that deep-seated emotional systems have a role in both the sharing of emotions and experiences with other individuals, and adaptive change in the growing brain and its cognitive capacities.

It is proposed that human beings have a specially adapted capacity for sympathy of brain activity that drives cultural learning. We need to understand the passions of this capacity if we are to appreciate normal child learning, and to recognize and alleviate the effects of deprivation, inadequate parenting, and psychopathology intrinsic to the child.

INTRODUCTION

In the intimacy of the family and in the less intimate company of people in the community, life, for all of us, depends on mutual awareness — on inter-subjectivity. We meet others as persons with intentions, consciousness, and feelings who interact with ourselves as friends or strangers. Persons may offer affection or antagonism, but their behavior is always in some sort of sympathy, never indifferent to perception of our presence.

A mirror offers a poor substitute for the living other we meet who meets us. A peculiar inversion in reflected light, its image lacks all psychological reciprocity. It cannot have sympathy. It can only show us how we move.

I offer "stepping away from the mirror" as a metaphor for a mind taking initiative in company — for a person asserting free will and independent curiosity. He or she may never be quite alone, may always be expecting to be active under real or imagined scrutiny by the attention of others, but should not wish to be dependent on their will. Infants are born with a bold self-consciousness of this kind; one that soon takes responsibility for independent acting and thinking, but that also may feel pleasure and pride in the approval of others, and shame at failure before them.

Taking initiative awakens a conscience that may bring joy or terrible regret. This is how we are able to belong in what the Italian psychiatrist Stanghellini (2001; Stanghellini and Ballerini 2002) calls "common sense," which is governed by complex affections and a sense of moral involvement. We can seek vain gratification in a mirror, and we can check our appearance, but the image in the mirror is not free, and it gives us no part in a friendship.

Vasu Reddy (2000) showed that a two- to three-month-old infant will look away with a "coy" smile when held up to face a mirror by the mother (Figure 4.1). Reddy notes that the behavior has the same form as that which regulates other humorous displays of self-consciousness with familiar others by young infants, i.e., in contexts of social attention by people whom the infant knows and likes (Reddy 2001a, 2003). Human relationships are motivated by innate emotions of affection, or of disaffection, that display and evaluate shared purposes and interests. These emotions of "attachment for companionship," innate affective systems for testing the opportunity and value of shared activity and experience, are as important for mental health as emotions of "attachment for care."

Intelligence is the product of animate activity, of being interested, making "experience." It depends upon what Panksepp (1998, 2000) identifies as "seeking" motives that prompt investigation and experiment (Table 4.1). Like other young mammals, infants are born with "investigative intelligence" (Wemelsfelder 1993), as well as with needs for parental care and protection of their

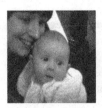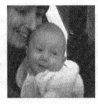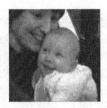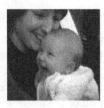

Figure 4.1 An 11-week-old infant shows a classic "coy" reaction when her mother holds her up to a mirror (Reddy 2000). (Photos reproduced with permission of Dr. Vasudevi Reddy.)

Table 4.1 Motives for regulation of the well-being of the body, for engagement with objects and the physical environment, and for communication with persons are necessarily different. In combination they regulate attachments, practical activities, and cooperation in the companionship by which knowledge and skills of culture are propagated. There are different physiological systems in the brain for these functions, and they are differently implicated in fields of scholarship, in technology and in social institutions.

Motives and Goals	Attachment and Care	Creative, Practical Consciousness	Companionship and Collaboration
Functions	• Seeking or giving care, comfort, and protection • Love • Sex • Nurturing, being nurtured • Therapeutic relationships	• Object cognition • Praxis, making things • Skills • Exploring nature and existence • Objective experience and knowledge	• Knowing/acting through communication, teaching/learning culture and language • Thinking theoretically, symbolically • Causing objects and actions to become meaningful
Academic and research field	Physiological and clinical psychology	S-R and learning theory, cognitive psychology	Intersubjective psychology
Application	• Parenting • Nursing • Socal work • Psychotherapy	• Science and engineering • Technology • Artificial intelligence	• Art and education • Business • Politics • Shared knowledge and skills
Affective system	• Consummation (well-being or contentedness) • Mutual pleasure	• Individual action and cognition • Seeking (anticipation or desire incentive)	• Both social and intellectual
Neurobiology	Trophotropic	Ergotropic	Integrating all systems

bodies. A young child makes games with the body and with what the world and other persons offer, imagining new tricks and solutions to problems that arise from acting on objects and in communication. This kind of information-seeking "assimilatory" intelligence builds the "object schemata" that Jean Piaget (1954) discovered. However, the rationalist Piaget gave little attention to the social aspect of the infant's search for experience.

From birth, a child's learning depends upon sharing his or her impulsive acting and thinking with other familiar persons, who themselves are experimenters, discoverers, and communicators, eager to share what they think and do (Trevarthen 1982). It is a serious deficiency of modern cognitive psychology that this interpersonal motivation for intelligence remains on the margins of the experimental psychology of early childhood, or a "special case" of consciousness of impersonal objects. The learning of meaning, of culture in all its forms, the getting to be part of "common sense," requires discovery in experimental or playful joint activities. What teachers call the child's "disposition to learn" is an urge of an inventive self that wants to be recognized by others, a self who teachers discover needs collaboration and encouragement from them (Bruner 1996; Rogoff 1998; Trevarthen 2001b).

In the discussion we are having about the importance of early attachments for mental health, I want to underline the two concerns we all have known from birth: to be both free in our hopes and enterprises, and to be accepted with approval by those who experience our acting (Trevarthen 2001a). We have always known who are the most important of our acquaintances, and we care what they think of us and how they receive the independence of our minds.

It is important to attend to the intellectual aspect of Freud's theory about the forces of emotional life and morality. I believe he, too, underestimated the innate capacity of a child to share understanding and to collaborate in intentions, and to have responsibility for them, without intellect. Thus his psychoanalytic explanation of anxieties and delusions of the self finds it simpler to attribute such failures of the spirit to lack of care and love, as if the child must have emotions molded by the responses of others to simple pleasures and pains of the self. I do not believe the infant's ego is unaware of the "alter" as a purposeful agent who may offer joy in collaboration.

THE NATURE OF SYMPATHETIC COMMUNICATION OF INITIATIVES, AND THEIR EMOTIONS

Animal agency is never just imitative, never just instructed, and never just protected. It does not just react to stimuli. There are emotionally charged negotiations of interest and purpose with every object or subject that attracts interest. Negotiations with objects, or in layout of the physical world within which we move, need prospective awareness of the "affordances" of things (Gibson 1979). This requires anticipatory guidance of the forces of the body in movement to fit environmental information (Lee 1998). Negotiations between active subjects or persons, depend on communication of states of vitality and consciousness between bodies, on socio-emotional affordances (Neisser 1993).

The intensity and aim of an animal's agency is communicated by the pulse, expressive form, and orientation of movement, even in invertebrates. As bodies have evolved more complex capacities for moving in, investigating about, and using the environment, they have gained in complexity, and the adaptive strength of the consciousness of the brain-regulated "self" has grown (Merker 2005). As social beings, animal bodies have evolved sympathetic detection between subjects of the motives inherent in one another's ways of moving (Rizzolatti et al. 2001; Trevarthen 1986a, 1997b). All social cooperation depends on this mysterious intersubjective sympathy (Trevarthen and Aitken 2001). Communication of emotions serves to increase the efficiency of cooperative action and the formation of dependable alliances in activity (Trevarthen 2004a). Impulses to move excite, not exactly "mirror" effects in the motor centers of other brains, but negotiable "sympathetic" impulses in the emotional systems of other individuals (Decety and Chaminade 2003). By this means the couple, family, group, or society gains the properties of an "organism" of higher adaptive order, the cohesion of which depends on the matching and mutually supportive emotions of its members. It depends on "sympathy."

My principal point is that care is but one form of cooperative behavior between subjects. Sympathy, from Greek *sympatheia*, means "moving and feeling with," in collaboration or in competition, not just solicitous concern, sensitivity, kindness, or help. It is not the effusion of emotion, described by the ancient Greek word *empatheia*, which is one-sided and suitable only to describe aesthetic contemplation of a passive object that is felt to inspire emotion. It is not as *empatheia* is in modern Greek, the deceitful projection onto another of malicious feelings of envy or hate. Respectful and responsive sympathy respects autonomy in its object, even when it disapproves; it is like an active form of Adam Smith's thinking "conscience," a "disinterested" presence that is firm in judgment about right and wrong in one's actions, but free to be indulgent, affectionate, and understanding (Smith 1759).

MOTIVES FOR COMPANIONSHIP IN THE EMOTIONS OF LEARNING

In my observations of the spontaneous communication of purposes, interests, and experiences of discovery between infants and their mothers or fathers, I see powerful innate motives and emotions on both sides that promote the shared pleasures and sometimes tough negotiations of *friendship* (Figure 4.2). These require more than just "rhythms of approach and withdrawal" (Winnicott 1960). A pleasure in discovering what more than one mind can conceive, seeking and finding approval for an original act or idea, is essential, and it grows rapidly with shared experiences in the life history of the relationship.

60

Figure 4.2 (a) At three months, Laura is a source of pleasure and pride to her family. Here we observe three degrees of intimacy in her presence: her mother seeks proto-conversation, her three-year-old sister wishes to be part of the game, and her father sits at a distance but is clearly admiring. On the right, Laura smiles and coos while "chatting" with her mother in the laboratory at the University of Edinburgh.
(b) Leanne is very curious about her mirror image at five months. At four months she tried to catch a ball presented by her mother, and enjoyed a musical game while her mother held her hands.
Photos by Colwyn Trevarthen.

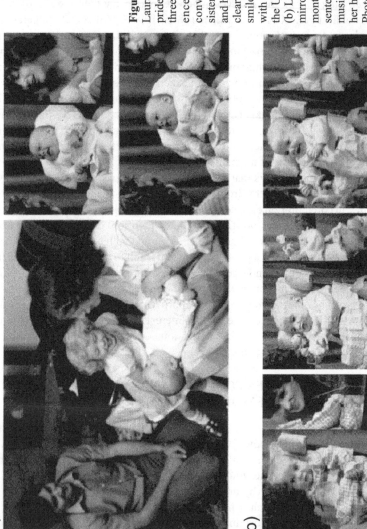

From birth to the beginning of language the child makes expressive moves to have adventures and ideas with known companions, to express impulses of thought that gain in meaning by being shared (Stern 2000; Trevarthen 1998, 2003). Memories and ideas are built in communication, in increasingly rich narratives of imaginative "mimesis" (Donald 2001). These intrinsically prompted developments have profound effects on the behavior of an affectionate, firmly "attached" parent, binding him or her to the life experience of the child. The child "educates" the adult how to discover meanings that make sense and joy for both of them.

It is increasingly realized that in effective psychotherapy a process has to be set in motion that is close to the dynamic relationship of mutual affection and trust that grows between a parent and child (Schore 2003a). When there is pain and suffering, there is need for compassion, supportive affection, and comfort. When there is the beginning of hope, there is need for praise and reflected pleasure, for fun and collaboration in a confident friendship.

Finally, a word has to be said about education and how it compares with therapy or "treatment," because I believe we have the same need to re-conceive the fundamental needs of children and their teachers for *collaborative learning* (Rogoff 1998; Trevarthen 2004c). It may be convenient for the management of a complex industrial society to plan education as a construction of skills according to curricular formulae that are "quality tested" at each prescribed stage. This is an artificial cultivation of the natural process by which children need to master cultural knowledge and for which adults give natural encouragement. The "intent participation" of the child in mastery of meaning with known and liked teachers must be respected (Rogoff et al. 2003).

THE ACHIEVEMENT AND LIMITS OF ATTACHMENT THEORY

The clinical observations of infants' and toddlers' distress after separation from parental care that led John Bowlby to his attachment theory required child psychiatrists and social workers to conceive more clearly what infants need from their mothers, and to change professional practices where these needs had been disregarded. It opened the way for a more coherent biological theory of how the emotions of the infant are open to maternal care (Bowlby 1988). Bowlby defined a form of emotional involvement that protects the young child in intimacy with a sensitive caregiver, and that leads to a kind of grieving when a parent's presence is lost. Approach behaviors of the child, and "imprinting" on the stimulations from parents (from eye contact, smiles, vocal signals of affection, body contact), became comprehensible as essential biological foundations for human relationships, and for the building of representations (working models) of a parent as a source of emotional strength and security.

The experimental investigations of Ainsworth (Ainsworth and Bell 1970) proved that different qualities of attachment between one-year-old children and their mothers could be rigorously identified, by recording the behavior of the child on reunion with the mother after a stressful separation. Main, who was also the first to draw attention to the fact that a child may actively distance itself from a parent (Main and Weston 1982), made the important discovery that the quality of a mother's relationship to her toddler could be correlated not only with a later stage of that relationship, and the child's social functioning, but also with the mother's thoughts and memories about her own childhood (Main and Goldwyn 1984). Thus a transgenerational transmission of emotional security in relationships, or of how these relationships are represented in person's minds, was demonstrated.

With advances in brain science, and especially in the understanding of emotional systems and their role in regulation not only of bodily well-being, but also of cognition and learning (Damasio 1999; Freeman 1999), the fundamental importance of subconsciously mediated affections in support of the development of a child's strong and confident self has become evident (Damasio 1999; Schore 1994, 2003b). Protection from the damaging effects of stress on the vulnerable infant brain can be demonstrated as one of the main benefits of close and consistent maternal contact and responsive care.

However, preoccupation with the support and protection a parent must give for the healthy development of a child's neurohumoral processes of alertness, stress-reduction, and energy recuperation does not address the more creative and positive needs of a human child who is motivated to explore meanings of experience in play with companions. Attachment theory, in its classical form, and especially in the form that has been tested experimentally with animals and through statistical analysis of socio-emotional developments in populations of children with different qualities and quantities of maternal care, does not explain the drive of young humans to invent new ways of behaving or thinking, and to discover new things to be interested in, and then to seek confirmation, praise, and practical cooperation from the minds of others. Though being given love, ease and food for living is necessary and good, affectionate human company, even for a very young infant, offers more than provision of comfort and sustenance. A "secure base" is not an appropriate metaphor for the "intuitive parenting" of a mentor or companion in play and learning (Papousek and Papousek 1987). We must also consider the biological foundations for imagination and thinking that makes a child's experience meaningful by giving it values and uses that other people have found to be important. We must comprehend the adaptive needs of human common sense, and the cruel suffering with diminished vitality that can be the effect of exclusion from meaning, whatever its cause.

Attachment theory has often been criticized for paying exclusive attention to maternal care. A mother has a unique importance for the nurturance of a newborn infant, and her loving presence gains a special power from its intimacy, which can remain as a lifeline for the child and for the adult, he or she becomes. No young child thrives without affectionate "mothering" from someone who cares consistently. However, the infant's pleasure in companionship and discovery can be shared with any playful partner, of any age, even a peer, and with more than one other (Belsky 1981; Fivaz-Depeursinge and Corboz-Wanery 1999). This point is forcefully presented by Selby and Bradley (2003) in a study of negotiations of mutual interest and emotion between infants communicating in triads, without any adult help. Human *sociability* innately seeks to build meaning by sharing the narratives implicit in adventurous activity, and by playing with ways of acting and experiencing. It is adapted to support exploration of life in a community that eventually extends over many generations, not just in parent–child dyads. The process of discovery in development of the imagination is best motivated in symmetric, or at least mutually valued, relationships where initiatives are exchanged between different identified persons and where stories with conventional meanings can be built. In addition, most loving mothers immediately become playmates and "best friends" as well as caregivers to infants.

It is perhaps a product of social organization and planning in industrial societies, and a reaction to the abuses of child labor as Rogoff et al. (2003) indicate, that mothers are seen as protectors or keepers of their infants, who may or may not be substituted by sufficiently sensitive surrogates, and teachers are seen as instructors, neither being understood as available friends and collaborators who benefit from the infant's or child's instinctive companionship and playfulness. The psychology we have created to support our society and measure its effects on individuals is one that attempts to assess the mental success of each person separately. We have come to think of ourselves as communicating just information about what each of us perceives is real and practical. Inevitably our conceptions of sympathetic and intuitive mental life have become over-cognitive and impoverished in emotional and imaginative aspects. Freud made a powerful effort to redress this imbalance, but left the unconscious mind at the mercy of language, the vehicle of clear thought. He did not have full confidence in the intuitive communication of purposes and concerns by nonverbal means. Like Piaget, he did not investigate how the process of communication begins in infancy (Bradley 1989).

CULTURAL LEARNING REQUIRES COLLECTIVE IMAGINING, CONSTANTLY INVENTED

Social animals communicate sensitively their immediate interests and impulses to action, and their young are playfully inventive in their movements. Play and humor, which may have a specific emotional/motive system in the brain, is obviously an adaptation for communicating motive impulses through exaggeration of movements, including movements to make contact with other individuals

(Bekoff and Byers 1998; Panksepp and Burgdorf 2003). In more restrained form, "play" movements may have a "serious" function for the individual or in interaction. Their messages are "meta-communicative," emphasizing why something is done by doing it more than is necessary (Bateson 1956). Adult humans play with the discoveries of the young. We continue to be playful, in varying degrees and with different goals, through adult life in ways no ape can match. Adult mammals are not often playful, though the young, especially those of socially cooperative species, are.

Monkeys and apes are highly sensitive of one another's moods and attentions, and apes learn skillful techniques of foraging by emulating the effects of what their companions do. They can take up strategies that engage with or outwit the inferred intentions of others in the social group. Human behavior is different in fundamental ways (Tomasello 1999). It displays a capacity for reflective thinking or the imaginative reconstruction of actions, events, and objects in a narrative history that extends into an imagined future with new events (Donald 2001). It also depends on the picking up of entirely novel knowledge and skill accumulated by transgenerational transmission of meanings.

Human cultural learning requires the young to have deep insight into the thinking behind the moves that elders make, and into the expressions of approval or disapproval that signal the value of experiences. The young learn an historically established cosmology and the meanings of behaviors and objects that have been invented and created among persons who were intensely aware of one another's interests and purposes. Discoveries of new ideas and ways of acting are especially attractive to human minds, even to those that are very young and inexperienced. This curiosity for meaning has innate motivation, and it needs an exceptional emotional sensitivity that goes far beyond the expression of immediate bodily needs (Trevarthen 1979b, 1982, 1988). The process can build with comfort, confidence, and confiding in a loving family and community, or it can fall prey to fear and distress, loneliness, and self-doubt. This is why infants crave the consistent sensitive company of an affectionate parent or other person who can be trusted to sustain the shared memories that have been discovered in their company.

Human knowledge is passed on by persons expressing to one another their dynamic inner state as well as their cognitive engagement with the "facts" of objective experience in a shared external world. Convergent relations of subjects with objects (overlapping "object concepts") are controlled by *joint attention*, mostly made evident by orientations of organs of perception or prehension, and may lead to shared practical actions or collaborations (Butterworth 1991; Scaife and Bruner 1975; Tomasello 1988). Interpenetrations of states of motivation depend upon on *mutual attention*, the sympathetic mimicry of affects that signal internal states and their changes and that govern both affectionate play and moral relationships as well as attachments (Reddy 2001b, 2003).

All such intersubjective coordination of actions or states of motivation between animals require *sympathetic mirroring of the dimensions of movement* as

well as physiognomic recognition of similarities or congruencies of body form
between perceiver and perceived (Trevarthen 2004a). Matching rhythm or pulse
of movement offers a powerful correspondence by which minds states may be
coupled and "march in step," but they are complemented by affect signaling gestural contours the accelerations of which are a standardized measure of power in
motivation (Trevarthen 1999). Daniel Stern (1993, 1999) describes the delicate
matching of expression between a mother and her infant as "attunement" of "vitality contours," which terms convey well the essential "musicality" of this signaling through modulations of the intensity of movement. Mechthild Papousek
(1996) has also described the essential musicality of intuitive parenting
communication.

THE ART AND EMOTION OF CULTURAL LEARNING

Victor Turner (1974) explains the community-building function of drama as
"the human seriousness of play." John Blacking (1971/1995, p. 31) accounted
for the universal place of music in human society as follows: "The function of
music is to enhance in some way the quality of individual experience and human
relationships; its structures are reflections of patterns of human relations, and
the value of a piece of music is inseparable from its value as an expression of human experience." The celebration of rituals in drama, music, and dance gives
support for social identities of individuals, and promotes solidarity in the group.
    Art is, as Ellen Dissanayake (2000) says, the product of human intimacy, and
that explains why it can be a source of solace for a troubled human spirit. These
are the factors of communication by nonverbal means that make improvisation
of music with a trained therapist such an effective means of bringing order into
confused feelings and harmony in relationships (Pavlicevic 1997). All human
cultural achievements arise in the intimacy of shared meaning, even when they
appear to be lonely products of dreaming. Thoughts, imagining experiences
generated by actions, gain value through sharing their originality and "truthful-
ness" with others, who judge their value and "significance." Human effort is directed to build relationships through cooperative and inventive works.
    A cognitive information processing, perception categorizing, memorizing
approach to human cumulative intelligence is unable to comprehend its social
motivation or its intersubjective psychological foundations in evolution. The
theory of cognitive modules in separate heads contrasts with a psychobiological
theory of culture as a product of human intentions to make and understand in relationships and communities (Donald 2001). Cultural learning is not just a cognitive achievement of the human mind. It is a new development in animal social
initiative, and in ways of relating intelligently. There are many features of the
human body and brain that are developed to enable this unique level of
cooperative awareness.

ADAPTATIONS OF THE HUMAN BODY AND BRAIN FOR COMPANIONSHIP IN EXPERIENCE

Human beings sense one another in unique ways by all modalities. Mammals take note of one another's eyes and regulate intimacy by shifts of looking. Only humans, with white sclera, depend upon accurate registration of other's changes of gaze to coordinate conscious awareness of shared surroundings and to receive information of others' emotional evaluation of objects, and their thinking moments of vacantly gazing reverie. Human eyes are adapted for communication of states of thinking (Kobayashi and Kohshima 2001). Loss of understanding for what another's eyes are signaling is one symptom of autism in a child. We need to know where other persons are looking to keep track of their thoughts and to detect the values they give to what they see, or imagine or remember seeing. Eye movements not only signal what a person is looking at in the present. They also convey evidence of the introspective retrieval from experience that Merlin Donald (2001) names "autocuing."

Only humans have this monitoring of momentary shifts of gaze, which serves an intersubjectivity, face to face, capable of detecting shifts of thought and feeling even when they indicate experiences of events of another time and place and with arbitrary meaning. The blind pick up intersubjective information from sounds of others' movements, from touch (the feel of hands reaching, grasping, and gesturing), and especially from changes in the direction and expression of the voice, or from reproductions of the vitality of the human spirit in music (Tønsberg and Hauge 1996). The fact that a blind person can compensate with these other senses for the information about activity of the mind that is signaled by intelligent eye movements proves that, however specialized human eyes are as organs of communication, it is the thinking and feeling of the intentional self behind the looks that is the sought for message.

Human hands are also uniquely adapted in their form and movements to transmit intentions and feelings, and they do so from birth (Trevarthen 1986b). The hands of infants are communicative before they are effective organs of manipulation, and they express subtle changes in alertness, directions of interest, and confident or hesitant purposes. Their movements can be cultivated as organs of sign languages as competent as speech by voice, and the intuitive expression of metaphoric ideas by hand gestures is unequaled by the voice (Goldin-Meadow and McNeill 1999). They can mimic expressions of the voice and the rhythms of body movement in mime, in dance, with musical instruments, and in graphical art. A deaf infant, whose mother is also deaf and skilled in hand signing, develops linguistic competence earlier than a blind baby who hears a mother's speech, but cannot see her gestures or the directions of her regard (Preisler 1995).

Speech and song turn rhythms and accents of the mind into events that can bridge space between distant human bodies. Versatility of human vocalization for expressions of feelings is exceptional (Scherer 1986; Zei Pollermann 2002), and sustained phonation by the uniquely adapted human respiratory mechanism makes it possible for rapid and infinitely varied time-controlled sequences of articulation by lips and tongue in speech (MacNeilage 1999).

By all these extraordinary means of expression, human subjects exchange their thoughts in making and announce rich evaluations of their hopes and fears concerning every detail of the narrative. Human relationships require sensitivity for these hopes and fears, and support for adventures in thought that can only be brought to fruition by close and sustained cooperation in confirmed relationships.

THE CIRCLE OF ATTACHMENTS

Minds active in awareness and the pursuit of experience undertake initiatives of three kinds: with the *body and its states*, with *physical objects and events*, and *with other subjects and their behavior.* These three kinds of purpose differ in their movements, senses, and emotions (Trevarthen 1993). The first is *interoceptive* and *proprioceptive*, monitoring the state of the body and the potential energy costs of acting, and regulating physiological processes with visceral muscle activity, breathing, and the pulses of the heart, skeletal muscle tonus of the whole body, and many means of chemical self-regulation and bodily defense that implicate the neurohumoral and immune systems. The second requires pragmatic, realistic intelligence, and *exteroceptive* awareness of place and situation, anticipation of events, object concepts and the like. The third requires volitional and emotional sympathy with other persons and their minds; by direct *alteroceptive* perception that is not reducible to "social cognition" and that does not require a declarative "theory of mind" (Figure 4.3 and Table 4.1).

A person can act voluntarily toward the world outside the body in two ways, with very different expectations. They can anticipate what will happen when they move about or when they act upon an object, or they can look and listen to what will happen from communicating with another person. They will have different emotions in anticipation in these two kinds of experience, and they will also evaluate their progress differently. The emotions that appraise objects empathically can be called "aesthetic," and those that engage with the potentialities for purposeful and self-regulated consciousness of other subjects are "moral." The third kind of emotional regulation concerned with internal states and feelings of the subject's body, which is sensed without reference to an outside reality, also has importance for relationships with other persons. "Autonomic" or "visceral" emotions of well-being or distress require sympathetic responses from others, who may feel they want to share, assist, exploit, or avoid what another is feeling in their body. There are differences between the anticipatory and regulatory functions of emotion when a subject is acting in these three different ways, with different expectations and different goals.

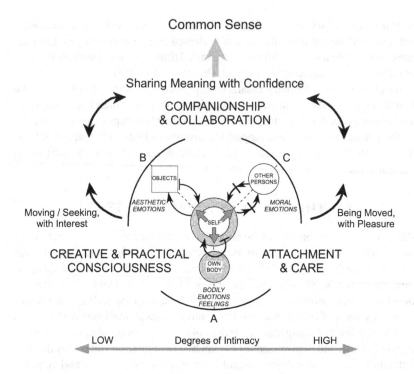

Figure 4.3   The "circle of attachments" to objects, to one's own body, and to other persons, and the different motive functions required for Attachment in Care, for Creative and Practical (Objective) Intelligence, and for Companionship and Collaboration with other persons, in "intersubjectivity."

However, this is just a first step in analyzing how emotions regulate an individual's experience and their position in relation to the world and in society. Initiatives of the three kinds — to gain protection for internal well-being, to move actively about in and use the external physical world, and to communicate with other independently motivated subjects — all work in combination. Emotional expressions of the body, and especially the hands, eyes, face, and voice, appear to be concerned with integrating across these three facets of the active self. The affective domains of purposeful psychological activity may be distinguished as Cognition, Attachment, and Companionship (Figure 4.3 and Table 4.1). Each of these mediates in transitions between two of the three facets of brain output concerned with things, persons, and the subject's body. Thus emotions signify transitional equilibria in the whole subject's changing motives and the accompanying internal autonomic processes, and in the expression of outwardly directed actions and interests that the motives are generating. They define three realms of psychological life: respectively, these integrate bodily self-regulation with "cognitive and practical action" on physical reality, "attachment" to persons that offer care and comfort to the body, and "companionship" with partners in experience and purposes.

In thriving relationships, all three of the modes of regulating experience by body activity — for places and things, for care for the self and others in the body, and for relationships of trust and cooperation with other persons — operate together, expressing the emotions that evaluate all prospects of success or frustration in initiatives of living. A comprehensive conception of emotional health and the building of a personal narrative that has confidence in understanding the world and communicating its meaning with other persons requires a single dynamic circle of motives and emotions.

DEVELOPMENTS OF COOPERATIVE INITIATIVES IN COMMUNICATION BEFORE LANGUAGE

The function of innate human initiative is neatly defined in a recent publication by Nagy and Molnar (2004). It is worth quoting the whole of the authors' abstract in which they summarize their discovery:

> Searching for the mechanism of neonatal imitation resulted in the discovery of neonatal initiative capacity, here called "provocation." Newborns spontaneously produced previously imitated gestures while waiting for the experimenter's response. A psychophysiological analysis revealed that *imitation* was accompanied by heart rate increase while gesture *initiation* was accompanied by heart rate deceleration, suggesting different underlying mechanisms. Results imply that infants are not only capable of responding to a model movement by imitating, but that they also have the capacity to provoke an imitative response, thus sustaining an interaction. These findings may constitute a laboratory demonstration of the first dialog and, according to our hypothetical model, they represent how human imprinting begins.

> [Emphasis added; "initiation" leads to "provocation" in communicative exchange.]

If this is how human imprinting begins immediately after birth, human attachment is perhaps first to a *conversational partner* who reciprocates motive states, not to a caregiver (Figure 4.4). Moreover this research shows that neonatal imitation is not just the affirmation of likeness of brain and body actions — it is an intersubjective invitation as well (Kugiumutzakis 1999; Trevarthen et al. 1999). Newborn infants show themselves sociable persons with minds of their own. The needs for sociability, even for a newborn, go beyond a seeking for regulation, care, protection, stress-regulation, etc., that the internal body needs. Bodies are active mind-driven agencies; there is also a need for support of interests or "purposes and concerns" (Donaldson 1992).

Infants certainly begin life with a well-functioning awareness of the sounds of another person's feelings in the voice, especially for that uniquely known other person, the mother, whose voice has familiar and preferred qualities

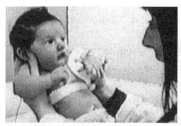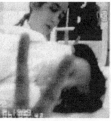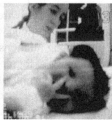

Figure 4.4 A newborn infant, a few days old, imitates a gesture made by two fingers. An attachment round the infant's chest records heart rate (photos by Dr. Emese Nagy in Szeged, Hungary).

learned before birth. There is no visual life before birth, but interest in a caregiver's face and eyes begins immediately and develops rapidly. In a few weeks a baby is watching the other's eyes with clear focus and reacting to their direct regard. A few months later the shifts of gaze of another occupied in seeking and acting can be followed easily. The mother is likely to be the principal and most effective caregiver for a young baby as well as the first companion, but soon she is not the only companion as others can share the infant's expressions of interest and anticipation (Figure 4.2).

Description of the behaviors of infants from birth and of changes at different ages shows steps by which human motivation seeks and learns meaningful ideas and ways of acting (Trevarthen and Aitken 2003). An infant's motives change his or her relationship with those persons who seek to communicate with the baby and who are ready to share the baby's experiences. There are both advances and vulnerable times. Each phase is characterized by particular initiatives and emotional responses in interaction with other persons, and in exploration and exploitation of places and objects. Infants develop increasingly adventurous initiatives, making more vigorous use of their growing bodies, seeking to explore and to form concepts of objects, negotiating purposes and the tempo of experience with others (Figures 4.2 and 4.5).

The developments in expressive body signs before speech — from proto-conversations of "primary intersubjectivity" with two-month-olds (Trevarthen 1979a), through games of the person and person–person–object games in the middle of the first year, to "secondary intersubjectivity" or "cooperative awareness" and protolanguage at the end of the first year (Trevarthen and Hubley 1978; Hubley and Trevarthen 1979) — show that communication of intentions, experiences, and feelings is the foundation on which the precise references and recollections of language are built (Trevarthen and Aitken 2001).

The coordination, in all modalities of sense at once, of a total awareness of the moving body of the self and of the movements made by other persons can be understood once it is observed that there are common temporal and energetic features of movement that inform all senses *in one time* (Trevarthen 1999). Research on the temporal foundations of expression and the development of

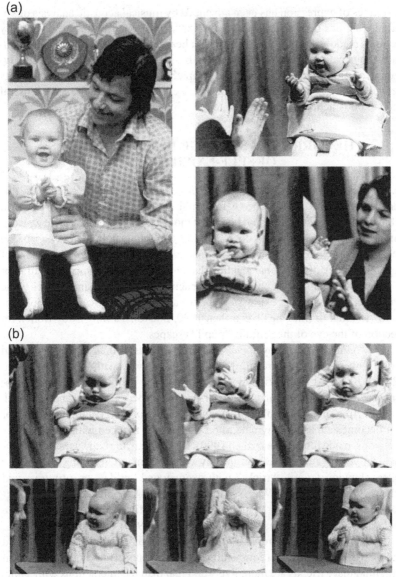

Figure 4.5   (a) Emma, six months, on the father's knee at home, is proud to show "clap-a-clap-a-handies" when prompted by her mother. She responds eagerly to imitate her mother in the laboratory at the University of Edinburgh and smiles to her image in the mirror of the camera window as she claps. (b) Emma, at the same age, is unhappy in the company of strangers and shows clear expressions of embarrassment or shame as she reacts to two other persons, a man and a woman, when they attempt to communicate, in the laboratory. She tries to show hand clapping, but the message fails. The woman in the bottom row of pictures, who first approaches timidly, expresses sympathetic expressions as Emma starts to cry (photos by Colwyn Trevarthen, University of Edinburgh).

narratives of expression has been advanced by musical acoustic analysis of vocal interactions between mothers and infants, and concurrent analysis of body gestures made as signals to be seen, felt, or heard. Malloch's theory of communicative musicality (Malloch 1999) gives a basis for understanding the innate dynamics of action and thinking and the sympathetic transmission of mental events between subjects. Infants are proved to be well equipped with the same sense of time in body action as that offered to them by adults.

THE MIRROR AS STRANGE PARTNER AND TEST OF SELF-EXPRESSION

Symptoms of the key changes in motives for engagement may be seen in the different ways babies behave when in front of the unnatural stimulation of a mirror, which reflects a visible face and body that moves with them in a strange way. An infant looking into a mirror does not find communication. There can be no "co-conscious" interaction with "coordinated interpersonal timing" and none of the contingency of emotional reaction that characterizes a protoconversation or game with a real other person. His or her reaction to the teasing immediacy of the image's movements and expressions is to stare, then look away or to look "inward" to think or imagine (Trevarthen 1990, 2004c). Turning away from a reflection of the eye of the self, the "pupil" escapes.

At two months, the baby appears to sense the mirror image as intrusive and looks with fascinated surprise, then turns shyly away with a coy expression (Reddy 2003). At four to five months an infant can see the mirror self at a distance, across a room, and may stare as if fascinated, becoming lost and detached, or "reflective" in "contemplation" (Figure 4.2). At six to eight months the mirror self becomes a teasing playmate to be challenged, mocked with clownish expressions, made fun of (Trevarthen 1990). By one year, the baby uses meta-communicative ways of expression to play with the image, recalling rivalries or jokes, showing favorite "tricks" with exaggerated "pride," or a timidity and "shame" (Reddy 2001a). We have found interesting differences in these reactions between boys and girls, indicating that in the first year, sex differences in sociability are well established (Trevarthen et al. 1999).

Toddlers may use a mirror as a stimulus to play but they never seem confused and treat the image as a real companion. Developments in play and conversation with imaginary friends are more lively and real than the interactions with a mirror. When the child passes the Gallup test of "grooming" the self by removing a spot of rouge on the face (Gallup and Suarez 1986), this is but a special interest in the body that does not really test "self-awareness" as this is important in communication with other "selves." Likewise the demonstrations of "shame" at being seen naked, which are seen in children even later than two, and the attainment of verbal skill in talking about thinking in one's own head or by others by a three- or four-year-old must be behaviors that depend upon social learning (Lewis 1995). I do not accept that they are *beginnings* of a sense of self or of the capacity to feel moral emotions. Reddy (2001c) argues that they are continuous with manifestations of self-consciousness in babies early in the first year. It appears as if "complex basic emotions" of relating develop elaborately in infancy (Draghi-Lorenz et al. 2000).

One-year-olds have not discovered that others have minds or "subjectivity." They have found new interest in sharing goals and purposes, probably because their own "seeking" has become systematic, better remembered, more precisely and constructively motivated. This "attracts" the interests of others and active purposefulness, changing the ways they address and respond to the infant (Figure 4.6).

A theory of mind is redundant to subconscious sympathy of motives and feelings. We no more need it than we need a theory of grammar to have a conversation. The intuitive subconscious collaboration of motives is clearly brought to light by a musical acoustic study of protoconversations that records the vocal gestural and facial moves (Malloch 1999; Trevarthen 1999).

The eagerness with which a toddler turns to a companion to share creations is surely more than an exploration *away from* a secure base. The evaluation of the other is necessary for an act to have any meaning. It is also important for the maker of meaning to defend his or her autonomy in finding things out or creating novelties. That is why there is so much discussion when toddlers are enjoying imaginative play, and when parents join in such play by becoming themselves challenging and self-conscious performers in the narrative of fantasies.

Research on the development of communication and cooperation in infancy indicates a different way of conceiving human teaching and learning and the propagation of cultural knowledge (Trevarthen 1988). It leads to surprising conclusions about the relationship between cultural learning, the form and movement of the human body, and the anatomical peculiarities of the human brain. The rich and rapidly developing sociability of infants and toddlers indicates that this brain has evolved for sharing knowledge and skill. The essential motivating and emotional systems are laid down long before birth as generators preparing the capacity of a human being for initiative in acting and experiencing, and for intersubjective communication.

INTRINSIC SYSTEMS OF THE BRAIN FOR MOTIVATING ATTACHMENTS AND FRIENDSHIP IN LEARNING

A most startling discovery of functional brain imaging in the last few years has been how much human brain tissue is given over to activity in support of expressing oneself to and being aware of other human bodies and their expressions (Adolphs 2003). Large territories of the frontal and parieto-temporal cortex are implicated in the simple sympathy of a conversation, with its gestures, vocalizations, and facial expressions (Adolphs et al. 2003; Decety and Chaminade

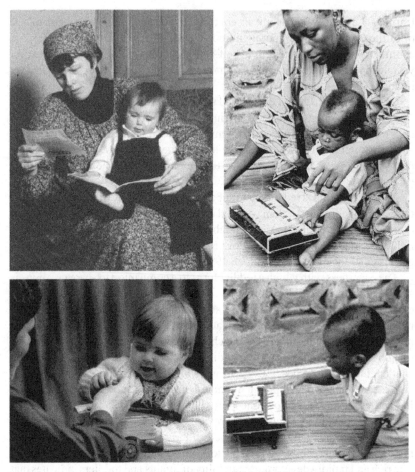

Figure 4.6 Left: In Scotland, Basilie (one year old) reads her book while her mother reads also (photo by John and Penelope Hubley). She enjoys cooperating in a task when her mother asks her to take a wooden doll and put it in the toy truck (photo by Colwyn Trevarthen). Right: In Lagos, Nigeria, Adegbenro (also one year old) shares his piano with his mother and happily "sings" and plays (photos by John and Penelope Hubley).

2003). These neocortical components of emotional and emotive systems have effective functional organization very early in infancy, if not from before birth (Tzourio-Mazoyer et al. 2002). Penfield's "homunculus" in the sensorimotor strip is largest for the organs of communication: face, hands, and vocal apparatus. These organs have evolved their emotion-communicating function from autonomic or visceral self-regulatory actions that are activated from the brainstem nuclei of the cranial nerves (Porges 1997). The parietal visual areas interconnected with the frontal eye fields are a great animator of a selective intelligence that also communicates. Emotion in the face and voice figure large in the

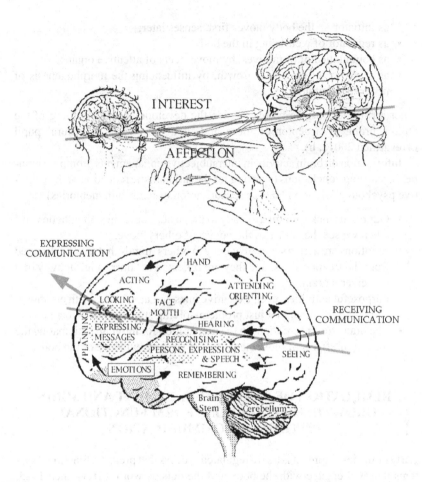

INTEREST

AFFECTION

EXPRESSING
COMMUNICATION

HAND

ACTING

ATTENDING
ORIENTING

LOOKING   FACE
MOUTH

RECEIVING
COMMUNICATION

EXPRESSING
MESSAGES

HEARING

RECOGNISING
PERSONS, EXPRESSIONS
& SPEECH

SEEING

PLANNING

EMOTIONS

REMEMBERING

Brain
Stem

Cerebellum

Figure 4.7 Mother and infant share expressions of interest and affection with pleasure in protoconversation. The human brain shows large territories of the cerebral cortex devoted to the functions of communication. These areas, which are functional from birth, are motivated and stimulated by inputs from subcortical centers (Trevarthen 2004b).

paralimbic neocortex, especially of the right hemisphere (Schore 2003a, b). All the neocortical regions found to be implicated in intersubjective awareness and communication are intensely and reciprocally interconnected with subcortical motive systems. We are discovering a new map of cortical functions, one that represents the functions of neural systems, both cortical and subcortical, that are designed to sustain our special awareness of one another, and of one another's thoughts (Figure 4.7).

The Intrinsic Motive Formation (IMF) of the subcortical brain (Trevarthen and Aitken 1994) can be identified with many essential integrative functions of the conscious subject:

- as initiator — the body moves first, senses later;
- as regulator of well-being in the body;
- as communicator of motives, by movements of attentive organs;
- as regulator of cognitive growth, by influencing the morphogenesis of neocortical circuits.

After birth, the intrinsic motives guide the development and learning of the child's brain, as acceptor of ideas and thoughts and as a cultural pupil (Trevarthen 2001a, b).

Information on brain activity in intersubjective engagements prompts a number of startling conclusions (startling for the rationalistic reduction of the cognitive psychology of individuals as sensorimotor systems with memories):

- Our brains make our minds ready to move our bodies in sympathetic ways when we see, hear, or feel the bodies of others move.
- Emotions are active states of agency in others' minds that may be detected from their expressions, and they are reflected in "mirroring" activity of a perceiver's brain.
- Purposeful activities, even executive ones, are adventures with emotional and emotive drama, not just problem-solving strategies or algorithms.
- The brain "feels" emotions in the preparation for moving, anticipating the feeling of effects of movements, not in sensory evidence of the body.

REGULATION OF BRAIN DEVELOPMENT AND MIND GROWTH: HOW NEURONS FORM FUNCTIONAL SYSTEMS OF COMMUNICATION

Early brain development is a self-regulated process that prepares functional systems that will engage with the body and the outside world (Trevarthen 1985, 2001b, 2004b; Trevarthen and Aitken 1994). Cells in the developing embryo brain and spinal cord gain affinities for molecules on the surface of glia cells and on other neurons. These direct cell migration as well as the paths that axons and dendrites follow in the late embryo (weeks 5 and 6). Neuroblasts divide around the ventricle of the neural tube, migrate out along radial glia fibers, and form layered arrangements in the hippocampus, cerebral cortex, and cerebellum. The tips of axons and dendrites are guided by "growth cones," sensorimotor structures that explore the intercellular terrain, sensing different molecular environments and laying down the path of the nerve cell extension. Finally, nerve terminals form intricate arrays of synaptic contacts on other nerve cells, with hundreds of contacts per cell. The formation and maintenance of effective synapses is affected by the excitations received from other neurons, and by growth factors and steroid hormones produced by endocrine glands. Building of brain systems involves enormous programmed loss of elements, sculpting functional systems, survival of nerve cells depending on genes that promote or inhibit cell death, and on protein growth factors.

Psychological functions of the mature brain depend on "activity-dependent patterning" or "plasticity" of synapses, shaped by stimuli from the world and from the body. The brain is most "plastic" in early childhood; even in the fetus, electrical impulse traffic triggered by excitation of receptors modifies the structures formed by spontaneous developmental processes. Nevertheless, the brain is at no stage a passive receiver of stimulus input, and major structural responses to epigenetic factors or the environment are regulated to occur at certain ages in critical periods.

In the mid-embryo stage (week 4), the nervous system is electrically inactive. The first generalized movements occur in week 8, but already in week 5 monoamine transmission pathways grow from the brainstem into the primordial cerebral hemispheres. Key components of the emotional motor system (hypothalamus, basal ganglia, and amygdala) are in place when the neocortex is unformed (Holstege et al. 1996). By the end of the second month the main components of the brain are in place; eyes, vestibular canals and cochlear, hands, nose, and mouth are rapidly differentiating their distinctive forms, each dedicated to the picking up of a particular form of physical information from the environment. Core regulatory mechanisms of the central nervous system — the periaqueductal grey of the midbrain, the hypothalamus, reticular formation, basal ganglia, and limbic system — are laid down in the first trimester, but the cognitive systems of the cerebral cortex do not appear until the second trimester. The motivating and life-maintaining structures form a link between regulation of gene instructions in prenatal brain morphogenesis and the acquired adaptations of the developing mind. Defects in this link are implicated in disorders of empathy and cognition, including autism and schizophrenia (Aitken and Trevarthen 1997; Trevarthen and Aitken 1994).

The neocortex and cerebellum make their first steps of anatomical differentiation in the fetus, and these steps are guided by the subcortex. Brainstem monoaminergic neurons penetrate the cortical plate at 13 weeks, before sensory thalamic axons arrive. Thus neural motive regulators of cortical activity mature ahead of those that are destined to bring in environmental information. At the mid-fetal stage (week 24) dopamine axons, important in coordination of innate motor patterns, are concentrated in the deep parts of the cortex, at the time when thalamic sensory afferents end their waiting to make their entry. Earlier formed, deeper neuron layers in the cortex linked with limbic structures mediate in the development of cognitive structures, which take inputs from sensory and cortico-cortical connections.

Research on the behavior, psychology, and physiology of the fetus indicates that in the last trimester functions are established in anticipation of an active postnatal life, and especially for assimilating maternal care (Lecanuet et al. 1995; Trevarthen 1997a). It is of particular interest that heart rate changes are integrated with phases of motor activity from 24 weeks. This is indicative of the formation of a prospective control of autonomic state coupled to readiness for muscular activity on the environment, a feature of brain function, which Jeannerod (1994) has cited as evidence for the formation of cerebral "motor images" underlying conscious awareness and purposeful movement.

The neurochemistry of the motor initiative that generates and explores experience (i.e., of *ergotrophic* motives) is complemented by more internally active movements that are adapted to maintain physiological well-being (the *trophotropic* motives) (Table 4.1). The former system operates particularly with the biogenic amines dopamine and noradrenalin; the latter invokes activity of a range of agents that include glutamate, neuropeptides, steroids, oxytocin, and others (Hess 1954; Luciana 2001; Panksepp 1998).

The link between expressive movements and reception of expressions, on the one hand, and core regulation of mind and behavior in the brain — and of brain systems and functions in development — identifies the mechanism that motivates communication of mental states between a child and others. This is the psychobiological system of cultural learning (Trevarthen 2004a).

CONCLUSIONS: HUMAN MOTIVES AND THEIR DISCONTENTS

I believe we have found a new set of conceptions regarding the evolutionary origins of human motivation and emotions — one that goes beyond concerns with organic well-being, regulation of arousal, and reduction of stress. I conclude that mental health issues must take into account the powerful motives of companionship in experience as we seek to understand the causes of severe failure of motivations and self-esteem that affect increasing numbers of young human beings in a world given over to the creation of material novelty without concern for the social relationships that make productivity of human effort meaningful.

In every human relationship, the pleasure of active discovery and the mastery of experience and skill are regulated by interpersonal or moral feelings. As long as essential needs are provided for and the child is not distressed, sick, or exhausted, these feelings are asserted powerfully in every young child. They guide the growth of experience, and they do so by emotional regulation of the growth of the brain. They are manifested out of control in disorders of mania and depression, and weakened in autism and schizophrenia.

I believe that the intensely shared pleasure of pride in knowledge and skill that others applaud as well as the feeling of shame in failure that threatens loss of relationship and hopeless isolation, are as important to the mental health of every human being as the emotions that seek comfort and care for the body (Figure 4.5). Indeed, I would suggest that attachment itself, if it is a friendship and not just the very asymmetric relationship between a weak and immature "patient" and a sensitive caregiver, is animated by emotions of shared discovery and the creation of inventive art. Even authoritative teaching requires a minimal mutual respect, or its purpose is totally defeated. I suggest we need a "circle of attachments" (Figure 4.3) — of emotionally charged relationships to caregivers and comfort-givers, to places and things that foster our discoveries and activities, and, above all, to friends who are; and companions in adventure, discovery, and invention; persons who share the impulses of our thinking and acting, and play with roles and meanings.

REFERENCES

Adolphs, R. 2003. Investigating the cognitive neuroscience of social behavior. *Neuropsychologia* **41**:119–126.

Adolphs, R., D. Tranel, and A.R. Damasio. 2003. Dissociable neural systems for recognizing emotions. *Brain Cogn.* **52**:61–69.

Ainsworth, M.DS., and S. Bell. 1970. Attachment, exploration, and separation illustrated by the behavior of one-year-olds in a strange situation. *Child Dev.* **41**:49–67.

Aitken, K.J., and C. Trevarthen. 1997. Self-other organization in human psychological development. *Dev. Psychopathol.* **9**:651–675.

Bateson, G. 1956. The message "This is play." In: Group Processes: Transactions of the Second Conference, ed. B. Schaffner, pp. 145–242. New York: Josiah Macy. (Republished in: Bateson, G. 1973. Steps to an Ecology of Mind. St Albans: Frogmore/ Paladin.)

Bekoff, M., and J.A. Byers. 1998. Animal Play: Evolutionary, Comparative and Ecological Approaches. New York: Cambridge Univ. Press.

Belsky, J. 1981. Early human experience: A family perspective. *Dev. Psychol.* **17**: 3–23.

Blacking, J. 1971/1995. The value of music in human experience. In: The 1969 Yearbook of the International Folk Music Council, vol. 1, pp. 33–71. (Republished in: Music, Culture and Experience: Selected Papers of John Blacking, ed. P. Bohlman and B. Nettl. 1995. Chicago: Univ. of Chicago Press.)

Bowlby, J. 1988. Developmental psychiatry comes of age. *Am. J. Psych.* **145**:1–10.

Bradley, B.S. 1989. Visions of Infancy. Cambridge: Polity.

Bruner, J.S. 1996. The Culture of Education. Cambridge, MA: Harvard Univ. Press.

Butterworth, G.E. 1991. The ontogeny and phylogeny of joint visual attention. In: Natural Theories of Mind, ed. A. Whiten, pp. 223–232. Oxford: Blackwell.

Damasio, A.R. 1999. The Feeling of What Happens: Body, Emotion and the Making of Consciousness. London: Heinemann.

Decety, J., and T. Chaminade. 2003. Neural correlates of feeling sympathy. *Neuropsychologia* **41**:127–138.

Dissanayake, E. 2000. Art and Intimacy: How the Arts Began. Seattle: Univ. of Washington Press.

Donald, M. 2001. A Mind So Rare: The Evolution of Human Consciousness. New York: Norton.

Donaldson, M. 1992. Human Minds: An Exploration. London: Allen Lane/Penguin.

Draghi-Lorenz, R., V. Reddy, and A. Costall. 2000. Rethinking the development of "non-basic" emotions: A critical review of existing theories. *Dev. Rev.* **21**:263–304.

Fivaz-Depeursinge, E., and A. Corboz-Warnery. 1999. The Primary Triangle: A Developmental Systems View of Mothers, Fathers and Infants. New York: Basic.

Freeman,W.J. 1999. How Brains Make up Their Minds. London: Weidenfeld and Nicolson.

Gallup, G.G., and S.D. Suarez. 1986. Self-awareness and the emergence of mind in humans and other primates. In: Psychological Perspectives on the Self, ed. J. Suls and A.G. Greenwald, vol. 3, pp. 3–26. Hillsdale, NJ: Erlbaum.

Gibson, J.J. 1979. The Ecological Approach to Visual Perception. Boston: Houghton Mifflin.

Goldin-Meadow, S., and D. McNeill. 1999. The role of gesture and mimetic representation in making language. In: The Descent of Mind: Psychological Perspectives on Hominid Evolution, ed. M.C. Corballis and E.G. Lea, pp. 155–172. Oxford: Oxford Univ. Press.

Hess, W.R. 1954. Diencephalon: Autonomic and Extrapyramidal Functions. Orlando, FL: Grune and Stratton.

Holstege, G., R. Bandler, and C.B. Saper, eds. 1996. The Emotional Motor System. Progress in Brain Research 107. Amsterdam: Elsevier.

Hubley, P. and C. Trevarthen. 1979. Sharing a task in infancy. In: Social Interaction during Infancy: New Directions for Child Development, ed. I. Uzgiris, pp. 57–80. San Francisco: Jossey-Bass.

Jeannerod, M. 1994. The representing brain: Neural correlates of motor intention and imagery. *Behav. Brain Sci.* **17**:187–245.

Kobayashi, H., and S. Kohshima. 2001. Evolution of the human eye as a device for communication. In: Primate Origins of Human Communication and Behavior, ed. T. Matsuzawa. pp. 383–401. Tokyo: Springer.

Kugiumutzakis, G. 1999. Genesis and development of early infant mimesis to facial and vocal models. In: Imitation in Infancy, ed. J. Nadel and G. Butterworth, pp. 36–59. Cambridge: Cambridge Univ. Press.

Lecanuet, J.-P., W.P. Fifer, N.A. Krasnegor, and W.P. Smotherman, eds. 1995. Fetal Development: A Psychobiological Perspective. Hillsdale, NJ: Erlbaum.

Lee, D.N. 1998. Guiding movement by coupling taus. *Ecol. Psychol.* **10**:221–250.

Lewis, M. 1995. Embarrassment: The emotion of self-exposure and evaluation. In: Self-conscious Emotions: The Psychology of Shame, Guilt, Pride and Embarrassment, ed. J.P. Tangney and K.W. Fischer, pp. 199–218. New York: Guilford.

Luciana, M. 2001. Dopamine-opiate modulations of reward-seeking behavior: Implications for the functional assessment of prefrontal development. In: Handbook of Developmental Cognitive Neuroscience, ed. C.A. Nelson and M. Luciana, pp. 647–662. Cambridge, MA: MIT Press.

MacNeilage, P.F. 1999. Whatever happened to articulate speech? In: The Descent of Mind: Psychological Perspectives on Hominid Evolution, ed. M.C. Corballis and E.G. Lea, pp. 116–137. Oxford: Oxford Univ. Press.

Main, M., and R. Goldwyn 1984. Predicting rejection of her infants from mother's representation of her own experience: Implications for the abused-abusing intergenerational cycle. *Intl. J. Child Abuse Negl.* **8**:203–217.

Main, M., and D.R. Weston. 1982. Avoidance of attachment figure in infancy. In: The Place of Attachment in Human Behaviour, ed. C.M. Parkes and J. Stevenson-Hinde, pp. 31–59. London: Tavistock.

Malloch, S. 1999. Mother and infants and communicative musicality. In: Rhythms, Musical Narrative, and the Origins of Human Communication, ed. I. Deliège, pp. 29–57. Musicae Scientiae, spec. iss. 1999–2000. Liège: Eur. Soc. Cognitive Sci. Music.

Merker, B. 2005. The liabilities of mobility: A selection pressure for the transition to consciousness in animal evolution. *Consciousness Cogn.*, in press.

Nagy, E., and P. Molnàr. 2004. Homo imitans or Homo provocans? Human imprinting model of neonatal imitation. *Infant Behav. Dev.* **27**:54-63.

Neisser, U. 1993. The self perceived. In: The Perceived Self: Ecological and Interpersonal Sources of Self-Knowledge, ed. U. Neisser, pp. 3–21. New York: Cambridge Univ. Press.

Panksepp, J. 1998. Affective Neuroscience: The Foundations of Human and Animal Emotions. New York: Oxford Univ. Press.

Panksepp, J. 2000. The neuro-evolutionary cusp between emotions and cognitions, implications for understanding consciousness and the emergence of a unified mind science. *Consciousness Emot.* **1**:17–56.

Panksepp, J., and J. Burgdorf. 2003. "Laughing" rats and the evolutionary antecedents of human joy? *Physiol. Behav.* **79**:533–547.

Papousek, H., and M. Papousek. 1987. Intuitive parenting: A dialectic counterpart to the infant's integrative competence. In: Handbook of Infant Development, 2nd ed., ed. J.D. Osofsky, pp. 669–720. New York: Wiley.

Papousek, M. 1996. Intuitive parenting: A hidden source of musical stimulation in infancy. In: Musical Beginnings: Origins and Development of Musical Competence, ed. I. Deliège and J. Sloboda, pp. 88–112. Oxford: Oxford Univ. Press.

Pavlicevic, M. 1997. Music Therapy in Context: Music Meaning and Relationship. London: Kingsley.

Piaget, J. 1954. The Construction of Reality in the Child (trans. M. Cook) New York: Basic.

Porges, S.W. 1997. Emotion: An evolutionary by-product of the neural regulation of the autonomic nervous system. In: The Integrative Neurobiology of Affiliation, ed. C.S. Carter, I.I. Lederhendler, and B. Kirkpatrick, pp. 62–78. New York: New York Academy of Sciences.

Preisler, G.M. 1995. The development of communication in blind and in deaf infants: Similarities and differences. *Child Care Hlth. Dev.* **21**:79–110.

Reddy, V. 2000. Coyness in early infancy. *Dev. Sci.* **3**:186–192.

Reddy, V. 2001a. Infant clowns: The interpersonal creation of humour in infancy. *Enfance* **3**:247–256.

Reddy, V. 2001b. Mind knowledge in infancy: Understanding attention and intention in the first year. In: Blackwell Handbook of Infancy Research, ed. G.J. Bremner and A. Fogel, pp. 241–264. Oxford: Blackwell.

Reddy, V. 2001c. Positively shy: Developmental continuities in the expression of shyness, coyness and embarrassment. In: International Handbook of Social Anxiety: Concepts, Research and Interventions Relating to the Self and Shyness, ed. W.R. Crozier and L.E. Alden, pp. 77–99. New York: Wiley.

Reddy, V. 2003. On being the object of attention: Implications for self–other consciousness. *Trends Cogn. Sci.* **7**:397–402.

Rizzolatti, G., L. Fogassi, and V. Gallese. 2001. Neurophysiological mechanisms underlying the understanding and imitation of action. *Nat. Rev. Neurosci.* **2**:661–670.

Rogoff, B. 1998. Cognition as a collaborative process. In: Handbook of Child Psychology, vol. 2, Cognition, Perception and Language, ed. D. Kuhn and R.S. Siegler, pp. 679–744. New York: Wiley.

Rogoff, B., R. Paradise, R.M. Arauz, M. Correa-Chávez, and C. Angelillo. 2003. Firsthand learning through intent participation. *Ann. Rev. Psychol.* **54**:175–203.

Scaife, M., and J.S. Bruner. 1975. The capacity for joint visual attention in the infant. *Nature* **253**:265–266.

Scherer, K.R. 1986. Vocal affect expression: A review and a model for future research. *Psychol. Bull.* **99**:143–165.

Schore, A.N. 1994. Affect Regulation and the Origin of the Self: The Neurobiology of Emotional Development. Hillsdale, NJ: Erlbaum.

Schore, A.N. 2003a. Affect Regulation and Disorders of the Self. New York: Norton.

Schore, A.N. 2003b. Affect Regulation and the Repair of the Self. New York: Norton.

Selby, J.M., and B.S. Bradley. 2003. Infants in groups: A paradigm for study of early social experience. *Hum. Dev.* **46**:197–221.

Smith, A. 1759/1976. Theory of Moral Sentiments. Edinburgh. (Modern ed.: D.D. Raphael and A.L. Macfie, eds., Glasgow ed. Oxford: Clarendon. Reprint, Indianapolis: Liberty Fund, 1984).

Stanghellini, G. 2001. Psychopathology of common sense. *Philos. Psychiat. Psychol.* **8**:201–218.

Stanghellini, G., and M. Ballerini. 2002. Dis-sociality: The phenomenological approach to social dysfunction in schizophrenia: WPA Section Report. *World Psychiatry* **1**:102–106.

Stern, D.N. 1993. The role of feelings for an interpersonal self. In: The Perceived Self: Ecological and Interpersonal Sources of Self-Knowledge, ed. U. Neisser, pp. 205–215. New York: Cambridge Univ. Press.

Stern, D.N. 1999. Vitality contours: The temporal contour of feelings as a basic unit for constructing the infant's social experience. In: Early Social Cognition: Understanding Others in the First Months of Life, ed. P. Rochat, pp. 67–90. Mahwah, NJ: Erlbaum.

Stern, D.N. 2000. The Interpersonal World of the Infant: A View from Psychoanalysis and Development Psychology. 2nd ed. New York: Basic.

Tomasello, M. 1988. The role of joint attentional processes in early language development. *Lang. Sci.* **10**:69–88.

Tomasello, M. 1999. The Cultural Origins of Human Cognition. Cambridge, MA: Harvard Univ. Press.

Tønsberg, G.H., and T.S. Hauge. 1996. The musical nature of prelinguistic interaction: The temporal structure and organisation in co-created interaction with congenital deaf-blinds. *Nord. J. Music Ther.* **5**:63–75.

Trevarthen, C. 1979a. Communication and cooperation in early infancy: A description of primary intersubjectivity. In: Before Speech: The Beginning of Human Communication, ed. M. Bullowa, pp. 321–347. London: Cambridge Univ. Press.

Trevarthen, C. 1979b. Instincts for human understanding and for cultural cooperation: Their development in infancy. In: Human Ethology: Claims and Limits of a New Discipline, ed. M. von Cranach, K. Foppa, W. Lepenies, and D. Ploog, pp. 530–571. Cambridge: Cambridge Univ. Press.

Trevarthen, C. 1982. The primary motives for cooperative understanding. In: Social Cognition: Studies of the Development of Understanding, ed. G. Butterworth and P. Light, pp. 77–109. Brighton: Harvester.

Trevarthen, C. 1985. Neuroembryology and the development of perceptual mechanisms. In: Human Growth, 2nd ed., ed. F. Falkner and J.M. Tanner, pp. 301–383. New York: Plenum.

Trevarthen, C. 1986a. Development of intersubjective motor control in infants. In: Motor Development in Children: Aspects of Coordination and Control, ed. M.G. Wade and H.T.A. Whiting, pp. 209–261. Dordrecht: Nijhof.

Trevarthen, C. 1986b. Form, significance and psychological potential of hand gestures of infants. In: The Biological Foundation of Gestures: Motor and Semiotic Aspects, ed. J.-L. Nespoulous, P. Perron, and A.R. Lecours, pp. 149–202. Hillsdale, NJ: Erlbaum.

Trevarthen, C. 1988. Universal cooperative motives: How infants begin to know language and skills of culture. In: Acquiring Culture: Ethnographic Perspectives on Cognitive Development, ed. G. Jahoda and I.M. Lewis, pp. 37–90. London: Croom Helm.

Trevarthen, C. 1990. Signs before speech. In: The Semiotic Web, 1989, ed. T.A. Sebeok and J. Umiker-Sebeok, pp. 689–755. Amsterdam: de Gruyter.

Trevarthen, C. 1993. The function of emotions in early infant communication and development. In: New Perspectives in Early Communicative Development, ed. J. Nadel and L. Camioni, pp. 48–81. London: Routledge.

Trevarthen, C. 1997a. Foetal and neonatal psychology: Intrinsic motives and learning behaviour. In: Advances in Perinatal Medicine, ed. F. Cockburn, pp. 282–291. New York: Parthenon.

Trevarthen, C. 1997b. The nature of motives for human consciousness. *Psychol. J. Hell. Psychol. Soc.* **4**:187–221.

Trevarthen, C. 1998. The concept and foundations of infant intersubjectivity. In: Intersubjective Communication and Emotion in Early Ontogeny, ed. S. Bråten, pp. 15–46. Cambridge: Cambridge Univ. Press.

Trevarthen, C. 1999. Musicality and the Intrinsic Motive Pulse: Evidence from human psychobiology and infant communication In: Rhythms, Musical Narrative, and the Origins of Human Communication, pp. 157–213. Musicae Scientiae, spec. iss. 1999–2000. Liège: Eur. Soc. Cognitive Sci. Music.

Trevarthen, C. 2001a. Intrinsic motives for companionship in understanding: Their origin, development and significance for infant mental health. *Infant Mental Hlth. J.* **22**: 95–131.

Trevarthen, C. 2001b. The neurobiology of early communication: Intersubjective regulations in human brain development. In: Handbook on Brain and Behavior in Human Development, ed. A.F. Kalverboer and A. Gramsbergen, pp. 841–882. Dordrecht: Kluwer.

Trevarthen, C. 2003. Language development: Mechanisms in the brain. In: Encyclopedia of Neuroscience, 3rd ed. with CD-ROM, ed. G. Adelman and B.H. Smith. Amsterdam: Elsevier.

Trevarthen, C. 2004a. Action and emotion in development of the human self, its sociability and cultural intelligence: Why infants have feelings like ours. In: Emotional Development, ed. J. Nadel and D. Muir. Oxford: Oxford Univ. Press.

Trevarthen, C. 2004b. Brain development. In: Oxford Companion to the Mind, ed. R. Gregory. 2nd ed. Oxford: Oxford Univ. Press.

Trevarthen, C. 2004c. Making common sense: Creative learning and teaching in infancy. In: A Learning Zone of One's Own, ed. M. Tokoro and L. Steels. SONY Future of Learning Series. Amsterdam: IOS Press.

Trevarthen, C., and K.J. Aitken. 1994. Brain development, infant communication, and empathy disorders: Intrinsic factors in child mental health. *Dev. Psychopathol.* **6**:599–635.

Trevarthen, C., and K.J. Aitken. 2001. Infant intersubjectivity: Research, theory, and clinical applications: Annual Research Review. *J. Child Psychol. Psychiat.* **42**:3–48.

Trevarthen, C., and K.J. Aitken. 2003. Regulation of brain development and age-related changes in infants' motives: The developmental function of "regressive" periods. In:

Regression Periods in Human Infancy, ed. M. Heimann and F. Plooij, pp. 107–184. Mahwah, NJ: Erlbaum.

Trevarthen, C., and P. Hubley. 1978. Secondary intersubjectivity: Confidence, confiding and acts of meaning in the first year. In: Action, Gesture and Symbol: The Emergence of Language, ed. A. Lock, pp. 183–229. London: Academic.

Trevarthen, C., T. Kokkinaki, and G.A. Fiamenghi, Jr. 1999. What infants' imitations communicate: With mothers, with fathers and with peers. In: Imitation in Infancy, ed. J. Nadel and G. Butterworth, pp. 127–185. Cambridge: Cambridge Univ. Press.

Turner, V. 1974. Dramas, Fields and Metaphors. Ithaca, NY: Cornell Univ. Press.

Tzourio-Mazoyer, N., S. De Schonen, F. Crivello et al. 2002. Neural correlates of woman face processing by 2-month-old infants. *NeuroImage* **15**:454–461.

Wemelsfelder, F. 1993. The concept of animal boredom and its relationship to stereotyped behaviour. In: Stereotypic Animal Behaviour, ed. A.B. Lawrence and J. Rushen, pp. 65–95. Wallingford, U.K.: CAB Intl.

Winnicott, D.W. 1960. The theory of the parent-infant relationship. *Intl. J. Psychoanal.* **41**:585–595. (Republished 1990 in: Winnicott, D.W., The Maturational Process and the Facilitating Environment. London: Inst. of Psychoanalysis/Karnak.)

Zei Pollermann, B. 2002. A place for prosody in a unified model of cognition and emotion. In: Proc. of Speech Prosody 2002, Laboratoire Parole et Langage, CNRS. Aix-en-Provence: Universitié de Provence. www.lpl.univ-aix.fr/sp2002/oral.htm.

5

Biological Perspectives on Social Attachment and Bonding

C. S. CARTER

Brain–Body Center, Department of Psychiatry, University of Illinois at Chicago,
Chicago, IL 60612, U.S.A.

ABSTRACT

The purpose of this review is to examine factors influencing both the development and expression of mammalian social bonds in the biological context of natural history, evolution, and neuroendocrinology. Animal research suggests that social bonding can be modulated by various hormones including oxytocin, vasopressin, opioids, corticotropin-releasing hormone (CRH), dopamine, and adrenal steroids, including corticosterone or cortisol. The effects of these hormones on social bond formation are especially apparent following periods of stress or anxiety. For example, social bonds are associated with birth or the introduction of a novel partner. Of possible relevance to behavioral attachment is the capacity of hormones, such as oxytocin and vasopressin, to overcome anxiety or fear. Brief exposure to oxytocin or vasopressin can facilitate social contact and in some species selective sociality. Neural systems associated with reward, including those that rely on dopamine and possibly the endogenous opioids, may help to regulate responses to the presence or absence of a preferred partner. The capacity to form social bonds emerges as a function of interactions among genetics and developmental experiences. Systems associated with sociality are designed to accommodate species and individual variations. Within a genetic background, social and hormonal experiences can reprogram the nervous system and thus potentially alter the tendency of individuals to form social bonds. An understanding of the physiological mechanisms responsible for social bonding may provide clues to the biological and psychological benefits of social support.

INTRODUCTION

Social relationships, including those structured around social bonds and emotional attachments, can be a source of life's greatest pleasures and deepest pain. The best described examples of social bonds, including parent–offspring and adult heterosexual relationships, are associated with reproduction and are most readily interpreted in the context of their evolution and adaptive functions (Bowlby 1969). The consequences of social bonds also extend beyond reproduction, with potential benefits for all aspects of life. Understanding the neurobiology of social bonds provides insights into the protective mechanisms underlying perceived social support (Carter 1998).

Adult pair bonds and bonds between mothers and their infants are based at least in part on shared neurobiological systems. Hormones and neural systems that are responsive to these hormones coordinate the formation of social bonds with other events such as birth or emotional states. There also is evidence that these same hormones may help to program the nervous system, especially during early life, contributing to individual and sex differences, and species-typical patterns of social behavior.

SOCIAL BONDS

What Is a Social Bond?

Social bonds are a subset of affiliative or positive social behaviors, which in turn are most simply defined by approach rather than avoidance or withdrawal. Positive sociality is sometimes defined by the absence of defensive or aggressive behavior. Social behaviors, including social bonds, are active processes that involve more than simply a failure to avoid another individual (Carter 1998).

Several features are common to most definitions of social bonds. Social engagement and individual recognition are the first steps in social bonding. Differential behavioral or emotional interactions in the presence or absence of the partner are most commonly used to define a social bond. Although the term "pair bond" implies only two partners, the tendency or willingness to form social bonds may extend to more than one partner. The capacity to form either one or more social bonds varies across species and, in some cases, may lead to extended family groups.

The most accessible operational definitions of social bonds are behavioral. Social bonds are often indexed experimentally by selective approach in partner preference tests. Such tests typically include a choice between a familiar partner or a stranger or the option to remain alone. Physical contact seems to be a particularly sensitive indicator of social bonding (Carter et al. 1995), although a choice between other types of social stimuli (such as odors) may be sufficient to detect preferences. In adult animals, there have been attempts to use sexual preferences to index pair bonding; however, these are complicated by the fact that some animals are more particular or exclusive in choosing their social partners than they are in selecting a mating partner.

Defense of the mate or territory can also be a defining feature of a social bond. For example, socially monogamous species tend to be aggressive toward strangers. Although aggression can occur toward familiar conspecifics, it is less common. Intense aggression, usually toward unfamiliar animals of the same sex, can be triggered by sexual experience (Winslow et al. 1993) and/or prolonged periods of cohabitation (Bowler et al. 2002). The selective aggression seen in socially monogamous species may serve to defend either the mate or family after a social bond has been established. Aggression is also seen in polygamous species; however, in such species, aggression may occur before mating, presumably in competition for resources or rank.

In some cases behavioral, autonomic, or other physiological responses to the presence or absence of a partner have been used to index social bonds. For example, heart rate or endocrine responses, such as increases in heart rate or adrenal hormone levels following separation, may reflect emotional changes associated with the absence of a preferred social partner. Physiological changes can be difficult to measure, especially during naturalistic behavioral interactions. Even more challenging are attempts to interpret physiological measures in behavioral or emotional terms (Hennessy 1997; Mason and Mendoza 1998; Porges 2001 and this volume). For example, changes in heart rate or stress hormones may occur as the result of mobilization, fear, changes in thermoregulation, or other processes that are not specifically related to emotions experienced during separation from a partner. Thus, without careful consideration of the context in which they occur, physiological measures may not be meaningful measures of social bonds.

Evolutionary Context

At the center of evolutionary theories is the concept of genetic survival or "fitness." Individual survival to at least reproductive age is a precondition for reproduction, and reproduction is essential for the transmission and survival of genes. Mammals produce young that are nutritionally dependent for at least some part of their lives on the mother. In most — but not all — mammals, milk and maternal behavior are both delivered primarily to the mother's genetic offspring. For the mammalian infant, the importance of the mother is clear. In addition, many benefits of the maternal or, where appropriate, paternal role may be provided by "alloparents," who are sometimes, but not always, genetically related to the young (Carter and Roberts 1997; Hrdy, this volume).

Parents and even alloparents can also benefit from interactions with young animals. In addition to genetic fitness, the mother may gain physically and emotionally from interactions with her own offspring. This is seen in the capacity of lactating women to be more resilient in the face of stressors (Carter and Altemus 1997; Carter et al. 2001). It is often difficult for a male to determine whether a female's young are his own offspring. Perhaps as a result it is rare for males to provide care for infants. However, in a limited number of mammalian species, both males and females exhibit selective social behaviors, sometimes termed "pair bonds," which may encourage the male and female to remain together after mating and even during nonreproductive periods. There also is a strong association between the tendency to form adult pair bonds and the expression of male parental behavior. The coincidence of these behaviors has been used to categorize species as "monogamous" (Kleiman 1977).

The term monogamy has also been used to describe sexual exclusivity or fidelity. The multiple uses of this word have created some confusion. It is now well-established that sexual exclusivity is not necessarily a reliable trait of "monogamous" species; i.e., those species that tend to live in pairs and show male parental behavior (Carter et al. 1995; Gowaty 1997). However, a male that remains with a female sexual partner and invests in her offspring may increase the chances that his own genetic offspring will survive. The advantages of one mating strategy over another in a particular situation are difficult to determine. However, as a lifestyle, polygamy, which does not demand either pair bonds or paternal behavior, can be successful under conditions when a single female can rear her offspring unaided by the father.

It is often argued that monogamy — or what is now sometimes called "social monogamy" — may be especially beneficial when two caretakers are necessary to rear a family. However, in apparent contradiction to Kleiman's original definition of monogamy (1977), Komers and Brotherton (1997) claim that social monogamy is observed more often in the absence of paternal care than in its presence. Thus, the latter propose that monogamy may have evolved first (for reasons other than the "need" for a second parent) and that the availability of a second parent as a caretaker is a secondary, but not essential, benefit of monogamy. Regardless of their evolutionary origins, socially monogamous species have provided a novel opportunity to understand the biological processes responsible for social bonds.

What Are the Proximate Causes of Social Bonding?

Social bonds are interwoven with the capacity to adapt to an ever-changing and challenging environment. Stable companionship may function to provide a sense of safety and reduce anxiety. Stressful experiences (such as pregnancy and parturition), anxiety, neophobia, and isolation often precede the formation of long-lasting social attachments (Bowlby 1969; Panksepp 1998; Carter. 1998).

Neurochemical changes that are capable of overcoming neophobia may also lead to a decrease in social inhibitions and increased sociality, a first step in social bond formation. However, under a variety of experimental conditions, animals may be indiscriminantly social. The tendency toward selectivity in social responses probably relies on mechanisms that promote both general sociality as well as specific neurophysiological processes necessary to reinforce or reward selective sociality (Insel 2003). In addition, inherent to the concept of a social bond is recognition memory. The neural substrates for nonselective social engagement and selective social bonding are related but not identical (Cho et al. 1999; Insel and Young 2001).

Transformations from behavioral avoidance to approach and the subsequent preferential or selective social behaviors are critical elements in the formation of social bonds. As described below, several hormones and receptor systems have been implicated in this transformation.

Table 5.1 Features of the neurobiology of oxytocin (OT) and arginine vasopressin (AVP). For details and exceptions, see Carter (1998) and Russell et al. (2003).

- Ancient origins prior to the separation between vertebrates and invertebrate
- Specific 9-amino acid structures of OT and AVP are novel to mammals
- OT is most abundant neuropeptide in the hypothalamus as indexed by mRNA
- Synthesized in largest cells in the CNS (magnocellular neurons) as well as other smaller cells
- Transported by neurosecretion to posterior pituitary, but also released in CNS
- Sibling hormones, OT and AVP, have consequences for each other's functions
- OT has only one known receptor but may bind to one or more of the three AVP receptors

Neuroendocrine Substrates for Social Bonding

Among the compounds that have been implicated in social engagement, social recognition, and bond formation are two uniquely mammalian peptide hormones: oxytocin and arginine vasopressin (Table 5.1). Vasopressin and oxytocin are closely related compounds that probably originated from a common gene. Both consist of nine amino acids. Oxytocin and vasopressin are present in many of the same regions of the brain, although usually not in the same cells (Russell et al. 2003). Oxytocin and vasopressin are made in and act on the brain, especially in the hypothalamus and areas of the nervous system that regulate the autonomic nervous system. Oxytocin has only one known receptor; however, vasopressin has three receptor subtypes, of which the V1a type has been implicated in social bonding (Young 1999). These two peptides have dynamic interactions that help to integrate emotional and autonomic states with social behaviors.

Oxytocin is associated with birth, lactation, and sexual behavior as well as modulation or down regulation of the hypothalamic–pituitary–adrenal (HPA) axis. It may help mammals to manage the stress of birth and the postpartum period (Carter et al. 2001), and remarkably, this same hormone has the capacity to produce behavioral and physiological calming (Uvnas-Moberg 1998). Oxytocin also has been implicated in various forms of positive social interactions including social bonding.

Model Systems

Early studies of the mechanisms associated with social bonds in animals focused primarily on primates, dogs, guinea pigs, and ungulates (reviewed by Hennessy 1997; Mason and Mendoza 1998; Panksepp 1998). Many of these studies were aimed at understanding the bonds between adults and infants and often emphasized the response to separation. For example, one of the first attempts to understand the regulation of separation distress in infant guinea pigs focused on opioids, suggesting that these endogenous peptides could modulate the crying normally associated with separation. Keverne and his colleagues, working with sheep, were the first to document a clear role for another neuropeptide hormone, oxytocin, in the formation of mother–infant bonds (Keverne et al. 1997).

Oxytocin

A more recent literature examining the neurobiology of adult–adult social bonding has come from socially monogamous rodents of the genus Microtus (voles). Several species from this genus (including prairie and pine voles) are capable of pair bonding as well as male parental behaviors, whereas others (including meadow and montane voles) that do not show pair bonds or male parental behavior are usually classified as nonmonogamous or polygamous. Among these species, prairie voles (*Microtus ochrogaster*) have been most extensively studied in the field as well as in the laboratory (Carter et al. 1995).

Treatment with oxytocin quickly facilitates positive social behaviors, including selective partner preferences and maternal behavior (Pedersen and Boccia 2002; Carter and Keverne 2002). Chronic exposure to oxytocin is capable of down regulating or buffering the response to stressors and the reactivity of the autonomic nervous system, including heart rate and blood pressure (Uvnas-Moberg 1998). Oxytocin is released during positive social interactions and may permit social interactions without fear (Porges, this volume). In rats, touch and massage (presumably in a context of perceived safety) can release oxytocin, which in turn may feed back on the nervous system to further enhance relaxation (Uvnas-Moberg 1998). Thus, oxytocin is an excellent candidate for the integration of emotional experiences with the physiological processes through which social bonds bestow benefits.

Vasopressin

Some of the effects of vasopressin on social behavior appear similar to those attributed to oxytocin. In particular, both peptides may have the capacity to reduce social anxiety and both can facilitate social bonding. In prairie voles, vasopressin that is administered into the central nervous system can increase social contact as well as facilitate the onset of a preference for a familiar partner (Cho et al. 1999). The effects of vasopressin on social behavior are blocked by pretreatment with a V1a vasopressin receptor antagonist (Winslow et al. 1993). In addition, when genes for the prairie vole vasopressin (V1a) receptor were transferred by a viral vector into the limbic system of male mice, these mice showed significant increases in affiliative contact, although this social behavior was not selective (Young 1999; Insel and Young 2001).

Complicating attempts to understand the separate effects of vasopressin and oxytocin is the fact that these structurally similar peptides are capable of binding to each other's receptors (Russell et al. 2003). However, the autonomic and possibly some of the emotional properties of the effects of vasopressin are different from those associated with oxytocin. Vasopressin is capable of increasing blood pressure and cardiovascular functions, and may facilitate the release of hormones of the HPA axis. Treatment with vasopressin is associated with alertness, behavioral reactivity, arousal, and in many cases the defense of both the individual and the family (Carter et al. 1995; Carter 1998). In certain areas of the brain, vasopressin is a sexually dimorphic hormone with males producing higher levels than females. This sex difference is due to the fact that vasopressin synthesis, especially within the limbic system, is facilitated by androgens (De Vries and Villalba 1997). Vasopressin may be especially important to the postcopulatory mate-guarding and male parental behavior that is typical of monogamous species (Winslow et al. 1993). The behavioral characteristics of vasopressin may permit males from socially monogamous species, such as prairie voles, to show necessary sexually dimorphic behaviors, such as mounting or even aggression toward strangers, while continuing to form social bonds and exhibiting high levels of social behavior within the family.

Other "Stress" Hormones

Another neuropeptide that has been implicated in stress and anxiety as well as pair bonding is corticotropin-releasing hormone (CRH). CRH is synthesized and released in several areas of the hypothalamus that are implicated in emotion and the regulation of autonomic responses. In male prairie voles there is also evidence that treatment with moderate, but not high, doses of CRH can facilitate pair bonding; pretreatment with a specific CRH antagonist blocked these effects (DeVries et al. 2002). Evidence from other species suggests that the actions of CRH may synergize with those of vasopressin to regulate the release of adrenal steroids. It is also possible that CRH and vasopressin work in synchrony to allow stressful experiences to facilitate pair bonding, especially in males. Whether CRH plays a role in pair bonding in females remains to be studied.

The relationship between anxiety or stress and social bonding also offers important clues to the identity of other hormones that may be associated with social attachment. At least some species of socially monogamous mammals have exceptionally high levels of adrenal steroids, and it is possible that these steroids have behavioral consequences related to the development and expression of the traits of monogamy (DeVries et al. 1996; Carter 1998; Carter and Keverne 2002). Also of possible relevance to the capacity of stressful experiences to facilitate social bonding is the fact that in rats the binding of oxytocin to its receptor is increased by the presence of adrenal steroids, especially in the amygdala (Liberzon and Young 1997).

Among the other hormones associated with stress and anxiety that have been implicated in pair bonding are the catecholamines, including dopamine and norepinephrine (Keverne et al. 1997). Norepinephrine, associated with arousal and activation, also helps to regulate oxytocin release (Russell et al. 2003).

Reward

The chemistry of reward, which involves dopamine, remains integral to the processes that allow attachments to form (Insel 2003). Among the possible roles for dopamine in social bond formation is enhancement of the perceived hedonic properties of the partner or stimuli associated with the partner. Both dopamine and opioid receptors are found in the nucleus accumbens, which (as described below) may be of relevance to the emotional states that accompany social bonding. In addition, in a yet to be determined manner, oxytocin and vasopressin may help to connect social stimuli to the reward system.

In prairie voles, dopamine–oxytocin interactions have been implicated in the formation of social bonds in both sexes (Aragona et al. 2003). Not all species of mammals have an anatomical association between dopamine and oxytocin; the co-localization — or alternatively lack of co-localization — of these chemicals may account in part for species differences in the capacity to form social bonds. Consistent with species differences in the tendency to show selective social behaviors is the fact that in rats and nonmonogamous voles, receptors for oxytocin and dopamine are not co-localized in classic reward pathways (Insel 2003). The rewarding effects of dopamine could serve to cement relationships and enhance emotional feelings associated with the formation of social bonds.

Addiction and Social Bonds

Early attempts to understand social bonds focused attention on possible parallels between the addictive properties of endogenous opioids and those of social bonds (Panksepp 1998). However, the effects of endogenous opioids on social behavior are complex and may vary as a function of species age, gender, and social rank. Evidence for opioid effects on social bonding came first from studies showing that blocking opioid receptors with naloxone increased separation cries in young guinea pigs, whereas morphine had the opposite effect. However, adult social behaviors are not readily blocked by naloxone treatments, leading Panksepp to conclude that although the endogenous opioids may play a role in separation distress, they are not essential for social reward. Endogenous opioids can, however, regulate oxytocin and vasopressin, including the capacity to release these peptides (Russell et al. 2003). Opioids also have been implicated in maternal behavior. For example, in sheep, blocking opioid receptors prevented both the release of oxytocin and the facilitatory effects of vaginal–cervical stimulation on social bonding (Keverne et al. 1997). It is possible that opioids have both direct and indirect modulatory effects on social behavior, although their role in social bonding is at present poorly defined (Panksepp 1998; Keverne, this volume).

Disruptions in or the absence of social bonds are associated with anxiety and vulnerability to substance abuse, and the most effective treatments for addiction often incorporate social support. As the identities of ancient and powerful neuroendocrine systems, including those that incorporate oxytocin, have become more apparent, knowledge of their properties helps us to understand causes and consequences of social bonds, including the mechanisms through which giving and receiving social support benefit health and well-being (Carter 1998; Uvnas-Moberg 1998). Oxytocin may be especially necessary for the selective and vulnerable immobility that is characteristic of social bonds and is necessary for birth, nursing, and orgasm (Porges, this volume).

Neuroanatomical Substrates of Social Bonding

The neural mechanisms for the actions of hormones that influence social bonding remain only superficially understood (reviewed Carter and Keverne 2002). It is known that the receptors for the hormones that have been implicated in social bonding, including oxytocin and vasopressin, are differentially distributed in regions of the nervous system, such as the olfactory system, the extended amygdala (including the nucleus accumbens and ventral pallidum), the lateral septum, and lower brainstem (Young 1999; Insel and Young 2001). In turn, these areas have been implicated in social behavior and social memory, anxiety, the regulation of autonomic and visceral responses, and reward (Carter and Keverne 2002; Insel 2003; Porges 2001 and this volume).

Summary

In pair-bonding species, biological changes associated with anxiety or fear set the stage for attachment. Oxytocin or vasopressin (or related hormones), released especially in the presence of or following exposure to stress hormones, could help to overcome anxiety or fear in the face of strangers. For example, we have recently observed in female prairie voles that brief exposure to an infant results in a rapid decline in corticosterone and can also facilitate the formation of subsequent adult social bonds, possibly through the release of endogenous oxytocin (Kim, Bales, and Carter, unpublished data). Oxytocin, especially in females but perhaps in males as well (Cho et al. 1999), may allow or encourage the social interactions and immobility which in turn permit social bonds to form. Other hormonal systems, including those classically associated with reward (e.g., dopamine and the endogenous opioids) may interact with oxytocin and vasopressin to specify a particular partner or regulate the response to the absence of a partner or other disruptions in social bonds.

HOW ARE INDIVIDUAL, GENDER, AND SPECIES VARIATIONS IN THE CAPACITY FOR SOCIAL BONDING PRODUCED?

Understanding differences in the tendency to form pair bonds requires an appreciation for interactions among genetic and epigenetic/developmental processes.

For example, a stressful or fearful experience, mediated in part by adrenal steroids, may have immediate consequences for social interactions and, in some cases, stress facilitates pair bonding (DeVries et al. 1996; Carter 1998). In addition, social experiences across the life span may also reprogram the later expression of peptide hormones and their receptors, further contributing to individual or species variation in the capacity or willingness to form pair bonds (Henry and Wang 1998; Pedersen and Boccia 2002). For example, in prairie voles, early handling, probably mediated by increased maternal stimulation of the pups, produces in those pups long-lasting increases in oxytocin within the brain. In separate studies we have found that exposure to oxytocin in early life increases the later production of oxytocin, especially in females, and also produces animals that form pair bonds more quickly than their untreated counterparts (reviewed Carter 2003).

The relationship between pair bonding and reproduction suggests a possible role for sex steroids. However, animals that are gonadectomized in adulthood are capable of forming pair bonds. Thus, in adult animals, gonadal steroids may not be essential for the formation of partner preferences (Carter et al. 1995). Sex steroids, however, may have a critical behavioral role during early development by altering the production of and adult responses to neuropeptides, including vasopressin and oxytocin. Over the life span of an individual, sex steroids regulate processes that lead to sexual differentiation and thus may help to explain sex differences in the tendency to form pair bonds (De Vries and Villalba 1997; Carter 2003). In addition, reproductive hormones such as estrogens and androgens can regulate the synthesis and actions of peptides, such as oxytocin and vasopressin, providing indirect effects on the ability of an individual to form social bonds.

Although gonadal hormones may not be essential for pair bonding, sex differences do exist in the capacity and mechanisms for pair bond formation (Carter 1998, 2003). For example, in prairie voles, stressful experiences and stress hormones from the adrenal gland tend to facilitate heterosexual pair bond formation in males; in contrast, in females comparable experiences or hormones inhibit female–male pair bonding (DeVries et al. 1996). However, following a stressful experience, females may form female–female bonds, suggesting that both physiological and social context must be taken into account in attempts to understand the mechanisms underlying pair bonding.

Mechanisms for sex differences in pair bond formation may involve sex differences in the behavioral effects of oxytocin and vasopressin (Carter 1998). Chronic exposure to oxytocin is associated with energy conservation and immobility, in part through interactions with the parasympathetic nervous system (Uvnas-Moberg 1998; Porges 1998, 2001, this volume). In contrast, vasopressin promotes sympathetic arousal, increases in blood pressure and cardiovascular activity, behavioral alertness, and physical mobilization. The best known functions of oxytocin (birth and lactation) are unique to females.

Estrogen tends to facilitate the synthesis and actions of oxytocin, although both males and females are capable of producing oxytocin. It is likely that the effects of vasopressin on pair bonding reflect the effects of this peptide within the limbic system, and vasopressin synthesis in the limbic system is especially androgen dependent (De Vries and Villalba 1997).

Relative differences between the production and effects of oxytocin versus vasopressin are compatible with sex differences in reproductive behaviors. However, the actions of these peptides may also differ as a function of the endocrine history of the individual. For example, castration in early life renders male prairie voles (in adulthood) less sensitive to the pair bond-facilitating effects of vasopressin (Cushing et al. 2003).

Recent breakthroughs in molecular genetics offer another perspective on the mechanisms for individual and species differences in the capacity to form social bonds. Species differences in the receptors for peptide hormones and their distributions in the nervous system, such as those seen in voles (Witt et al. 1991; Insel and Young 2001), are now widely accepted. However, both the synthesis of both peptide hormones and their receptors can also be altered by early social and hormonal experiences. Such processes create variations in the nervous system and may be responsible for subsequent behavioral differences among species, between males and females within a species, and among individuals (Carter 2003). For example, interspecific variations in the regulatory regions of the gene for the vasopressin V1a receptor have been implicated in social behavior (Young 1999; Insel and Young 2001).

Working within genetic constraints, early exposure to hormones, including peptides and steroids, has the capacity to reprogram the developing nervous system. In addition, early experiences can alter the capacity of the nervous system to produce hormones, including oxytocin (Carter et al. 2003). Such changes can produce adaptive and, in some cases, long-lasting changes in physiology and behavior. Patterns of social behaviors seem to be especially sensitive to the effects of early experience (Pedersen and Boccia 2002; Carter 2003). It is likely that differences in the capacity to form social bonds reflect the social and endocrine history of the individual, the consequences of sexual differentiation, as well as species variations in neuroendocrinology and neuroanatomy.

HUMAN SOCIAL BONDS

What Is Known regarding the Biological Basis of Human Social Bonding?

Studies directly investigating the biological basis of human social bonds are uncommon. However, the physiological circumstances associated with social bond formation are probably similar in humans and other mammals. The basic hormones and neural mechanisms responsible for social behaviors are also conserved among mammals, and thus shared by humans and other mammals.

As in other mammals, human physiology is usually capable of accommodating the demands of birth and lactation. However, there is considerable variation in the birth process among individuals, and the large size of human infants and their skulls relative to the human cervix/pelvis presents special challenges to the birth process. In this context, humans, along with a few domestic animals, are unique in the fact that they may experience hormonally assisted and/or surgical delivery of their young. The effects of a recently introduced oxytocin-antagonist (Atosiban) as a method for preventing premature labor remain to be studied in humans; however, in other species, blocking oxytocin in early life can disrupt social behavior (Carter 2003). Furthermore, human females may or may not nurse their own offspring. In those women who do breastfeed, patterns and durations of nursing/lactation are extremely variable. Finally, human infants are raised under extremely variable conditions (Hrdy, this volume), which based on our experience with animals, might be expected to have effects on the subsequent sociality of the infant. The consequences for the parent–infant bond of such variations and modifications in labor, lactation, and parental behavior have received little attention.

It is known that lactating women may be protected from psychological and physiological stressors, and breastfeeding women are in general less reactive to stressful experiences than women who give birth but do not lactate (Carter and Altemus 1997; Carter et al. 2001). Human pregnancy and birth are associated with transient elevations in CRH, cortisol, estrogen, catecholamines, prolactin, vasopressin, and oxytocin. Furthermore, gonadal steroids decline following parturition. Dramatic hormonal shifts which occur during pregnancy, birth, and the postpartum period may affect the emotional state of the mother and indirectly influence the child (Carter 2003). Impairments in the capacity to manage these shifts could predispose some women to emotional instability, including a vulnerability to depression or in rare cases psychosis (Carter et al. 2001). The emotional status of the mother could of course also affect the baby. Lactation may help to buffer the new mother from these hormonal and autonomic shifts, including dramatic changes in the HPA axis and other hormonal systems. The HPA axis has been implicated in depression. However, the relationship between lactation and postpartum depression is poorly understood, and this literature is both incomplete and difficult to interpret, complicating any attempts to draw strong conclusions. Even in the face of this complexity, there is evidence that the emotional reactions of both mothers and fathers to their infants may correlate with hormonal levels in late pregnancy (Storey et al. 2000; Fleming, this volume).

Of particular relevance to the mother–infant interaction may be the pulsatile release of oxytocin that normally induces uterine contractions and is necessary for milk ejection (Russell et al. 2003). Women who deliver by caesarian section, especially if the surgery occurs before the onset of labor, may not experience the birth-related pulses of oxytocin and may have difficulty in establishing lactation, in part because they do not readily produce a pulsatile pattern of oxytocin release in the immediate postpartum period (Uvnas-Moberg 1998).

It is plausible that the physiological conditions that lead to parental bonding in humans are related to those that are associated with social bond formation in other species. Based on the literature in nonhuman animals, we can postulate that a woman (and her partner or other companions) who experiences high levels of emotional arousal and HPA axis activity, in the prenatal period, or even during labor, might be especially primed to form a new social bond with a child. Birth, lactation, and stimuli from a newborn may be powerful releasers of hormones such as oxytocin and dopamine, which could in turn reinforce social bonds during this period (Insel 2003). The relationship between oxytocin and dopamine might be especially relevant to social bonding if the postpartum period were accompanied by arousal followed by a sense of emotional safety. As in other mammals, human lactation and perhaps even the hormonal milieu associated with birth has, at least in theory, the potential to be emotionally protective and perhaps to predispose the mother to form a bond with her infant.

What Mechanisms Exist to Permit Fathers or Other Caretakers to Form Social Bonds with Children?

The capacity to form strong social bonds is not limited to mothers and infants. As described by Hrdy (this volume) and Keverne (this volume), the historical tendency of humans and other primates to show patterns of communal rearing of offspring would demand mechanisms to support social bonds between nonmaternal caretakers and infants. Because the hormones associated with social bonding are not unique to birth or lactation, we can postulate that the same or related hormones that are associated with maternal attachment might have the potential to encourage the formation of social bonds between children and their nonmaternal caretakers, including fathers, adoptive parents, and grandparents. For example, although less well-studied, the hormonal changes experienced by fathers may be in partial synchrony with their domestic partners (Storey et al. 2000; Fleming, this volume). Furthermore, as suggested by studies of pair bonding in animals, it is possible that a uniquely masculine hormonal cocktail, including centrally active vasopressin, predisposes the prospective father or other male caretaker to form social bonds with offspring (De Vries and Villalba 1997). Included in the features of a paternal bond may be a particular need for a father to attempt to protect his own children or acquire the resources necessary to support his family. The role of testosterone in male social attachment has not been well studied even in animal models. Testosterone does produce relatively long-lasting increases in vasopressin in areas of the nervous system, such as the amygdala, which may be of importance to the capacity of parents to respond appropriately to stimuli from an infant. Furthermore, transient declines in androgens may accompany the birth of a child or perhaps exposure to stimuli from an infant (Storey et al. 2000). Androgens can interfere in some cases with the release or actions of oxytocin, and it is possible that temporarily lower levels of sex steroids around the time of birth could be adaptive, permitting males as well as females to experience the behavioral consequences of oxytocin. Whether oxytocin plays a role in paternal behavior remains to be determined, but the capacity of oxytocin and vasopressin to influence each other's receptors provides yet another possible explanation for the tendency of fathers or other males who are exposed to children to develop strong emotional attachments.

SUMMARY

The nervous system of modern humans is constructed from ancient neural and endocrine components that are shared among mammals. The patterns of emotion and behavior that humans call "social bonds" emerge from neurobiological roots. Even rather unsophisticated creatures, such as prairie voles, can develop lifelong social relationships with properties apparently similar to human social attachments. We now recognize that behavior is sculpted by genetic and epigenetic processes producing differences that are labeled as "species," "gender," and "individuality." Knowledge of the origins and properties of these systems does not totally explain social behavior. However, this knowledge does give us an exciting new perspective with far-reaching implications for understanding this essential aspect of human nature.

ACKNOWLEDGMENTS

I wish to express gratitude to my colleagues and students whose insights and hard work have been essential to this paper. I am especially grateful to Stephen Porges for many discussions and editorial suggestions that have guided this research. Grants from NICHD (PO1 HD 38490), NIMH, NSF, DOD, the National Alliance for Autism Research, and the Institute for Research on Unlimited Love have supported studies described here that originated in my laboratory.

REFERENCES

Aragona, B.J., Y. Liu, J.T. Curtis, F.K. Stephan, and Z. Wang. 2003. A critical role for nucleus accumbens dopamine in partner-preference formation in male prairie voles. *J. Neurosci.* **23**:3483–3490.

Bowlby, J. 1969. Attachment. Attachment and Loss, vol. 1. London: Hogarth.

Bowler, C.M., B.S. Cushing, and C.S. Carter. 2002. Social factors regulate female–female aggression and affiliation in prairie voles. *Physiol. Behav.* **76**:559–566.

Carter, C.S. 1998. Neuroendocrine perspectives on social attachment and love. *Psychoneuroendocrin.* **23**:779–818.

Carter, C.S. 2003. The developmental consequences of oxytocin. *Physiol. Behav.* **79**:383–397.

Carter, C.S., and M. Altemus. 1997. Integrative functions of lactational hormones in social behavior and stress management. *Ann. NY Acad. Sci.* **807**:164–174.

Carter, C.S., M. Altemus, and G. Chrousos. 2001. Neuroendocrine and emotional changes in the postpartum period. *Prog. Brain Res.* **133**:241–249.

Carter, C.S., A.C. DeVries, and L.L Getz. 1995. Physiological substrates of mammalian monogamy: The prairie vole model. *Neurosci. Biobehav. Rev.* **19**:303–314.

Carter, C.S., and E.B. Keverne. 2002. The neurobiology of social affiliation and pair bonding. In: Hormones, Brain, and Behavior, ed. D.W. Pfaff, vol. 1. pp. 299–337. San Diego: Academic.

Carter, C.S., and R.L. Roberts. 1997. The psychobiological basis of cooperative breeding. In: Cooperative Breeding in Mammals, ed. N.G. Solomon and J.A. French, pp. 231–266. New York: Cambridge Univ. Press.

Cho, M.M., A.C. DeVries, J.R. Williams, and C.S. Carter. 1999. The effects of oxytocin and vasopressin on partner preferences in male and female prairie voles (*Microtus ochrogaster*). *Behav. Neurosci.* **113**:1071–1080.

Cushing, B.S., U. Okorie, and L.J. Young. 2003. The effects of neonatal castration on the subsequent behavioral response to arginine vasopressin and the expression of V1a receptors in adult male prairie voles. *J. Neuroendocrin.* **15**:1021–1026.

DeVries, A.C., M.B. DeVries, S.E. Taymans, and C.S. Carter. 1996. Stress has sexually dimorphic effects on pair bonding in prairie voles. *PNAS* **93**:11,980–11,984.

DeVries, A.C., T. Guptaa, S. Cardillo, M. Cho, and C.S. Carter. 2002. Corticotropin-releasing factor induces social preferences in male prairie voles. *Psychoneuroendocrin.* **27**:705–714.

De Vries, G., and C. Villalba. 1997. Brain sexual dimorphism and sex differences in parental and other social behaviors *Ann. NY Acad. Sci.* **807**:273–286.

Gowaty, P.A., ed. 1997. Feminism and Evolutionary Biology. New York: Chapman and Hall.

Hennessy, M.B. 1997. Hypothalamic–pituitary–adrenal responses to brief social separation. *Neurosci. Biobehav. Rev.* **21**:11–29.

Henry, J.P., and S. Wang. 1998. Effects of early stress on adult affiliative behavior. *Psychoneuroendocrin.* **23**:863–876.

Insel, T.R. 2003. Is social attachment an addictive disorder? *Physiol. Behav.* **79**:351–357.

Insel, T.R., and L.J. Young. 2001. The neurobiology of attachment. *Nat. Rev. Neurosci.* **2**:129–136.

Keverne, E.B., C.M. Nevison, and F.L. Martel. 1997. Early learning and the social bond. *Ann. NY Acad. Sci.* **807**:329–339.

Kleiman, D. 1977. Monogamy in mammals. *Qtly. Rev. Biol.* **52**:39–69.

Komers, P.E., and P.N.M. Brotherton. 1997. Female space use is the best predictor of monogamy in mammals. *Proc. Roy. Soc. Lond. B* **264**:1261–1270.

Liberzon, I., and E.A. Young. 1997. Effects of stress and glucocorticoids on CNS oxytocin receptor binding. *Psychoneuroendocrin.* **22**:411–422.

Mason, W.A., and S.P. Mendoza. 1998. Generic aspects of primate attachments: Parents, offspring, and mates. *Psychoneuroendocrin.* **23**:765–778.

Panksepp, J. 1998. Affective Neuroscience. New York: Oxford Univ. Press.

Pedersen, C.A., and M.L. Boccia. 2002. Oxytocin links mothering received, mothering bestowed and adult stress responses. *Stress* **5**:259–267.

Porges, S.W. 1998. Love: An emergent property of the mammalian autonomic nervous system. *Psychoneuroendocrin.* **23**:837–861.

Porges, S.W. 2001. The polyvagal theory: Phylogenetic substrates of a social nervous system. *Intl. J. Psychophysiol.* **42**:123–146.

Russell, J.A., G. Leng, and A.J. Douglas. 2003. The magnocellular oxytocin system, the fount of maternity: Adaptations in pregnanacy. *Front. Neuroendocrin.* **24**:27–61.

Storey, A., C.J. Walsh, R.L. Quinton, and K.E. Wynne-Edwards. 2000. Hormonal correlates of paternal responsiveness in new and expectant father. *Evol. Human Behav.* **21**:79–95.

Uvnas-Moberg, K. 1998. Oxytocin may mediate the benefits of positive social interaction and emotions. *Psychoneuroendocrin.* **23**:819–835.

Winslow, J.T., N. Hastings, C.S. Carter, C.R. Harbaugh, and T.R. Insel. 1993. A role for central vasopressin in pair bonding in monogamous prairie voles. *Nature* **365**:545–548.

Witt, D.M., C.S. Carter, and T.R. Insel. 1991. Oxytocin receptor binding in female prairie voles: Endogenous and exogenous oestradiol stimulation. *J. Neuroendocrin.* **3**:155–161.

Young, L.J. 1999. Oxytocin and vasopressin receptors and species-typical social behaviors. *Horm. Behav.* **36**:212–221.

6

Neurobiological and Molecular Approaches to Attachment and Bonding

E. B. KEVERNE

Animal Behaviour Department, University of Cambridge, Madingley,
Cambridge CB3 8AA, U.K.

ABSTRACT

Bonding and attachment refer to an aspect of close relationships that develop primarily between mother and infant. The existence of other special relationships which embrace male–female pair bonding and social kin bonding in a variety of mammalian species raises the question as to whether or not similar neural mechanisms underpin the development of such relationships. At the level of the limbic brain, there are common neural mechanisms involving both classical transmitter and neuropeptidergic transmitter systems which are activated by peripheral hormonal and visceral autonomic inputs. These limbic mechanisms are probably common to all mammalian species, but how they are addressed has substantially changed with the brain's evolution.

Bonding and attachment often involve a component of recognition that is integral to the deployment of the mechanisms that underpin these special relationships. In small-brained mammals this recognition process is primarily dependent on olfaction, which is dimorphically hardwired into the brain of males and females. Moreover, the olfactory recognition that deploys the behavior is itself dependent on pregnancy and parturition, events which simultaneously activate the limbic mechanisms for bonding. In primates with large executive brains, the relative contribution of olfaction and physiology in determining the behavioral output has diminished. There are still biological constraints on maternalism in large-brained primates through lactation, but bonding and parental care can be activated via cognitive mechanisms. Cognitive capacity increases with larger executive brains, the development and growth of which extends substantially into the postpartum period, which in turn necessitates extended parental care. This has been facilitated by the emancipation of maternal behavior in humans from hormonal homeostatic determinants. Such executive control not only permits a mother to extend her caregiving beyond the weaning period, but also enables fathers, older siblings, and grandparents — none of whom have been required to experience pregnancy or parturition — to participate in caregiving and extended family bonding.

INTRODUCTION

"Bonding" is a concept that embraces special affectional relationships, and although it is perfectly acceptable to apply this term to behavior of all members of the animal kingdom, it is important to realize that the neural mechanisms which subserve these behavioral events may both differ and have similarities across different mammalian species. To gain some perspective on these similarities and differences requires an understanding of how the brain has evolved. While it is generally accepted that the brain has enlarged relative to body size over evolutionary time, a more detailed examination of its component parts reveals that a remodeling also occurred. Some parts have become larger while others have diminished in size, as determined from comparative studies on modern-day phylogenies. This in turn has had a considerable impact on how the brain handles sensory information and how the brain functions to regulate behavioral outcomes, both of which are relevant to the understanding of bonding.

BRAIN EVOLUTION

Allometric scaling and a large comparative database on mammalian brains has enabled assessments of brain evolution based on the widely accepted assumption that modern-day phylogenies represent evolutionary progression (Harvey and Pagel 1991). Most hypotheses of brain evolution have suggested larger brain size correlates with greater cognitive ability, and selection pressures for such abilities have come from ecological variables where the knowledge of available food sources in time and space requires complex cognitive maps. Equally important has been the complex nature of primate social life and the cognitive skills required to process and store this social information. Although the size of the brain as a whole has been linked to different lifestyles or ecological features, this approach fails to take into account the different functions served by its component parts. For example, the hippocampus is concerned with processing spatial information and is remarkably enlarged in species which store food, whereas the neocortex is enlarged in social living primates, with those living in larger groups having the larger neocortex (Dunbar 1992). In terms of function, the frontal cortex is essential for anticipation and forward planning and is intimately related to the striatum, which interfaces with other cortical areas for calling these plans into action. For the purpose of this chapter, I group these cortical/striatal brain regions together and refer to them as the "executive" brain. This executive brain is, however, constantly in communication with those brain regions which generate emotions.

From a behavioral viewpoint, other parts of the brain might be considered to conflict potentially with the functioning of the executive brain. Certain areas of the limbic brain (hypothalamus, medial preoptic area) are important for primary motivated behavior such as maternal care, feeding, sexual and aggressive behavior. These areas of the brain are under strong hormonal and visceral influences and in small-brained mammals are primarily activated by olfactory cues. Most mammals only show maternal care after pregnancy and parturition while sexual behavior responds to the demands of the gonadal hormones which determine sexual motivation. However, large-brained primates are spontaneously maternal while most sexual activity is nonreproductive and emancipated from gonadal determinants. How then, do these evolutionary changes in the brain influence differing behavioral strategies?

While certain regions of the primate "executive" brain have expanded relative to the rest of the brain, regions of the brain that regulate primary motivated behavior (hunger, sex, aggression, maternal care) have contracted (Keverne et al. 1996). Areas of the cortex that are concerned with forward planning have increased exponentially while those regions which respond to gonadal and visceral hormones have decreased in size (Figure 6.1). This does not mean that

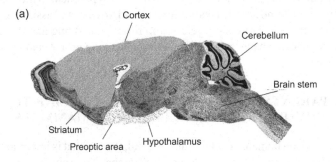

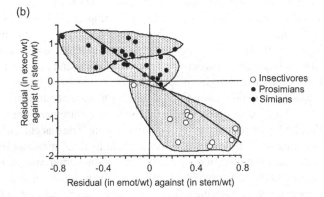

Figure 6.1   (a) Sagittal section of mammalian brain. Gray area (executive brain) includes neocortex and striatum; white area (motivational brain) includes septum, preoptic area and hippothalamus. (b) Comparison of these brain regions (controlling for body weight) against the phylogentically older region of the brain (brain stem) for three mammalian phylogenies. Those mammals with the larger "executive brain" tend to have the smaller "motivational" brain, and vice versa for smaller "executive" brains.

motivated behavior has also declined in large-brained primates, but the controlling mechanisms for the behavior have shifted away from tight linkage with
physiological determinants in favor of deployment of intelligent behavioral
strategies (Keverne et al. 1996). One important consequence of these evolutionary trends can be seen in the way the brain processes sensory information
(Barton et al. 1995), with a move away from olfactory regulation of behavior to
greater dependence on visual cues in species with a large executive brain (Zhang
and Webb 2003). It is generally accepted that small-brained mammals rely
strongly on olfactory information not only for regulating maternal and sexual
behavior but also for making the individual recognition that is integral to bonding. Primates, on the other hand, including humans, have all of their senses well
developed and with the evolutionary enlargement of the executive brain, they
have the capacity to assimilate and integrate information rapidly from a number
of sensory channels simultaneously. More to the point, primates possess the
ability to attend to whichever sensory channel is most pertinent to the context in
which the animal finds itself. This ability to attend to detail and assimilate multiple features may be particularly relevant to maternal bonding and the need to
continually update changes in the infant through a long post-weaning dependency period.

PARENTAL CARE AND BONDING: THE LINK TO
PHYSIOLOGY IN SMALL-BRAINED MAMMALS

Invasive work on humans is not permissible and, therefore, it is important to understand how working with animals might tell us something about the neural basis of attachment and bonding (Carter and Keverne 2002). Bowlby, who was interested in evolutionary biology, was struck by the imprinting work of Konrad
Lorenz; it influenced his own thinking about "sensitive periods" of human infant development. If, as Bowlby suggested, an infant's attachment behavior
evolved jointly with maternal caregiving behavior (George and Solomon 1999),
then are there common underlying mechanisms?

In mammals, the female is committed to the major share of parental care. By
virtue of internal fertilization and viviparity, the female mammal commits considerable time and resources to the developing offspring. The placenta, a lifeline
for the developing fetus, produces hormones which increase maternal food intake, shut down sexual motivation, prime the brain for maternal care, and prime
the mammary gland for milk production contingent on the timing of birth. These
aspects of maternalism are an integral part of physiology which not only provides for the immediate energetic requirements of the offspring, but has the capacity to plan ahead physiologically for postpartum needs. In sheep, parturition
is itself the trigger for maternal care, milk letdown, and maternal recognition of
the infant. Progesterone levels during pregnancy increase and promote oxytocin
synthesis (Kendrick and Keverne 1992). Toward the end of the pregnancy

progesterone levels decrease and estrogen levels rise to promote synthesis of oxytocin receptors. The massive release of oxytocin caused by parturition provides the hormonal signal which synchronizes neural systems for promoting maternal care, decreasing appetite so that maternal motivation is prioritized, reducing pain and activating neural networks in the olfactory bulb and ventral striatum that are integral to offspring recognition and bonding (Keverne 1995). In the postpartum period, suckling activates the release of oxytocin and prolactin. The former insures delivery of the current meal, whereas prolactin stimulates synthesis of milk for the next meal, and both hormones sustain maternal behavior until the infant is self-sufficient at obtaining food. Removing the tactile stimulation of suckling terminates maternal care, milk synthesis, and milk letdown, and the accompanying endocrine changes re-engage sexual motivation. Hence the onset, sustainability, and termination of maternal care are synchronized with the mother's ability to provide both nutrition and sustain maternalism until the offspring is able to fend for itself. How does bonding match with these biological needs?

One of the most intensive studies of the neurobiology of bonding has been undertaken on sheep, which are seasonal breeding mammals that live in large social groups and produce few offspring, each being well developed at birth (precocial). These infants quickly become mobile, and it is thus biologically important for the mother to insure that she only allows her own offspring to suckle. In these mammals, selective bonding occurs and involves a recognition mechanism that insures only her own lamb is allowed to suckle. This early recognition bonding is initially entirely dependent on olfactory cues and occurs during a critical period contingent on birth itself. Visual and auditory cues are subsequently incorporated into the recognition process. Not only does this selective bonding insure that the mother suckles only her own offspring, but if they get separated, the mother shows detachment distress and vocalizes loudly to attract the infant. Bonding, although integral to maternal behavior, can be distinguished from this. This distinction is most obvious in the postpartum mother that is highly maternal but rejects her offspring through a failure to bond (Keverne and Kendrick 1992).

Neural Mechanisms of Bonding

A number of findings indicate that endogenous opioids are active during late pregnancy and parturition. Plasma concentrations of β-endorphin increase during labor and birth in humans, and in the rat brain β-endorphin concentrations are elevated in the hypothalamus, midbrain, and amygdala during pregnancy and parturition (Wardlaw and Frantz 1983). Proopiomelanocortin, the precursor peptide for β-endorphin, shows an increased synthesis in ewes following estradiol or progesterone replacement therapy, which mimics the effects of pregnancy hormones. The terminal areas of distribution for endorphin neurons have much in common with oxytocin neurons, and in certain areas of the brain the release of oxytocin is strongly regulated by β-endorphin, suggesting it may regulate presynaptic release of oxytocin. Taken together, these findings provide an anatomical basis for opioid–oxytocin interactions during pregnancy and lactation. A functional relationship between these peptides has also been demonstrated in the context of maternal behavior.

Studies with sheep have shown that intracerebral administration of the opioid receptor blocker, naltrexone, reduces the ability of vaginal–cervical stimulation to stimulate maternal bonding, and ewes continue to be aggressive to the lamb, with head butts and withdrawals, as though they had not received this somatosensory stimulation. The behaviors that normally result in acceptance of the lamb all decrease when vaginal–cervical stimulation is preceded by naltrexone treatment, and ewes fail to bond with the lamb (Figure 6.2). Moreover, central naltrexone administration directly to the brain blocks the release of oxytocin that normally occurs following vaginal–cervical stimulation. Hence, although opioid receptor blockade has little effect on cerebrospinal fluid levels of oxytocin during baseline conditions, in the context of parturition (vaginal–cervical stimulation) similar receptor blockade causes failure of oxytocin levels to increase in cerebrospinal fluid but not in plasma. The failure in maternal responsiveness and bonding could therefore be due to a failure of oxytocin release, and hence be a secondary consequence to the effects of opioid receptor blockade itself. The converse study, namely opioid agonist administration, fails to promote maternal acceptance or bonding when given outside the context of vaginal–cervical stimulation but reduces the level of overt aggression (head

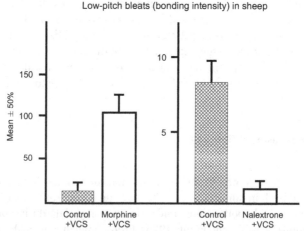

Figure 6.2 Behavior of ewes stimulated to show maternal behavior by vaginal–cervical stimulation (VCS). Frequency of low-pitch bleats, which is an indicator of maternal bonding, decrease with opiate receptor blocker (naltrexone) and is facilitated by opiate receptor agonists (morphine).

butts to lambs) (Keverne and Kendrick 1991). Together with vaginocervical stimulation, the opioid agonist not only eliminates rejection behavior, but also greatly potentiates the amount of licking and low-pitch bleats the ewe makes with the lamb, behaviors which are crucial to bonding (Figure 6.2). Vaginal–cervical stimulation given to morphine-treated ewes produces an intense and focused display of maternal behavior that is qualitatively and quantitatively indistinguishable from that of the postparturient ewe. Evidence of firm bonding is seen when the lamb is removed and the ewe protests vocally with high-pitched bleats. This potentiation in bonding is in line with a number of studies that have suggested a role for opioids in social attachment and affiliative behavior and is probably a part of the neural "reward" mechanism for these behaviors (Panksepp et al. 1997). The potentiating effects of opioids producing intensity and focus in the mother–infant interaction probably involve the ventral striatum, an area of the brain concerned with reward of both natural and conditioned olfactory cues (Kippen et al. 2003).

Why Is Parenting Primarily a Female Role in Small-brained Mammals?

In most mammals, the mother is the only individual guaranteed to be present when infants are born, so it is no biological surprise that she has the primary parental role. In social living mammals, female kin may also participate in parenting and in monogamous mammals, where the male and female stay together, the male also makes an active contribution to the caring. However, even in these cases, the mother is always the exclusive provider of nourishment prior to weaning. Male mammals cannot take over the role of pregnancy or lactation for their mates, and males, rather than providing parenting, frequently choose to seek reproductive opportunities elsewhere. Not only is the male's reproductive priority different from that of the female, but their brain is wired together in a different way to that of females, a feature that is pertinent to the issue of recognition bonding and parental care in small-brained mammals.

Behavior of small-brained mammals is strongly influenced by the perinatal action of gonadal hormones in the developing limbic brain. Castration on neonatal day one in rats increases the likelihood of males showing maternal behavior when adult, whereas neonatal exposure to testosterone in females reduces their maternal care and facilitates infanticide. In both rats and mice, studies on the position of females in the uterus have shown that maternal behavior onset is delayed if the female spent her intrauterine life between two males. This early influence of gonadal hormones on maternal behavior and infanticide is partially determined by the differential wiring of the chemosensory system into the developing limbic brain (Keverne 2002) (Figure 6.3). The critical timing for testosterone production in sexual differentiation of the rodent brain is determined by GnRH neurons, which themselves originate in the olfactory placode. Hence the maturational events in the developing neuroendocrine system are

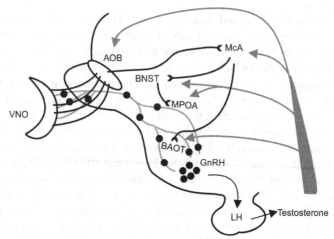

Figure 6.3   The GnRH and VNO neurons take their origin in the olfactory placode. GnRH neurons migrate to the hypothalamus and make neural connections with the blood supply to the pituitary and through the pathway regulate testosterone release. Sensory projections from the VNO neurons relay in various limbic brain nuclei (black labeling) prior to terminating on the medial preoptic area (MPOA). If this nucleus is lesioned in the adult female, maternal care is abolished. The hormonal cascade from the GnRH neurons initiates the perinatal testosterone surge (gray arrows) which produces the sexual dimorphism in the relays for the VNO projection pathway.

synchronized with the masculinization of the developing accessory olfactory projection pathway, which thereby exhibits sexual dimorphism at all its neural relays (Segovia and Guillamon 1996) (Figure 6.3). Lesions in discrete parts of this projection pathway in males enhance components of female behavior, including maternal behavior in male rats. Recently, targeted mutagenesis of a specific ion channel (TRP2–/–) that blocks signaling in this chemosensory pathway in a mouse renders them gender blind (Stowers et al. 2002). This genetic lesion results in males failing to show aggressive behavior and increases mating with other males; in females it results in failure to respond with postpartum aggression to an intruder male, but has no effect on the levels of gonadal hormones.

Small-brained mammals have their maternal care strongly tied into physiological mechanisms. Steroid hormones play a primary role not only in initiating the behavior according to the appropriate signals, but in hardwiring this signaling system to the sexually dimorphic regions of the brain during early "critical period" development. Interestingly, lesioning this system or parts of this system in adults does facilitate male parental care, and prolonged exposure of this system to the odor of infants will also facilitate male parental care, should they stay around and not choose to look for other mates. When female bonding does occur in small-brained mammals, it often involves olfactory signaling since lesions of the olfactory system prevent selective bonding and, in many cases, also impair adult maternal care. My interpretation of these findings is that bonding in small-brained mammals is primarily tied into sexual dimorphisms in the limbic brain that relate to olfactory signaling.

The advantages of such lower level olfactory processing via direct projections to the amygdala and hypothalamus is that it tends to be automatic and fast and has evolved to meet the needs of biologically relevant signaling for behavior. Moreover, it is relatively easy to switch motivational priorities through hormonal signaling. For example, when progesterone is high and estrogen is low during pregnancy, feeding behavior is upregulated, sexual behavior is inhibited, and the brain is primed for maternal care. At parturition, progesterone falls and estrogen rises promoting maternal care and postpartum estrus, while feeding is temporally inhibited. The sexually dimorphic wiring of the brain and the sustained release of testosterone postpubertally in the male maintains the continuous potential for sexual or aggressive behavior throughout reproductive life depending on the appropriate olfactory signaling. Males are most likely to show parental care and inhibit infanticide if they are familiar with offspring olfactory signals. Likewise, the female is most likely to tolerate the male's presence and inhibit postpartum aggression if the male smell is familiar.

MATERNAL BONDING IN LARGE-BRAINED PRIMATES

Old World primates are characterized by their large executive brain, and one consequence of this enlargement has been the emancipation of maternal behavior from the determining actions of hormones. In line with this is the diminished sexual dimorphisms of the hypothalamus (medial preoptic area, MPOA) compared with the rodent brain (Figure 6.4), while the sexually dimorphic chemosensory projections are nonexistent. Humans do not possess a vomeronasal organ or vomeronasal receptors, and the olfactory receptor genes are themselves between 60–70% nonfunctional pseudogenes. These evolutionary events have had a large impact on all primary motivated behavior, including parental care where pregnancy and parturition are not an essential prerequisite for good parenting or indeed for bonding with infants. What is, therefore, important for good parenting among primates with a complex social organization?

Most of the primate executive brain development is postponed to the postnatal period (neotany), and this neocortical development continues throughout the time infants experience maternal care and experience the skills necessary to cope with social living. This includes interactions with peers, younger siblings, and infants. Play mothering occurs with juveniles of both sexes, indeed some male primates may also participate in maternal care. Early experiences with their own mother are also crucially important, and it is well recognized that the prognosis for good mothering is poor if that infant received inadequate mothering herself (Harlow 1971; Kraemer et al. 1991). What is it then that early socialization and attachment have in common to promote good

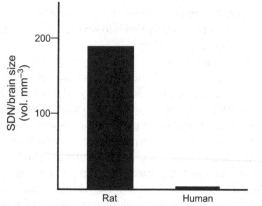

Figure 6.4   Relative decrease in the size of the medial preoptic area (MPOA) sexually dimorphic nucleus (SDN) in a large-brained (human) versus a small-brained mammal (rat).

mothering? Related to this question is the importance of how the relationship of maternal bonding reciprocated by infant attachment is served at the neural level. Clearly there are strong cognitive components involving social learning in primates as well as strong emotional components in both the infant attachment and maternal bonding. However, if adult social relationships are to be structured on the foundations of early secure attachment, it is pertinent to ask whether there are common underlying mechanisms that serve "socialization" just as there are common mechanisms that underpin the reward for primary motivated behavior.

Opioids and Primate Infant Attachment

The early development (first 10 weeks) of social behavior in monkeys occurs exclusively in the context of interactions with the mother. These early social interactions are almost totally under the mother's control, in terms of both the amount and kinds of interaction permitted. By 40 weeks of age, infants are considerably more independent from their mother, and much of their behavior is oriented toward peers. Nevertheless, mothers continue to monitor their infants and quickly intervene in response to risks arising during play (Simpson et al. 1989). The mother serves as a secure base from which the infant can obtain contact and grooming while developing and strengthening its social bonds with peers and other kin.

Administration of opioids has been shown to reduce the distress shown by infants of various species when separated from their mothers. For example, the opiate agonist morphine reduces distress vocalization rates in chicks, puppies, and rhesus monkeys. Processes involving opioid reward may therefore play a role in infant attachment, but is this same mechanism deployed in development of social behavior as well as in maternal bonding? This has been investigated in a study of young rhesus monkeys given acute treatment with the opioid receptor blocker, naloxone, and observed in their natal group (Martel et al. 1995). Naloxone increases the duration of affiliative infant–mother contact and the amount of time the infants spend on the nipple. This occurs even at one year of age, when the mothers are no longer lactating. Indeed, feeding is unaffected by naloxone treatment of infants, but play activity decreases and their distress vocalizations increase. Moreover, the opioid system in both infant and mother coordinates intimate contact during reunion (Kalin et al. 1995). These results may be interpreted in terms of opiate receptor blockade reducing the "positive affect" that accrues from the developing attachment relationship with mother, as a result of which the young infant returns to mother as an established secure base.

Prior to puberty, the effects of opioid blockade on infant attachment is the same in males and females: both increase contact with their mother. At puberty, males tend to leave their natal social group whereas females stay with the group. This type of social organization in Old World monkeys is referred to as being "female bonded." Why do we find this sex difference in social bonding, and if the mechanisms serving maternal bonding and infant attachment extend to social bonding, why should it differ between males and females? In males entering puberty, opioid receptor blockade results in significant increases in the time these males spend with mother and decreases the time they spend with others. At the same age, females tend to spend more time alone than males, but when subjected to opioid receptor blockade they spend more time with other females, not their mother. This suggests that at puberty, females have developed other socially meaningful relations and have expanded their secure base beyond the mother, although these social relationships are invariably with matrilineal kin. Postpubertal males running to mother would not be favorably tolerated by dominant males, would invite aggression, and hence the peripheralization and subsequent mobility of males from the natal social group. The attachment that rhesus monkey infants develop with the matriline is especially enduring in females, lasting a lifetime, whereas in males it rarely lasts beyond puberty.

Opioids and Maternal Bonding

It has been suggested that the activation of the endogenous opioid system at parturition and during suckling promotes the positive affect arising from maternal behavior. In the early postpartum period, a mother's social interactions are almost exclusively with her infant, and opiate receptor blockade in the mother has marked effects on this relationship.

Studies on naloxone treatment of postpartum rhesus monkey mothers living in social groups have addressed the importance of opioids in maternal bonding. Naloxone treatment reduces the mothers' caregiving and protective behavior shown toward their infants. In the first weeks of life when infant retrieval is normally very high, naloxone-treated mothers neglect their infants and show little

E. B. Keverne

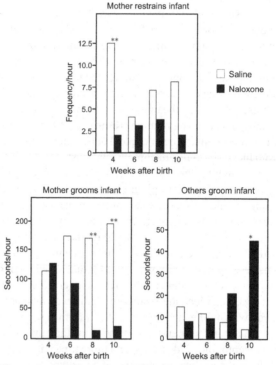

Figure 6.5   Effects of opioid blockade on mother–infant behavior (restraining maternal grooming and permitting others to groom infant) in the rhesus monkey.
* = p < 0.05; ** = p < 0.01.

retrieval even when the infant moves a distance away. As the infants approach eight weeks of age, when a strong grooming relationship normally develops between mother and infant, mothers treated with naloxone fail to develop such a grooming relationship. Moreover, they permit other females to groom their infants, while saline-treated controls are very possessive and protective of their infants (Figure 6.5) (Martel et al. 1993).

The infant is not rejected from suckling, but the mother's possessive preoccupation with the infant declines. She is not the normal attentive caregiver, and mother–infant interactions are invariably initiated by the infant. It is clear, therefore, that primates and other mammals have in common opioid involvement in maternal care, but the consequences of opioid blockade in small-brained mammals are much greater for the biological aspects of maternal behavior. In rodents and sheep, interference with the endogenous opioid system severely impairs maternal behavior, including suckling, whereas monkeys neglect their bonding but still permit suckling. These differences may reflect the degree of emancipation from endocrine determinants that maternal behavior has undergone in primates, and the importance of "emotional reward" for the bonding mechanism. If the endogenous opioid system in the monkey is positively linked to mother–infant bonding, then heroin addiction, which acts on the same opioid receptor, would be predicted to have severe consequences for human maternal bonding. Women who are addicted to heroin have many aspects of their social and economic life disrupted, making the data difficult to disentangle. Nevertheless, the facts are that by one year of age, nearly 50% of children are living away from their biological mothers, and by school age only 12% remain with their biological mother (Mayes 1995). These infants have been abandoned for adoption or are taken into the care of their grandparents and other female kin. Moreover, in a follow up of 57 methadone-maintained mothers compared with controls matched for ethnicity, socio-economic status, infant birth weight, and gestational age, opiate-addicted mothers were far less likely to have remained the child's primary parent and the children were significantly more likely to have been referred to child protective care or special service agencies for neglect, abandonment, or abuse.

Integral to the bonding process in primates is the brain's endogenous opioid system, which has been shown to act on naloxone-binding receptors in the ventral striatum. This area of the brain is involved in "reward" as is the mesolimbic dopamine system, which detects rewarding stimuli and ways they occur differently from prediction to enable "updating." Primates attend to all sensory cues, the integration of which requires neocortical integration in prefrontal association cortex in order for rapid bonding to occur. The down regulation of olfaction for recognition and the importance of auditory and visual recognition in activating emotional reward is reflected in the obsessive grooming given especially to hands, face, and genitalia, which are the phenotypic traits that show greatest individual and sex differences. Primates also show extended postpartum care, which requires continual updating of the infants morphological and behavioral development, again engaging prefrontal–ventral striatal reward pathways and their intimate connections with the emotional brain via the amygdala. Emotional activity that infants generate in female primates enables parental care to occur without the continual priming of pregnancy or parturition that is needed to engage emotional affect associated with caregiving in small-brained mammals.

EVOLUTIONARY GENETICS OF CAREGIVING

Because mammalian females have an obligatory greater investment of time and resources in offspring, which sets a limit on their lifetime reproductive success, the most successful reproductive strategy for them is to insure survival of these offspring to a reproductive age. The male strategy for optimal reproductive success is to mate with as many fertile females as possible. For this to succeed for the male, there needs to be some sort of biological guarantee that the female he mates will provide good nurturing of his offspring. Recent studies have identified a category of mammalian genes (imprinted genes) that are autosomal haploid but expressed according to parent of origin. Interestingly, many of these genes which are paternally expressed have an important function ensuring maternal care and provisioning for offspring both pre- and postnatally (Keverne 2001). Hence a number of these paternally expressed genes promote growth and enlargement of the placenta (Peg3, Peg1, Igf2, Dlk1, Ins1, Pl1v), nutrient transfer through the placenta (Igf2), milk letdown (Peg3), maternal care (Peg1, Peg3), placentophagia (Peg1), suckling (Peg3, Gnas), and pre-weaning offspring growth (Peg3, Peg1, Gnas, Igf2, Grf1). The paternal genome is therefore ensuring good maternal care across the biologically relevant parameters and this is especially important for small-brained mammals. In primates with a large executive brain, however, progression away from the obligatory synchronization of maternal behavior with the hormones of pregnancy to a system of cognitive and emotional control requires exceptional cognitive abilities. Indeed, it is claimed that the push for evolving an exceptionally large executive brain has developed from a complex social lifestyle that requires the ability to construct a "theory of mind" and involves internalized working models of self and others. In Old World monkeys, where this complex social organization is described as "female bonded," it is the females which provide social stability and group cohesion (Wrangham 1980). Females are more affiliative and maintain continuity of the group over successive generations, while males deploy aggressive strategies and show mobility from the group. Females are the primary caregivers, and social rank of daughters, but not sons, is related to the matriline. This kind of matrilineal selection pressure is also compatible with genomic imprinting, which not only results in the development of a larger executive forebrain from maternally expressed alleles, but the advantages of such development being passed on to both sons and daughters (Keverne 2001). Asymmetries between the sexes in the context of parental care and in the context of social behavior (Keverne 1993) have provided differential selection pressures through which imprinted genes might operate (Haig 1997). In addition, the evolution of a larger executive brain has been essential for emancipation from endocrine determinants of behavior and in enabling lifetime attachments like those that occur in humans.

As young children develop, their knowledge base expands, especially in regard to the changing ways in which their mother responds to them and, more importantly, how each is likely to respond to the other. Not surprisingly, the executive brain and its connections are developing extensively during this time period. Indeed, evolution of a large neocortex which develops postnatally would not have been possible if parental and alloparental care had not extended way beyond the biological dictates of hormonal factors. The child's knowledge base steadily becomes organized in the form of internal working models of self and mother, encompassing and understanding both her moods and intentions. Building on this early knowledge provides the infant an ability to simulate happenings in an expanding world of relationships. Forward planning may occur with all the advantages gained from foresight and security. Because these working models are in constant daily use, their influence on thought, emotions, and behavior becomes routine and all-pervasive.

It is important to note that in these early years, when the neocortex is forming and making its connections and associations with other parts of the brain, the limbic emotional brain is already well developed. The large emotional repertoire of very young infants bears testimony to this. Understanding, curbing, and channeling these emotions for beneficial purposes must represent an important phase in brain development. These cognitive abilities have undoubtedly prospered from interactions with the limbic brain, especially in the context of emotional interplay between mother and child. The subsequent expansion of social relationships, based on this secure attachment, provides a second cushion for the emotional turmoil of puberty. The child's need for an attachment figure and the mother's predisposition to bond provides an optimal social environment in which the human executive brain can develop. Weaning and expansion of the child's social world have not only coincided but are made easier by having a secure base from which to explore this world (Bretherton and Munholland 1999).

With the evolutionary increases in executive brain power, maternalism has shifted from being primarily a component of physiological determinism perfected to match the biology of pregnancy and parturition, to being heavily dependent on cognitive control. Such cognition is itself dependent on social and emotional learning. The human mother has both biology and emotional cognition to facilitate her bonding, which makes her the primary figure for infant attachment. However, the lengthy dependence of children on parental care is also aided by the participation of nonparturient family members (fathers and grandparents). Since these kin have not been primed by the hormones of pregnancy, then such participation has been facilitated by the evolutionary emancipation of infant care from hormonal determinants.

REFERENCES

Barton, R.A., A. Purvis, and P.H. Harvey. 1995. Evolutionary radiation of visual and olfactory brain systems in primates, bats and insectivores. *Phil. Trans. Roy. Soc. Lond. B* **348**:381–392.

Bretherton, I., and D.A. Munholland. 1999. Internal working models in attachment relationships: A construct revisited. In: Handbook of Attachment: Theory, Research, and Clinical Applications, ed. J. Cassidy and P.R. Shaver, pp. 89–111. New York: Guilford.

Carter, C.S., and E.B. Keverne. 2002. The neurobiology of social affiliation and pair bonding. In: Hormones, Brain and Behavior, ed. D.W. Pfaff, A.P. Arnold, A.M. Etgen et al., vol. 1, pp. 299–335. San Diego: Academic.

Dunbar, R.I.M. 1992. Neocortex size as a constraint on group size in primates. *J. Hum. Evol.* **20**:469–493.

116 *E. B. Keverne*

George, C., and J. Solomon. 1999. Attachment and caregiving. In: Handbook of Attachment: Theory, Research, and Clinical Applications, ed. J. Cassidy and P.R. Shaver, pp. 649–670. New York: Guilford.

Haig, D. 1997. Parental antagonism, relatedness asymmetries, and genomic imprinting. *Proc. Roy. Soc. Lond. B* **264**:1657–1662.

Harlow, H.F. 1971. Learning to Love. San Francisco: Albion.

Harvey, P.H., and M.D. Pagel. 1991. The Comparative Method in Evolutionary Biology. Oxford: Oxford Univ. Press.

Kalin, N.H., S.E. Sheldon, and D.E. Lynn. 1995. Opiate systems in mother and infant primates coordinate intimate contact during reunion. *Psychoneuroendocrin.* **7**:735–742.

Kendrick, K.M., and E.B. Keverne. 1992. Control of synthesis and release of oxytocin in the sheep brain. *Ann. NY Acad. Sci.* **652**:102–121.

Keverne, E.B. 1993. Sex differences in primate social behavior. In: The Development of Sex Differences and Similarities in Behavior, ed. M. Haug, R.E. Whalen, C. Aron, and K.L. Olsen, pp. 227–240. Dordrecht: Kluwer.

Keverne, E.B. 1995. Olfactory learning. *Curr. Opin. Neurobiol.* **5**:482–488.

Keverne, E.B. 2001. Genomic imprinting, maternal care, and brain evolution. *Horm. Behav.* **40**:146–155.

Keverne, E.B. 2002. Pheromones, vomeronasal function, and gender-specific behavior. *Cell* **108**:735–738.

Keverne, E.B., and K.M. Kendrick. 1991. Morphine and corticotropin releasing factor potentiates maternal acceptance in multiparous ewes after vaginocervical stimulation. *Brain Res.* **540**:55–62.

Keverne, E.B., and K.M. Kendrick. 1992. Oxytocin facilitation of maternal behavior. *Ann. NY Acad. Sci.* **652**:83–101.

Keverne, E.B., F.L. Martel, and C.M. Nevison. 1996. Primate brain evolution: Genetic and functional considerations. *Proc. Roy. Soc. Lond. B* **262**:689–696.

Kippen, T.E., S.W. Cain, and J.G. Pfaus. 2003. Estrous odours and sexually conditional neutral odours activate separate neural pathways in the male rat. *Neurosci.* **117**:971–979.

Kraemer, G.W., M.H. Ebert, D.E. Schmidt, and W.T. McKinney. 1991. Strangers in a strange land: A psychobiological study of infant monkeys before and after separation from real or inanimate mothers. *Child Dev.* **62**:548–566.

Martel, F.L., C.M. Nevison, F.D. Rayment et al. 1993. Opioid receptor blockade reduces maternal affect and social grooming in rhesus monkeys. *Psychoneuroendocrin.* **18**:307–321.

Martel, F.L., C.M. Nevison, M.D.A. Simpson, and E.B. Keverne. 1995. Effects of opioid receptor blockade on the social behavior of rhesus monkeys living in large family groups. *Dev. Psychobiol.* **28**:71–84.

Mayes, L.C. 1995. Substance abuse and parenting. In: Handbook of Parenting: Applied and Practical Parenting, ed. M.H. Bornstein, vol. 4, pp. 101–126. Mahwah, NJ: Erlbaum.

Panksepp, J., E. Nelson, and M. Bekkedal. 1997. Brain systems for the mediation of social separation-distress and social reward. *Ann. NY Acad. Sci.* **807**:78–100.

Segovia, S., and A. Guillamon. 1996. Searching for sex differences in the vomeronasal pathway. *Horm. Behav.* **30**:618–626.

Simpson, M.J.A., M.A. Gore, M. Janus, and F.D. Rayment. 1989. Prior experience of risk and individual differences in enterprise shown by rhesus monkey infants in the second half of their first year. *Primates* **30**:493–509.

Stowers, L., T.E. Holy, M. Markus et al. 2002. Loss of sex discrimination and male–male aggression in mice deficient for TRP2. *Science* **295**:1493–1500.
Wardlaw, S.L., and A.G. Franz. 1983. Brain β-endorphin during pregnancy, parturition, and the postpartum period. *Endocrinology* (Baltimore) **113**:1664–1668.
Wrangham, R.W. 1980. An ecological model of female-bonded primate groups. *Behaviour* **75**:262–300.
Zhang, J., and D.M. Webb. 2003. Evolutionary deterioration in the vomeronasal pheromone transduction pathway in catarrhine primates. *PNAS* **100**:8337–8341.

7

Adult Social Bonding

Insights from Studies in Nonhuman Mammals

N. SACHSER

Department of Behavioural Biology, University of Münster, 48149 Münster, Germany

ABSTRACT

Social bonds between adult individuals constitute a major aspect of many mammalian social systems. Based on the analysis of adult social bonds in a well-studied animal system, five general insights are derived: (1) Social bonds result from behavioral strategies of individuals that were brought about by natural selection and help the individual to adapt to its environment and ultimately maximize its reproductive success. Changes in the social and physical surroundings, however, may lead to the emergence or disappearance of adult social bonding when alternative behavioral strategies yield higher reproductive success. Thus, even if the ability evolved to establish this trait, it will not necessarily be realized under a particular environmental condition. (2) The process of domestication does not reduce the ability to form adult social bonds. When the wild ancestor is characterized by this trait, we can also expect its existence in the domesticated form. (3) The ability to establish adult social bonds depends on social experiences during ontogeny. Requirements might be a sense of security during an early phase as well as the learning of significant behavioral patterns around puberty. (4) Stress responses can be ameliorated by the presence of members of the same species. This phenomenon is called "social support." Frequently, however, such social support cannot be provided by just any conspecific; the ability to give social support is restricted to bonding partners. Thus, bonding partners function as security-conferring figures, promoting well-being and health. (5) Adult social bonds contribute in a fundamental way to the generation of stable social networks. If individuals are socially integrated, and if social stability exists, good welfare and health will be achieved. Under conditions of social disintegration and social instability, however, significant increases are found in disease susceptibility mediated by hormonal and immunological responses.

INTRODUCTION

Social bonds are not an exclusive trait of humans, but rather are found in many nonhuman mammals as well. Furthermore, the variety of social bonds that exists in our own species — ranging from mother–infant to bonds between adult males and females, subadults of both sexes, and homosexual bonds — also occur in animals. It is reasonable to assume that the motivational and behavioral systems underlying social bonds are evolutionarily ancient traits that were brought about by natural selection. The study of social bonding in nonhuman mammals can therefore provide insights not only into the nature of this phenomenon in these animals, but also in our own species. A comprehensive understanding of behavioral phenomena, such as social bonding, encompasses the knowledge of the genesis, control, and consequences of this trait. The study of the genesis involves the effects of evolution, domestication, culture, and ontogeny. Control refers to short-term regulation by external stimuli impinging on the animals and by internal physiological and mental events. The consequences concern the effects on the organism itself (e.g., its health), on its social and physical environment, and on its Darwinian fitness, that is, its reproductive success. (This classification follows Dewsbury [1992] in most points.) Until now, social bonding in either human or nonhuman mammals has rarely been analyzed in a way that gives equal attention to these different levels of analysis. Thus, at present we are far from understanding social bonding in a comprehensive way.

In this chapter, I address primarily social bonding between adult individuals in nonhuman mammals. First, I discuss the characteristic traits of social bonds and its occurrence in this systematic group. Then a multilevel analysis is presented on the genesis and consequences of social bonding in a well-studied animal model: wild and domestic guinea pigs. Based on this, general insights into the phenomenon of social bonding in nonhuman mammals are derived and conclusions for the understanding of social bonding in humans are drawn. I do not focus on the control of social bonding, that is, the interplay of internal (e.g., hormones) and external (e.g., olfactory stimuli) factors in the formation and maintenance of social bonding, as a detailed understanding of the control of mother–infant bonding (e.g., in sheep) and of male–female bonding (e.g., in prairie voles) has been achieved (see reviews of this in Carter and Keverne 2002).

ADULT SOCIAL BONDING IN NONHUMAN MAMMALS: CHARACTERISTIC TRAITS AND OCCURRENCE

In mammalian social systems, a wide range of social relationships can be found. In almost all species, dominance relationships exist that are established and maintained by agonistic behaviors. As a result, members of a social system are characterized by differences in dominance status. Affiliative social relationships may also exist which are established and maintained by sociopositive behaviors. The intensity of affiliative relationships can vary distinctly. For instance, interactions with familiar individuals may take place in a generally positive manner; "friends" for whom the positive social interactions are somewhat more pronounced may also be present; and there can be one or a few bonding partners for whom a strong attachment is shown. In many mammals, such intense affiliative relations can be found between mothers and infants. In some species they also occur between adult individuals, for example, when a monogamous social organization exists (Sachser et al. 1998). In this chapter, social bonds are viewed as particularly intense affiliative social relationships rather than as any social interaction characterized by sociopositive behaviors.

How can social bonds be recognized at a behavioral level? Although no single measure has gained universal acceptance (Carter and Keverne 2002), bonding partners are usually characterized by proximity in space over a period of time and often by synchronization of their behaviors as well as by frequencies and types of positive social behavior among them, which differ from their contacts with other individuals (Wickler 1976). Loss of, or separation from, a bonding partner will elicit behavioral signs of stress (e.g., restlessness and contact vocalizations) and physiological stress responses; correspondingly, reunion with the bonding partner will bring about the opposite effect. The presence of a bonding partner in a challenging situation may attenuate or suppress behavioral and physiological stress responses (Sachser et al. 1998; Hennessy 1999; Carter and Keverne 2002). In addition, preference tests, in which an experimental animal is allowed a choice between different individuals, can be used to detect social bonds (Carter and Keverne 2002). Remarkably, social bonds among adult individuals are not always dependent on mating behavior. Mate preferences can be different from social preferences. Even in species that organize in socially monogamous pairs or small harems, sexual exclusivity is not necessarily found (see below).

Bonds between adult individuals constitute a major aspect of many mammalian social systems, though the animals of most species live a solitary life, in the sense that no adult social bonds exist. In such species, like the tiger or hamster, adult individuals meet only for mating, and the offspring leave their mothers around puberty. Other species form stable social units consisting of two or more permanently bonded adult individuals: gibbons and beavers, for example, live in monogamous pairs, a social system that is found in about 5% of all mammals. Hamadryas baboons and plains zebras establish harems of one male and several females, a system that frequently occurs in primates, rodents, and ungulates. Saddled-backed tamarins may live in polyandric groups of one female and two males, a system that has only rarely been described. Elephants, like many other ungulates, establish stable groups of related females, and in a few species like cheetahs, a strong permanent company is formed between several adult males (for references, see Sachser et al. 1998). Social bonds toward adult conspecifics of the opposite sex are normally established after sexual maturity; female–female bonds frequently develop from mother–daughter relationships, particularly when daughters do not leave their natal group. Male–male bonds are found between brothers, though not exclusively. Although typical basic forms of social organization can be assigned to many species, a high intraspecific degree of flexibility in social structure exists. When, for example, population density increases, a dominance-structured system without adult bonding may shift to an organization in which this character becomes the predominant trait (see below). Although social flexibility does not mean "anything goes" socially, the answer to the question, "What is the social organization of a given species?" must not necessarily be fixed.

In the following section, the genesis and consequences of adult social bonding in wild and domestic guinea pigs will be addressed. Wild guinea pigs (Caviinae) provide a suitable group to study the behavioral ecology of social bonding in a comparative way because much variation exists concerning this trait even in closely related species. Domestic guinea pigs (*Cavia aperea f. porcellus*) were derived from wild cavies (*Cavia aperea*). Since the wild form is characterized by adult social bonds and because both forms can be easily kept in the lab, they are especially suitable animals for studying the effects of domestication on this behavioral trait. Domestic guinea pigs build up stable social organizations involving dominance relationships and adult social bonds, even under spatially restricted conditions. Thus, domestic guinea pigs allow the experimental analysis of adult social bonding in the context of a complex social network.

ADULT SOCIAL BONDS: A STUDY IN WILD AND DOMESTIC GUINEA PIGS

The Behavioral Ecology of Social Bonding in Wild Guinea Pigs

In populations with low density in southeast Brazil, the wild cavy (*Cavia aperea*) lives in pairs or small harems and occupies stable home ranges that overlap only slightly with home ranges of adjacent groups. A male chases away every rival that approaches "his" females, and first investigations of paternity indicate that he is the father of the offspring in his group (Asher et al. 2004). In contrast, the big cavy (*Cavia magna*) in Uruguay shows no indications of social bonding and space use reveals highly overlapping home ranges of different males and females (Kraus et al. 2003). This striking difference in social relationships between species is related to differences in their habitats: The big cavy dwells in an unpredictable habitat in which flooding after heavy rainfall is common. High rates of immigration and emigration occur, and a high turnover of social partners takes place. Under these conditions an almost nonsocial, solitary way of living and promiscuous mating seems adaptive (Kraus et al. 2003). In contrast, wild cavies inhabit a stable, predictable grassland habitat with abundant food supplies. The females occupy small home ranges with almost no competition for food. This constellation enables a male to monopolize one or several females. Here, living in social monogamy or in a small harem seems a most suitable way to maximize reproductive success (Asher et al. 2004).

It was originally assumed that the social system of the wild cavy is exclusively the results of the behavioral incompatibility of the adult males (Sachser et al. 1999). However, experiments in which every female is given free choice among four different unfamiliar males in a mate-choice apparatus reveal her active role in the formation of social bonds. Each female displays clear social preferences for a single male, which then becomes the favorite mating partner. Half of the females mate with additional males but multiple paternity does not occur. Exclusively, the female's favorite social and mating partner is proven to be the father. Furthermore, reproductive success of females that mate with more than one male decreases in that more of their offspring are stillborn. Thus, the polyandrous mating strategy is assumed to be followed only in case of doubts about the quality of the partner (Hohoff 2002). Currently there are no indications as to what underlies this compatibility between individual males and females.

A completely different picture emerges, however, in the closely related yellow-toothed cavy (*Galea musteloides*). This species from central Argentina does not form adult social bonds. Accordingly, the females do not show social preferences for a single male in the mate-choice apparatus but actively seek copulations with more than one male. Moreover, their mating behavior is displayed in a way that favors the mixing of sperm (Hohoff et al. 2003). As a result, an extremely high degree of multiple paternity (> 80%) occurs, and females have greater offspring viability after mating multiple males (Sachser et al. 1999). Thus, the females of both species utilize behavioral strategies that maximize their individual reproductive success. Since these strategies differ significantly between species, significant variation in the social and mating systems of wild and yellow-toothed cavies exists.

Differences in social and mating systems have major consequences for the males' certainty about their paternity. In wild cavies, a male can be relatively certain that he indeed is the father of his bonding partner's offspring. The same seems to be true for males of a recently discovered species of wild guinea pigs from Bolivia (*Galea sp.*), which shows all traits of monogamy (Hohoff et al. 2002). In contrast, in yellow-toothed cavies a high uncertainty about paternity exists (see above). It is assumed that such variation results in different paternal investments by the males. In wild guinea pigs, paternal behaviors consist primarily in playing with the offspring and grooming them. Indeed, males of the monogamous Bolivian cavy exhibit the greatest amount of paternal care and show the least offspring-directed aggression. Males of the wild cavy also care for their young, and little aggression occurs. In contrast, males of the promiscuous yellow-toothed cavy never display paternal behaviors but frequently direct aggression toward the offspring (Adrian et al. 2005). Thus, males establish social bonds with the young and invest time and energy in their care only when they are certain about their paternity.

A Behavioral Comparison of Wild and Domestic Guinea Pigs

The wild cavy is the feral ancestor of the domestic guinea pig which was domesticated about 3000–6000 years ago. Behavioral patterns are similar in both the domesticated and the wild animals; distinct differences, however, occur in behavioral frequencies and thresholds. Domestic guinea pigs are distinctly less aggressive than their wild ancestors, and they display more sociopositive behaviors (Künzl and Sachser 1999). Owing to these differences, social interactions between members of the domesticated form proceed in a more sociopositive and tolerant way than in wild cavies. The ability to establish adult social bonds was not affected by the process of domestication. As in the wild ancestor, formation of long-term male–female bonds is a characteristic trait of the domestic guinea pig.

Adult Social Bonds in Domestic Guinea Pigs: Causes and Consequences

The social structure of domestic guinea pigs is highly flexible. The change in social organization from a strictly dominance-structured system at low individual numbers to a system in which long-lasting bonds are predominant at high numbers makes these animals eminently suitable for analyzing causes and consequences of adult social bonding. When a small number of guinea pigs (e.g., three males and three females) is placed into an enclosure, social organization is characterized mainly by a linear dominance hierarchy among the adult males (Figure 7.1). Subordinate males retreat whenever a higher-ranking conspecific approaches. Individuals of identical rank are never found. The highest-ranking male shows much more courtship behavior toward each of the females than any other male, and he probably is the father of the offspring. Social bonds do not exist between males and females. Females also construct a linear dominance hierarchy. However, compared to males, their agonistic behavior is less pronounced. Between the sexes, fighting and threat displays do not occur (Sachser 1986).

When population numbers increase, guinea pigs change their social organization (Figure 7.1). Groups of 10–15 or more split into subunits, each consisting

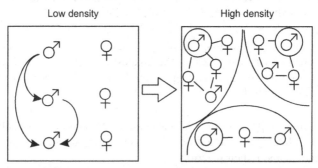

Figure 7.1 Social organization of guinea pigs at high and low population densities. Low density: arrows among males indicate direction of aggressive behaviors. High density: lines between males and females indicate individual social bonds. Alphas (circled males) dominate non-alphas (uncircled males). Broken lines: the borders of "territories." For reference and original data see Sachser (1986).

of one to four males and one to seven females. The highest-ranking male of each subunit, the alpha, establishes long-lasting social bonds with all of the females in his subunit. He guards and defends these females around estrus, and more than 85% of the offspring are sired by him. Lower-ranking males also have bonds with the females of their subunits. Alphas of different subunits respect each other's bondings, that is, they do not court the females of other alphas even if they are receptive. Remarkably, the attainment of an alpha status is not merely a result of high dominance position. Instead, building up a social bond toward an individual female leads to the alpha status. For instance, all juvenile males that form bondings toward individual females around puberty eventually attain an alpha's status as adults. In addition, females can change their allegiance from alphas to subdominant males that have established long-term bonds with them by directing sociopositive and courtship behavior toward them. Some time later, these males will be high-ranking alphas themselves. In general, individuals belonging to a given subunit live in non-overlapping areas. It is in these areas that most of the social interactions are displayed and where the individuals have their resting and sleeping places. The alphas defend the borders of these areas near the time of their females' estrus (Sachser 1986). In addition to bonds between males and females, homosexual bonds can be found. In a group of about 50 animals, 4 out of 29 males established bonds toward individual adult males, that is, they directed their affiliative, courtship, and sexual behavior nearly exclusively toward their male partners and did not show any sexual interest in females (Sachser 1994). If such a male was transferred to an unfamiliar colony he maintained his homosexual orientation by choosing again one single male to whom he displayed all his sociopositive and sexual behavior (Sachser and Renninger 1993). There are no indications, however, as to the conditions that might have led to the homosexual orientation of these males. In summary, the social organization at high individual numbers is characterized as follows: (a) the whole group splits into subunits, providing all individuals with social and spatial orientation; (b) escalated fighting is rare because alphas respect the male–female bonds of other alphas; and (c) the individuals' different social positions are stable over months. Thus, the change in social organization can be regarded as a mechanism for facilitating adjustment to increasing population density.

What causes this change? At low density, the highest-ranking male monopolizes all females. However, the costs, for example, in time and energy spent in agonistic encounters and in maintaining the exclusive access to all females within the whole area, increases with the population of competitors and females. It is economical to defend all females only as long as the net benefits (in terms of reproductive success) exceed net costs. When the relationship between benefits and costs becomes unprofitable, an alternative behavior yielding a higher reproductive success is preferable, that is, controlling a certain number of females within a certain area and respecting the same behavior pattern displayed by other males. Thus, the cause for change in social organization is considered to be the highest-ranking male's change in reproductive strategy for maximizing his fitness (Sachser 1986).

A comparison of guinea pigs living at different population numbers reveals that the activity of the hypothalamic–pituitary–adrenal (HPA) system — one of the organism's major stress axes — is not at all affected by population numbers; that is, a male living in a large colony does not show higher cortisol concentrations than a male living in a small group or with only one female. These endocrinological data support the behavioral findings: it appears that a change in density does not necessarily mean an increase in stress for the individuals as long as a stable social environment is maintained by species-typical mechanisms. Correspondingly, the reproductive success of females (i.e., the number of surviving offspring/time) does not decline at high population density.

At high and low population numbers males take different social positions, which remain stable over months. Alphas always clearly dominate non-alphas of the same subunit. These clear differences in status are reflected by higher hypothalamic catecholaminergic activities and a trend toward higher blood concentrations of testosterone in alphas as compared to non-alphas (Sachser 1990). However, both categories of males do not differ significantly in indices of HPA activities, that is, having low social status does not necessarily entail a higher degree of social stress than having high social status. Established social relationships resulting in predictable behavior are seen as a main reason for this finding (Sachser et al. 1998).

The question arises, which factors enable guinea pigs to arrange in a nonstressful and nonaggressive way even at high densities? The answer is: a great tolerance toward conspecifics as well as the ability to establish and respect dominance relationships and social bonds. Interestingly, the ability to establish dominance relationships with unfamiliar animals is not related to early social experiences; it is acquired in agonistic encounters with older dominant males around the time of puberty (Sachser et al. 1994). Likewise, some data suggest that the ability to respect adult social bonds may also be dependent on social rearing conditions around this time: For example, when two adult males that have grown up in different large mixed-sex colonies are placed into an unfamiliar enclosure in the presence of an unfamiliar female, they quickly establish dominance relationships without displaying overt aggression, and no significant changes in stress hormones are found in either the dominant or in the subdominant male. Remarkably, the males do not court the female earlier than several hours after the onset of the experiment. In contrast, when two males that had grown up either singly or as a pair with a single female are confronted in the same way, high levels of aggressive behavior are displayed, and both males begin to court the female immediately (Sachser et al. 1994).

Male–female bonding is very prominent in colonies of guinea pigs. There are three categories of females for an individual colony-living male: (a) "his" bonded females with whom most amicable interactions take place, (b) females

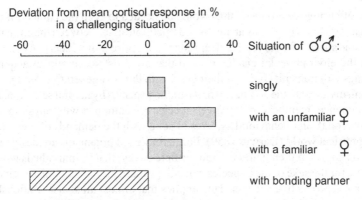

Figure 7.2   Social support from bonding partner. Male guinea pigs (N = 10) were tested in four situations. They were placed into an unfamiliar enclosure (i.e., challenging situation) singly, together with an unfamiliar female, together with a familiar female with whom no bonding existed, or together with the female bonding partner. Plasma cortisol concentrations increased significantly in all four situations (from this a mean cortisol response was calculated); however, significant variations were found between groups (p < 0.002): cortisol titers were lowest in 9 out of 10 males when they were tested together with their bonding partners. For reference and original data see Sachser et al. (1998).

which live in the same colony, and with whom he is familiar but has no social ties, and (c) unfamiliar females which live in a different colony, and which he has never before encountered. When placed in an unfamiliar cage, the male's endocrine stress response (i.e., increase in serum cortisol concentrations) is sharply reduced when the bonded female is present. In contrast, presence of a strange female, or one with whom he is merely acquainted, has little effect (Figure 7.2). Thus the effect of various types of relationships differs remarkably, and substantial social support is given only by the bonded partner (Sachser et al. 1998). Moreover, in female guinea pigs, presence of the male bonding partner leads to a sharp reduction in the acute stress response. Thus, social support can be provided by social partners in females as well. In contrast to males, however, the female's stress responses can be reduced not only by the bonding partner but also by a familiar conspecific, though in a less effective way (Kaiser et al. 2003).

What general conclusion can be drawn from these studies in wild and domestic guinea pig? When we look at the relevant literature in a comparative fashion, contributions to five different fields can be made, as discussed below.

ADULT SOCIAL BONDING: SOME GENERAL TRENDS IN NONHUMAN MAMMALS

Biological Evolution and Social Bonding

In the long-term, the number of individuals comprising a population of a given species typically is more or less the same. In every generation, though, many more offspring are produced than would be needed to keep the number of individuals constant. From this an intense competition arises between the animals of the same species for survival and reproduction. Those individuals that cope best with the environmental challenges and that are most successful in acquiring matings will transmit copies of their genes into the next generation. In this way, organisms adapt to the ecological niche of their species by natural selection. As a consequence, members of any given species are equipped with physiological, motivational, and behavioral systems to cope with the demands of their social and physical world (Darwin 1859). Furthermore, all organisms are designed to pass on copies of their genes in a most efficient way; that is, individuals will not behave for the sake of their species, but will primarily try to maximize their own lifetime reproductive success. This implies that almost all social relationships lead to conflicts of interests between individuals. Such conflicts are obvious when, for example, males compete for the access to females, but they also exist between the sexes as well as between parents and their offspring, though frequently in a less conspicuous way (Clutton-Brock 1989).

Whether or not adult social bonds are a characteristic trait of a given species is related to the environmental conditions under which the animals live, as can be seen very clearly from the comparison of different species of wild guinea pigs (see above). Generally speaking, social bonds will be formed only if the individuals involved profit from them. That is, whether or not the motivational and behavioral systems to establish social bonds were brought about by natural selection depends on whether or not these systems helped the individual to adapt to its environment and ultimately maximized its reproductive success. Thus, it is not surprising that social monogamy, for example, occurs usually in species where, for physiological or ecological reasons, male assistance is required for successful rearing of offspring, as is the case in marmosets and many canid species. Here, males presumably can achieve higher breeding success by guarding a single female and helping her rear their joint young than by attempting to breed with several females (Clutton-Brock 1989). (Note, however, that social monogamy occurs also in species in which male care for infants is not required or male care is absent. The assumption is that monogamy precedes male care in evolution.) It is, however, by no means always the male's decision as to whether a male–female bond is formed. In the wild cavy, the female's behavior allows adult social bonds to exist, whereas in the yellow-toothed cavy the female's behavior makes this form of social relationship impossible. Although the females of both species behave in a completely different way, they both maximize their reproductive success (see above). Correspondingly, a male wild guinea pig will only invest time and energy in the care of young if he is the father (see above). Thus, social bonds result from behavioral strategies of individuals that represent adaptations to their social and nonsocial world and ultimately aim to pass on copies of their genes in a most efficient way.

We should not expect that any given species possesses the ability to form adult social bonds (e.g., Mendoza and Mason 1986). Only if natural selection has brought about this ability will adult social bonding occur. Even if the motivational and behavioral systems to establish adult social bonds evolved, this trait will not necessarily be established under any environmental condition. Guinea pigs, for example, have the potential to form strong adult social bonds. This trait is manifested, however, only at high population numbers (Figure 7.1), probably because the highest-ranking males change their behavioral strategies in order to maximize their fitness under these conditions. In general, even for individuals of the same species, sex, and age, a sole fixed strategy cannot necessarily be defined as being the optimal way to behave: what is optimal in terms of maximizing reproductive success depends on the environmental conditions as well as on the behavioral strategies of the other individuals. Thus, variation in environmental conditions will frequently cause changes in the propensity to establish social bonds, and forming a social bond will not necessarily be superior to living in a solitary, nonbonded way.

Domestication and Social Bonding

During domestication, wild animals have to adapt over a period of many generations to their new conditions in captivity and human care, and this results in long-term genetic changes. Domestication, therefore, involves an evolutionary process based on the shift in selective pressures. As a consequence, distinct changes in morphology, physiology, and behavior will occur. On a behavioral level, domesticated animals are usually characterized by certain behavioral traits — reduced aggressiveness, increased social tolerance, and sexual behavior — when compared to their wild ancestors (see above). On a physiological level, a less intense hormonal response to stressors is usually found (Künzl and Sachser 1999). Concerning social bonds, it was argued that the requirement for this behavioral trait may be reduced in the process of domestication. Correspondingly, selective social bonds may be rare or absent in domestic species (Carter and Keverne 2002). However, the social life of domesticated guinea pigs clearly contradicts this view: adult social bonds exist in the wild ancestor as well as in the domesticated form (see above). Likewise, dogs were derived from wolves, a species with strong social bonds among group members. As in the wild ancestor, the domesticated animals still form long-term adult social bonds if a potential bonding partner is available — this can be a member of the same species or a human. In contrast, laboratory mice or cats do not form adult social bonds. This, however, does not seem to be caused by domestication, rather it reflects the absence of this behavioral trait in the wild ancestors of these species. Thus, in terms of adult social bonds, domestic animals apparently bear the heritage of their wild counterparts: when the wild species is characterized by adult social bonding, it is reasonable to expect this trait in the domesticated form as well.

Ontogeny and Social Bonding

Nearly fifty years ago, experiments with rhesus monkeys (Harlow and Harlow 1962) clearly demonstrated for the first time that experiences during ontogeny with the attachment figure significantly influence behavioral patterns in adulthood. Monkeys raised in isolation are fearful and depressed in new situations, while they are hyperaggressive in response to unfamiliar members of the same species and cannot form "normal" social relationships. These findings are not restricted to primates. All mammals probably require adequate socialization to be able to communicate and interact successfully with members of the same species. In many mammals, close contact with conspecifics, predominantly the mother, provides the young with a sense of security. Only if this secure base is available can they explore the environment and new objects in a nonanxious way (Bowlby 1972; Gandelmann 1992). It is generally believed that such early experiences in mother–offspring and/or sibling–sibling interactions are of primary importance for the development of behavioral strategies and good welfare in later life. Recent studies, in addition, point to the importance of social interactions around puberty. During this time, social relationships change dramatically. Conspecifics of the same sex frequently become rivals, and animals of the opposite sex become attractive as mating and bonding partners. Thus, it is not surprising that the time around puberty is also crucial for the acquisition of significant coping patterns needed during the animal's future life. Male guinea pigs, for example, raised in large mixed-sex colonies experience agonistic encounters with older dominant males around puberty, whereby they acquire the social skills needed to adapt to conspecifics in a nonaggressive and nonstressful way (Sachser et al. 1994). Similarly, it might be speculated that the ability to form and maintain adult social bonds also depends on social experiences at about this time. Some data, indeed, point in this direction: the "respect" that males show for the social bonds of other males does not seem to develop without certain social experiences around puberty (see above). To date, no extant experimental animal studies relate social experiences during both the early postnatal period and puberty to the ability to establish and maintain adult social bonds. Moreover no systematic data exist to assess the relative weight of influences in these different phases of life. A promising hypothesis might be that the requirements to establish social bonds in adulthood are (a) the experience of security during early life and (b) the learning of significant behavioral patterns near puberty.

Consequence of Social Bonds for the Individual: Social Support

Stress responses can be ameliorated by the presence of members of the same species (Henry and Stephens 1977). This phenomenon is called "social support." Frequently such social support cannot be provided by any conspecific (Mendoza et al. 1991), but rather the ability to give social support is restricted to bonding partners (Figure 7.2) (Sachser et al. 1998). In many mammalian species, mothers are important bonding partners for their infants. As a general rule, mothers provide social support to their offspring in a very effective way (Mendoza et al. 1991; Hennessy 1999).

Most experimental data in animals show that social support is related to well-being for individuals under stress and can weaken the influence of a stressor. In such cases, social support is a kind of buffer for the state of health (Figure 7.2). In addition, some data exist that bonding partners may also confer beneficial effects regardless of whether individuals are under stress or not. In these cases, social support can act directly on the physical condition of an individual, so that health is improved. An impressive example is described for tree shrews (von Holst 1998). These animals usually live in pairs in the wild. Putting a male and a female together, however, does not inevitably lead to the formation of a pair bond. In not more than 20% of all pairings is contact between an unfamiliar male and female characterized from the onset by amicable behavior, conveying the strong impression of "love at first sight." In these harmonious pairs, a lasting decrease in heart rate of up to 20% and an improvement of the immunological state of both partners are found (von Holst 1998). Whatever the mechanism by which a bonding partner acts on the organism, it will promote well-being and health in a significant way.

The positive effects of a bonding partner on the organism's physiological state are reflected by the reduced activity of the pituitary–adrenocortical and the sympathetic–adrenomedullary axes. Changes in the activation of the first system may indicate changes in an individual's degree of security, whereas changes in the activity of the latter system may reflect changes in the degree of arousal. On a psychological level the bonding partner, therefore, functions as a "security-giving and arousal-reducing structure" (Sachser et al. 1998). This is true irrespective of whether the bonding partner is the mother, in the case of an infant, or a male or a female, in the case of an adult individual.

Consequence of Social Bonding for the Group: A Stable Social Network

Group-living mammals frequently build up complex social networks which involve dominance hierarchies and/or different types of affiliative social relationships. If dominance relationships are settled, and if affiliative social relationships exist in the form of long-lasting social bonds, this network will be characterized by a high degree of social stability. In such stable systems, established social relationships result in predictable behavior and, thereby, provide all members of the system with social orientation and high security. As a consequence, changes in population parameters (e.g., a rise in population numbers and stratification in different social positions) do not seem to affect aversely the animals' welfare and health. In addition, differences in social status do not lead to differences in endocrine stress responses so that both high- and low-ranking individuals can live in a nonstressful way. This has not only been shown for guinea pigs (see above) but for many mammalian species (Henry and Stephens 1977; Sachser et al. 1998; von Holst 1998).

The relevance of a successful integration into a stable social network is especially evident from work on wild rabbits. In parts of southern Germany, only an average of 5% of the young survive the winter. Young animals leave their natal groups in autumn and attempt to join other groups. In this process, all immigrants are initially attacked and chased away. However, some juveniles are tolerated after a while and integrated into the group: friendly interactions with adults occur and social bonds are formed. As a result of successful integration, these animals show an improved immune state and a reduced parasitic infestation, and only these juveniles actually survive the winter (von Holst 1998).

If instability exists in the whole social system, high degrees of stress will be found in all individuals. At extreme population densities, for example, dramatic increases in aggressive behavior, a disruption of social bonds, and a breakdown of the social organization regularly occur. As a general rule, individuals living in such unstable conditions show distinct increases in pituitary–adrenocortical and sympathetic–adrenomedullary activities and, thereby, are subjected to a higher disease susceptibility and mortality than conspecifics living in stable ones (Henry and Stephens 1977; von Holst 1998). In the laboratory, instability can easily be evoked by periodically changing group memberships. Hereby agonistic encounters are intensified and affiliative interactions between individuals are disrupted. When, for example, the group composition of Cynomolgus monkeys is changed experimentally, a consistent increase in aggressive behavior occurs and the development of permanent social bonds is hindered. This situation is particularly stressful for the dominant animals, which must always be active in order to establish new social bonds and to maintain their high social rank. If a high-cholesterol diet is fed in such an unstable social system, the frequency of arteriosclerosis increases in the high-ranking animals. In a stable social system in which the group composition is not changed, however, all animals remain healthy, even when they are fed the same cholesterol-containing food (Kaplan et al. 1982).

To summarize, social bonds contribute in a fundamental way to establish stable social networks. If individuals are socially integrated therein, good welfare and health will be achieved. Under conditions of social disintegration and social instability, however, significant increases in disease susceptibility mediated by hormonal and immunological responses exist.

CONCLUSION

Our everyday experiences confirm that the ability to form social bonds between adult individuals exists in contemporary humans. In theory, the motivational and behavioral systems to establish such bonds might have developed only recently, particularly, because male–female bonding does not seem to be a basic trait of all recent hominoids (e.g., orangutan). Studies on domestication in non-human mammals, however, suggest that adult social bonds exist in the domesti-cated form only if they were present in the feral ancestor. Modern humans can no longer be considered a feral species and hominization resembles, in many ways, a domestication-like process. Thus, it seems reasonable to assume that in our species, adult social bonds represent an ancient trait that existed in our "feral ancestors" and was brought about by natural selection.

If so, adult social bonding emerged in our ancestors due to behavioral strate-gies that helped the individual to adapt to his or her environment, and ultimately maximized his or her reproductive success. If, in addition, we still bear the an-cient motivational systems underlying the formation of adult social bonds — a key assumption of evolutionary psychology (Laland and Brown 2002) — the following predictions can be made in the same way as for nonhuman mammals: (a) adult social bonds will not necessarily be established under all environmen-tal conditions; (b) changes in the social and physical environment may cause changes in adult social bonding patterns; (c) living in a social organization char-acterized by social bonds may not necessarily be superior to living in a solitary, nonbonded way. It would be interesting to elucidate which modern-life environ-mental conditions may favor adult social bonding and which might promote an alternative way to live.

Nonhuman mammals require adequate socialization to be able to communi-cate and interact successfully with members of the same species. The same ap-plies to humans, but to a much greater extent. The formation and maintenance of normal adult social bonds require particular experiences during behavioral de-velopment. Given that basic processes are similar in human and nonhuman mammals, it might be hypothesized for humans as well that normal adult social bonds require both: (a) the experience of security during an early phase and (b) the learning of specific behavioral patterns around puberty.

The physiological consequences of adult social bonding for the individual as well as for the society in which the individual lives seem to be comparable for human and nonhuman mammals in many important aspects (as was already pointed out by Henry and Stephens more than 25 years ago): the presence of the bonding partner gives social security and ameliorates the organism's physiolog-ical stress responses. Thus, the bonding partner promotes well-being and health, at least when a harmonious relationship exists, although there is some evidence in humans for gender-related differences in providing social support (Kirschbaum et al. 1995). Likewise in human and nonhuman mammals, adult social bonds contribute to the generation of stable social networks. If individu-als are socially integrated, and if social stability exists, good welfare and health will be achieved. Under conditions of social disintegration and social instability, however, significant increases in disease susceptibility mediated by hormonal and immunological responses are found (Henry and Stephens 1977). Though these insights are of paramount importance concerning well-being and health in human and nonhuman animals, they have not yet been appreciated in the way they deserve.

ACKNOWLEDGMENTS

I thank Michael B. Hennessy, Dietrich von Holst, Gustl Anzenberger, and the participants of the Dahlem Workshop for valuable comments on the manuscript.

REFERENCES

Adrian, O., I. Brockmann, C. Hohoff, and N. Sachser. 2005. Paternal behaviour in wild guinea pigs: A comparative study in three closely related species with different social and mating systems. *J. Zool.*, in press.
Asher, M., E. Spinelli de Oliveira, and N. Sachser. 2004. Social system and spatial organization of wild guinea pigs (*Cavia aperea*) in a natural low density population. *J. Mammalogy* **85**:788-796.
Bowlby, J. 1972. Attachment. Attachment and Loss, vol. 1. Middlesex: Penguin.
Carter, C.S., and E.B. Keverne. 2002. The neurobiology of social affiliation and pair bonding. In: Hormones, Brain, and Behavior, ed. D.W. Pfaff, A.P. Arnold, A.M. Etgen, S.E. Fahrbach, and R.T. Rubin, vol. 1, pp. 299–335. San Diego: Academic.
Clutton-Brock, T.H. 1989. Mammalian mating systems. *Proc. Roy. Soc. Lond. B* **236**:339–372.
Darwin, C. 1859. The Origin of Species. London: Murray.
Dewsbury, D. 1992. On the problems studied in ethology, comparative psychology, and animal behaviour. *Ethology* **92**:89–107.
Gandelmann, R. 1992. Psychobiology of Behavioral Development. New York: Oxford Univ. Press.
Harlow, H.F., and M.K. Harlow. 1962. Social deprivation in monkeys. *Sci. Am.* **207**:136–146.
Hennessy, M.B. 1999. Social influences on endocrine activity in guinea pigs, with comparisons to findings in nonhuman primates. *Neurosci. Biobehav. Rev.* **23**:687–698.
Henry, J.P., and P.M. Stephens. 1977. Stress, Health, and the Social Environment: A Sociobiologic Approach to Medicine. New York: Springer.
Hohoff, C. 2002. Female Choice in Three Species of Wild Guinea Pigs. Ph.D. thesis, Univ. of Münster, Germany.
Hohoff, C., K. Franzen, and N. Sachser. 2003. Female choice in a promiscuous wild guinea pig, the yellow toothed cavy (*Galea musteloides*). *Behav. Ecol. Sociobiol.* **53**:341–349.
Hohoff, C., K. Solmsdorff, P. Löttker et al. 2002. Monogamy in a new species of wild guinea pigs (*Galea sp.*) *Naturwiss.* **89**:462–465.
Kaiser, S., M. Kirtzeck, G. Hornschuh, and N. Sachser. 2003. Sex-specific difference in social support: A study in female guinea pigs. *Physiol. Behav.* **79**:297–303.
Kaplan, J.R., S.B. Manuck, T.B. Clarkson, F.M. Lusso, and D.M. Taub. 1982. Social status, environment, and atherosclerosis in cynomolgus monkeys. *Arteriosclerosis* **2**:359–368.
Kirschbaum, C., T. Klauer, S.H. Filipp, and D.H. Hellhammer. 1995. Sex-specific effects of social support on cortisol and subjective response to acute psychological stress. *Psychosom. Med.* **57**:23–31.

Kraus, C., J. Künkele, and F. Trillmich. 2003. Spacing behaviour and its implications for the mating system of a precocial small mammal: An almost asocial cavy *Cavia magna? Anim. Behav.* **66**:225–238.

Künzl, C., and N. Sachser. 1999. The behavioral endocrinology of domestication: A comparison between the domestic guinea pig (*Cavia aperea f. porcellus*) and its wild ancestor, the cavy (*Cavia aperea*). *Horm. Behav.* **35**:28–37.

Laland, K.N., and G.R. Brown. 2002. Sense and Nonsense: Evolutionary Perspectives on Human Behaviour. Oxford: Oxford Univ. Press.

Mendoza, S.P., D.M. Lyons, and W. Saltzman. 1991. Sociophysiology of squirrel monkeys. *Am. J. Primatol.* **23**:37–54.

Mendoza, S.P., and W.A. Mason. 1986. Contrasting responses to intruders and to involuntary separation by monogamous and polygynous new world monkeys. *Physiol. Behav.* **38**:795–801.

Sachser, N. 1986. Different forms of social organization at high and low population densities in guinea pigs. *Behaviour* **97**:253–272.

Sachser, N. 1990. Social organization, social status, behavioural strategies and endocrine responses in male guinea pigs. In: Hormones, Brain and Behaviour in Vertebrates. 2. Behavioural Activation in Males and Females: Social Interaction and Reproductive Endocrinology, Comp. Physiol., ed. J. Balthazart, vol. 9, pp. 176–187. Basel: Karger.

Sachser, N. 1994. Sozialphysiologische Untersuchungen an Hausmeerschweinchen. Hamburg: Parey.

Sachser, N., D. Hierzel, and M. Dürschlag. 1998. Social relationships and the management of stress. *Psychoneuroendocrin.* **23**:891–904.

Sachser, N., C. Lick, and K. Stanzel. 1994. The environment, hormones and aggressive behaviour: A five-year-study in guinea pigs. *Psychoneuroendocrin.* **19**:697–707.

Sachser, N., and S.V. Renninger. 1993. Coping with new social situations: The role of social rearing in guinea pigs. *Ethol. Ecol. Evol.* **5**:65–74.

Sachser, N., E. Schwarz-Weig, A. Keil, and J.T. Epplen. 1999. Behavioural strategies, testis size, and reproductive success in two caviomorph rodents with different mating systems. *Behaviour* **136**:1203–1217.

von Holst, D. 1998. The concept of stress and its relevance for animal behavior. *Adv. Stud. Behav.* **27**:1–131.

Wickler, W. 1976. The ethological analysis of attachment. *Z. Tierpsychologie* **42**:12–28.

8

Plasticity of Innate Behavior

Experiences throughout Life Affect Maternal Behavior and Its Neurobiology

A. S. FLEMING

Department of Psychology, University of Toronto, Mississauga, Ontario L5L1C6, Canada

ABSTRACT

In many litter-bearing mammalian species, mothers express responsiveness and nurturance to entire litters and do not become attached to single offspring. In others that give birth to singletons or twins, mothers become selectively attached to individuals. In both situations, postpartum experiences occur and are encoded by brain mechanisms, producing long-term changes in behavior. Although different brain mechanisms may mediate these experience effects, there are also some striking similarities, and the impact of these experiences can be seen in rats, sheep, and humans, alike.

Although species-characteristic and often quite stereotyped in form, maternal behavior and its neurobiology do not emerge *de novo* at the time of parturition; it also has developmental and experiential precursors. One of these precursors is the experience that animals have had with their own mothers and in their home of origin. These early experiences have an impact during the pre-weaning period, as well as later on, and affect the psychobiological mechanisms which later mediate maternal behavior. Included among these are effects on behavior (attention, fear, prosocial behavior, learning), endocrine function (the hypothalamic–pituitary–adrenal [HPA] axis, estrogen receptor systems), the brain (olfactory bulbs, medial preoptic area, limbic system), and neurochemistry (catecholamines, oxytocin).

It is quite likely that plasticity and experience are important in nonhuman mammals as in humans; however, until we understand more about the neurobiology of maternal behavior in humans and how experience affects this neurobiology, comparisons are analogous at best. Given the known cross-species similarities in underlying endocrine and brain mechanisms, animal models may provide a useful roadmap for the analysis of human maternal behavior.

INTRODUCTION

In most mammals, the expression of maternal behavior is both highly stereotyped in form and predictable in its timing. Although there are many aspects of maternal behavior that are species specific, there are commonalities that cross almost all mammalian species; however, among primates, and especially humans, there may be more variability in the form of behavior exhibited (see Hrdy, this volume). Among these are: some form of nest-building or "home" preparation in advance of the birth, signaling behaviors that function to bring the young in proximity to the mother, some form of hygienic grooming or licking of the young, a particular posture or behavior that facilitates nursing of the young, a means of retrieving and transporting offspring, and a means of locating and identifying offspring.

Mammalian maternal behaviors appear at or shortly after giving birth. This is a time of heightened maternal responsiveness, when the mother first has the opportunity to form a bond with her litter or with an individual infant and, through learning, may then show individual recognition and bonding. Maternal behaviors are expressed in response to hormonal changes associated with gestation and parturition. In most species, the steroids estrogen, and/or progesterone are involved as well as a variety of pituitary (prolactin) and brain (neuro) hormones (oxytocin, vasopressin, opioids) (Carter, this volume; Keverne, this volume). In some species, and under certain conditions, maternal behavior can be expressed toward infants in the absence of hormones (as in inexperienced virgin mice, multiparous, nonpartum rats, in some nonhuman primates, and humans). In fact, in some primates and in humans, allomothering is often essential to the health and survival of offspring (Hrdy, this volume; Ahnert, this volume). Under most common conditions and circumstances, however, the precise timing of the expression of maternal behavior depends on the coordinated change in hormones that occurs at the time of parturition (Rosenblatt 2002; Numan and Insel 2003).

The site of action of hormones that induce maternal behavior has been studied in rodents and a few other species. The primary site includes a circuit or system of olfactory–limbic–hypothalamic and midbrain structures. The medial preoptic area (MPOA) of the hypothalamus is the hub, or essential nuclear group, where many of the "maternal" hormone receptors reside and where the hormones act. In the rat, for example, the MPOA must be activated for maternal behavior to be expressed. The fact that the MPOA is critical for the expression of maternal behavior in many animal species suggests that this is part of a phylogenetically old and highly selected system (Numan and Insel 2003; Fleming and Li 2002; Gonzalez-Mariscal and Poindron 2002). Confirmation of the universality of this "maternal circuit" awaits important studies in humans and other primates, using fMRI and PET to image the brains of parents and allomothers while caring for infants (Lorberbaum et al. 2002; Leckman et al., this volume).

At one level of analysis it may appear that maternal behavior is usually expressed under tight biological constraints. However, in every species that has been studied, large individual differences in a mother's motivation to be maternal have been observed. This is expressed in the intensity or quality of behavior exhibited and, in some cases, even in whether or not maternal behavior is expressed at all in first-time mothers. That maternal behavior varies in relation to environmental and experiential factors, or can even fail, indicates that there is considerably more plasticity in the mechanisms regulating the timing, form, and intensity of the behavior than is generally recognized.

In this chapter I discuss the contributions of environment and experience to the variability in expression of adult maternal behavior as it occurs during the pre-weaning period. I focus both on factors that affect the "motivation" to be nurturant or "maternal responsiveness" as well as on learning that is involved in the development of a selective bond to an individual offspring or the litter. In this context, the use of the term *attachment* will only be used when discussing the infants' responses to their caregivers, and the term *bond* will be restricted to the mothers' selective responsiveness to her offspring. My primary focus will be on one altricial species: the rat. Beyond this, comparative analyses of experience effects in other species, particularly in humans, will be provided. A comparative approach helps us to understand the foundations of human maternal behavior. I begin by describing the phenomenology of maternal responsiveness and selective bonding and underlying sensory, endocrine, and brain mechanisms that mediate their plasticity in rat, sheep, and human mothers. Reviews that relate to much of the research described herein include Numan and Insel (2003), Rosenblatt (2002), Fleming and Li (2002), Levy et al. (1996), Gonzalez-Mariscal and Poindron (2002), and Corter and Fleming (2002). Many relevant chapters may also be found in Bornstein (2002).

Thereafter, we consider the effects of early experiences of being mothered (or not), in a particular context or environment, on the form and quality of maternal behavior that emerges in adulthood and on the adult endocrine, neurochemical, and neural mechanisms that mediate adult maternal behavior and its plasticity. I attempt to address, mechanistically, the "transmission gap" between early experiences with mother and siblings and possible attachments formed at that time and later responses to own offspring. Review papers that describe many of the developmental studies include Hofer and Sullivan (2001), Fleming and Li (2002), Fleming et al. (1999), and Fleming et al. (2002).

EFFECTS OF POSTPARTUM EXPERIENCE WITH YOUNG ON THE EXPRESSION AND MAINTENANCE OF MATERNAL BEHAVIOR

Animals

Maternal learning improves the survival rate of offspring, and hence the fitness of the mother. Comparisons of primiparous and multiparous rat and mice mothers indicate that multiparous mothers are better able to respond sensitively to infant cues and rear offspring that will achieve reproductive maturity (Noirot 1972; Fleming and Li 2002). Experience thus alters the form of expression of a set of behaviors that seem to be under considerable species-specific constraint.

How experience can alter a hormonally primed and stereotyped set of behaviors has received some attention, but there is still much to learn. In addition, virtually nothing is known about the individual differences in susceptibility to the effects of experience and the interactive effects of these experiences with the genotype. That is, we know very little about the epigenesis of maternal behavior.

The demonstrable (measurable) value of parity differences emerges and is probably most significant when the mother is challenged by environmental adversity. Multiparous, as opposed to primiparous, rat mothers are more likely to continue caring for young under conditions of crowding, food deprivation, nest disruption, after caesarian section, lesions, and so forth (Fleming and Li 2002). In some species, like sheep, we see that the priming of maternal responsiveness with gestational hormones and vaginocervical stimulation, which is so effective in nonpartum multiparous animals, cannot be produced in nulliparous animals (Poindron and Le Neindre 1980). Something about the earlier experience (parity) has altered the nervous system so that subsequent stimuli have an effect that they would not have otherwise. Giving birth, however, is not the only issue surrounding maternal learning. In combination with parity effects (the simple case of having given birth or not), there are exposure effects. Prior experiences caring for infants (allomothering as juveniles or as adults) enhance subsequent responsiveness in rats, social nonhuman primates, and humans (Fleming and Li 2002; Corter and Fleming 2002; Hrdy, this volume; Ahnert, this volume). In rats, maternal responding toward younger siblings or foster pups ("babysitting") among juveniles is common and can enhance responsiveness to foster pups in the virgin adult (Fleming and Li 2002). Interestingly, these juvenile effects are less clear, and sometimes opposite, in rats that experienced separation from their own mothers earlier (Rees and Fleming 2001), indicating that experiences acquired early in life can affect susceptibility to later experiences.

Humans

In humans, prior maternal experience is the single most substantial predictor of positive responsiveness to offspring. For instance, in comparison to primiparous human mothers, multiparous mothers with previous maternal experience are more attracted to the body odors of newborn infants. They respond more sympathetically to pain than to hunger cries (primiparous mothers are equally responsive to the two cry types) and have more positive attitudes to infants in general (Corter and Fleming 2002). In addition, primiparous mothers with more prior infant exposure (e.g., as babysitters or with siblings) feel more adequate as mothers. They also like children more, engage in more *en face* behavior, and maintain more proximal contact when holding their firstborn infants (Corter and Fleming 2002). This beneficial effect of caregiving experience in humans may help to explain why in many cultures, allomothering among nonrelated individuals is common and where inclusive fitness of the allomother would not be enhanced (Hrdy, this volume).

NATURE OF THE EXPERIENCE

What aspects of earlier experiences with offspring contribute to the later "enhanced" responsiveness? With a previous parity, animals experience not only an earlier interactive experience with the young, and all that that entails, but also a set of endocrine experiences associated with a previous pregnancy and parturition. Bridges, Fleming, and colleagues have explored the mechanisms that underlie the enhancement of maternal behavior shown by an animal that obtains an experience interacting with pups (Bridges 1977; Cohen and Bridges 1981; Orpen and Fleming 1987; Orpen et al. 1987). Studies show that once the parturitional hormones have exerted their effects and maternal behavior has been displayed, a particular set of psychological and brain mechanisms are activated. These mechanisms maintain responsiveness throughout the lactational period and enhance the responsiveness in mothers who have had a previous parity and experience with offspring (Fleming et al. 1996) (see Figure 8.1).

To identify the psychobiological mechanisms underlying the maternal experience effect, a paradigm was developed in which new primiparous mother rats are (a) initially restricted from contact with their offspring at parturition (dam is caesarian sectioned or pups are removed as they emerge from the birth canal); (b) the mother is then provided with varying amounts and kinds of contact with neonatal pups; (c) the mother is thereafter separated from pups for varying periods; (d) the mother is finally tested with foster pups to assess the retention of her maternal responsiveness. Using this paradigm, Bridges and colleagues (Bridges 1977; Cohen and Bridges 1981) and Orpen and Fleming (1987; Orpen et al. 1987) demonstrated that if new mothers interact with their young for a brief postpartum period (e.g., 1/2 to 24 hrs during the first 24 hrs postpartum), they exhibit a reduced latency to retrieve and crouch over foster pups, in the absence of the "maternal" hormones, for up to three weeks or more.

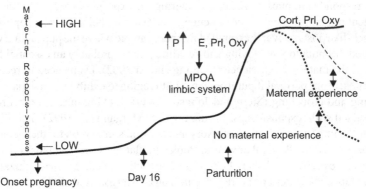

Figure 8.1 Schematic of changes in maternal responsiveness across pregnancy and postpartum in the rat. After parturition, maternal responsiveness is sustained during lactation and beyond through interactive experiences with the litter. P: progesterone; E: estrogen; Prl: prolactin; Oxy: oxytocin; CORT: corticosterone.

We know that this "memory" is not hormonally mediated since animals begin to show normal estrous cycles during the separation period. Reduced latency in days to retrieve and crouch over foster pups is evidence of maternal memory related to maternal experience. It is a "memory" phenomenon, but it occurs within the context of a hormonally mediated "innate" behavior, which also shares many characteristics with other forms of both social and nonsocial learning studied in the laboratory (Fleming and Li 2002). This maternal experience effect has now been demonstrated in other species: in the rabbit by Gonzalez-Mariscal and Poindron (2002); in sheep by Levy et al. (1991) and Keller et al. (2003).

STIMULUS-DEPENDENT BASES OF EXPERIENCE

Animals

Although it is clear that interactive experience is important for the long-term retention of behavior, which aspect of the experience is important is not known. As will become apparent, for an experience to be acquired, a mother rat has to exhibit crouching behavior and, while doing so, receive somatosensory and chemosensory input. If the mother is prevented from crouching over her young postpartum, but receives other distal inputs, her responsiveness declines more rapidly with earlier weaning (Morgan et al. 1992; Fleming and Li 2002). Thus, the subsequent exhibition of "learning" involves not just exposure to the events, but also responses to them (this is not a latent memory phenomenon).

Orpen and Fleming (1987) found that if mothers were separated from their litters by a perforated clear plastic floor during the one-hour postpartum exposure phase, such that they could see, hear, and distally smell pups but receive no tactile or proximal chemosensory input, they showed no long-term benefit of maternal experience, as measured by tests performed ten days later. Instead, they responded to pups as virgins do. During the exposure phase, there was an evident attempt by the mother to engage in maternal behavior by adopting a crouch-like posture over the rounded floor area above where the pup huddle was located. Stimulation by moving and suckling pups is probably an essential feature of the maternal experience (Fleming and Li 2002). Dams need to receive somatosensory perioral input from the mouth region to exhibit normal maternal licking and crouching (Stern and Johnson 1989). Licking during exposure is correlated with responsiveness during the test (Morgan et al. 1992). This highlights the importance of chemosensory and perioral stimulation for the maternal experience effect. Perioral or ventral trunk stimulation is sufficient to produce a maternal experience. When both inputs are eliminated, by desensitization procedures, the experience effect is eliminated (Morgan et al. 1992).

Olfaction is not necessary for the formation of a maternal experience (Fleming and Li 2002). Nevertheless, during interactions with pups, dams will learn about specific olfactory and chemosensory features of the pups, as also occurs during the formation of bonds in other rodent species (Keverne, this volume). In rats, if pups are scented with an artificial odorant during the exposure phase, on test ten days later, mother rats respond more rapidly to pups labeled with the same scent than to those labeled with a discrepant scent. That this effect depends on the association of the odors with the pups is shown by an additional observation. Pre-exposure to the odor on its own (in the absence of pups) does not result in the same facilitation of responsiveness to similarly scented pups (Fleming et al. 2002). In some contexts involving social learning, it appears that artificial odorants work much like biological odorants, whereas in others it does not (Pedersen et al., this volume). What happens to an animal when it is re-exposed to a familiar (learned) pup stimulus is unclear, although animals are not avoidant when presented with pups and may well be actively attracted to them. We know that this combination of affective change normally occurs at parturition (Fleming and Li 2002).

Although maternal experience and parity effects occur in other animals, more salient for some species is the learning about individual offspring, rather than about entire litters, or about how to interact with young. In precocial sheep, lambs must be recognized by the mother within hours of birth if she is not to lose them in the herd. Sheep have very specialized mechanisms that enable the ewe to discriminate the olfactory and vocal characteristics of her own lamb. Poindron, Levy, Kendrick, and others have determined in large measure how ewes know their lambs (Levy, Kendrick et al. 1995; Gonzalez-Mariscal and Poindron 2002): by the ewe's willingness to let their own, but not alien, lambs suckle at their udder. Own and alien lambs were presented consecutively at different postpartum periods ranging from birth to four hours postpartum (Keller et al. 2003). A high proportion (33/51) of ewes showed selectivity at nursing as early as 30 minutes after parturition. After two hours of contact, the majority of ewes (42/50) were selective. With four hours of exposure to lambs, most ewes show selectivity at 36 hours but not at 72 hours later; with seven days of contact, selectivity was retained up to 72 hours, but no longer. These data suggest that recognition for nursing is a very rapid learning process that takes place at parturition (Levy et al. 1992; Keller et al. 2003). Interestingly, unlike the long-term retention of responsiveness found with maternal experience in the rat, the olfactory recognition of individual offspring in sheep is quite short lived (no longer than three days regardless of the duration of the initial experience) and certainly does not persist into the next parturition.

Numerous observational and experimental studies indicate that the sense of smell plays a primary role in ewes' selective acceptance of lambs for nursing. When ewes are rendered "anosmic" by experimental manipulation of the olfactory system, they subsequently show no selective preference for their own young, but will nurse alien young as well as their own. In related experiments, manipulation of access to a lamb's smell (placing a lamb at a distance out of olfactory range vs. in close proximity but within an opaque enclosure), rather than of the mother's sensory modality, produced similar effects (see Gonza-lez-Mariscal and Poindron 2002). Although ewes depend primarily on olfactory cues to recognize their lambs at suckling, they are also able to recognize their neonate from a distance > 1 m without olfactory cues, using auditory and visual cues (Ferreira et al. 2000; Keller et al. 2003; Terrazas et al. 1999). The nonolfactory recognition that develops later on is already effective as early as eight hours postpartum (Ferreira et al. 2000; Keller et al. 2003), but clearly not as early as is olfactory recognition. Interestingly, there is some evidence that anosmic ewes which showed no initial suckling selectivity can come to recognize their lambs at suckling at one month postpartum, which suggest that ewes can compensate for their loss of olfaction by using the auditory/visual cues from their lambs (Ferreira et al. 2000).

Humans

Some human mothers, like sheep mothers, are also able to recognize their own infants using olfactory, touch, and auditory cues (Corter and Fleming 2002). This identification is probably not critical during the early postpartum period, when mother and altricial young remain in close contact with one another. Nevertheless, the ability to discriminate exists very early on and, although not necessary for infant survival, may be part of a more general kin recognition system. Porter et al. (1983) and Schaal et al. (1980) demonstrated that within a couple of days of birth, mothers can discriminate their own infants' soiled T-shirts from the T-shirts of same-age infants. That recognition learning of own infants' odors is based on experience is indicated by the additional observations that mothers who were better at recognizing their own infants' odors had earlier and longer contact with their infants after birth and had spent more time in close proximal contact with their infants during interactions (Fleming et al. 1993). The effective identifiable odors are probably derived from the sweat and sebaceous glands on the baby's body and back. Alternatively, and not tested in this context, mothers may more easily come to recognize their own infants based on similarities between their own odors and the odors of their infants; odor cues are influenced by major histocompatibility (MHC) molecules (see Singh 2001); there are now numerous studies showing that the MHC genotype is associated with the production of distinctive odors used in individual discriminations and may be involved in phenotype matching (Hepper and Cleland 1999). Human mothers are not likely to "lose" their infants, as are ewes. Their recognition likely functions to enhance the mothers' feelings of nurturance and attachment and, hence, her responsiveness to the infant (Corter and Fleming 2002).

Recognition of a mother's own infant's cries versus other infants' cries has also been a focus in studies of human mothers. Valanne et al. (1967) and Formby (1967) showed that mothers could identify crying samples belonging to their own infants; Wisenfeld and Malatesta (1982) showed that patterns of maternal heart rate change differed in response to audiotapes of their own versus another's baby, even though these tapes were presented without identification to the mothers. In the latter study, heart rate acceleration, interpreted as arousal preparatory to active coping, followed cries of other infants. Formby (1967) also reported findings consistent with preparatory arousal to the mother's own infant's cries. The ecologic relevance of these studies is suggested by the observations that among mothers who roomed together in the hospital with their infants and with several other infant–mother pairs, 58% reported awakening to their infants cries on the first few nights, whereas thereafter the percentage rose to 96%.

ENDOCRINE BASES AND EFFECTS OF EXPERIENCE ON BIOLOGICAL MECHANISMS

Recent work on the neuroendocrinology of parity and maternal experience indicates that the endocrine systems and the brain are clearly changed by a previous parity and experience and in ways that probably enhance subsequent maternal responsiveness.

Animals

Studies in rodents and sheep suggest that a previous parity and experience alters the underlying endocrine, neuroendocrine, and neural mechanisms to render them more responsive to physiological factors with subsequent exposure to offspring. In both rats and humans there is evidence for parity effects on circulating hormones. In rats, Bridges and Hammer (1992) have found lower circulating prolactin in multiparous- as opposed to primiparous-lactating dams. The fact that multiparous animals have more milk than primiparous animals suggests that with a previous lactation the mammary gland galactophores become considerably more responsive to the stimulating effects of prolactin (Mann and Bridges 2002). In humans, first births are associated with higher levels of baseline cortisol than observed following subsequent births, an effect that has been associated with elevated postpartum anxiety in first-time mothers, and which may also affect lactational performance (Corter and Fleming 2002). Thus with parity, the molecular signaling of the body changes and the brain changes as well.

Parity effects on brain and circulating hormones are also seen for hormone receptors. For instance, the number of estrogen receptors in olfactory cortices is higher in multiparous than primiparous nonpartum mice (Ehret and Buckenmaier 1994; Koch 1990) and postpartum sheep (Poindron et al. 2003). This may explain why, in comparison to primiparous nonpartum animals, multiparous rats and sheep are more maternally responsive to exogenous steroids (Byrnes et al. 2001; Bridges, pers. comm.; Gonzalez-Mariscal and Poindron 2002). In sheep, on the other hand, parity enhances oxytocin receptor mRNA in the paraventricular nucleus (Broad et al. 1999) which has been implicated at the time of parturition in the rapid onset of maternal behavior and in maternal memory (Keverne and Kendrick 1992). Finally, in partum sheep, the brain release of a variety of neurotransmitters and neuropeptides involved in maternal recognition learning is higher in multiparous than in primiparous animals (Keverne et al. 1993; Levy et al. 1993; Levy, Locatelli et al. 1995).

In the rat, the maternal experience effect is not due to hormones of parturition but it is most certainly affected by them. Parturitional hormones influence the robustness of maternal learning. Animals which acquire maternal experience under the influence of parturitional hormones (whether postpartum animals or virgins given hormone replacement with progesterone and estrogen) exhibit better retention of maternal behavior thirty days later than do animals who have not been stimulated with hormones at the time of the maternal experience (virgins or nonparous but experienced animals). Moreover, the optimal condition for the expression of maternal behavior occurs when both the initial experience and the test occur during a period of hormonal priming (Fleming and Li 2002), a type of state dependency if you will.

In addition to the ovarian hormones, adrenal hormones are also implicated both in the formation of maternal experience and in the extent of licking that mother rats give to their offspring. However, effects of HPA axis are bimodal, depending on the "reason" for their elevation and the context in which HPA system is being activated. Removal of the adrenals during late pregnancy reduces the retention of maternal behavior ten days after a maternal experience, whereas glucocorticoid replacement at the time of the experience reverses these effects, and animals respond more rapidly and more intensively to pups (Graham et al., in prep.). As indicated below, where postpartum corticosterone is elevated as a result of disrupted early parenting, high levels of corticosterone are related to less, rather than more, maternal licking and grooming (Rees et al., in prep.).

Humans

In light of these HPA axis results, it is of interest to note that in human mothers, those who have higher levels of salivary cortisol on Days 2 and 3 postpartum engage in more close contact affectionate interactions with their infants, are more attracted to infant body odors (Corter and Fleming 2002), are more sympathetic to infant hunger cries and make greater distinctions between pain and hunger cries (Stallings et al. 2001), and are better able to recognize the body odor of their own, versus another, infant (Fleming et al. 1997). Many of these facilitatory effects of glucocorticoids are more evident in primiparous mothers where the overall levels of glucocorticoids are higher than in multiparous mothers (Corter and Fleming 2002). As indicated below (under early experience effects), where cortisols are elevated in either depressed mothers or mothers with inconsistent early care experiences, levels of cortisol hormones are associated with negative, rather than positive, maternal feelings (Krpan et al. 2005; Gonzalez et al., in prep.) (see Figure 8.2). Based on these and other data (Gunnar, this

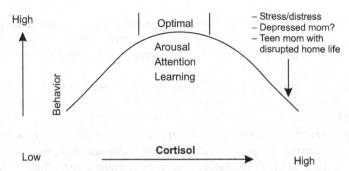

Figure 8.2 Hypothetical relation between HPA axis (hypothalamic–pituitary–adrenal) activity and behavior. Both high and low cortisol are associated with less optimal behavior.

volume; Carter, this volume), it is clear that elevated glucocorticoids or HPA activity have different effects under different circumstances and that there is an optimal level of HPA activity for optimal functioning. For instance, high sustained levels, which grow out of chronic and stressful life experiences or very low levels that can also reflect early trauma-induced stress, are deleterious to the individual and result in negative behavioral outcomes. Moderate levels or acute high levels released in a particular context may instead produce elevations in information-processing, alertness, and overall positive adaptations to the proximal environment (Wang 1997).

NEUROCHEMICAL BASES OF EXPERIENCE

In addition to hormones, there is now growing evidence that brain neurochemicals and peptides may also be implicated in maternal learning. Intra-cerebro-ventricular (ICV) administration of protein synthesis inhibitors affect retention of a maternal memory. We found that if cycloheximide was administered either immediately before or immediately after the experience, but not at a later point, animals responded like inexperienced animals during tests ten days later (Fleming et al. 1996). This short-term, reversible manipulation suggests that brain proteins must be synthesized at the time of the experience for the experience to be laid down or consolidated. Which proteins are relevant is not known. A growing body of evidence implicates both neuropeptides as well as classic neurotransmitter systems. Manipulations of the noradrenergic (NE), dopamine (DA), opioid, and oxytocin systems all affect maternal memory (see Li and Fleming 2003; Keverne and Kendrick 1992).They also affect the initial motivation to be maternal (Numan and Insel 2003; Fleming and Li 2002). Recent work on mice homozygous for the Dbh mutation (Dbh–/–), which do not synthesize NE or epinephrine, show deficits in both mothering and the ability of offspring to elicit care; which of the pair (mother or young) contributes more substantially to the disrupted relationship is not presently known (see Leckman et al., this volume). Together, these systems are likely to be involved in all phases of maternal experience and probably interact differently at different stages, on different aspects of the learning process, and in different sites within the maternal neural circuit.

There are a number of psychobiological mechanisms through which hormones and neurochemicals could act to enhance learning and experience effects. They could increase the animals' arousal, attentional, and/or perceptual function and hence the ability to process information; they could increase the salience (throughput) of associative cues, most likely unconditioned pup cues (e.g., proximal tactile or olfactory) during the learning phase. They could increase the hedonic value of those cues and hence their reinforcing properties. They could act to facilitate or strengthen the association between the conditioned and unconditioned pup-associated cues. Finally, they could produce internal cues which themselves act as conditioned stimuli, a mechanism that could explain the apparent state dependency of the maternal-hormone interactions described above.

NEURAL MECHANISMS UNDERLYING EXPERIENCE AND THE TRANSLATION TO MATERNAL RESPONSIVENESS

Animals

Which brain systems mediate these experience effects? In the rat, at least, there seem to be two mechanisms. The first is specific to maternal learning and includes the "final common path," the MPOA. This nuclear group, which mediates the expression of the behavior, as described earlier, is also changed by maternal experience; it is changed in its neurochemistry, in its responsiveness to hormones, in its structure, and in its pattern of activation and the proliferation and survival of new neurons (c-fos: Fleming et al. 1996; gfap: Featherstone et al. 2000; neurogenesis: Mohebat et al., in prep.; Kinsley et al. 1999). These changes are similar in some respects to the change in the hippocampus that occurs with spatial learning or in the amygdala that occurs with fear conditioning.

The second set of structures includes systems and structures that are nonspecific, that are activated in many learning contexts during either the acquisition of the learning/experience (basolateral amygdala) or its consolidation (nucleus accumbens, shell region), and that have interconnections with the MPOA (Li and Fleming 2003). In addition, mesolimbic dopamine systems involved in pup stimulus salience and "reinforcement" are also recruited during the associative process (Li and Fleming 2003). In the maternal context, we believe that these latter systems are activated early in learning but are then no longer relevant once "memory" is encoded and the MPOA system altered (for extensive discussion of these systems, see Fleming and Li 2002; Li and Fleming 2003).

What we have yet to add to this picture in rats is a better understanding of the role of the main and accessory olfactory bulbs. These are known to be involved in maternal experience and lamb recognition learning in sheep (Poindron and Le Neindre 1980; Keverne 1995) and in social recognition learning in rats and mice (Levy et al. 2003; Keverne, this volume), two processes that are heavily dependent on olfactory function. In fact, in sheep the primary central nervous system structure, which undergoes change with individual lamb recognition learning, is the olfactory bulbs.

Humans

Until now, we have uncovered very little about the brain mechanisms mediating maternal behavior and maternal memory in humans. This situation is likely to change dramatically with the advent of functional imaging technologies. A number of recent fMRI studies show, for instance, activation of the cingulate cortex and other limbic and hypothalamic regions with exposure to infant cues (Lorberbaum et al. 2002). Some evidence indicates that in mothers, brain size may increase 6–8 weeks postpartum when compared to the size during the third trimester of pregnancy (Oatridge et al. 2002). Whether the change results from the production of new neurons or glial cells, or to the enlargement of cells, we do not know. Also unknown is whether these changes in humans are due to interactive social experiences, to the experience of hormones of pregnancy, endocrine, and somatosensory experiences associated with parturition or lactation, or to the suckling stimulation itself. In rats, however, we know that the psychological experiences are primary, since the experiences of pregnancy alone will not enhance responsiveness to pups weeks later (Fleming and Li 2002).

PSYCHOLOGICAL EFFECTS OF EXPERIENCE

Animals

Hormones, neurochemicals, and brain function mediate and affect the efficacy of experience. But how is the new mother changed psychologically by her experience with young, what kind of learning actually occurs, and how do these changes impact on her subsequent maternal behavior? In animals, motor learning probably is only minimally involved. In the rat, experience has very little effect on the actual topography of the stereotyped motor responses in the maternal behavior repertoire. Movements are changed only in the speed with which pups are retrieved and in where on the body the mother grasps the pup to retrieve it. More likely the maternal experience involves a form of perceptual learning, where the mother develops a familiarity with pup associated stimuli and when she re-encounters them, she recognizes them. This then has the subsequent effect of reducing her natural "neophobic" tendency to withdraw from novel, new stimuli; when she encounters pups again they no longer induce a fear-withdrawal state. We know that with maternal experience pups acquire heightened reinforcing properties which further motivate the mother to approach and respond nurturantly to them (Fleming and Li 2002).

Humans

In humans, maternal experience has multiple psychological effects. It involves developing an increased ability to both perceive and then discriminate infant cues. Successful maternal behavior is also associated with heightened self-esteem, positive affect, and greater feelings of maternal competence. In fact, mothers who are better able to recognize and then discriminate their infants' cues from others also report more positive maternal feelings and attitudes. Finally, in humans, experience with infants also provides the mother with actual, as opposed to imagined, practice in breastfeeding, changing the diaper, and doing general maternal behaviors (Corter and Fleming 2002). Despite the clear "positive" parity effects, it would not be hard to imagine that the benefits of experience would, at some point, asymptote and that with too many offspring, more negative reactions could also occur.

Of clear importance in biparental species, but not addressed in this chapter, is the issue of fathering or paternal behavior. In humans, this occurs and caregiving experience can play an even greater role than in mothers. Fathers tend to have had fewer life experiences caring for young babies prior to becoming fathers; hence, the experiences they acquire are quite powerful and underlie their heightened responsiveness to infant cues (reflected in attraction to infant odors and sympathy in response to infant cries) (Fleming et al. 2002; Storey et al. 2000; Corter and Fleming 2002).

EARLY EXPERIENCES AND INTERGENERATIONAL TRANSMISSION OF MOTHERING STYLE

Although experiences during adulthood clearly have an impact on behavior in adulthood, the efficacy of the adult experience depends on the sensitivity of a substrate or systems that has been molded by earlier experiences acquired in interaction with mother and siblings during the pre-weaning period (Hofer and Sullivan 2001).

Stimulus-dependent Bases of Experience

Animals

The mother rat and maternal nest provide a host of stimuli for the young to learn, which in turn can form the basis of their later behavior. The newborn pups preferentially approach and learn to recognize the mother and the nest site based on their unique odors (Polan and Hofer 1998). Their first attachments to the teats are guided and activated by the odor and taste of amniotic fluid first experienced by the young *in utero* (Pederson and Blass 1981; Smotherman and Robinson 1988) in ambient temperature with the birth, and licking stimulation provided by the mother (Abel et al. 1998).

Subsequent attraction to a mother's odor helps the infant orient itself to the mother and, in some species, locate a nipple position. It provides a basis for later food preferences and results from the pairing of a mother's odors with the licking stimulation provided by the mother prior to a nursing bout (Wilson and Sullivan 1994; Hofer and Sullivan 2001). The neurobiology of this early conditioning has been determined and involves neural and neurochemical systems that are also involved in later learning (Hofer and Sullivan 2001; Wilson and Sullivan 1994).

Odors. Until recently, the long-term effects of this learned attraction to a mother's odors on female offspring were not known. However, we found (Fleming et al. 2002) that mother rats respond preferentially to pups scented with the same odors that they experienced earlier on their own mothers than to pups that carried a different scent. Simple exposure to odorants early in life, not in association with mother, produced no such preference in adulthood. Pilot data indicate that if young are deprived of their mothers' odors during their early development, by being reared artificially on a pump, they also lose their conditioned preference for mothers' nest odors at weaning (but instead may develop a preference for the odor of the gloves worn by the experimenter maternal "surrogates"), which indicates again that considerable olfactory learning occurs during the pre-weaning period and contributes to the early attachments between mother and offspring (Levy and Fleming, in prep.). Although, as indicated below, we know that early exposure to odorants alters structural and chemical properties of the olfactory bulb in the neonate, whether these effects persist into adulthood and mediate adult behavior, is unknown.

Licking. The early experiences of being licked have long-term (and intergenerational) effects on the quality of mothering offspring will show toward their offspring when they mature. The experience of receiving more somatosensory stimulation and a more varied nest experience, while in the presence of the natural mother, siblings, and nest odor, may directly affect the animals' physiology and maturational processes; active associative processes may not be involved (Hofer and Sullivan 2001). Francis et al. (1999), however, demonstrated that when young receive more licking from their mothers, they grow up to show higher levels of licking toward their own offspring in comparison to those who received low licking. This effect was also found if the young from high- and low-licking mothers were cross-fostered to a mother who showed the opposite pattern of licking from their biological mothers; this indicates that the effect is based on experiential processes and not on genetics.

Long-term licking effects can also be demonstrated experimentally by altering the characteristics of the mother and nest to enhance or reduce the amount of licking the offspring will receive. The amount of licking experienced by pups is reduced if the mother is rendered anosmic through olfactory bulbectomy, or if pups are raised in a large litter (Fleming et al. 2002; Liu et al. 1997). Total licking by mothers on Day 6 postpartum and total licking by their adult offspring at the same time period postpartum were positively and significantly correlated. Hence, differential experiences of being licked had effects on expression of that behavior in offspring when they became mothers (Gonzalez et al. 2001). This result occurred even though the daughters could smell their litters and had litters of intermediate size. The "reasons" or causes for more or less licking, however, had demonstrably changed across the two generations. More specifically, an "event" occurring in one generation (e.g., having a large or small litter) can later alter maternal behavior somewhat independently of context. The proof is that you can produce two dams that lick their offspring more or less based on their own neonatal experience, and not on the size of their litters.

The most effective period for intergenerational effects seems to be during the very early postpartum period. Significant correlations between mother–daughter behavior occurred when comparing behaviors exhibited during the first postpartum week but not after that period. This cross-generational effect of licking provides a nongenomic mechanism for the transmission of behavioral phenotypes. It is clear from the work of Francis et al. (1999) that enhanced licking is associated with multiple receptors and hippocampal effects (in the "licking" animal and their offspring; see below). Whether these transgenerational behavioral effects are reflected in effects on "maternal" brain systems specifically involved in licking itself or in other maternal behaviors is still under investigation.

Maternal and stimulus deprivation.   One way of manipulating the maternal system is to alter the consistency and reliability of the mother's behavior toward her pups by separating mothers and offspring during the nesting period (Fleming et al. 2002; Hofer and Sullivan 2001). In a series of maternal deprivation studies, pups were either left with their own mothers for the entire pre-weaning period (controls) or separated from their mothers for 15 minutes, for 3 hours daily (from Days 1–9), or for 5 or 24 hours daily during the first 18 days of life and placed in a warm chamber. In some cases, entire litters were removed and separated together; in others, only some pups were removed and separated, either alone or together. In all cases, pup temperatures were maintained during the separation period. The most severe deprivation paradigm (24 hours) involved raising pups artificially in a variant on Hall's "pup-in-a-cup" environment and comparing these to mother-reared sibling controls. Unlike the limited deprivation procedures, which really involve separations and reunions, the "pup-in-the-cup" procedure involves a continuous separation, where pups never know their mothers and littermates. In all of these studies, animals were pair-weaned until adulthood when they were mated, gave birth, and observed for maternal behavior.

The offspring of the artificially reared (AR) females (F1 generation) were themselves reared to adulthood, mated, and tested with their own offspring (F2 generation). Using these deprivation procedures, we found that maternal behavior deficits in the offspring were related to the degree of earlier maternal deprivation. Offspring that had experienced the least deprivation (3 hours daily for 9 days) showed no deficits in adult maternal behavior in comparison to controls; those that experienced somewhat longer periods of daily deprivation (5 hours daily for 18 days) showed initial deficits in licking behavior compared to controls, and once they were fully maternal these deficits persisted in both licking and crouching by comparison to controls (Fleming et al. 2002). Given their clear proximal effects on a variety of homeostatic systems (Hofer and Sullivan 2001), we were surprised to find that variations in the social conditions of deprivation, whether in terms of the mother or the separated pups, did not reliably alter the quality of maternal behavior shown by the pups during either the juvenile period or in adulthood (Rees et al., in prep.). Mothers experiencing as pups the most extreme periods of maternal deprivation (24 hours daily over 18 days) exhibited even greater reductions in pup body-licking, genital licking, and crouching as adults (Fleming et al. 2002), although it should be noted that all mothers did care for their young. The intergenerational effect of licking pattern was also demonstrated when the female offspring of AR and maternally reared (MR) mothers were tested with their own offspring; hence in this F2 generation, offspring of MR mothers showed more licking toward their own offspring than did offspring of AR mothers (Fleming et al. 2002) (Figure 8.3).

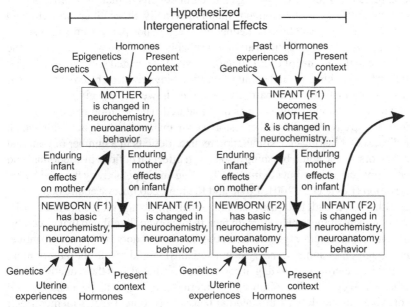

Figure 8.3 Hypothesized relation between mother's effect on her offspring and the offspring's effect on the mother. Both are changed behaviorally and neurobiologically by the other (from Fleming et al. 1999).

Stimulus replacement and reversal of maternal deprivation effects. To determine whether the deleterious effects on adult maternal behavior of more extended pre-weaning maternal deprivation (24-hr separation) could be remedied or reversed by providing additional licking-like somatosensory stimulation, which is known to influence a variety of metabolic, endocrine, and homeostatic systems (see Hofer and Sullivan 2001), we reared pups artificially and then determined the effects of more or less stimulation during the pre-weaning. AR pups require a minimum of two anogenital swabbings a day to facilitate urination and defecation. Without this amount of stimulation, pups will not survive. One group of AR animals (MIN group) were stroked twice a day (the required minimum) with a warm, wet paintbrush swiping their anogenital regions for approximately 45 seconds to stimulate urination and defecation. A second group of AR pups (MAX group) was stroked five times a day both anogenital and overall body stimulation, the stimulation lasted two minutes per pup. To determine whether additional social stimulation normally provided by littermates may also make a contribution, we included a group of AR animals reared in the cups in pairs (Fleming et al. 2002).

These stimulations were carried out from the day pups were placed on the pumps (postnatal Day 4) to the day of weaning (Day 20 postnatal). Animals were assessed for their pup-directed behaviors as adults, with their own litters, culled to 8 pups, starting on the day of parturition through Day 18 postpartum. Complete privation of mothering resulted in deficits in many maternal behaviors but not in the motivation to respond maternally. Since all groups retrieved young, the usual reduction in "neophobia" seen in postpartum animals also occurred in AR groups. Deficits are thus probably associated with changes in the salience to the mother of cues (olfactory, taste?) associated with the young. Deficient body licking, genital licking, and crouching produced by complete privation of mothering were partially restored, however, by giving AR pups maximum brushing stimulation as they matured. The addition of a conspecific into the cup environment further restored adult maternal licking behavior, which indicates that licking-like stimulation reduces deficits in a number of maternal behaviors. In the adult, brushing also had an effect on deficits in attentional and emotional behaviors; but not in social learning and hyperactivity induced by deprivation (Lovic et al. 2001; Lovic and Fleming 2003; Levy et al. 2003).

Other as yet undefined aspects of maternal stimulation must contribute to the development of these behaviors. In fact, there is every likelihood that a "combination" replacement regime (simulating mothers' odors, temperature, movement, and other somatosensory characteristics) would result not only in more complete maternal responding in adult offspring, but also in the reduction of the other social deficits that follow early maternal deprivation and which may well contribute to the deficits in maternal behavior (Moore 1995; Kraemer 1992; Wilson and Sullivan 1994; Hofer and Sullivan 2001). In addition, initial results indicate that the pattern of stimulation provided by conspecifics (their movement, warmth, and tactile characteristics) also contributes to the normal development of behavior.

Reversals of deprivation effects can occur if the ecologically appropriate stimulation is provided at the biologically relevant time, that is, during the pre-weaning period. However, the question also arises as to whether other "therapies" or "enrichments" following weaning can reverse the deficits in behavior produced by early deprivation. This has not been attempted in the study of maternal behavior. However, post-weaning environmental enrichment does reverse the negative effects of maternal separation on HPA axis function, but without reversing many of the molecular changes that are associated with the altered HPA function (Francis et al. 2002). This suggests that post-weaning "therapies" may hone or tune-up the expression or development of other mechanisms that compensate for the disrupted mechanisms and that could normalize HPA function. Whether these effects are fragile and would dissociate with subsequent stressors is not known.

It is clear that in the absence of added stimulation, either pre- or post-weaning, maternally deprived mothers show deficits in their ability to gain lasting benefits from their postpartum interactions with pups (Levy et al. 2003). If MR animals were exposed to pups during the first few postpartum hours (exposure phase) and then separated from them, they show enhanced responsiveness to pups when tested after a 15-day separation (retention phase). Maternally deprived animals seemed less affected by a similar experience and took considerably longer to respond maternally to foster pups; hence, their ability to learn from their pup-related experiences was compromised. It is not surprising that "learning" deficits of artificial rearing are not restricted to the maternal context. They extend and propagate to other social experiences acquired throughout later development (Kraemer 1992; Levy et al. 2003).

Humans

We take for granted the idea that early experiences with mother, father, and the home of origin affect human offspring (Bowlby 1969; Plomin 1989). In fact, there is a growing literature that shows that humans, like other animals, learn individual characteristics of their mothers' voice *in utero* and, postnatally, will come to orient to both natural and artificial odors previously associated with their own mothers (Hofer and Sullivan 2001; Schaal and Porter 1991). Young infants clearly learn all sorts of things about their mothers and home environments and in that process either develop secure attachments, ambivalent attachments, or avoidant behaviors in relation to their caregivers (Ainsworth 1979; Belsky, this volume). However, longitudinal studies that track reasonable biological variables are lacking to contrast the quality of parenting received by infants to the quality of caregiving they provide to their own young some 15 to 30 years later. There are, however, numerous short-term longitudinal studies connecting consecutive pairs of relations: the sensitivity of mothers (F1) with attachment status in their infants (F2); attachment status in their infants (F2) with the infants' later adult attachment status (F2); the infants' later adult attachment status (F2) with the infants' later maternal sensitivity (F2), and, into the next generation, infants' later maternal sensitivity (F2) with the attachment status of the F3 infants and so on (van IJzendoorn 1995). Based on van IJzendoorn's meta-analyses of studies exploring these relations, it is statistically probable that the quality of parenting one receives would be related to the quality of parenting one gives offspring, barring major intervening disruptions and stresses to disrupt positive parenting or therapeutic interventions to improve negative parenting (Belsky, this volume).

Early family instability or dysfunctional parenting. In low socio-economic status, high-risk groups, these intergenerational effects are even more pronounced when more severely dysfunctional parenting is evaluated. Intergenerational effects are seen among women whose early lives were disrupted by abuse, maternal depression, and poor family functioning early in adolescence (Weinfield et al. 2000). For instance, 30% of mothers who were abused as children abuse their own children later in life, whereas only 5% of mothers who were not abused abuse their infants (Knutson 1995). Consistent with the epidemiological data, in retrospective studies, Main and Goldwyn (1984) report that the experience of maternal rejection as a child is related to the rejection of offspring later in life. This intergenerational effect may account for the cyclic occurrence of premature motherhood among teenagers who have often received inadequate or inappropriate parenting (de Paul and Domenech 2000). These children go on to raise poorly adjusted children who tend to become teen parents themselves (Geronimous 1987; Furstenberg et al. 1987; Maynard 1996).

In a recent series of studies of high-risk "teen" and depressed mothers, we explored, using retrospective data, the relation between early experiences being cared for and quality of care mothers provide to their offspring. We compared the role of hormones and early life experiences in the regulation of the actual maternal behavior toward the infant in teen and adult mothers (Krpan et al. 2005). Primiparous mothers, including teen mothers 18 years or less, young mothers 19–25 years, and mature mothers over 25 years, were assessed for their maternal feelings, attitudes, salivary cortisol profile, and behavior through interview, questionnaires, and observations of videotaped interactions with their infants. Groups were compared on the basis of age and of early life experience (consistent vs. inconsistent parenting during the first 12 years of life). Mothers who as children and adolescents received consistent care engaged in significantly more affectionate and less instrumental caretaking behaviors toward their infants as compared to mothers with multiple and changing caregivers. Two younger groups of mothers showed early experience effects most strongly. When all age groups were combined, more frequent changes in caregivers during childhood were related to higher levels of cortisol, which in turn was related to negative affect and then to reduced affectionate behavior (Figures 8.4–8.6).

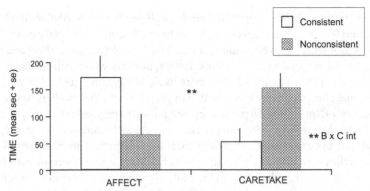

Figure 8.4 Effects of early experiences (inconsistent vs. consistent) in family of origin on affectionate and caretaking behavior in teenage mothers (Krpan et al. 2005).

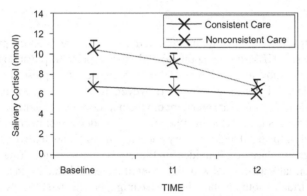

Figure 8.5 The effects of early experiences (inconsistent vs. consistent) in family of origin on salivary cortisol levels in postpartum depressed mothers.

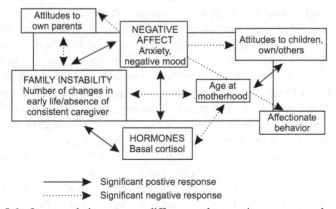

Figure 8.6 Intercorrelations among different early experiences, maternal attitudes, mood, salivary cortisol, and behavior in three-month postpartum mothers.

Consistent with these results, in a study of clinically depressed older mothers we found the same basic direct relation between "inconsistent" early parenting and cortisol levels, as well as indirect relations between negative affect and behavioral interactions with the infants. Hence, mothers who received less early consistent care prior to age 12 were more likely to have high cortisol levels and to become clinically depressed. We do not yet know whether mothers' sensitivity to their offspring and, in particular, their ability to respond affectively to and recognize their infants' odor and cry cues are related to mothers' earlier prepubertal and pubertal experiences with their own parents. The implications of these studies are that early family instability has long-lasting effects on maternal behavior by altering the offspring's adult affective state. However, whether these relations are mediated by the mother in the family of origin remains open.

Endocrine Effects of Experience

Animals

We know that the early pre-weaning period has many effects on the pups' cardiac responses, HPA stress responses, and other aspects of physiological homeostasis. We know also that some of these effects are also expressed in physiological vulnerabilities in adulthood. However, it is not clear whether these effects impact adult maternal behavior or whether the ability to gain from subsequent experiences is reflected in either disrupted endocrine or neural responses to pups and/or to social and olfactory cues in general in the deprived animals.

Although we have a clear idea of the endocrine and endocrine-receptor changes normally associated with the onset of maternal behavior in adulthood, we know virtually nothing about how these might be affected by early maternal deprivation. In a preliminary study, we have found differences between AR and MR animals in the density of estrogen and oxytocin receptors (two receptor systems clearly activated in the maternal animal) in the MPOA, with MR animals showing higher densities (Rees et al., in prep.). These effects have, of course, also been found in studies comparing offspring of high- and low-licking dams (Champagne et al. 2001). Interestingly, AR animals receiving additional stroking stimulation had levels equivalent or even higher than MR females. In light of these findings, it is interesting that we were unable to find AR–MR differences in the effects of exogenous estrogen and progesterone steroids on maternal behavior in virgin female rats. It is possible, however, that if we had titrated the exogenous hormone concentrations, we may have found differences in sensitivities to the hormones as a function of early rearing experiences.

Another possible endocrine effect of deprivation that may influence adult maternal behavior is in the demonstrated effects on the stress system and HPA axis, both during the early pre-weaning period and later in adulthood (Suchecki et al. 1995; van Oers et al. 1998; Vazquez et al. 1996; Liu et al. 1997). Early deprivation may well produce dysregulations of the HPA axis, such that the basal and/or stress levels of corticotropin-releasing hormone (CRH) or corticosterone (CORT) during the early postpartum period are not being maintained within the optimal regulated range to enhance maternal memory or licking; it may be that due to early deprivation, CRH or CORT levels are quite erratic and elevated, producing instead disrupted behavior. In a first study exploring this possibility, we found that in comparison to MR animals, AR rearing resulted in quite elevated levels of basal CORT in adulthood during the postpartum period and these were inversely related to pup-licking shown by the mothers (Rees et al., in prep., see also Suchecki et al. 1993).

Humans

Results with new mothers map onto these HPA findings quite directly. In two different studies, we have now found that mothers who are at risk — either teen or clinically depressed — are more likely to show disrupted interactions with their infants and to have elevated basal cortisol levels. Although we find no direct relation between cortisol levels and negative maternal behavior, there is clearly an indirect relation, where higher cortisol is associated with more depression/negative affect and higher dysphoria is associated with less adapted maternal behavior. Not known, of course, is whether the elevated cortisol levels found in high-risk mothers are restricted to the postpartum period, or whether as youngsters these mothers also had elevated baseline and/or stress cortisol levels. Based on findings by Spangler et al. (1994; Spangler and Schieche 1998), which show that in certain contexts cortisol levels are elevated in infants who are insecurely attached and/or who have intrusive caregivers, it would not be surprising to learn that these high-risk mothers have a history of an over-responsive HPA axis, much as has been described for "maternally deprived" rat pups. Taken together, it is clear that the relation of adult maternal behavior to glucocorticoid levels is a complex one, bimodal at best (see Figures 8.2, 8.5, and 8.6).

Neural and Neurochemical Effects of Experience

There is now substantial evidence that the experience of exposure to mothers' odors in association with her licking is encoded by the brain and produces changes in the brain lasting into the juvenile period, at least. Whether these changes persist into adulthood is not known. Formation of the association between licking and maternal odor produces changes in the olfactory bulbs, altering their neurochemical and structural properties, and depends on the activation of the noradrenergic system that originates in the midbrain and terminates in the olfactory bulbs (Wilson and Sullivan 1994; Najbauer and Leon 1995). In addition to olfactory mechanisms, substantial data indicate that additional environmental manipulations during the pre-weaning period (including somatosensory stimulation) produce changes in cortex, hippocampus, other limbic areas, and in the MPOA (Post et al. 1998; Rosenzweig and Bennett 1996; Pascual and

Figueroa 1996; Cramer 1988; Liu et al. 2000). Finally, with early experience and
separation manipulations, alterations also occur in a number of biogenic amine
systems, relevant to maternal behavior and maternal experience effects in adulthood including the noradrenergic and dopamine systems (Hall et al. 1998;
Hansen 1994; Stern and Keer 1999). At present we do not know whether
changes in these systems through early experience manipulations are
responsible for the changes in adult maternal behavior.

Psychological Effects of Experience

Animals

The intergenerational transmission of maternal behavior in animals seems quite
clear at this point. What is less clear is how these effects are transmitted. Since
we know they are not genetically inheritable, they might be based on experience. Experience has long-term effects on behavioral systems that normally
contribute to the motivation to be maternal or to the quality of maternal behavior
an animal exhibits. For instance, maternal deprivation also affects the development of fear and emotionality (Francis et al. 1999), attentional systems (Lovic et
al. 2001; Lovic and Fleming 2003), conspecific social learning, and learning
about new odors. Oddly enough, it does not disrupt performance on numerous
other cognitive, nonsocial tasks, where in some cases the deprived animals excel
(Levy et al. 2003). This dissociation between the effects of early deprivation on
social and nonsocial learning likely derives from the fact that during social
learning, the animal has to learn about individual characteristics of other initially unfamiliar, unpredictable, and behaving conspecifics, and, as a result, animals are probably more easily distracted from attending to the cues to be processed during the learning. If the primary deficit in learning in the deprived
animal is, in fact, an attentional one, then learning about a social stimulus as opposed to a static environmental stimulus should be considerably more difficult.
Moreover, the known involvement of affective and attentional systems in the expression of maternal behavior suggests that early experience-based changes in
these behavioral systems likely contribute to the deficits in adult maternal
behavior (Fleming et al. 2002; Fleming and Li 2002).

Humans

There is strong evidence to suggest transmission of attachment styles in both
mothers and offspring. Although the issue of mediation has not been extensively
explored, Belsky (this volume) provides a thoughtful analysis of the possible
mediators of these relations, including in the equation a consideration of how
mothers talk about their infants (their "mind-mindedness"), the quality of the
marriage and home environment, and the acquired emotional bias used by infants to process their world. This latter "affect-memory" mechanism finds its

analogy in the animal work, in early experience effects on attention, sociability, emotion, and memory.

SUMMARY

Mammals living in a changing and sometimes unpredictable environment possess mechanisms that permit them to alter their behavior to accommodate such variation. These mechanisms underlie experience, learning, and memory.

In this chapter we have explored the extent to which experiences both in adulthood and early life influence the initial expression of maternal behavior which, in most animals, is a highly stereotyped species-characteristic behavior. The distinction was made between factors influencing the "motivation" to mother, or maternal responsiveness, and the processes involved in the formation of a bond toward the litter (if there exists no individual recognition) or an individual offspring (in the case of selectivity). I do not use the term *attachment* in the context of the mother, but instead use it to refer to the individual recognition and learned selectivity expressed by the offspring toward the caregiver.

These experience effects are by no means restricted to "higher" mammals but occur at all phyletic levels of these animals. I described what is known at present about the underlying sensory, endocrine, and neural mechanisms of experience, revealing both their specificity of action and their general properties. Further, I discussed the behavioral and physiological effects of experience that mediate the change in subsequent maternal responsiveness. Mechanisms of attachment were contrasted in the infant and in the mother; in some instances, those mechanisms are the same, in others clearly different. Finally, I contrasted maternal behavior and its regulatory mechanisms in a variety of mammals, differing in developmental precocity at birth and in complexity of cognitive function. I took a psychobiological perspective and emphasized the similarities, rather than the more obvious cognitive differences between rat and human mothers, in an attempt to illustrate the heuristic value of using animal models to develop questions relating to human maternal behavior.

Although we have learned quite a bit about the mechanisms that mediate maternal behavior in the rat, there is still much to learn. This is clearly the case for the many other species that have not been mentioned in this brief review and even more so for humans. Below I list five issues that were raised during this Dahlem Workshop, which I feel should be addressed in the years to come.

1. Among many primate species and humans, juveniles, aunts, and other adults are often called upon to care for infants and are motivated to do so and, under some circumstances, young grow attached to allomothers; in others they do not (see Hrdy, this volume; Ahnert, this volume; Grossmann and Grossmann, this volume). What are the mechanisms that underlie alloparenting in terms of the role of hormones and of experience? In some cases, hormones may indeed be involved; in others, not. In

some cases the neural structures mediating postpartum maternal behavior and parental behavior in alloparents are the same; in other cases, they are not. What accounts for these differences?

2. Striking in our discussions of maternal behavior and mother–infant attachment is a disturbing absence of any discussions of fathering or, indeed, of family systems altogether. With respect to animal models for fathers, there is now quite elegant work on the neurobiology of fathering in biparental rodent species, and these constitute good models to guide the future psychobiological analysis of human paternal behavior (see Sachser, this volume; Carter, this volume; Young et al. 2001).

3. Within recent years and with the ease of salivary assays, many attachment and bonding researchers have used salivary cortisol as a marker of stress responsiveness and comfort level in the infant under a variety of contexts. However, the "meaning" of elevations in cortisol is not always clear and often contradictory. In some cases, high cortisol is a positive and healthy response associated with "approach" responding; in other cases, it is maladaptive physiologically and negative. This same can be said for the relation between behavior and very low levels of the HPA hormones. Over the next few years, with the use of multiple measures of HPA, autonomic function, and a closer analysis of the earlier experiences and present context, we should get a better handle on the subtleties in this "stress" system and the nonlinearity in the relation between HPA function and behavior.

4. Although we have made substantial progress in our understanding of the neuroanatomy of maternal behavior, only one study has explored this neuroanatomy in human mothers, fathers, and alloparents. With the use of fMRI, the next ten years should prove very productive in this respect.

5. Finally, the role of epigenetics in the regulation of parental behavior and of the effects of experience on individual differences in development is totally unchartered territory in nonhuman mammals or humans. The question arises as to why the same stressful early experiences can have such different effects on different individuals. How do subsequent experiences modulate the effects of earlier experiences, and how do both interact with the genetic and neurochemical profile of the offspring to influence subsequent development and the adult phenotype?

Taken together, with new technology and the new interdisciplinary approaches to the science, this next decade promises to be a very exciting one for the study of attachment and bonding.

ACKNOWLEDGMENTS

Many thanks to Jodie Cox for her editorial contributions and to the Natural Sciences and Engineering Research Council of Canada and the Canadian Institutes of Health Research for supporting the work reported herein. Some of the ideas expressed here may also be found in Corter and Fleming (2002) and Fleming and Li (2002).

REFERENCES

Abel, R.A., A.E. Ronca, and J.R. Alberts. 1998. Perinatal stimulation facilitates suckling onset in newborn rats. *Dev. Psychobiol.* **32**:91–99.

Ainsworth, M. 1979. Attachment as related to mother–infant interaction. *Adv. Stud. Behav.* **9**:1–49.

Bornstein, M.H. 2002. Handbook of Parenting (vols. 1–5). Mahwah, NJ.: Erlbaum.

Bowlby, J. 1969. Attachment. Attachment and Loss, vol. 1. London: Hogarth.

Bridges, R.S. 1977. Parturition: Its role in the long term retention of maternal behavior in the rat. *Physiol. Behav.* **18**:487–490.

Bridges, R.S., and R.P. Hammer. 1992. Parity-associated alterations of medial preoptic opiate receptors in female rats. *Brain Res.* **578**:269–274.

Broad, K.D., F. Levy, G. Evans et al. 1999. Previous maternal experience potentiates the effect of parturition on oxytocin receptor mRNA expression in the paraventricular nucleus. *Eur. J. Neurosci.* **11**:3725–3737.

Byrnes, E.M., J.J. Byrnes, and R.S. Bridges. 2001. Increased sensitivity of dopamine systems following reproductive experience in rat. *Pharmacol. Biochem. Behav.* **68**: 481–489.

Champagne, F., J. Diorio, S. Sharme, and M.J. Meaney. 2001. Naturally occurring variations in maternal behavior in the rat are associated with differences in estrogen-inducible central oxytocin receptors. *PNAS* **98**:12,736–12,741.

Cohen, J., and R.S. Bridges. 1981. Retention of maternal behavior in nulliparous and primiparous rats: Effects of duration of previous maternal experience. *J. Comp. Physiol. Psychol.* **95**:450–459.

Corter, C., and A.S. Fleming. 2002. Psychobiology of maternal behavior in human beings. In: Handbook of Parenting: Biology and Ecology of Parenting, ed. M.H. Bornstein, pp. 141–182. Mahwah, NJ: Erlbaum.

Cramer, C.P. 1988. Experience during suckling increases weight and volume of rat hippocampus. *Brain Res.* **470**:151–155.

de Paul, J., and L. Domenech. 2000. Childhood history of abuse and child abuse potential in adolescent mothers: A longitudinal study. *Child Abuse* **24**:701–713.

Ehret, G., and J. Buckenmaier. 1994. Estrogen-receptor occurance in the female mouse brain: Effects of maternal experience, ovariectomy, estrogen and anosmia. *J. Physiol. (Paris)* **88**:315–329.

Featherstone, R.E., A.S. Fleming, and G.O. Ivy. 2000. Plasticity in the maternal circuit: Effects of experience and partum condition on brain astrocyte number in female rats. *Behav. Neurosci.* **114**:158–172.

Ferreira, G., A. Terrazas, P. Poindron et al. 2000. Learning of olfactory cues is not necessary for early lamb recognition by the mother. *Physiol. Behav.* **69**:405–412.

Fleming, A.S., C. Corter, P. Franks et al. 1993. Postpartum factors related to mother's attraction to newborn infant odors. *Dev. Psychobiol.* **26**:115–132.

Fleming, A.S., G.W. Kraemer, A. Gonzalez et al. 2002. Mothering begets mothering: The transmission of behavior and its neurobiology across generations. *Pharmacol. Biochem. Behav.* **73**:61–75.

Fleming, A.S., and M. Li. 2002. Psychobiology of maternal behavior and its early determinants in nonhuman mammals. In: Handbook of Parenting, ed. M.H. Bornstein, pp. 61–97. Mahwah, NJ: Erlbaum.

Fleming, A.S., H.D. Morgan, and C. Walsh. 1996. Experiential factors in postpartum regulation of maternal care. *Adv. Stud. Behav.* **25**:295–332.

Fleming, A.S., D.H. O'Day, and G.W. Kraemer. 1999. Neurobiology of mother–infant interactions: Experience and central nervous system plasticity across development and generations. *Neurosci. Biobehav. Rev.* **23**:673–685.

Fleming, A.S., D. Ruble, H. Krieger, and P.Y. Wong. 1997. Hormonal and experiential correlates of maternal responsiveness during pregnancy and the puerperium in human mothers. *Horm. Behav.* **31**:145–158.

Formby, D. 1967. Maternal recognition of infant's cry. *Dev. Med. Child Neurol.* **9**: 292–298.

Francis, D., J. Diorio, D. Liu, and M.J. Meaney. 1999. Nongenomic transmission across generations of maternal behavior and stress responses in the rat. *Science* **286**:1155–1158.

Francis, D., J. Diorio, P. Plotsky, and M.J. Meaney. 2002. Environmental enrichment reverses the effects of maternal separation on stress reactivity. *J. Neurosci.* **22**: 7840–7843.

Furstenberg, F.F., J. Brooks-Gunn, and S.P. Morgan. 1987. Adolescent mothers and their children in later life. *Fam. Plan. Perspect.* **19**:142–151.

Geronimous, A.T. 1987. On teenage childbearing and neonatal mortality in the United States. *Pop. Dev. Rev.* **13**:245–279.

Gonzalez, A., V. Lovic, G.R. Ward, P.E. Wainwright, and A.S. Fleming. 2001. Intergenerational effects of complete maternal deprivation and replacement stimulation on maternal behavior and emotionality in female rats. *Dev. Psychobiol.* **38**:11–32.

Gonzalez-Mariscal, G., and P. Poindron. 2002. Parental care in mammals: Immediate internal and sensory factors of control. In: Hormones, Brain and Behavior, ed. D.W. Pfaff, A.P. Arnold, A.M. Etgen, S.F. Fahrbach, and R.T. Rubin, pp. 215–298. New York: Academic.

Hall, F.S., L.S. Wilkinson, T. Humby et al. 1998. Isolation rearing in rats: Pre- and postsynaptic changes in striatal dopaminergic systems. *Pharmacol. Biochem. Behav.* **59**:859–872.

Hansen, S. 1994. Maternal behavior of female rats with 6-OHDA lesions in the ventral striatum: Characterization of the pup retrieval deficit. *Physiol. Behav.* **55**:615–620.

Hepper, P.G., and J. Cleland. 1999. Developmental aspects of kin recognition. *Genetica* **104**:199–205.

Hofer, M.A., and R.M. Sullivan. 2001. Toward a neurobiology of attachment. In: Handbook of Developmental Cognitive Neuroscience, ed. C.A. Nelson and M. Luciana, pp. 599–616. Cambridge, MA: MIT Press.

Keller, M., M. Meurisse, P. Poindron et al. 2003. Maternal experience influences the establishment of visual/auditory, but not of olfactory recognition of the newborn baby lamb by ewes at parturition. *Dev. Psychobiol.* **43**:167–176.

Keverne, E.B. 1995. Neurochemical changes accompanying the reproductive process: Their significance for maternal care in primates and other mammals. In: Motherhood in Human and Nonhuman Primates: Biosocial Determinants, ed. C.R. Pryce, R.D. Martin, and D. Skuse, pp. 69–77. Basel: Karger.

Keverne, E.B., and K.M. Kendrick. 1992. Oxytocin facilitation of maternal behavior in sheep. *Ann. NY Acad. Sci.* **652**:83–101.

Keverne, E.B., F. Levy, R. Guevara-Guzman, and K.M. Kendrick. 1993. Influence of birth and maternal experience on olfactory bulb neurotransmitter release. *Neurosci.* **56**:557–565.

Kinsley, C.H., L. Madonia, G.W. Gifford et al. 1999. Motherhood improves learning and memory. *Nature* **402**:137–138.

Knutson, J.R. 1995. Psychological characteristics of maltreated children: Putative risk factors and consequences. *Ann. Rev. Psychol.* **46**:401–431.

Koch, M. 1990. Effects of treatment with estradiol and parental experience on the number and distribution of estrogen-binding neurons in the ovariectomized mouse brain. *Neuroendocrinology* **51**:505–514.

Kraemer, G.W. 1992. A psychobiological theory of attachment. *Behav. Brain Sci.* **15**: 493–541.

Krpan, K., R. Coombs, D. Zinga, M. Steiner, and A.S. Fleming. 2005. Experiential and hormonal correlates of maternal behaviour in teen and adult mothers. *Horm. Behav.*, in press.

Levy, F., R. Gervais, U. Kindermann et al. 1991. Effects of early postpartum separation on maintenance of maternal responsiveness and selectivity in parturient ewes. *Appl. Anim. Behav. Sci.* **31**:101–110.

Levy, F., R. Guevara-Guzman, M.R. Hinton, K.M. Kendrick, and E.B. Keverne. 1993. Effects of parturition and maternal experience on noradrenaline and acetylcholine release in the olfactory bulb in sheep. *Behav. Neurosci.* **107**:662–668.

Levy, F., K.M. Kendrick, J.A. Goode, R. Guevara-Guzman, and E.B. Keverne. 1995. Oxytocin and vasopressin release in the olfactory bulb of parturient ewes: Changes with maternal experience and effects on acetylcholine, gamma-aminobutyric acid, glutamte and noradrenaline release. *Brain Res.* **669**:197–206.

Levy, F., K.M. Kendrick, E.B. Keverne, V. Piketty, and P. Poindron. 1992. Intracerebral oxytocin is important for the onset of maternal behavior in inexperienced ewes delivered under peridural anesthesia. *Behav. Neurosci.* **106**:427–432.

Levy, F., K.M. Kendrick, E.B. Keverne, R.H. Porter, and A. Romeyer. 1996. Physiological, sensory, and experiential factors of prenatal care in sheep. In: Advances in the Study of Behavior, ed. J.S. Rosenblatt and C.T. Snowdon, pp. 385–416. San Diego: Academic.

Levy, F., A. Locatelli, V. Piketty, Y. Tillet, and P. Poindron. 1995. Involvement of the main but not the accessory olfactory system in maternal behavior of primiparious and multiparious care in sheep. *Adv. Stud. Behav.* **57**:97–104.

Levy, F., A.I. Melo, B.G. Galef, M. Madden, and A.S. Fleming. 2003. Complete maternal depreivation affects social, but not spatial, learning in adult rats. *Dev. Psychobiol.* **43**: 177–191.

Li, M., and A.S. Fleming. 2003. Differential involvement of nucleus accumbens shell and core in subregions in maternal memory in postpartum rats. *Behav. Neurosci.* **117**: 426–445.

Liu, D., J. Diorio, J.C. Day, D.D. Francis, and M.J. Meaney. 2000. Maternal care, hippocampal synaptogenesis and cognitive development in rats. *Nature Neurosci.* **3**: 799–806.

Liu, D., J. Diorio, B. Tannenbaum et al. 1997. Maternal care, hippocampal glucocorticoid receptors, and hypothalamic–pituitary–adrenal responses to stress [see comments]. *Science* **277**:1659–1662.

Lorberbaum, J.P., J.D. Newman, A.R. Horwitz et al. 2002. A potential role for thalamocingulate circuitry in human maternal behavior. *Biol. Psych.* **51**:431–445.

Lovic, V., and A.S. Fleming. 2003. Artificially reared female rats show reduced prepulse inhibition and deficits in the attentional set shifting task-reversal of effects with maternal-like licking stimulation. *Behav. Brain Res.* **148**:209–219.

Lovic, V., A. Gonzalez, and A.S. Fleming. 2001. Maternally separated rats show deficits in maternal care in adulthood. *Dev. Psychobiol.* **39**:19-33.

Main, M., and R. Goldwyn. 1984. Predicting rejection of her infant from mother's representation of her own experience: Implications for the abused-abusing intergerational cycle. *Child Abuse* **8**:203–217.

Mann, P.E., and R.S. Bridges. 2002. Prolactin receptor gene expression in the forebrain of pregnant and lactating rats. *Molec. Brain Res.* **105**:136–145.

Maynard, R.A. 1996. Kids Having Kids: A Robin Hood Foundation Special Report on the Costs of Adolescent Childbearing. New York: Robin Hood Foundation.

Moore, C. 1995. Maternal contributions to mammalian reproductive development and the divergence of males and females. In: Advances in the Study of Behavior, ed. P.J.B. Slater, J. Rosenblatt, C. Snowdon, M. Milinski, pp. 47–118. San Diego: Academic.

Morgan, H.D., A.S. Fleming, and J.M. Stern. 1992. Somatosensory control of the onset and retention of maternal responsiveness in primiparous Sprague-Dawley rats. *Physiol. Behav.* **51**:541–555.

Najbauer, J., and M. Leon. 1995. Olfactory experience modulated apoptosis in the developing olfactory bulb. *Brain Res.* **674**:245–251.

Noirot, E. 1972. The onset of maternal behavior in rats, hamsters, and mice. In: Advances in the Study of Behavior, ed. D.S. Lehrman, R.A. Hinde, and E. Shaw, pp. 1569–1645. New York: Academic.

Numan, M., and T.R. Insel. 2003. The Neurobiology of Parental Behavior. Berlin: Springer.

Oatridge A, A. Holdcroft, N. Saeed et al. 2002. Change in brain size during and after pregnancy: Study in healthy women and women with preeclampsia. *Am. J. Neuroradiol.* **23**:19–26.

Orpen, B.G., and A.S. Fleming. 1987. Experience with pups sustains maternal responding in postpartum rats. *Physiol. Behav.* **40**:47–54.

Orpen, B.G., N. Furman, P.Y. Wong, and A.S. Fleming. 1987. Hormonal influences on the duration of postpartum maternal responsiveness in the rat. *Physiol. Behav.* **40**:307–315.

Pascual, R., and H. Figueroa. 1996. Effects of pre-weaning sensorimotor stimulation on behavioral and neuronal development in motor and visual cortex of the rat. *Biol. Neonate* **69**:399–404.

Pederson, P.E., and E.M. Blass. 1981. Olfactory control over suckling in albino rats. In: Development of Perception: Psychobiological Persepectives, ed. R.N. Aslin, J.R. Alberts, and M.R. Peterson, pp. 349–381. New York: Academic.

Plomin, R. 1989. Environment and genes: Determinants of behaviour. *Am. Psychol.* **44**:105–111.

Poindron, P., G. Gilling, H. Hernandez, N. Serafin, and A. Terrazas. 2003. Early recognition of newborn goat kids by their mother. I. Nonolfactory discrimination. *Dev. Psychobiol.* **43**:82–89.

Poindron, P., and P. Le Neindre. 1980. Endocrine and sensory regulation of maternal behavior in the ewe. In: Advances in the Study of Behavior, ed. J.S. Rosenblatt, R.A. Hinde, and C. Beer, pp. 75–119. New York: Academic.

Polan, H.J., and M.A. Hofer. 1998. Olfactory preference for mother over home nest havings by newborn rats. *Dev. Psychobiol.* **33**:5–20.

Porter, R.H., J.M. Cernock, and F. McLaughlin. 1983. Maternal recognition of neonates through olfactory cues. *Physiol. Behav.* **30**:151–154.

Post, R.M., S.R. Weiss, H. Li et al. 1998. Neural plasticity and emotional memory. *Dev. Psychopathol.* **10**:829–855.

Rees, S., and A. Fleming. 2001. How early maternal separation and juvenile experience with pups affect maternal behavior and emotionality in adult postpartum rats. *Anim. Learn. Behav.* **29**:221–233.

Rosenblatt, J.S. 2002. Hormonal bases of parenting in mammals. In: Handbook of Parenting, ed. M.H. Bornstein, pp. 31–60. Mahwah, NJ: Erlbaum.

Rosenzweig, M.R., and E.L. Bennett. 1996. Psychobiology of plasticity: Effects of training and experience on brain and behavior. *Behav. Brain Res.* **78**:57–65.

Schaal, B., H. Montagner, E. Hertling et al. 1980. Les stimulations olfactives dans les relations entre l'enfant et la mère. *Reprod. Nutr. Dev.* **20**:843–858.

Schaal, B., and R.H. Porter. 1991. "Microsmatic humans" revisited: The generation and perception of chemical signals. *Adv. Stud. Behav.* **20**:135–199.

Singh, P.B. 2001. Chemosensation and genetic individuality. *Reproduction* **121**: 529–539.

Smotherman, W.P., and S.R. Robinson. 1988. The uterus as environment: The ecology of fetal behavior. In: Handbook of Behavioral Neurobiology: Development Psychobiology and Behavioral Ecology, ed. E.M. Blass, pp. 149–196. New York: Plenum.

Spangler, G., and M. Schieche. 1998. Emotional and adrenocortical responses of infants to the strange situation: The differential function of emotional expression. *Intl. J. Behav. Dev.* **22**:681–706.

Spangler, G., M. Schieche, U. Ilg, U. Maier, and C. Ackerman. 1994. Maternal sensitivity as an external organizer for biobehavioral regulation in infancy. *Dev. Psychobiol.* **27**:425–427.

Stallings, J., A.S. Fleming, C. Corter, C. Worthman, and M. Steiner. 2001. The effects of infant cries and odors on sympathy, cortisol, and autonomic responses in new mothers and nonpostpartum women. *Parenting Sci. Prac.* **1**:71–100.

Stern, J.M., and S.K. Johnson. 1989. Perioral somatosensory determinants of nursing behavior in Norway rats, *Rattus norvegicus*. *J. Comp. Psychol.* **103**:269–280.

Stern, J.M., and S.E. Keer. 1999. Maternal motivation of lactating rats is disrupted by low dosages of haloperidol. *Behav. Brain Res.* **99**:231–239.

Storey, A.E., C.J. Walsh, R.L. Quinton, and K.E. Wynne-Edwards. 2000. Hormonal correlates of paternal responsiveness in new and expectant fathers. *Evol. Hum. Behav.* **21**:79–95.

Suchecki, D., D.Y. Nelson, H. van Oers, and S. Levine. 1995. Activation and inhibition of the hypothalamic–pituitary–adrenal axis of the neonatal rat: Effects of maternal deprivation. *Psychoneuroendocrin.* **20**:169–182.

Suchecki, D., P. Rosenfeld, and S. Levine. 1993. Maternal regulation of the hypothalamic–pituitary–adrenal axis in the infant rat: The roles of feeding and stroking. *Dev. Brain Res.* **75**:185–192.

Terrazas, A., G. Ferreira, F. Levy et al. 1999. Do ewes recognize their lambs within the first day postpartum without the help of olfactory cues? *Behav. Proc.* **47**:19–29.

Valanne, E., V. Vurenkowski, T. Partanen, J. Lind, and O. Wasz-Hockert. 1967. The ability of human mothers to identify the hunger cry signals of their own new-born infants during the lying-in-period. *Experientia* **23**:768–769.

van IJzendoorn, M.H. 1995. Adult attachment representations, parental responsiveness, and infant attachment: A meta-analysis on the predictive validity of Adult Attachment. *Psychonomic Bull.* **117**:387–403.

van Oers, H.J.J., E.R. de Kloet, T. Whelan, and S. Levine. 1998. Maternal deprivation effect on the infant's neural stress markers is reversed by tactile stimulation and feeding but not by suppressing corticosterone. *J. Neurosci.* **18**:10,171–10,179.

Vazquez, D.M., H. van Oers, S. Levine, and H. Akil. 1996. Regulation of the glucocorticoid and mineralocorticoid receptor mRNA in the hippocampus of the maternally deprived infant rat. *Brain Res.* **131**:79–90.

Wang, S. 1997. Traumatic stress and attachment. *Acta Physiologia Scand.* **161**:164–169.

Weinfield, N.S., L.A. Sroufe, and B. Egeland. 2000. Attachment from infancy to early adulthood in a high-risk sample: Continuity, discontinuity, and their correlates. *Development* **71**:695–702.

Wilson, D.A., and R.M. Sullivan. 1994. Review: Neurobiology of associative learning in the neonate: Early olfactory learning. *Behav. Neur. Biol.* **61**:1–18.

Wisenfeld, A., and C.Z. Malatesta. 1982. Infant distress: Variable affecting responses of caregivers and others. In: Parenting: Its Causes and Consequences, ed. L.W. Hoffman, R. Gandelman, and H.R. Schiffman, pp. 123–139. Hillsdale, NJ: Erlbaum.

Young, L.J., M.M. Lim, B. Gingrich, and T.R. Insel. 2001. Cellular mechanisms of social attachment. *Horm. Behav.* **40**:133–148.

9

The Developmental and Evolutionary Psychology of Intergenerational Transmission of Attachment

J. BELSKY

Birkbeck University of London, Institute for the Study of Children,
Families and Social Issues, London WC1B 3RA, U.K.

ABSTRACT

Developmental psychologists studying attachment security have theorized that the parent's security of attachment should be systematically related to the attachment the child establishes with the parent. Thus, a parent who has a secure state of mind regarding attachment is (probabilistically) expected to rear children who develop secure attachments to the parent in question, whereas a parent who has an insecure state of mind regarding attachment is (probabilistically) expected to rear children who develop insecure attachments. What developmentalists have not addressed is *why*, from an evolutionary perspective, one would expect attachment security to be intergenerationally transmitted in the first place. Three plausible answers to this question are thus considered in the first section of this chapter — one suggesting that intergenerational transmission should not be expected, a second suggesting that it should be, and a third suggesting that it both should and should not be. In view of these diverse possibilities, available evidence on the subject of intergenerational transmission is examined. It reveals that even though the parent's state of mind regarding attachment is systematically related to the child's attachment security, the strength of the association is modest. Attention is then turned to various developmental mechanisms which have been found to — or might — account for *how* attachment comes to be transmitted from parent to child. These emphasize the quality of parenting, the general emotional climate of the family, and the parent's capacity to see the child as an individual with a separate mind. The conclusion is drawn that although much still needs to be learned about how attachment is intergenerationally transmitted, the available evidence is consistent with the third evolutionary perspective considered, namely, that in some cases attachment should and in other cases it should not be intergenerationally transmitted. This may be due to the fact that children vary in their susceptibility to rearing influence, such that for some, attachment security will be a function of rearing experience (which is itself probabilistically shaped by parental state of mind regarding attachment), whereas for others it is a function of biological inheritance.

INTRODUCTION

Within the discipline of developmental psychology and the subfield of child development, contemporary theorizing about attachment relations (i.e., about close, emotionally charged, security-inducing bonds between parent and child) grew out of psychoanalytic theory. John Bowlby, the eminent British psychiatrist rightfully regarded as the father of attachment theory, was disaffected with a variety of aspects of Freudian theory. Bowlby was particularly disenchanted with the emphasis in classical psychoanalysis on the importance and developmental influence of the child's fantasy life, regarding as he did the child's actual lived experiences as far more important when it came to understanding the course of individual psychological development. Despite diverging in this and other ways from his original theoretical roots, Bowlby's (1973) ethological theory of attachment which emphasized, among other things, the survival value for the infant of developing a close emotional tie to his/her principle caregiver, nevertheless remained true in certain respects to its psychoanalytic foundation. Most notable for purposes of this chapter is the shared view that, under normal circumstances, the mother integrates her experiences with her child into her pre-existing mental model of close relationships (Fonagy 1999). That is, the mother (unconsciously) interprets the behavior of the child through a lens shaped by her own experiences in close relationships while growing up in her family of origin, especially with her parents. In consequence, her manner of relating to and interacting with her child is presumed to be an expression of her own attachment history.

It is on the basis of this "assimilation" model of mothering that it is postulated — in both psychoanalytic and attachment theory — that the quality of social bonds between child and parent are intergenerationally transmitted (George and Solomon 1999): Parents who have experienced transactions with responsive, accepting attachment figures in childhood are considered to be better able themselves to respond to their own children's distress with empathy and emotional support, in the course of providing nurturing care, than are parents who have not had such developmental experiences. As a result, these parents who were themselves emotionally supported and nurtured as children have children who themselves feel understood, valued, and competent and who have developed positive and secure representations of their parents and their relationships with them. Such thinking led Bowlby (1973, pp. 322–323) to speculate that "the inheritance of mental health and mental ill health through the medium of family microculture…may well be far more important than is their inheritance through the medium of genes."

In this chapter, three major issues are addressed:

1. *Why* intergenerational transmission should or should not be expected to characterize the process of human development.

2. *Whether* there is evidence that individual differences in attachment are transmitted across generations.
3. *How* intergenerational transmission may actually take place.

The first issue pertains to ultimate causation and thus focuses attention on the evolutionary reasons why intergenerational transmission might or might not be expected. The second issue is one of data rather than of theory; thus the second major section of this chapter summarizes what is currently known about whether patterns of attachment are intergenerationally transmitted and, if so, to what extent. The third issue is concerned with proximate causation, and it is such processes that are central to the field of developmental psychology.

THE EVOLUTIONARY PSYCHOLOGY QUESTION: *WHY* ATTACHMENT SHOULD (OR SHOULD NOT) BE INTERGENERATIONALLY TRANSMITTED

It is perhaps not unreasonable to claim that John Bowlby was the first evolutionary psychologist (after Darwin). Trained in traditional psychoanalysis, Bowlby found himself disenchanted with Freud's view that the baby's tie to its mother was a product of, essentially, classical conditioning: Because the mother feeds the baby with her breast, an experience that is inherently pleasurable, the baby comes to associate the positive experience of having its hunger sated with the mother and so comes to develop strong urges to be with the mother (irrespective of its need to feed). Informed as he was by Darwinian thinking, Bowlby posited another cause of the infant's strong tie to its mother — natural selection.

More specifically, Bowlby (1973) argued that in the "environment of evolutionary adaptedness," that is, the ecological conditions under which the human species evolved, infants who were not able to evoke and maintain contact with their mothers were at high risk of an early death (e.g., by failing to maintain thermoregulation, by falling in a fire, by wandering away from the home base and getting lost or eaten by a predator). In contrast, those infants able to call and cling to their mothers, to follow them, and to otherwise attract and maintain their principal caregiver's attention would have been more likely to survive. Their genes, including those responsible for such attachment behaviors, would therefore have passed down through the generations, whereas those infants whose behavioral repertoire did not include such attachment behaviors would have been less successful in passing their biological legacy down the generations. As a result, the human species came to possess a capacity, at the earliest stages of postnatal life, to attract the attention and ministrations of the caregiver, to evoke and maintain contact with the caregiver, and thus to promote parental investment. This, according to Bowlby, is the attachment behavioral system.

Much has changed in evolutionary thinking since the time Bowlby developed attachment theory. Perhaps most notable for purposes of the current analysis is the emphasis on individual reproductive success. Where Bowlby emphasized the importance of behavior that promoted "survival of the species," modern evolutionary thinking regards the reproductive success (rather than survival) of the individual (rather than the species) as central to the process of natural selection. What might be considered striking in light of the dramatic changes that have taken place in thinking about evolution and natural selection since Bowlby first advanced his theory is how little modern evolutionary thinking has shaped developmental psychology, in general, and thinking about attachment, in particular (cf. Belsky [1999] and Simpson [1999] for evidence that things are changing). As a result, while Bowlby, like psychoanalysts before him and even most students of attachment theory today, embraced the notion that attachment would be intergenerationally transmitted and offered explanations of *how* such a transmission process operates (see below), there has been virtually no discussion as to *why*, from an evolutionary perspective, one might expect human developmental processes to evolve to accommodate the intergenerational transmission of attachment in the first place.

A reasonable starting point, however, is Belsky, Steinberg, and Draper's (1991) evolutionary theory of socialization, which conceptualizes individual differences in attachment security (and much more) as part and parcel of evolved and facultatively (i.e., environmentally) shaped reproductive strategies. In attempting to integrate life-history thinking by Darwinian anthropologists with the probabilistic developmental thinking of attachment and social learning theorists, as well as life-course sociologists, Belsky et al. (1991) theorized that attachment may serve as an evolved psychological mechanism by which the developmental experiences of parents that shape their sense of what the inevitably uncertain future will be like are passed on — probabalistically — to children to guide their own developmental trajectory and reproductive strategy (see also Chisholm 1999). Under conditions in which the future is regarded as precarious (i.e., risk and high uncertainty), based upon the experiences of parents and transmitted to children through parenting behavior and the nature of family relationships more generally, the child will (probabilistically) develop an insecure attachment, leading — again probabilistically — to patterns of psychological, behavioral, and even somatic development reflecting a quantity-oriented reproductive strategy, including earlier physical maturation, earlier onset of sexual activity, more mating partners, more offspring, and less parental investment. In contrast, under conditions in which the future is regarded as promising and hopeful (i.e., less risk and uncertainty) based on the experiences of parents, secure attachments will probabilistically develop and this will lead — again probabilistically — to patterns of development reflecting a quality-oriented reproductive strategy, including later physical maturation, later onset of sexual activity, fewer mating partners, fewer offspring, and greater parental investment. To the extent that such reproductive strategies end up reproducing themselves intergenerationally through this process, there would be grounds for expecting the intergenerational transmission of attachment. In actuality, however, it would seem possible to use evolutionary reasoning to advance three somewhat competing ideas about the intergenerational transmission of attachment. Each are considered briefly in turn, one suggesting that intergenerational transmission should be the exception rather than the rule, a second suggesting that intergenerational transmission should be the rule rather than the exception, and a third which postulates that intergenerational transmission of attachment should *and* should not characterize the human condition.

Why Not to Expect Intergenerational Transmission

As will be elaborated below, most students of attachment theory presume that the attachment which the child develops with his/her parent will show evidence of intergenerational transmission because the child's attachment to the parent is assumed to be probabilistically affected by the parent's "state of mind regarding attachment," which is itself probabilistically derived from the parent's own history of attachment dating back to early childhood. In essence, then, attachment theory stipulates, more or less, that the attachment bond between parent and grandparent at the time when the parent was a child will be probabilistically related to the attachment bond that the child establishes with the parent. It seems arguable, from the standpoint of evolutionary thinking, that this should be unlikely, at least if other assumptions of attachment theory are taken into account.

Central to attachment theory is the notion that the attachment which the child establishes to his/her principal caregiver(s) in infancy and early childhood will shape, to some not insubstantial degree, the child's future development, in particular his/her emotional development, social development, and, perhaps in particular, development in close relationships, including parenting behavior in adulthood. If, however, the ultimate goal of all living things is, in general, to maximize reproductive fitness, as currently presumed by modern evolutionary theory, and the nature of one's emotional, social, and especially close-relationship development will play significant roles in the bearing and rearing of offspring, then there are strong grounds for questioning the working hypothesis within attachment theory that attachment security will be transmitted across generations. This is because what it takes to reproduce and rear children successfully to maturity, so that they, too, can eventually reproduce, may be different from one generation to the next.

Imagine, for sake of argument, growing up in a world in which trust, cooperation, and working for the mutual benefit of self and others pays off highly when it comes to successfully bearing and rearing children. Continuing with this thought experiment, imagine just the opposite occurring in the next generation. Perhaps due to war, famine, or a host of other contextual and ecological conditions, it is radical self-centeredness and opportunistic advantage taking which now pays off the most, reproductively speaking. Were this to characterize the life courses of parent and child generations, how could the older parent generation realize its (not necessarily conscious) biological goals (i.e., increased reproductive fitness) if intergenerational transmission was the rule rather than the exception? After all, what "worked" — in terms of promoting reproductive fitness — in one generation would be distinctly different from what would work in the subsequent generation.

On the basis of theory and evidence regarding the developmental sequelae of attachment security, there would be little reason to expect that a secure child who grows up to be a secure parent would be advantaging his/her offspring by transmitting security to them in a world in which *in*security would seem not only to be the norm, but perhaps an advantage. The argument, of course, works the other way around as well. Would a parent who had developed a mistrusting, deceitful, and advantage-taking orientation due to his/her insecure attachment be enhancing the prospects of his/her progeny by intergenerationally transmitting such insecurity if the child was to encounter a substantially different world, one in which trust and working for the mutual benefit of self and others was rewarded — socially, economically, and reproductively?

Although it is truly impossible to know exactly what the environments of evolutionary adaptation were like, it is certainly plausible that ecological circumstances changed substantially over time — due to hostilities (or peacemaking) with neighbors, patterns of migration, and the weather, among other factors — so that what worked in terms of promoting reproductive success for one generation simply would not necessarily do so for the next. Were this commonly the case, it is hard to see that the benefits of intergenerational transmission would have outweighed its costs with sufficient frequency such that natural selection would have shaped the process of human development to foster intergenerational transmission. Consistent with attachment theory, this analysis presumes, of course, that the intergenerational transmission process is experiential (rather than genetic) and that early attachment does indeed shape emotional, social, and especially close-relationship development.

Why to Expect Intergenerational Transmission

Once we entertain the proposition that a core assumption built into the preceding analysis may be factually wrong — something that we simply do not and cannot know — the evolutionary analysis of intergenerational transmission changes dramatically, and that potentially mistaken presumption concerns the stability of contextual conditions across *adjacent* generations. Because it seems conceivable that stability of such conditions across such modest time spans would have been more the rule rather than the exception in the long period of time that it took evolution to sculpt human development, there are (bio)logical grounds for challenging the analysis offered in the preceding section as to why we should not expect there to be intergenerational transmission.

Contrary to the earlier analysis, if we assume that contextual and ecological conditions were far more stable than unstable across adjacent generations, then intergenerationally transmitting attachment might make evolutionary sense. A parent who has developed an insecure orientation toward attachments, based upon early and later experiences in life, especially with parents and other close relationships, might reap rewards in terms of increased reproductive fitness if such an orientation could be intergenerationally transmitted through experiential mechanisms. After all, if that orientation — or some other, including its opposite — reflected the best developmental fit which this individual could make to the context of development, why would not that be the case for his/her offspring as well, especially if that child's context of development were going to be reasonably similar to that of the parent? In other words, if one assumes that adjacent generations were substantially more rather than less likely to develop under similar ecological conditions in Bowlby's (1973) environment of evolutionary adaptation, then natural selection may have designed an attachment system so that it could be intergenerationally transmitted through environmental means (rather than through direct biological inheritance).

It should be noted that it may be just because perfect stability in contextual conditions did not characterize the ancestral environments of humans that natural selection designed an attachment system that could be intergenerationally transmitted via experiential processes. After all, that way there could be some flexibility in the system when contextual conditions changed markedly, even if not routinely, between adjacent generations, so that intergenerational transmission no longer operated as might typically be the case.

Why Both Views May Be Correct

Implicit in the preceding analyses, as well as in almost all research on attachment, is the notion that all infants and children are affected by the quality of care they receive — and in the same manner and to the same degree. Although, when pushed, most developmentalists would probably eschew this view and call attention to noteworthy work on gene–environment or treatment–X–aptitude interactions as evidence to the contrary, there is very little developmental theory which explicitly contends that children *should* vary in their susceptibility to rearing, especially children within a family. However, were it the case that only some children were expected to be affected by their rearing and others not (or at least less so), then one might expect, derivatively, that in some cases attachment should be intergenerationally transmitted whereas in other cases it should not (and for reasons different than those just delineated, having to do with [infrequently] changing ecological conditions across adjacent generations).

The fact that the future is uncertain dictates, from both an evolutionary and financial perspective, that hedged bets and thus diversification of investments tend to optimize long-term returns. This suggests that it may make biological and developmental sense for parents to bear progeny who are more and less susceptible to rearing influence and thus more and less likely to show evidence of the intergenerational transmission of attachment. After all, if all children in a family were equally affected by their parents' proclivities to have them develop and behave in one way or another, then families, and parental reproductive success, would face devastation if, for reasons that could not have been anticipated nor controlled, those ways proved to be highly counterproductive in the future.

Consider as a dramatic example of such a process the killing fields of Cambodia. Among the first to be consigned to an early death once the Khmer Rouge came to power following the withdrawal of American forces from Southeast Asia in the last century were individuals who wore glasses or otherwise appeared to be educated (e.g., smooth rather than calloused hands) or were known to be highly educated. It is likely that those who were educated had been encouraged to pursue education by their parents. Here we have a clear case of something highly valued and promoted by parents leading to a literal biological dead end. Were there some children in such families who resisted parental entreaties to become educated, chances of survival in the face of the uncertain future that turned out to be the killing fields of Cambodia would have been measurably increased relative to siblings who were highly susceptible to the rearing influences of their parents and pursued (successfully) a formal education.

Although this is a rather dramatic example of how, in the face of an ever uncertain future, the reproductive success of individual parents might benefit from children not all being equally susceptible to the rearing influence of parents, it serves to make the point that, from an evolutionary perspective, natural selection may have shaped parents to bear children who differ in how responsive they are to parental behavior (or at least some parental behaviors) because of the extremely high (biological) costs (in terms of reproductive fitness) of not doing so. Because the future is inherently uncertain, the goals that parents have for their children, whether held consciously or unconsciously, could turn out to have huge reproductive costs if (a) realized by all their children and (b) future conditions turn out to be highly unlike those that parents, again consciously or unconsciously, anticipate. For this reason it seems to make evolutionary sense for children, especially within a family, to vary in their susceptibility to parental rearing (or at least some aspects of it), with some being highly responsive and others being less responsive and perhaps not responsive at all. A growing body of evidence, which is not inconsistent with this view, suggests interestingly that it may be highly negatively emotional infants who are most susceptible to parental influence — for better (when receiving emotionally supportive care) or for worse (when receiving less supportive care), at least with respect to certain developmental outcomes (for a review, see Belsky 1999).

This latter observation raises the possibility that children may differ more generally in their susceptibility to aspects of parental behavior and rearing. Whereas one child might be more susceptible to emotional socialization, for example, and another less so, susceptibility could conceiveably be different with respect to the development of athletic prowess or some other behavioral development. In other words, this discussion of the possibility that children differ in their susceptibility to rearing should not (necessarily) be read to imply that some children are more and less susceptible to all aspects of rearing and all aspects of development.

If, in fact, children do vary in their susceptibility to rearing influence, whether due to forces of natural selection as argued by Belsky (1999, 2000) or for other reasons, then one would not necessarily expect the intergenerational transmission of attachment to be the norm. This is because, as will be shown below, the intergenerational transmission process is currently understood to be mediated by the quality of care that parents provide their children and its effect upon attachment security. In sum, it can be argued, from an evolutionary perspective, that the intergenerational transmission process should *and* should not characterize the process of human development. That is, it should characterize it for some individuals who are more susceptible to rearing influence (at least with respect to attachment), but not for others who are less susceptible to rearing influence. Below, evidence pertaining to the actual degree of documented intergenerational transmission is considered.

A QUESTION OF DATA: IS ATTACHMENT INTERGENERATIONALLY TRANSMITTED?

Within the field of child development, students of attachment theory have examined questions of intergenerational transmission by determining the extent to which assessments of infant–mother attachment security made during infancy or early childhood are related to parents' state of mind regarding attachment. Before examining the findings of this body of research, it is necessary to review the primary methods by which attachment in infancy and in adulthood has been assessed.

Measuring Attachment Security in Infants and Adults

The development of methods to assess infant attachment security occurred well before methods of measuring state of mind regarding attachment in adults. The development of the latter measurements, however, were very much informed by the former, as should become apparent when each set of assessments is described.

Infant Attachment Security

Infant and even early childhood assessments are based on the classic work of Ainsworth and Wittig (1969) who developed a laboratory procedure known as the Strange Situation, which was designed to exert an increasing amount of mild stress on the infant and, thereby, arouse the attachment behavioral system and evoke attachment behavior. This is accomplished by exposing the child to a series of progressive stressors: an unfamiliar place, an unfamiliar person, separations from parent/caregiver, and the experience of being alone. On two occasions following separation, the child is reunited with the parent.

To evaluate the child's attachment security based upon his/her behavior in the Strange Situation, the videotape of the procedure is carefully examined and ratings are made of each of the eight distinct episodes (e.g., mother and child together, child and stranger, child alone), of the degree to which the child seeks proximity with the caregiver (e.g., follows, moves toward), maintains physical contact with the caregiver (e.g., clings), avoids the caregiver (e.g., averts gaze, moves away), resists contact with the caregiver (e.g., pushes away), and evinces distress. In determining an infant's categorical attachment status, emphasis is placed on the infant's behavior with the caregiver during the two reunion episodes (i.e., episodes 5 and 8), although the organization of the infant's behavior during and across all eight episodes of the Strange Situation is taken into account.

Important to appreciate is that eventual classifications of security of attachment or insecurity is not a direct function of the degree to which the child becomes distressed, as both secure and insecure infants can evince high and low levels of negative emotion in the Strange Situation. Of critical importance is how the infant co-regulates his/her emotions and behavior with the caregiver. Having said this, it needs to be pointed out that the behavior of the parent in the Strange Situation is purposefully controlled (via directions to her), and it is only the behavior of the child that is used to appraise the child's attachment security. As such, the Strange Situation does not provide an evaluation of the mother's bond to the baby nor of the relationship as an entity in and of itself. What is being evaluated instead is the child's attachment to his mother and thus the security/insecurity of the relationship as experienced by the child.

Infants who are classified as *secure* typically use the caregiver as a secure base for exploring the environment. If distressed, secure infants actively seek proximity and contact with the caregiver and are comforted by the caregiver. If not overtly distressed, secure infants explore toys avidly and actively engage in affective sharing and interaction with the caregiver (e.g., showing toys, vocalizing, smiling). In contrast, infants categorized as *insecure-avoidant* engage in little affective sharing with the caregiver, show little preference for the caregiver over the stranger, and actively avoid and exhibit neutral or dampened affect with the caregiver on reunion. Infants categorized as *insecure-resistant* exhibit impoverished exploration, are vigilant of the caregiver's whereabouts, wary of the stranger, and tend to become highly distressed during separation. Upon reunion with the caregiver, insecure-resistant infants typically mix contact seeking with contact resistance and have difficulty settling; for this reason, they are sometimes labeled insecure-ambivalent. In most samples studied around the world, and there have now been thousands of children observed in the Strange Situation as part of published scientific reports, approximately two-thirds to three-quarters of children are classified as secure, with about twice as many typically classified as insecure-avoidant as insecure-resistant (van IJzendoorn and Kroonenberg 1988). Some have questioned the wisdom of scoring security categorically rather than continuously (Fraley and Spieker 2003).

Adult State of Mind regarding Attachment

When it comes to assessing state of mind regarding, or internal working models of, attachment in adulthood, two general approaches have been used: one by developmental psychologists interested in issues like parenting and intergenerational transmission, and the other by social psychologists with primary interest in romantic relationships. The former approach involves a lengthy clinical interview, called the Adult Attachment Interview (AAI), whereas the second involves a brief series of forced-choice questions (designed for use in survey research) and is thus far less time consuming. Because the two approaches do not yield identical results and the more intensive approach has been central to the study of intergenerational transmission, it is this one that will be described.

The AAI consists of 18 questions and is structured entirely around the topic of attachment, principally the individual's relationship to the mother and father during childhood (see Hesse 1999). Interviewees are instructed to describe their relationships with their parents and to provide specific biographical episodes to substantiate global evaluations. Thus, if an individual reports that the parent was very generous or highly affectionate, he is asked to recall specific incidents of such behavior. Interviewees are asked directly about childhood experiences of rejection, being upset, ill, and hurt, as well as about loss, abuse, and separations. They are also asked to offer explanations for parents' behavior and to describe the current relationships with their parents and the influence they consider their childhood experiences exerted on their development. The interview is designed not so much to evoke the adult's actual, veridical experiences in childhood but, rather, their reconstructions of the meaning and mental representations of early experiences.

The tape-recorded interview is transcribed by a typist and, on the basis of the information obtained from the AAI, a specially trained evaluator rates the subject on a series of rating scales (e.g., role reversal: the extent to which the respondent parented the parent during childhood; idealization: the extent to which the respondent idealizes his/her parent(s); preoccupying anger: the extent to which the respondent is still very angry at the parent; inability to recall: the extent to which the respondent cannot remember events and experiences from childhood). These ratings, coupled with the evaluator's general sense of the entire transcript, especially how coherent (i.e., organized and integrated) it is, leads the evaluator to characterize the respondent's state of mind regarding attachment (i.e., internal working model) using a limited set of classification categories. Ultimately, the coding of AAI transcripts is based not on the participant's description of childhood experiences per se, but on the way in which these experiences and their effects on current functioning are reflected on and evaluated. It is significant that attachment classifications based on the AAI have been found to be independent of general intelligence and verbal ability (see Hesse 1999).

The *secure-autonomous* state of mind is reflected in an individual's inclination to value attachment relationships and regard attachment-related experiences as developmentally influential. In the course of the AAI, such persons appear self reliant, objective, and nondefensive. It is noteworthy that persons receiving this classification either convincingly describe a history of emotionally supportive relationship experiences or provide evidence that they have come to terms with a childhood lacking in them, thus permitting a balanced view of relationships.

Adults classified as *insecure-dismissing* have a tendency to deny negative experiences and emotions or to dismiss their developmental significance. These individuals can remember little and seem unable to re-evoke the feelings associated with the experiences they do recall. Often they offer an idealized picture of parent or parents but, in response to probes eliciting evidence to substantiate generalizations, may recall experiences quite inconsistent with their positive, global appraisals. For example, in response to a follow-up query from the interview asking for details about how a parent was generous, the respondent ends up talking about a parent's failure to attend their birthday party or their disappointment with a present received from a parent. Insecure-dismissing individuals present themselves as strong, independent people for whom closeness and attachment mean little. The defensive flavor of the detached pattern is reminiscent of the insecure-avoidant infant pattern.

Adults classified as *insecure-preoccupied* demonstrate a continuing involvement of preoccupation with their parents. They appear confused, incoherent, and unobjective regarding relationships and their influences upon them. Anger over the past and present seems not to be resolved but, instead, to be a major organizing theme of their relationships with their parents. These individuals seem caught up in their early relationships with little ability to move beyond them.

Concordance of Adult and Child Attachment

From a conceptual standpoint, attachment classifications based on the Strange Situation and the AAI have much in common, with the child's attachment manifested in attachment behavior (i.e., proximity seeking, contact maintaining, avoidance of contact, resistance of contact) and the adult's attachment manifested in verbal representation. More specifically and with respect to the balance between exploration and attachment, children who are attached avoidantly to their parents minimize or deactivate attachment behavior, whereas ambivalently attached children maximize or amplify attachment behavior at the expense of exploration. Securely attached children strike a balance between attachment behavior (e.g., seeking comfort) immediately after reunion and return to exploration after some time. Similarly, the AAI classifications are based on verbal communications about emotions in attachment relations. Autonomous individuals are characterized by an open and unbiased reflection on their attachment experiences, dismissing individuals minimize the influence of early attachment experiences on their adult personalities, and preoccupied individuals are still absorbed with their childhood experiences or the present relationship with their parents.

Theoretically, it is anticipated that a parent's state of mind regarding attachment, as measured in the AAI, should be probabilistically related to the security of attachment which the child establishes with the parent, as assessed in the Strange Situation. As will become apparent when we consider the developmental psychology question, "How is attachment transmitted across generations?," students of attachment theory presume that the anticipated association between parent and child attachment is mediated principally, if not exclusively, by the quality of parenting experienced by the child, as the parent's state of mind regarding attachment shapes parenting which, in turn, shapes the child's attachment security.

To determine whether, and to which extent, attachment might be intergenerationally transmitted, van IJzendoorn (1995) carried out a meta-analysis of research in which both adult and child attachment were measured, drawing upon 18 samples included in 14 studies, which collectively comprised 854 parent–child dyads. Although most studies were restricted to mother and child, some focused upon fathers. To be noted, as well, is that at least one study was restricted to adolescent mothers, though others focused upon economically disadvantaged families. In some studies, data collected on adult attachment were measured many months before the child's attachment was assessed, in fact, before the child was even born, though this was not routinely the case. The general proposition guiding the meta-analysis was that autonomous parents would rear children who developed secure attachments, whereas children of dismissing and preoccupied parents would develop insecure-avoidant and insecure-resistant attachments, respectively.

As a first step in exploring this prediction, van IJzendoorn (1995) tested whether security/insecurity of parental attachment was related to security/insecurity of child attachment, irrespective of the manner in which insecurity was manifest (i.e., dismissing/avoidant or preoccupied/resistant). The relation between parent and child attachment proved "quite strong" (p. 392), with parent attachment accounting for 22% of the variance in child attachment (or 35% on the basis of a biserial correlation). Follow-up analyses revealed that the intergenerational association of attachment was stronger for mothers (effect size

$d = 1.14$, $r = 0.50$) than for fathers ($d = 0.80$, $r = 0.37$), though not generally affected by variation in other study design features (e.g., whether adult attachment was measured before, at the same time, or after child attachment; age of child).

As a second step in his meta-analysis, van IJzendoorn (1995) focused upon the dismissing/resistant attachment classification, finding that dismissing attachment in the parent predicted insecure-avoidant attachment in the child ($d = 1.02$, $r = 0.45$). Once again, the cross-generational association varied by parent, with maternal dismissing attachment more strongly related to children's avoidance ($d = 1.17$, $r = 0.50$) than paternal dismissing attachment ($d = 0.68$, $r = 0.32$). When the meta-analysis focused upon the preoccupied/resistant association, evidence emerged, consistent with expectations, that preoccupied parents were disproportionately likely to have children with insecure-resistant attachments ($d = 0.93$, $r = 0.42$). Finally, when a single analysis, which included 661 cases in which both the three-category AAI and 3-category Strange Situation scoring systems were utilized, was conducted to determine the extent to which autonomous, dismissing, and preoccupied AAI classifications predicted, *respectively*, secure, insecure-avoidant, and insecure-resistant classifications in the Strange Situation, a 70% rate of adult–child attachment concordance was discerned.

In sum, the results of this meta-analysis provide clear evidence of concordance of parent and child attachment and thus of the intergenerational transmission of attachment — via mechanisms that remain to be explored — in contemporary Western society. What remains unknown, of course, is the extent to which — if at all — the aforementioned findings would be replicated if parents and children from dramatically different societies were the subject of study. In any event, because concordance was by no means perfect, it would be inappropriate to conclude that intergenerational transmission of attachment is inevitable. The findings remain noteworthy, nevertheless, not only because they are consistent with theory, but because of the dramatic differences in the way in which parent and child attachment are assessed. Recall that whereas the measurement of adult attachment is based upon a semi-structured interview involving the coding of discourse characteristics, the assessment of child attachment is based upon a structured laboratory procedure involving the coding of infants' behavioral responses to reunions with their attachment figure.

THE DEVELOPMENTAL PSYCHOLOGY QUESTION: HOW IS ATTACHMENT INTERGENERATIONALLY TRANSMITTED?

Now that it has been demonstrated that there is a substantial degree of intergenerational transmission of attachment in contemporary Western society, consideration is turned to the question of mechanisms that could account for how such transmission takes place. As mentioned earlier, when discussing evolutionary rationales as to why intergenerational transmission should and/or should not characterize human development, a central assumption of contemporary attachment theory is that the process of intergenerational transmission is experiential in nature. More specifically, students of attachment theory presume, consistent with Bowlby's (1973) aforementioned emphasis on the microculture of the family, (a) that the quality of parenting which the child experiences strongly influences whether a young child establishes a secure or insecure attachment to his/her parent; (b) that security/insecurity established in the early years remains more or less stable over time (unless contextual conditions change markedly, as development remains an open-ended process), thereby leading to security or insecurity in adulthood; and (c) that security/insecurity in adulthood shapes parenting behavior specifically and perhaps family relationships more generally and, thereby, fosters security/insecurity in offspring. As we will see shortly, there is an abundance of evidence, obtained in mostly modern Western societies, that is consistent with this most general developmental model.

The fact that most, if not all, of the relevant evidence is correlational in nature means that the drawing of any causal inferences from the results of even longitudinal studies is precarious at best. Indeed, in the face of an ever-burgeoning behavior-genetic literature, which indicates that genetic variation makes a substantial contribution to phenotypic variation for virtually all behavioral domains, there are certainly grounds for questioning the presumed environmentally mediated processes postulated by attachment theorists to account for the already documented concordance in attachment security across generations. After all, it could be the case that the evidence cited below, highlighting environmental and specifically parenting "influences" on the development of attachment security and thus environmental explanations of the intergenerational transmission of attachment, is little more than heritability masquerading as rearing effects. The same genes that shape adult attachment could shape child attachment and even parenting as well as other family processes presumed to account for intergenerational concordance in attachment security.

Until recently, there was rather limited evidence on this subject, given that so few studies have been conducted of the attachments that twins or even siblings forge with their parents. That is, most attachment research has not incorporated genetically informed research designs, but rather has focused upon one child in a family. The few investigations that have included twins have been relatively small in terms of sample sizes. In perhaps the first test of the heritability of attachment security, Ricciuti (1992) combined data from three such twin samples and, after comparing concordance of attachment security across monozygotic and dizygotic twins, concluded that attachment security was not demonstrably heritable, at least in the case of 12–22 month olds. More recently, O'Connor and Croft (2001) employed behavior-genetic modeling of attachment data collected on 110 identical and fraternal twin pairs seen in the Strange Situation as preschoolers and detected only modest genetic influence, but substantial environmental influence.

The largest and most comprehensive study of the heritability of attachment security conducted to date provides further evidence of the disproportionate role of environmental factors in shaping attachment security. Indeed, when Bokhorst and associates (2004) subjected to analysis data on more than 150 pairs of twins seen in the Strange Situation as infants, they discovered that biological inheritance did not play a role in determining whether children were classified as secure or insecure in their attachment to mother, or even whether children evinced high or low levels of avoidance and resistance, two key aspects of behavior central to determining a child's attachment classification (and especially type of insecure attachment). More specifically, 52% of the variance in attachment security was explained by shared environmental influences and 48% by unique environmental influence and measurement error. Unpublished analyses that also included data on siblings and unrelated pairs of children further revealed (a) that in the case of avoidant and resistant behavior, 98% of the variance was explained by shared environment and (b) that similar findings highlighting the role of shared environment and very little evidence of genetic effects emerged when the focus of attention was security (vs. insecurity) of attachment to father, as measured not by the Strange Situation, but using q-sort methodology in which the baby's behavior toward the father was reported by mother.

In light of this evidence, which indicates that attachment security, at least in the early years, is not principally, if at all, heritable, this alternative explanation of the intergenerational transmission of attachment can be largely discounted. This, of course, leaves us to consider in more detail the developmental mechanisms that might explain how attachment in the parent, as measured using the AAI, comes to be systematically related to the infant/child's attachment to his/her parent, as measured by means of the Strange Situation. Below, we consider evidence pertaining to the several steps in the developmental process that is widely presumed by students of attachment theory to account for intergenerational transmission. For purposes of this analysis, the following terms need to be defined: "G1" will refer to the parent generation and "G2" to the child generation. Thus, "G2 security" refers to the attachment security of the child. Attachment security will be labeled as "early" or "later," in order to distinguish the security of the child early in life from the security of the teenager/adult later in life.

Step 1: G1Early Security → G1Later Security → G2Early Security

Evidence summarized above showing that adult working models of attachment, as measured by means of the AAI, are systematically related to the attachments that children establish with these adults (i.e., G1Later Security → G2Early Security) has been interpreted as evidence of the intergenerational transmission of attachment. To substantiate this interpretation, especially in its standard version, which presumes that adult internal working models themselves derive from childhood histories of security/insecurity, it needs to be demonstrated that adult working models of attachment are themselves systematically related to the security of attachment during childhood. Until very recently, this has been impossible to demonstrate, if only because of the constraints of time. After all, longitudinal studies measuring attachment security in infancy were only initiated in the mid- to late 1970s, so before the issue of whether attachment security in infancy and/or childhood was related to internal working models of attachment in adulthood could be researched, enough time had to pass for children participating in longitudinal studies to grow up.

Fraley (2002) recently subjected to meta-analysis data on 218 cases, drawn from five longitudinal studies which, to date, have presented data directly pertaining to cross-time linkages in attachment assessments. The participants in these investigations were seen in the Strange Situation when 12 months of age and then assessed using the AAI at ages ranging from 16–21 years. Stability coefficients ranged from a low of –0.14 to a high of 0.50 in the individual studies, yielding a weighted (for sample size) cross-time correlation of 0.27 (and an unweighted correlation of 0.30). These data, along with related data included in the meta-analysis from many more individual studies pertaining to attachment stability across much shorter time intervals (e.g., from 1.0 to 1.5 years of age, from 1.0 to 6 years of age), led Fraley (2002, p. 135) to conclude that "there is a moderate degree of stability in attachment from infancy to adulthood."

When it comes to making meaning of these results, one is left wondering what to make of evidence of "moderate" stability. For some, especially devotees of attachment theory, the glass of stability will surely be regarded as "half full," whereas for others, it will be regarded as "half empty." In considering the relative modesty of the stability coefficient from infancy to young adulthood, it must be appreciated that even Bowlby (1973) contended that experiences subsequent to infancy and early childhood could modify earlier established developmental trajectories. Thus, one should not necessarily expect very high levels of stability, except perhaps in the most stable of environments.

To explore this issue, Fraley (2002) tested the hypothesis that cross-time continuity would be attenuated under conditions of relational discord, economic hardship, and child abuse, after categorizing studies in terms of whether they focused upon high- or low-risk samples. Results indicated, as expected, that under the aforementioned conditions presumed to disrupt parent–child relations, stability was substantially attenuated. More specifically, the point-biserial correlation between the risk status of the study sample (i.e., $0 = $ low, $1 = $ high) and the stability-of-attachment coefficient of the individual study was –0.23, indicating that study samples characterized by such risk factors exhibited less stability than did other study samples. In fact, whereas the stability coefficient for the subset of samples classified as at-risk was 0.27, the corresponding figure was almost twice as large (i.e., 0.48) for samples not so classified. Such results led Fraley (2002, p. 138) to conclude that "environmental risks and changes appear to reduce the degree to which people can exert an influence on their environment but do not appear to alter the underlying dynamics of continuity and change."

Step 2: G1Early Security → G1Later Security → G1Sensitive Parenting →
G2Early Security

The fact that early security predicts later security and that later security (in the parent generation, G1) predicts child security (i.e., G2) raises a second process-oriented question: How does security in the parent lead to security in the child? As already noted, central to attachment theory is the proposition that it is via the quality of care that the parent provides on a day-to-day basis that adult state of mind regarding attachment comes to be related to child attachment. More specifically, it is the sensitive responsiveness of parental care that is theorized to mediate the association between G1Later Security and G2Early Security. Evidence pertaining to this process is discussed below delineating the link between adult attachment and parenting, the link between the quality of mothering and the security of the child, and actual mediation.

G1Later Security → G1Sensitive Parenting

Because attachment theory posits (a) that the primary determinant of whether a child establishes a secure or insecure attachment to his/her parent is the child's day-to-day experience in being cared for by the parent and (b) that attachment security is, in the main, intergenerationally transmitted, it was not very much of a theoretic leap to hypothesize that adult state of mind regarding attachment should predict parenting. Van IJzendoorn (1995) assembled data from ten studies, which included 389 parent–child dyads to subject this core theoretical proposition to meta-analysis. Each of the investigations included in the meta-analysis measured adult attachment by means of the AAI and obtained some index of parenting theorized to be related to the child's attachment security. Thus, some investigators assessed the extent to which parents provided help and comfort to a stressed child, behaved in confusing/controlling ways, and/or were sensitive or supportive or warm in their interactions with the child, whereas other researchers measured the parents' expressions of positive and negative affect, their flexibility, involvement, and/or organization. Some of these investigations gathered parenting data when mothers were at home going about their everyday household routines, whereas others studied parenting after mothers had been instructed to read their child a story, help him with a drawing, or just play with the child, either in the home or in the laboratory.

Consistent with theoretical expectations, van IJzendoorn (1995) found that effects sizes for the relation between parental attachment representations and parental responsiveness/support/sensitivity ranged from $d = 0.35$ ($r = 0.17$) to $d = 1.37$ ($r = 0.57$), yielding a combined effect size of $d = 0.72$ ($r = 0.34$). The association proved sufficiently robust that it was concluded that it would take more than 155 studies with null results to bring the collective effect size down to a level of statistical insignificance. Parental attachment appeared to account for about 12% of the variation in parental responsiveness. In sum, then, parents classified as autonomous-secure on the AAI evinced (somewhat and significantly) greater parental responsiveness, sensitivity, and supportiveness when interacting with their infants and young children than did parents classified as dismissing or preoccupied.

G1Sensitive Parenting → *G2Early Security*

Linkages between parenting and the child's attachment to his/her parents have been investigated for more than three decades now. The theoretical proposition guiding this work is that secure attachment is fostered when parents provide sensitive responsive care to their infants and young children, whereas the provision of harsh, interfering, unresponsive, or inconsistently responsive care promotes attachment insecurity. A meta-analysis of correlational evidence, collected as part of 66 studies involving more than 4,000 cases, provides indisputable support for this claim (De Wolff and van IJzendoorn 1997). When the analysis was restricted to 21 studies involving more than 1,000 mother–infant dyads, which used the Strange Situation to assess infant–mother attachment security and measured maternal sensitivity either concurrently or at some point prior to the attachment assessment, a "moderately strong" effect size was detected of maternal sensitivity on infant attachment security ($r = 0.24$). Importantly, the effects of mothering on attachment security did not vary as a function of how maternal behavior or mother–infant interaction was measured. Investigations focused upon interactional synchrony, mutuality in the interaction, emotional support, positive attitudes, and stimulation all revealed, in the main, the theoretically anticipated association. Further, a follow-up meta-analysis of a smaller number of studies ($n = 8$) comprising more than 500 cases revealed the anticipated association between parenting and infant attachment when the focus was upon fathering and the infant–father relationship, though it was somewhat smaller than that for mother and infant ($r = 0.13$) (van IJzendoorn and De Wolff 1997).

The fact that the data subject to analysis in the meta-analyses was correlational in nature does not afford the drawing of strong causal conclusions. After all, infant behavior that is either a reflection of attachment security or a direct contributor to attachment security could influence the quality of parenting, leaving open the possibility that the results of the meta-analysis reflect as much the impact of security on parenting as the reverse. Fortunately, a related meta-analysis of experimental studies designed to promote attachment security yields evidence that systematic and theoretically guided manipulations of infants' experiences do, in fact, contribute to attachment in an indisputably causal manner (van IJzendoorn et al. 1995). So, too, does a recently published updating of this meta-analysis (Bakermans-Kranenburg et al. 2003). Perhaps the most compelling evidence that this is so comes from van den Boom's (1994) experimental manipulation of mothering, which revealed that efforts to foster maternal responsiveness to both positive and negative infant cues not only succeeded in promoting maternal sensitivity, but infant–mother attachment security as well. That is, although low-income Dutch mothers of irritable infants randomly assigned to experimental and control groups did not differ in the quality of their parenting when observed prior to the experimental treatment at six months of age, the experimental mothers evinced greater sensitivity than the controls at nine months of age following a brief intervention geared toward promoting maternal sensitivity. Moreover, when infants were seen in the Strange Situation at 12 months of age, the rate of security in the experimental group was almost three times greater than that of the control group (62% vs. 22%)!

The Mediational Role of Maternal Sensitivity

Having discovered that adult attachment predicts mothering and that mothering predicts infant attachment security, the fundamental question of mediation remains, as construct A (i.e., G1Security) could predict construct B (i.e., mothering) and construct B could predict construct C (i.e., G2Security) without construct B actually mediating the association between A and C. To address this issue, van IJzendoorn (1995) built upon his aforementioned meta-analyses which chronicled linkages (a) between adult and child attachment and (b) between adult attachment and parenting. More specifically, he integrated his meta-analytic results and found that a correlation of 0.47 characterizes the combined direct and indirect effect of state of mind regarding attachment on the attachment security of the child, with about 25% of that total explained by the mediational effect of sensitive-responsive parenting. Were the data assembled by van IJzendoorn (1995) adjusted to take into account De Wolff and van IJzendoorn's (1997) more recent estimate of the magnitude of the relation between parental sensitive responsiveness and child attachment security, somewhat less than 20% of the total effect of parental attachment on child attachment would be accounted for by parenting, at least as measured in most studies examining the origins of attachment security in infancy and childhood. Although neither of these figures estimating the magnitude of the mediational effect of parenting is particularly large, the fact that they are substantially greater than zero confirms the theoretical expectation that G1Later Security → Sensitive-Responsive Parenting → G2Early Security.

Step 3: The Transmission Gap and Additional Mediators

Although van IJzendoorn (1995) found in his meta-analysis that maternal sensitivity mediated the relation between parental and infant attachment security, he drew attention to the presence of a "transmission gap." That is, most of the interrelation between parent and child attachment could not be accounted for by the theorized mediator, maternal sensitivity. This gap seems even larger now that behavior-genetic research indicates that attachment is only modestly, if at all, heritable, as it remained possible in the face of van IJzendoorn's (1995) findings that shared genes might be responsible for the overlap in parent and infant attachment not explained by maternal sensitivity. As that seems less likely now, two additional processes which might account for some part of the transmission gap are considered.

Mind-mindedness

In seeking to further illuminate the determinants of child attachment security, Meins and her associates (2001) have recently highlighted a developmental mechanism in addition to maternal sensitivity, which they label "mind mindedness," to account for at least some of van IJzendoorn's (1995) transmission gap, though these investigators have yet to test its role in bridging the gap. Moreover, this mechanism has not been investigated in non-Western cultures so it remains unclear the extent to which the results to be considered are generalized beyond current study populations. Nevertheless, what Meins et al. (2001) discovered is that this potential mediator between parent and child attachment, when measured at six months of age, is related to the infant's security measured in the Strange Situation six months later, even with maternal sensitivity taken into account, thus affording it credibility as a plausible additional mediator.

Because Ainsworth (1973) originally emphasized not just prompt responsiveness to the infant's cues and needs in her conception of sensitivity, but also *appropriate* responsiveness, Meins et al. (2001) postulated, as did Ainsworth, that the mother's capacity to see things from the child's point of view and to regard the child as a separate person — that is, mind-mindedness — might be especially important to the developing child's attachment security. According to Meins et al., a mother who evinces mind-mindedness is inclined "to treat her infant as an individual with a mind, rather than merely as a creature with needs that must be satisfied" (p. 638).

Support for the Meins et al. (2001) hypothesis that mind-mindedness contributes to the development of attachment security comes from work showing that mothers of secure infants are more likely than mothers of insecure infants to make appropriate mind-minded comments when interacting with their infants. Such comments take the form of maternal remarks about the child's mental state during the course of interaction that seem appropriately reflective of that state. Thus, highly mind-minded mothers make comments about the infant's psychological state that are consistent — rather than at odds — with the infant's mood, behavior, and/or desire (e.g., kicking feet to signal desire to be put down when held); make comments that link current activity with similar events in the past or future (e.g., "Do you remember seeing this toy before?"); and/or make comments that serve to clarify how to proceed when there is a lull in the interaction between mother and child (e.g., "Do you want to look at posters?" after the infant had been gazing around the room and not focused upon anything for a period of time). In contrast, mothers showing low levels of mind-mindedness make comments that misinterpret the child's psychological state (e.g., stating that the infant is bored with a toy when he/she is still actively engaged in playing with it); make comments which refer to past or future events that have no obvious relation to ongoing events; and/or endeavor to redirect the child's attention and activity when the child appears clearly interested in on-going events.

In sum, Meins et al.'s work clearly demonstrates — at least in the restricted samples studied to date — that the mother's capacity to represent the mental and emotional state of her infant contributes to the infant's security. As such, it could play a role in the transmission of attachment security from one generation to the next, should future work further reveal mind-mindedness to be related to adult attachment.

Marital Quality and the Emotional Atmosphere of the Home

Whether one considers maternal sensitivity or mind-mindedness, the emphasis through this point in explaining the intergenerational tranmission process has been on the infant's direct experience *in interaction with* the mother. It seems reasonable, however, that attachment security could also be affected by the more general emotional atmosphere of the home in which a child develops (or even in the surrounding communal living arrangements in societies that are less nuclear-family oriented). It is not difficult to imagine, for example, how a home characterized by frequent, intense, and loud conflicts could be emotionally distressing to a child and, thereby, undermine his felt security, including the security of his attachment to mother or father. Indeed, Davies and Cummings (1994) advanced their "emotional security hypothesis" in support of such a view. This hypothesis stipulates, among other things, that a child's sense of security is not exclusively rooted in his interactions with parents, as assumed by attachment theory. Rather, children also develop their own specific sense of security in the context of the interparental relationship that is distinct from the effects of interparental relationships on parenting. Growing up in a household in which parents have a harmonious loving relationship should directly foster emotional security in the child, whereas being raised in one in which parents are constantly squabbling or refusing to communicate with one another should instead promote insecurity. Of note is that this view (i.e., the quality of the marital relationship could directly affect the child's felt security) grew out of extensive research showing that marital conflict is distressingly arousing to children, especially when it is frequent, intense, and remains unresolved (for a review, see Cummings and Davies 1994).

Although there has been no research linking marital conflict, marital quality, or the more general emotional climate of the home directly to the intergenerational transmission of attachment, it seems reasonable to posit such a process in view of the fact that (a) the quality of the marriage is associated with adult attachment, (b) the quality of the marriage is associated with infant–parent attachment, and (c) the quality of the marriage is associated with the very qualities of parenting known to predict attachment security (i.e., sensitive responsiveness). Illustrative evidence of the first point can be found in work showing that individuals with secure working models, as measured by the AAI, exhibit better functioning in marital or romantic relationships than those individuals with an insecure attachment, as revealed by patterns of conflict resolution during marital interaction (Paley et al. 2002). Isabella and Belsky's (1985) work showing that deterioration of the marriage across the first year of life is related to the development of insecure infant–mother attachment provided some of the first evidence in support of the second point — that marital quality and infant attachment are related. Thus, when both relevant bodies of work are considered together, one showing a link between adult attachment and marital processes and the other between marital processes and infant attachment, a transmission mechanism involving adult attachment affecting marital processes and, thereby, infant/child attachment is highlighted as another possible process by which attachment security could be intergenerationally transmitted, perhaps accounting for part of the transmission gap.

This three-step process (i.e., G1Security → marital quality → G2Security) is, however, not the only one that comes to mind on the basis of the available data. Because a large body of research indicates that both mothers and fathers are more likely to provide sensitive, responsive, developmentally appropriate, and growth-promoting parenting from infancy through adolescence when marriages are more rather than less harmonious and satisfying (i.e., third point in above paragraph; for a review, see Belsky and Jaffee 2005), this three-step process can also be revised into a four-step one to account, theoretically at least, for the intergenerational transmission of attachment: G1Security → marital quality → sensitive parenting → G2Security. Consider in this regard Lundy's (2002) data showing that marital dissatisfaction adversely affected the quality of fathering and, thereby, infant–father attachment security. In light of the three- and four-step processes just outlined, it seems appropriate to conclude that the quality of the marital relationship probably affects the child's security both directly (i.e., via emotional atmospherics) and indirectly (i.e., via parenting). As such, we can now entertain four distinctive, though not necessarily independent processes by which attachment could be intergenerationally transmitted:

1. G1Security → sensitive parenting → G2Security,
2. G1Security → parental mind-mindedness → G2Security,
3. G1Security → marital quality → G2Security, and
4. G1Security → marital quality → sensitive parenting → G2Security.

A Still Missing Link: Internal Working Model Processes

Central to Bowlby's (1973) theory of attachment is the view that secure and insecure children actively and differentially filter information selectively, evoke responses form other people, and select niches in a manner consistent with their secure or insecure attachment relationships (Belsky and Cassidy 1994; Bretherton and Munholland 1999). The construct of the internal working model forms the core of the theory's account of *how* early infant–mother relations come to influence the child's perceptions of the world, the responses he/she evokes from other people, the relationships and experiences that attract or fail to attract him/her, and, thereby, continuity in development, including the intergenerational transmission of attachment. The internal working model is conceptualized as an affective-cognitive mechanism that guides the processing of information:

> Internal working models of relationships provide rules and rule systems for the direction of behavior and the felt appraisal of experience. Internal working models of relationships will provide rules for the direction and organization of attention and memory, rules that permit or limit the individual's access to certain forms of knowledge....Many [internal rules] will be unconscious...Internal working models are best conceived as structured processes serving to obtain or to limit access to information (Main et al. 1985, p. 77).

Although the internal working model is routinely invoked to explain why anticipated relations obtain between early measurements of attachment security (i.e., G1 Early Security) and subsequent assessments of behavioral functioning, including state of mind regarding attachment (i.e., G1 Later Security), it remains the case that internal working model *processes*, such as those highlighted in the above quote from Main et al. (1985), have not been well studied by developmentalists (cf. Kirsh and Cassidy [1997] studying children, and recent efforts by Zeijlmans van Emmichoven and associates [2005] studying adults using the AAI, and Shaver and Mikulincer [2002] using survey measurements to study attachment in the context of romantic relationships). That is, even though it has been repeatedly demonstrated that early attachment predicts phenomena such as peer relations, frustration tolerance, and even emotion regulation (for a review, see Thompson 1999), the experientially induced, internal, psychological, affective-cognitive processes that mediate linkages between past and present remain relatively unexamined in attachment research. Thus, although we know that early attachment predicts later attachment, the intrapsychic mechanisms responsible for such continuity in development remain relatively unexplored, with the same being true of linkages between adult attachment and parenting, though Meins et al.'s (2001) work on mind-mindedness certainly presents movement in that direction. As such, much remains to be understood about the intergenerational transmission process, even that for which there is no transmission gap. After all, discovering that adult attachment contributes to sensitive parenting which contributes to infant attachment security still leaves unaddressed the question of psychological processes responsible for linking adult attachment to the very parenting which at least partially accounts for the transmission of attachment security across generations. The same is true about how early attachment comes to predict later attachment.

In one of the few studies to endeavor to unpack the internal working model while studying young children, Belsky et al. (1996) tested the hypothesis, derived directly from Main et al.'s (1985) above-cited process analysis of the internal working model construct, that 36-month olds with secure and insecure attachment histories would process affectively laden information, designed into a series of puppet shows, differently. Although no evidence emerged that children with histories of secure and insecure attachments differentially attended to these positive and negative events, children with secure histories were found to remember positive events more accurately than negative ones, with the reverse being true of children with insecure histories, when the young children were tested 30 minutes after watching the puppet shows.

To the extent that such results reflect some of the differential information processing of secure and insecure children, these data suggest that the very same experience may register differently with children with varying attachment histories, and in ways that could contribute to continuity in development. After all, a child whose memory emphasizes the positive over the negative may likely respond to both negative and positive experiences encountered in the future differently than one whose memory emphasizes the negative over the positive. By being relatively poor at recollecting negative events, for example, the secure child might not respond to future negative events as adversely as another might and, in so doing, could be less likely to generate more negative experiences in the future. As such, a secure attachment early in childhood could "bias" the child to disproportionately attend to positive events in the parent–child relationship over negative ones and thereby promote further enjoyable experiences. This could be one subprocess by which continuity from early security to later security might arise. Not to be discounted is also the very real possibility that such "biased" and affectively laden information-processing processes could be neurally instantiated.

The findings and extrapolation from the Belsky et al. (1996) investigation should be regarded as only illustrative of the kind of research and thinking that is required to elaborate fully the rich notion of an internal working model and *how* it operates to shape development. It is just such "how" questions that are at the core of much developmental inquiry. That is, although it is one thing to know that early attachment predicts later attachment and that later attachment in the parent predicts early attachment in the child, it is quite something else to know what is really happening inside the child's and adult's mind and how intrapsychic affective-cognitive information processing contributes to the cross-time and even cross-generational linkages under discussion. It must be acknowledged, then, that even though we have evidence that attachment is intergenerationally transmitted in contemporary Western society, and apparently by nonheritable means, and know a substantial amount about how intergenerational transmission operates, there is much we do not know about the processes involved, even beyond the transmission gap that van IJzendoorn (1995) has astutely pointed out.

CONCLUSION

The analysis of the evolutionary and developmental psychology of the intergenerational transmission of attachment presented in this chapter began by considering reasons why natural selection may have shaped the process of human development to transmit attachment across generations, to not transmit attachment across generations, or to do both (but in different individuals). The summary of empirical evidence presented on the concordance of parent and child attachment — assessed in quite different, even if conceptually similar ways — revealed a substantial degree of support for the claim that attachment is intergenerationally transmitted, at least in contemporary Western culture in which the topic has been virtually exclusively studied. Furthermore, the developmental psychology evidence considered also showed, consistent with contemporary attachment theory, that sensitive-responsive parenting (in its many measurable variations) mediates, to some extent, the linkage between parent and child attachment. Finally, consideration of additional plausible mediators (i.e., mind-mindedness, emotional atmosphere of the home, marital quality) raised the possibility that the substantial "transmission gap," which van IJzendoorn (1995) identified, might be bridged in the not too distant future once more research on these potential mechanisms of influence is conducted.

However, even if this proves to be the case, it must be acknowledged that the detected degree of intergenerational transmission is far from perfect. The absence of intergenerational transmission reflected in the data could be the result of a variety of factors, including simple measurement error, though it needs to be recalled that discontinuity in attachment within and across generations is theoretically anticipated by attachment theory, given the role that lived experiences play in the mediational process. When events and experience conspire to promote changes in the individual's internal working model of attachment, whether that person be a young child, teenager, or adult, discontinuity of attachment, both inter- and intragenerationally, can be expected.

This theoretical proposition within attachment theory, along with the evidence reviewed of the imperfect environmental mediation of attachment across generations, is consistent with the evolutionary argument advanced early in this chapter: natural selection could have shaped an attachment system that would be susceptible to intergenerational transmission through experiential mechanisms. At the same time, all of the evidence considered is consistent with the view, also argued from an evolutionary perspective, that individuals are differentially susceptible to rearing influence. After all, the data considered indicated that (a) intergenerational transmission is far from perfect and (b) that there is a substantial transmission gap when it comes to accounting for how attachment gets transmitted across generations, suggesting perhaps that the theorized process of intergenerational transmission might hold for some individuals and not for others. Unfortunately, no investigators have explored this possibility, so it is difficult to know whether the imperfect prediction repeatedly documented in the course of this chapter is a function of error of measurement or, among many other possibilities, the fact that not all individuals are actually susceptible to the environmentally mediated processes that lie at the heart of attachment theory's account of how intergenerational transmission takes place.

The possibility that intergenerational transmission via experiential processes may describe the developmental prospects of only some individuals and not others raises some interesting issues about gene frequencies and population genetics. If we presume for sake of argument that differential susceptibility to rearing influence is itself a function of biological inheritance (i.e., genes), even if this is clearly not the only possibility, then there is reason to wonder whether populations vary in the proportion of children who are more and less susceptible to rearing influence and, thus, in the extent to which one might expect attachment to be intergenerationally transmitted. For reasons of contextual history, it seems possible that some populations living under more frequently changing environmental conditions could have been selected to resist — more than other populations — parental influence and thus environmentally mediated intergenerational transmission, if only because following in the psychological footsteps of parents in such contexts would not have paid off reproductively to the extent that it might have in perhaps more environmentally stable ecological niches. Were this the case, then one might expect the probability of environmentally mediated intergenerational transmission of attachment to vary across time and even place, with some populations showing more of it than others. Such a prospect is not something most developmentalists and certainly not most students of attachment theory think about and this may be but one reason why cross-cultural work on intergenerational transmission has not yet been conducted. Once again the error may be in thinking that while we of the human species are so very much alike in so many ways, in many other, perhaps more subtle ways, we may be rather different. Thinking about the intergenerational transmission of attachment from an evolutionary *and* developmental perspective would seem to add scope to the questions one can ask and the discoveries one might be able to make about human development.

PROBLEMS, QUESTIONS, AND ISSUES

- Are patterns of attachment part and parcel of facultative reproductive strategies?
- To what extent are rearing contexts and the broader ecological context stable over time, especially across adjacent generations?
- Do children vary in their susceptibility to rearing influences? And, if so, is such differential susceptibility domain specific or domain general? That is, are some children more susceptible to rearing across all aspects of development (e.g., social, emotional, cognitive) and some less so, or might it

be the case that a child susceptible to emotion socialization is less susceptible to cognitive socialization, with the reverse being true of another child?
- How much of the noncorcordance of parent and child attachment is simply
  a function measurement error?
- What about hunter–gatherer societies: the distribution of attachment security, parent–child concordance, and stability from childhood to adulthood?
- What other processes mediate the linkage between parent and child attachment security?
- What are the intrapsychic processes which mediate linkages between adult
  attachment and parenting and between child and adult attachment?
- Could different populations be more and less susceptible to the intergenerational transmission, via experiential means, of attachment — and for
  genetic reasons?

REFERENCES

Ainsworth, M. 1973. The development of infant–mother attachment. In: Review of Child
  Development Research, ed. B. Caldwell and H.N. Ricciuti, pp. 1–94. Chicago: Univ.
  of Chicago Press.
Ainsworth, M., and B. Wittig. 1969. Attachment and exploratory behavior of one-year
  olds in a strange situation. In: Determinants of Infant Behavior, ed. B.M. Foss, vol. 4,
  pp. 27–49. London: Methuen.
Bakermans-Kranenburg, M.J., M. van IJzendoorn, and F. Juffer. 2003. Less is more:
  Meta-analysis of sensitivity and attachment interventions in early childhood.
  Psychol. Bull. **129**:195–215.
Belsky, J. 1999. Modern evolutionary theory and patterns of attachment. In: Handbook
  of Attachment: Theory, Research, and Clinical Applications, ed. J. Cassidy and P.R.
  Shaver, pp. 151–173. New York: Guilford.
Belsky, J. 2000. Conditional and alternative reproductive strategies: Individual differ-
  ences in susceptibility to rearing experience. In: Genetic Influences on Human Fertil-
  ity and Sexuality: Theoretical and Empirical Contributions from the Biological and
  Behavioral Sciences, ed. J. Rodgers, D. Rowe, and W. Miller, pp. 127–146. Boston:
  Kluwer.
Belsky, J., and J. Cassidy. 1994. Attachment: Theory and evidence. In: Development
  through Life: A Handbook for Clinicians, ed. M. Rutter and D.F. Hay, pp. 373–403.
  Oxford: Blackwell.
Belsky, J., and S. Jaffee. 2005. The multiple determinants of parenting. In: Handbook of
  Psychopathology, ed. D. Cicchetti and D.J. Cohen, 2nd ed. New York: Wiley, in press.
Belsky, J., B. Spritz, and K. Crnic. 1996. Infant attachment security and affective-cogni-
  tive information processing at age 3. *Psychol. Sci.* **7**:111–114.
Belsky, J., L. Steinberg, and P. Draper. 1991. Childhood experience, interpersonal devel-
  opment and reproductive strategy: An evolutionary theory of socialization. *Child
  Dev.* **62**:647–670.
Bokhorst, C., M. Bakermans-Kranenburg, P. Fearon et al. 2004. The importance of
  shared environment in mother–infant attachment: A behavior-genetic study. *Child
  Dev.* **74**:1769–1782.

Bowlby, J. 1973. Separation: Anxiety, and Anger. Attachment and Loss, vol. 2. New York: Basic.

Bretherton, I., and K. Munholland. 1999. Internal working models in attachment relationships: A construct revisited. In: Handbook of Attachment: Theory, Research, and Clinical Applications, ed. J. Cassidy and P.R. Shaver, pp. 89–111. New York: Guilford.

Chisholm, J. 1999. Death, Hope and Sex: Steps to an Evolutionary Ecology of the Mind and Morality. New York: Cambridge Univ. Press.

Cummings, E.M., and P. Davies. 1994. Children and Marital Conflict: The Impact of Family Dispute and Resolution. New York: Guilford.

Davies, P., and E.M. Cummings. 1994. Marital conflict and child adjustment: An emotional security hypothesis. *Psychol. Bull.* **116**:387–411.

De Wolff, M., and M. van IJzendoorn. 1997. Sensitivity and attachment: A meta-analysis on parental antecedents of infant attachment. *Child Dev.* **68**:571–591.

Fonagy, P. 1999. Psychoanalytic theory from the viewpoint of attachment theory and research. In: Handbook of Attachment: Theory, Research, and Clinical Applications, ed. J. Cassidy and P.R. Shaver, pp. 595–624. New York: Guilford.

Fraley, R.C. 2002. Attachment stability from infancy to adulthood: A meta-analysis and dynamic modelling of developmental mechanisms. *Pers. Soc. Psych. Rev.* **6**: 123–151.

Fraley, R.C., and S. Spieker. 2003. Are infant attachment patterns continuously or categorically distributed? A taxometric analysis of Strange Situation behaviour. *Dev. Psychol.* **39**:387–404.

George, C., and J. Solomon. 1999. Attachment and caregiving: The caregiving behavioural system. In: Handbook of Attachment: Theory, Research, and Clinical Applications, ed. J. Cassidy and P.R. Shaver, pp. 649–670. New York: Guilford.

Hesse, E. 1999. The Adult Attachment Interview. In: Handbook of Attachment: Theory, Research, and Clinical Applications, ed. J. Cassidy and P.R. Shaver, pp. 395–433. New York: Guilford.

Isabella, R., and J. Belsky. 1985. Marital change during the transition to parenthood and security of infant–parent attachment. *J. Fam. Iss.* **6**:505–522.

Kirsh, S., and J. Cassidy. 1997. Preschoolers' attention to and memory for attachment-relevant information. *Child Dev.* **68**:1143–1153.

Lundy, B. 2002. Paternal socio-psychological factors and infant attachment: The mediating role of synchrony in father–infant interactions. *Infant Behav. Dev.* **25**:221–236.

Main, M., N. Kaplan, and J. Cassidy. 1985. Security in infancy, childhood and adulthood: A move to the level of representation. *Mono. Soc. Res. Child Dev.* **50**:66–104.

Meins, E., C. Fernyhough, E. Fradley, and M. Tuckey. 2001. Rethinking maternal sensitivity: Mothers' comments on infants' mental processes predict security of attachment at 12 months. *J. Child Psychol. Psychiat.* **42**:637–648.

O'Connor, T., and C. Croft. 2001. A twin study of attachment in preschool children. *Child Dev.* **72**:1501–1511.

Paley, B., M. Cox., K. Harter, and N. Margand. 2002. Adult attachment stance and spouses' marital perceptions during the transition to parenthood. *Attach. Hum. Dev.* **4**:340–360.

Ricciuti, A. 1992. Child–mother attachment: A twin study. *Diss. Abstr. Intl.* **54**: 3364–3364. (Univ. Microfilms No. 9324873).

Shaver, P., and M. Mikulincer. 2002. Attachment-related psychodynamics. *Attach. Hum. Dev.* **4**:133–161.

Simpson, J. 1999. Attachment theory in modern evolutionary perspective. In: Handbook of Attachment: Theory, Research, and Clinical Applications, ed. J. Cassidy and P.R. Shaver, pp. 115–140. New York: Guilford.

Thompson, R. 1999. Early attachment and later development. In: Handbook of Attachment: Theory, Research, and Clinical Applications, ed. J. Cassidy and P.R. Shaver, pp. 265–286. New York: Guilford.

van den Boom, D. 1994. The influence of temperament and mothering on attachment and exploration: An experimental manipulation of sensitive responsiveness among lower-class mothers with irritable infants. *Child Dev.* **65**:1449–1469.

van IJzendoorn, M. 1995. Adult attachment representations, parental responsiveness, and infant attachment: A meta-analysis on the predictive validity of the Adult Attachment Interview. *Psychol. Bull.* **117**:387–403.

van IJzendoorn, M., and M. De Wolff. 1997. In search of the absent father: Meta-analysis of infant–father attachment. *Child Dev.* **68**:604–609.

van IJzendoorn, M., F. Juffer, and M. Duyvesteyn. 1995. Breaking the intergenerational cycle of insecure attachment: A review of the effects of attachment-based interventions on maternal sensitivity and infant security. *J. Child Psychol. Psychiat.* **36**: 225–248.

van IJzendoorn, M., and P. Kroonenberg. 1988. Cross-cultural patterns of attachment: A meta-analysis of the strange situation. *Child Dev.* **59**:147–156.

Zeijlmans van Emmichoven, I.A., M. van IJzendoorn., C. De Ruiter, and J. Brosschot. 2005. Selective processing of treating information: Effects of attachment representation and anxiety disorder on attention and memory. *Dev. Psychopathol.* **15**:219–238.

10

Universality of Human Social Attachment as an Adaptive Process

K. E. GROSSMANN and K. GROSSMANN

Institut für Psychologie, Universität Regensburg, 93040 Regensburg, Germany

ABSTRACT

Attachment is the phylogenetically programmed propensity of a human child to form a special relationship with responsive caregivers as part of the infant–parent bond. Attachment theory is rooted in traditional ethology as well as in psychoanalysis. Infants' actively seeking protection and care has most likely been one of the selective forces. Other bonds between individuals may contain certain elements of attachment. During ontogenesis, individual differences in the organization of emotions and integration into a coherent internal working model throughout the years of immaturity is particularly prominent in human individual development. Secure and insecure patterns of attachment result from different qualities of interaction between infants' expressions and adults' responses to them. In adulthood, secure attachment representations reflect a sense of being worthy of help, free access to supportive attachment figures when needed, and appropriate, partnership-oriented evaluations of challenging social situations. Secure internal working models constantly integrate coherently and adaptively emotional and relevant cognitive aspects across lifetime. Secure attachment and secure exploration serve "psychological security" and quality of adaptation to life in the mental health sense. A longitudinal study conducted in northern Germany demonstrates that children's experience with both parents influenced their psychological security in representation of attachment as well as partnership representation at age 22 years. Currently, traditional attachment theory is on its way to being integrated into modern sociobiology and physiology. A future synthesis of attachment and bonding could benefit from addressing Tinbergen's four questions about the evolution, function, causation, and development of attachment and bonding.

ATTACHMENT, BONDING, AND RELATED ISSUES

Historical Notes

Attachment theory, as conceptualized by John Bowlby (1987), focuses on the nature of the child's tie to the mother. It posits a pre-programmed propensity in the young child to develop attachments to a very few, special adults who are willing and able to care for, support, and invest resources in the young individual. It was designed to serve as a theoretical concept for human emotional and social development and to explain qualitative individual differences in the ontogenesis of psychological adaptation and mental health, depending on the quality of care received. Stated within the framework of modern sociobiology that was unknown to Bowlby, attachment theory focuses on the "gene-selfish" interest of the child to receive as much of his parents' (physical as well as psychological) resources as needed to become an emotionally and socially healthy and competent individual in his social group. In terms of Trivers' (1974) parent–offspring conflict, attachment theory focuses on the offspring's side of that conflict as well as on the parent's willingness or unwillingness to invest in *this* individual offspring. In the case of parental unwillingness, infant survival is at stake. For example, among the langurs of Abu, allomothering is abundant, but "no mother was ever seen to allow any infant but her own to suckle" (Hrdy 1977, p. 211). Therefore, it is vitally important for an infant to be able to identify and seek out its mother extremely soon; otherwise, it will find no other source of nourishment. In support of this assumption, Hrdy observes that an infant langur knows its mother very well despite extant allomothering. "An infant that has been quietly holding its mother may begin to whine soon after being taken by some other female. Conversely, an infant that has been struggling and complaining will usually grow quiet when retrieved by the mother" (Hrdy, 1977, p. 215). From the maternal perspective in this conflict, rejecting an infant carries a much lesser cost to the mother, as she can expect another offspring.

In four interdisciplinary meetings of the World Health Organization Study Group on the Psychobiological Development of the Child (Geneva 1953, 1955, 1956 and London 1954) John Bowlby encountered ethology of the 1950s as Lorenz (1960) and Tinbergen (1951) formulated it (Tanner and Inhelder 1960). Bowlby was tutored in this new discipline by the comparative biologist Robert Hinde (Bowlby 1991; Hinde 2005). Bowlby aimed at providing a theoretical frame for a new synthesis of phylogeny, ontogeny, psychoanalytic insights, inner control systems (e.g., schemata, equilibration sensu Piaget; Bowlby 1960) and Darwinian thinking. Attachment theory was formulated by Bowlby to encourage empirical examination of the right questions of psychoanalysis — to which the psychoanalysts, as he believed, often gave the wrong answers — according to modern scientific standards. He perceived a need to study prospectively healthy as well as maladaptive social-emotional development of individuals "from the cradle to the grave" (Bowlby 1979).

One of the central observations that paved the way for the concept of behavioral systems in attachment theory was the behavioral response patterns demonstrated by Harlow's rhesus monkeys, which were dependent on their emotional state. In the presence of their surrogate mother and when calm, infant monkeys would play freely in an open field. However, when alarmed and frightened, they did not run away from the frightening object but rather fled to their surrogate mother figure as a safe haven, where they could calm down. In the absence of the mother figure, no calming down was observable. Other vivid examples of the functioning of the aroused attachment system in mammals have been provided by Robert B. Cairns (1979, p. 47), who described the abrupt transformation of a one-month-old monkey from a relaxed, content infant into a restless, crying, and sometimes extremely agitated organism through forced separation from its mother. Lambs separated from other sheep run full speed around the isolation chamber, sometimes against the door or wall; this behavior is repeated "with groggy redundancy."

The co-regulation of the attachment need of the young and its corresponding maternal caregiving system was termed "affectionate system" by Harry Harlow (1961, 1971). The behavioral systems are "fitted" to each other and have been phylogenetically selected as a unit of age-specific adaptive behaviors of infants and mothers *if*, as modern sociobiology would suggest, the mother has decided to invest in this infant.

The child's need is expressed through attachment behaviors accompanied by expressions of emotions (Darwin 1872/1998), which function to increase close proximity to the caregiver. The caregiving behavioral system is expressed by protecting and caring for the attached individual. The need for care and protection of a dependent or weaker individual — which may also be an adult in times of ill health, adversity, or old age — by a "stronger and wiser" adult is central to Bowlby's conceptualization. Because care and protection are vital needs of "weaker and inexperienced younger" individuals, the attachment behavioral system is driven by strong motivations. "Many of the most intense emotions arise during the formation, the maintenance, the disruption and the renewal of attachment relationships" (Bowlby 1979, Lecture 7). This concept was certainly influenced by Bowlby's training as a psychotherapist, as well as by having seen the misery of many children throughout Europe who were separated from or had lost their parents after World War II (Bowlby 1951).

Of course, human beings also form affectional bonds with others in the course of their life. Ainsworth (1985, p. 199) highlighted the difference between attachment of infants to their mothers and affectional bonds in other social relations as follows: "An *attachment* is an affectional bond in which the attachment figures are never wholly interchangeable with or replaceable by another, even though there be another to whom one is also attached." In addition, she refers to "developmental changes in the way in which a child's attachment to parents manifests itself beyond the infancy period ..., that one's attachment to parents tends to persist throughout life rather than attenuating and eventually disappearing — as many believe...."

In comparison, *"bonds* are also relatively long-lived ties to unique individuals....A bond is to be distinguished from other long-term relationships (attachments) in which it is the *role* of the other that is significant, so that with

separation or loss there would be at most some regret, tempered by an expectation of soon finding another to play the same role in one's life" (Ainsworth 1985,
p. 799). Later, Ainsworth adds, "There is one criterion of attachment that is not
necessarily present in other affectional bonds. This is a seeking to obtain an experience of security and comfort in the relationship with the partner. If and when
such security and comfort is available, the individual is able to move off from the
secure base provided by the partner, *with confidence* to engage in other activities" (Ainsworth 1991, p. 38).

Among those "other affectional bonds throughout the life span" she lists the
bond of *mother to infant* (as contrasted to the phylogenetically programmed process of infants forming attachments to individual caregivers), the bond of father
to child, bonds resulting from sexual behavior, friendships, companionships, as
well as bonds between siblings and other kin. All of these bonds may develop
into attachment relationships, and they appear to be somehow influenced by attachment experiences. These other relationships, however, are characterized by
properties of their own, which may be well "beyond" attachment (Hinde 1976;
Dunn 1993). We view attachment as the developmental process during which
infants' genetic programs become phenotypically manifest, observable, and
testable as a function of caretakers' responsiveness.

Historically, the concept of bonding entered developmental psychology
through the work of Klaus and Kennell (1976). They argued for an imprinting
type of *maternal* readiness to establish a close relationship to the infant in the human mother, as in ungulates, that has to be triggered within the first hour(s) after
delivery. The process by which a mother comes to feel close to her infant has
been termed *bonding* in the developmental psychology literature ever since.

We have tested this assumption by providing a group of 24 German mothers
with "early contact" for the first hour after birth and compared their tender behavior toward their newborn with 25 mothers who did not receive "early contact." Results showed that non-early contact mothers reached the level of
tenderness of the early contact mothers by the second week, and that later quality of maternal sensitivity or infant–mother attachment was not affected by our
experimental manipulation of "maternal bonding" (Grossmann, K. et al. 1981).

Below, we present our arguments on the universality of human social attachment as an adaptive process using the following framework:

1. Development of the attachment system in human infants.
2. Different qualities of secure and insecure attachment patterns.
3. Attachment development from infancy to adulthood.
4. Interrelations between sociocultural and cognititive development within
   attachment development as the infant learns about the motivations, intentions, and perspectives of their mothers and incorporates them "naturally" into their own cultural world views.

In the second section, we present the idea, first developed by Lorenz (1967), that
attachment is a universal genetic program valid in all cultures, despite clearly

observable variations in parental caregiving behaviors between existing cultures and within cultures in different epochs. This will be augmented by results of studies using the separation–reunion procedure with infants and their mothers in various cultures that support the universality claim of attachment theory. In the third section, some of the primary results from our German longitudinal studies are discussed as an example for variations in attachment development in a group of children growing up in their families of origin. Finally, new theoretical considerations are presented that appear to be important for a new synthesis of attachment and bonding.

Development of the Attachment System

Although human infants are physically premature at birth, they are equipped with communicative competencies inherent in the child's emotional expressions and behaviors; under most circumstances these are recognized by the caregiver as bodily and social needs and are responded to appropriately (Ainsworth and Bell 1974; Trevarthen, this volume). The infant is not born with an attachment to his mother; this begins to develop after birth. Still, development of an attachment is pre-programmed such that given a caregiver who is reliably available over a long period, an infant will necessarily develop an attachment to that particular adult independent of the quality of caregiving, even to a nonresponsive surrogate mother (Harlow 1971) or abusive mother (Hennighausen and Lyons-Ruth, this volume). The quality of care, however, will have a major influence on certain aspects of the personality development of that infant and child (e.g., how behaviors and intentions of others are perceived and responded to).

Ainsworth and her team spent many hours observing infants and mothers in their natural environment. Their results showed that prompt and appropriate responsiveness to all the infant's behaviors shaped the infant's attachment development toward a secure individual attachment from early on, whereas unresponsive, uncooperative, inappropriate care paved the way for an insecure attachment. Mothers who responded promptly and sensitively to their infants' crying and other emotional expressions more frequently experienced infants who cried less toward the end of the first year and who were more compliant with their mother. Likewise, giving the baby close bodily contact *when he signaled for it* was associated both with secure attachment and the growth of self-reliance (Ainsworth et al. 1974; Grossmann, K. et al. 1985).

In contrast to the prevailing learning theory at that time, Ainsworth and Bell (1977) offered an ethological interpretation, which corresponded to a shift toward a new phylogenetic paradigm: If all infant behaviors are seen as acts of communication instead of accidental "operant" behaviors, then qualitatively different responsiveness by the adult will lead to qualitatively different communicative competencies and developmental consequences for the child rather than just changing the frequency of certain specific behaviors (Ainsworth and Bell 1974).

Individual Qualities or Patterns of Attachment of Mother–Child Dyads

Ainsworth tested the validity of her home observations in the so-called "strange situation" (Ainsworth and Wittig 1969). Because an infant will not show attachment behaviors under conditions of well-being, Ainsworth devised a standardized procedure to arouse the infant's attachment system. The Strange Situation assessment of attachment relationship emphasizes the infant's responses to mild stress induced by a novel environment, novel person, and two brief separations from the mother. During separations from the attachment figure, infants usually limit or stop their exploratory activities (later we will point to the universality of this phenomenon). A pattern of attachment behaviors throughout the Strange Situation was considered "secure" if the attachment person functioned well as a haven of safety calming the infant and alleviating anxiety and distress, and as a secure base from which the infant resumed exploratory and playful orientation to the world beyond the attachment figure after the aroused attachment system had been calmed (see Figure 10.1).

Attachment behavior patterns were considered "insecure" if an infant showed behavioral restrictions or limitations when using the mother as a safe haven by not seeking bodily proximity to her or when using the mother as a secure base by not wanting to move off and explore again after separation. Subsequently, three major patterns of an infant's behavioral strategy in response to separation from and reunion with the attachment figure were distinguished: secure, insecure-avoidant, and insecure-resistant. The most general marker of the three patterns is appropriate expression, hypo- or hyperactivation of attachment relevant behaviors. Ainsworth's home studies suggested that infants' patterns of attachment in the Strange Situation procedure were a consequence of variations in sensitivity of maternal responsiveness to their baby's attachment signals and their signals of wanting to explore during the first year.

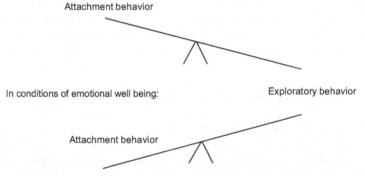

Figure 10.1 The concept of the attachment–exploration balance. The attachment and exploratory behavioral systems are linked to each other. When one system is activated the other is deactivated.

Studies of attachment development, spanning from preschool age to old age, included the symbolic and representational level of perceiving, feeling, thinking, and discussing attachment. Secure and insecure patterns of behaving or thinking were reliably found in response to the aroused attachment system and in relation to attachment figures (see Cassidy and Shaver 1999). Individuals responding with a secure strategy to distress show a free, uninhibited access to an attachment figure when alarmed and explore readily when the attachment figure is (mentally) present and responsive. The studies neither under- nor overemphasize attachment behaviors, exploration, or their mental representations. The patterns can be shown in narrations, reflecting an internalization of such processes. The secure pattern has been considered by Ainsworth as psychologically more adaptive because reliance on the trusting support of significant others increases the chances of mastering new challenges.

The three major patterns of attachment have been confirmed and validated in many studies across many countries (van IJzendoorn and Kroonenberg 1988; van IJzendoorn and Sagi 1999). In addition, Main and Solomon (1986) described the behavior of infants who either could not be classified or who showed signs of extreme disturbance such as fear of the attachment figure. They were classified as *insecure disorganized and disoriented in their attachment*. Evidence for attachment insecurity of this group came from an analysis of the cortisol level of these infants. Spangler and Grossmann (1993) showed that *all* infants with signs of disorganization had elevated cortisol levels after the Strange Situation as compared to infants with a secure pattern of attachment that showed no increase in cortisol level. Disorganization in response to distress plays an increasingly important role in clinical and otherwise psychologically maladapted samples (Hennighausen and Lyons-Ruth, this volume).

Attachment across the Life Course

Attachment development has been conceptualized as a continuous process not only in infancy, but well into adolescence. "Principal determinants of the pathway along which an individual's attachment behavior develops, and of the pattern in which it becomes organized, are the experiences he has with his attachment figures during his years of immaturity — infancy, childhood and adolescence" (Bowlby 1980, p. 41). This quotation cautions those who perceive attachment theory and research as relating only to infancy and early childhood. Attachment theory posits instead that attachment experiences result in internal working models (IWMs) or expectations, which begin from an early age: how the attachment figures will respond when the person finds herself in conditions of adversity which evoke feelings of anger, fear, and sadness. IWMs of attachment are thought of as a set of rules and filters regulating the perception of the social world. Working models of attachment can be secure or confident to be worthy of help, insecure and dismissing of the importance of attachment, or insecure and enmeshed/confused about the meaning of attachment experiences.

IWMs of attachment are assessed through interviews about current thoughts on the person's own attachment experiences in childhood and adolescence (Hesse 1999).

Longitudinal studies in attachment development spanning from infancy to young adulthood, such as our Bielefeld and Regensburg studies (Grossmann, K.E. et al. 2005), the Minnesota study (Sroufe et al. 2005), and the Berkeley study (Main et al. 2005), leave no doubt that there are many long-lasting influences of attachment experiences with parents in childhood and adolescence on social and personality development (Thompson 2000; Waters and Cummings 2000).

During attachment development, sensitivity to the infant's attachment signals is important, as are sensitivity to exploratory intentions and behaviors that support a balanced organization of behavior. According to Konrad Lorenz (1967, p. 383), exploration means *Forschung* (i.e., research), which needs a relaxed atmosphere free from anxiety or other pressures. Exploration is necessary for adaptation to the wider social and material world as new and increasingly complex experiences have to be integrated throughout development. The indispensable role of exploration for healthy personality development has been part of attachment theory right from the onset (Bowlby 1979, p. 133). Playful exploration of the physical and mainly cultural world at large and the people in it profits from a secure base or a secure IWM of attachment that needs to be constantly updated during development to function adaptively.

The markers of psychological security, as described by most attachment researchers, are physical or mental access to others in times of distress as well as the ability to clarify and manage complex and unhappy social–emotional challenges by developing realistic solutions, including open communication with others and seeking and accepting their help; in short, the capacity to overcome anxiety and fear through proximity and with the help of others. It should be noted, however, that without the arousal of the attachment system, everyday routine problem solving will prevail. Psychological security is most relevant in emotional "testing the limits" situations, which require "updates" of IWMs as in psychological adaptation in the elderly (Kliegl et al. 1989).

Attachment relationships as the first and often only relationships in infancy are pivotal to an individual's social relationships and their evaluations, to partnership-oriented planning, and particularly to finding goals worth pursuing (Minsky 1987, p. 175). Later attachment relationships and IWMs of attachment seem to influence the person's view about the world, whether perceived as being threatening or benevolent. This has been shown for all age periods from childhood (Suess et al. 1992) to old age (Wensauer and Grossmann 1998). Quality of attachment and quality of support during exploration, in our view, function jointly as a new system with novel and special qualities resulting in psychological security or insecurity. The quality of psychological security organizes and integrates emotions, cognition, and communicative discourse for intricate adaptations to special other people.

In summary, attachment refers primarily to the young child's need for protection, care, and support for adaptation to his social and nonsocial environment. Attachments are the "natural" prerequisite for becoming emotionally and socially "acculturated." Attachment relationships set the stage for cognitive interpretation of experiences and for acquiring meaning about self and others in complex social situations that are vital in infancy but continue to be important throughout life.

Attachment and Sociocultural Cognition

The acquisition of meaning relies on more knowledgeable persons providing an interpretation of the world within a child's context of immediate action and experience. Language, as the obvious carrier of meaning, is learned and functions best in situations of "joint attention" of young and older humans (Tomasello 1999). Joint attention for the sake of acculturation is prominent only in the human species. In situations of joint experiences, infants approaching their first birthday come to be aware of the other's mind. The adult partner will most certainly be an attachment figure or another familiar and trusted person, because, by that age, fear of strangers will be functioning strongly. It seems as if nature wanted to make sure that infants begin their lifelong education by first learning about the values of their own people. The subsequent stages of joint attention, following and guiding attention of the adult partner, appear around 11 to 13 months of age, closely linked to language development. These might already be shared with more interactive partners. In any case, *Forschung* in exploration and in joint attention is inseparably linked to cognitive as well as emotional development. In addition, discourses during joint attention and narratives about joint and observed experiences help to link inner states and feelings cognitively to external events (Grossmann, K.E. 1999; Nelson 1999). According to Bowlby (1982, p. 355), "by sharing a common set-goal and participating in a joint plan to achieve it, partners have a rewarding sense of common purpose; and they are likely also to identify with one another."

From a cognitive perspective, psychologically adaptive or "secure" behavior strategies in face of adversity are the result of undistorted perceptions of relevant situations that demand well planned, goal-corrected actions. Robert Sternberg (1997), an intelligence researcher, sees adaptive intelligence as a cognitive correspondence between a complex outside reality and its coherent representation in the human mind ("internal coherence and external correspondence"). In attachment theory, "reality" often refers to close other people's minds, feelings and intentions, and "internal coherence" to the organization of one's emotions as well as one's knowledgeable insights and reflections. Sternberg's concept of adaptive intelligence helps us understand how the historical–cultural dimension, with its cultural artifacts and its culture-specific meanings, pre-programmed during evolution, is transmitted during ontogenesis. "The overall model is thus that human beings have cognitive skills that result from biological inheritance working in phylogenetic time; they use these skills to exploit cultural resources that have evolved over historical time; and they do this during ontogenetic time" (Tomasello 1999, p. 48).

Strong and emotional identification with the values of one's culture requires persons that are respected and loved by the child (Lorenz 1967, 1977); it needs attachment learning (Minsky 1987), meaning conveyed through narrative discourses (Bruner 1990), social mediation (Cole 1996), and community participation (Rogoff 2003). The emotional organization established in the early years seems to be a basic component of an adaptive synthesis of the cognitive system and the emotional system especially in challenging situations (Grossmann, K.E et al. 2002; Sroufe 2000). "Man's capacity to use language and other symbols, his capacities to plan and build models, his capacities for long-lasting collaboration with others and for interminable strife, these make man what he is. All these processes have their origin during the first three years of life, and all, moreover, are from their earliest days enlisted in the organization of attachment behavior" (Bowlby 1982, p. 358).

EVIDENCE FOR THE UNIVERSAL NATURE OF ATTACHMENT

Relevant specific endowments for attachment as well as cultural development in humans are seen in a number of behavioral and mental programs:

- the organization of emotions (Cosmides and Tooby 2000),
- joint attention (Tomasello 1999),
- language and the creation of meaning (Bruner 1982, 1983, 1990),
- awareness of other's minds including the ability to see events from the perspective of another person (Ainsworth et al. 1974; Meins 1999),
- the ability to consider another person's wishes and goals when pursuing own goals ("goal-corrected partnership," Bowlby 1982),
- self-cognition (Cassidy 1988), and
- autobiographical narrative constructions (Nelson 1996, 1999).

With development, these universal mental and representational programs become increasingly individualized and differentiated in the course of interactions with special individuals, who are the transmitters of cultural meaning.

Nature has programmed human beings as cultural beings. Cultural learning begins within the attachment relationship. Attachment is not an option with which culture can freely "play." It is a universal necessity for individual human development. History has shown that there are definite limits of human adaptability to "inhumane" child-rearing conditions that disregard attachment. Examples can be seen in the legendary sad outcomes of infants raised in large de-individualized groups, as described by René Spitz (1945), or in the German

Nazi Project *"Lebensborn,"* a project intended to produce a purely Aryan race but which removed infants from their mothers (Lilienthal 1993; Abe 2003), or, more recently, in Romanian orphanages (O'Connor, this volume). The following concepts may serve to exemplify the universal nature of attachment.

First, the universality concept of attachment states that all infants become attached to at least one primary caregiver. Infants and young children may become attached to more than one person, such as fathers and regular caregivers (Sagi et al. 1995), but not to many. As regular interactive partners, additional familiar persons may become secondary attachment figures in the hierarchy of attachment figures. Although the attachment system operates independently of genetic kinship, the biological mother is usually the primary attachment figure as she is typically the primary caregiver. Sleeping together may be an important experience in attachment development. A survey of 90 non-Western cultures revealed that, in every one, infants and toddlers slept in the same bed with the mother or a closely related adult (Barry and Paxson 1971). By comparison, a study of Israeli infants showed that the majority of infants sleeping in community houses, instead of their parents' home, showed disorganized attachment behaviors (Sagi et al. 1994). This was also found for infants of divorced parents if, as a result of joint custody, the infant slept alternately at the mother's and father's homes (Solomon and George 1999).

Affectionate responsiveness, attentive protection, sensitive support, and challenges during joint play seem to suffice for attachment formation and become highly influential across the life span (Grossmann, K.E. et al. 2002; Thompson 2000). A person has become an attachment figure to a child if three universal criteria are met: (a) the young child seeks closeness to and protection from that person when it perceives danger or experiences distressed (the "haven of safety" function); (b) the young child uses that person as a "secure base" from which it explores the environment, and (c) the young child will experience emotional as well as physiological distress when separated from that figure (separation distress). By the end of the second year, the toddlers of our Bielefeld longitudinal study had up to three attachment figures, comparable to the toddlers in the Glasgow study (Schaffer and Emerson 1964).

Next, the concept of the attachment–exploration balance implies that when the attachment behavioral system is active or aroused, the exploratory behavioral system is less active and vice versa (see Figure 10.1). This activation and deactivation does not to seem be complete, however, to the degree of closing down one or the other system completely. Environmental clues to danger are continuously monitored as are events stimulating curiosity. Arousal of the attachment system is best calmed by close bodily proximity ("tender loving care"). Nonarousal of the attachment system can be taken as an index of emotional well-being, which favors playful exploration in the service of competent social and cultural adaptation to the complexities of human life. The universal functioning of the attachment–exploration balance is experienced most likely by anyone who comes too close to an unfamiliar toddler in any culture. The toddler will often flee in panic to her mother or other familiar figure. This functioning has been systematically and empirically demonstrated in many cultures (van IJzendoorn and Sagi 1999).

We inspected and collected data gained from Strange Situation studies from four very different cultures. In each group of toddlers, exploratory activity declined markedly when a stranger entered the room and wanted to interact with the toddler and separation from the mother was enforced. This decline in exploration with increasing distress was shown by toddlers in Baltimore, U.S.A. (Ainsworth et al. 1978), by German toddlers in various cities (Grossmann, K. et al. 1985; Grossmann, K.E. 1999), by Japanese toddlers (Miyake et al. 1985), and by Trobriand toddlers (Grossmann, K.E. et al. 2005). Exploration was dominant when the U.S./German/Japanese/Trobriand toddler was with her mother; the entrance of a stranger reduced exploration to a certain degree, and it declined further or remained at a low level after the mother departed. The mother's return resulted in some increase of exploratory activity, although not nearly to the level that was observed prior to separation. Thus, even short separations (maximum of 3 min) from the secure base made all toddlers wary or anxious. Separations from the mother had a lasting dampening effect on infant exploratory activity in a strange environment in all of the observed toddlers from four continents, regardless of their pattern of attachment.

Third, the normativity hypothesis states that the secure pattern of attachment is — with very few exceptions — the most frequent pattern in all samples of uncompromised infants observed in many cultures. Ainsworth (1979, p. 44) proposed that the secure pattern is to be considered as normative and the optimal adaptive developmental outcome for human infants. Subsequently, there have been many studies of infant patterns of attachment to mother, father, and sometimes to a permanent nonparental caregiver. The Strange Situation procedure has been conducted with infants from many cultural backgrounds in the Western and Eastern hemispheres, from agriculturally oriented to industrialized peoples. Almost all confirmed this proposition (van IJzendoorn and Sagi 1999). Only two exceptions have been published: (a) in our northern German sample, but not in several southern German samples, the insecure-avoidant pattern was found to be dominant (Grossmann, K. et al. 1985); (b) in an Israeli sample of infants with out-of-home sleeping arrangements, the insecure-ambivalent pattern and even disorganized attachment behaviors were dominant (Sagi et al. 1994).

Finally, the sensitivity hypothesis states that the quality of attachment depends on the attachment figure's sensitivity to the child's attachment and exploratory behaviors, that is, the quality of care received. Quality of care even extends to being given enough food under poor economic living conditions (Valenzuela 1997). Secure or insecure patterns of attachment are not genetically determined, as qualities of attachment to two or even three attachment figures are largely independent of each other (van IJzendoorn et al. 1992). Studies investigating antecedents of security of attachment conducted in the U.S.A., Europe, and in other cultures all demonstrated a significant relationship between maternal sensitivity and a secure pattern of infant attachment. Although each research team defined maternal sensitivity in a somewhat different way, no study yielded contradictory evidence (De Wolff and van IJzendoorn 1997).

Some cultural institutions, however, clearly hinder parents in providing sensitive and cooperative care. General cultural beliefs that "crying strengthens the lungs" or "responding to crying spoils a child and creates a tyrant in the house" have dominated child-rearing customs in Germany in the past and have kept many a mother from responding to her crying infant (Grossmann, K. et al. 1985). Some social groups may even limit parents' access to their children, as formerly in some traditional Israeli kibbutzim (Aviezer and Sagi 1999).

DEVELOPMENT OF PSYCHOLOGICAL SECURITY: A NORTHERN GERMAN LONGITUDINAL STUDY OF ATTACHMENT DEVELOPMENT IN THE FAMILY

Attachment theory posits a causal relationship between an individual's experience with his/her parents and his/her later capacity to make affectional bonds. Enduring and supportive bonds between adult partners, together with the capacity to care and make affectional bonds with one's own infants, are optimal preconditions for a joint and successful upbringing of one's offspring. This is interpreted as the adaptive value of attachment and sensitive caregiving.

Evidence supporting this hypothesis can be found within one of our longitudinal studies of a group of 38 young German adults, whom we observed since birth as they grew up in their nonrisk families of origin. At 22 years of age, the young adults' representations of partnership, including markers of attachment, were assessed based on a German adaptation of the "current relationship interview" by Crowell and Owens (see Crowell and Waters 2005). A secure partnership representation describes a person who values an intimate relationship as a reliable source of comfort, who has a mutual "secure-base" relationship with the partner, and who has an easy access to partnership-related thoughts and feelings without denying unfavorable aspects of that partnership. Trained evaluators rated "security" versus "insecurity" of partnership representation on one dimension and "quality of discourse" about partnership on another. Quality of discourse was an important marker of the capacity to make affectional bonds for those young adults who did not experience a mutually supportive partnership but could still present a clear and coherent discourse about his/her disappointing partnership experiences, be open and competent in his/her discourse about partnership and address freely attachment aspects within a partnership. Security and quality of discourse were correlated significantly ($r = 0.42$).

Longitudinal analyses revealed three major influences on the quality of partnership representation in childhood experiences with both parents starting from the early years: (a) maternal sensitivity, (b) the child's quality of discourse when interviewed about attachment and friendship issues, and (c) the quality of father's sensitive and challenging interactions during play with his toddler (Grossmann, K. et al. 2005; Grossmann, K.E. et al. 2002).

Maternal sensitivity was observed and assessed in situations appropriate to the child's development during the first year, at 24 months, and at age six. Later, mothers and children/adolescents were interviewed, and maternal support, acceptance, and empathic understanding of the child, as reported by each side, was rated. Aggregation of maternal sensitivity ratings with ratings of maternal support for each age of assessment yielded aggregated scores for the age periods infancy, childhood, and adolescence. These scores revealed a significant influence for each aggregated score on security of partnership representation and quality of discourse about partnership. In particular and surprisingly, a significant relationship emerged between observed maternal sensitivity and support for exploration during the infancy years and quality of discourse about partnership. We interpret these results as reinforcing the assumption that interactive experiences with the mother serve as a model for interactions with close others.

When interviewed about attachment and friendship issues, the child's quality of discourse emerged as the second most important influence on the quality of partnership representation. The interviews were conducted with the children at the ages of six, ten, and sixteen. They were analyzed for their coherency, clarity, and openness with which a child described and discussed his/her emotions and motives during social interactions with family and friends, as well as for his/her attachment orientation when presenting solutions for their problems in distressing situations or when having negative feelings.

Partnership representation at age 22 had as significant predictors each of the assessments of discourse quality starting from the age of six years. In turn, discourse quality in adolescence could be predicted by discourse quality in childhood as well as by maternal sensitivity during childhood. The quality of discursive language when talking about close relationships seems to play a major role in the development of IWMs of attachment.

We also applied the traditional assessments of quality of attachment to the children. In infancy, quality of attachment to the mother and father were assessed with the Strange Situation procedure: six-year-olds were given a projective picture test — the separation anxiety test — to assess their security of attachment representation; at adolescence, the Adult Attachment Interview was used. Compared to maternal and paternal sensitivity and support as well as, somewhat later, the child's quality of discourse about attachment issues, traditional attachment measures yielded fewer and much weaker relations to later partnership representation in this longitudinal study as well as in our second longitudinal study presented elsewhere (Grossmann, K. et al. 2005).

The third major influence on partnership representation came from the child's experiences with his/her father. When the children were two and six years of age, fathers were observed in playful interactions with the child and rated on a scale for their "Sensitive and Challenging Interactive Play" (SCIP Scale; Grossmann, K. et al. 2002). This rating of the quality of their interactions was a significant predictor of later security of attachment representation at the ages of 10, 16, and 22 years, and it was a significant predictor of quality of later discourse about friendship representation at the age of 16 years and partnership representation at the age of 22 years. Later assessments of paternal sensitivity during play and paternal support, acceptance and empathic understanding of the child as reported by each side at age 10 also contributed significantly to later partnership representation (Grossmann, K. et al. 2005).

Figure 10.2 presents the major results of the analyses of early influences on partnership representation at age 22. Maternal and paternal sensitivity and appropriate challenges while interacting with the preschool child were the two most important predictors. Traditional measures of security of attachment contributed very little, if anything at all. The quality of child discourse about attachment and friendship is not part of the graph because it was closely related to earlier maternal and paternal sensitivity.

A wider view of attachment, which includes a child's experiences with both parents as havens of safety and secure bases in the domain of secure and playful exploration, was advocated quite early in the formulation of attachment theory (Bowlby 1982). Important for the development of a secure IWM of attachment is not only the extent to which a child's parents provide a secure base, but also the extent to which they encourage the child to explore from it. We fully endorse this wider view of attachment as it may yield a more comprehensive picture of the roots of a person's IWM of attachment. In modern sociobiological terms, these results indicate that quality of parental investment during the preschool years strongly affects a child's mental state with respect to the value of a close and supportive partnership many years later.

Fathers as Trusted Companions during Exploration

For a long time, attachment research has neglected the role of fathers as attachment figures and the child's negative emotions during exploration (e.g., wariness of mild fear). One reason for this may be that fathers challenge their young children's competencies, leaving the task of providing tender loving physical care and contact comfort to the mother (Parke 1996). This appeared true for the group of fathers that we studied in Germany: If a father wanted to be with his infant or toddler, they usually spent time exploring and playing. A supportive father who was neither overly demanding nor dominated their joint play seemed to provide the exploring young child with sufficient security through his supportive presence, while at the same time challenging the child's competencies. This appeared to motivate the toddler to master the challenges without anxiety. Positive, sensitive, and appropriate playful interactions often looked like vivid

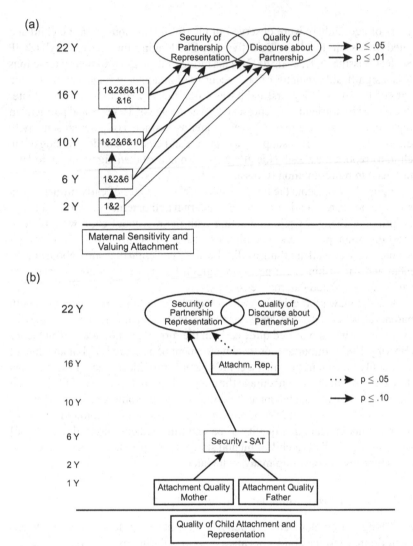

Figure 10.2   (a, b) Relationships between maternal sensitivity and valuing of attachment and children's later partnership representation. SAT = security anxiety test.

examples of a father knowing about Vygotsky' zone of proximal development as the best way to foster his child's cognitive development. Therefore, when meeting difficulties, the children with their father at their side did not need to interrupt their concentration during exploratory and constructive play. The supportive, sensitively challenging companionship of fathers was found to have long-lasting effects on the child's socio-emotional and attachment development. Our findings suggest that infants develop attachment relationships to their mothers and fathers through distinctive pathways.

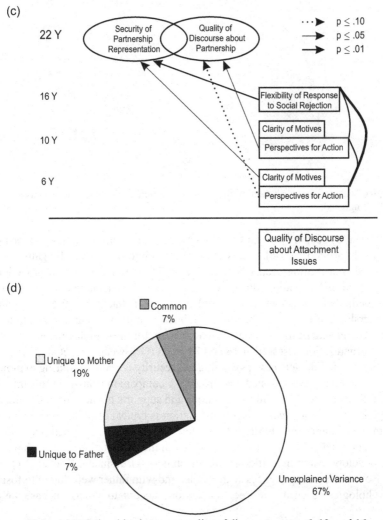

Figure 10.2 (c) Relationships between quality of discourse at age 6, 10, and 16 years and children's later partnership representation. (d) Explained variance in predicting partnership representation at 22 years: influences from mothers, fathers, and both parents (common).

In Figures 10.3 and 10.4, the two kinds of security are contrasted for the purpose of demonstration in two pictures drawn by our team member, Sue Kellinghaus (Grossmann, K. and Grossmann, K.E. 2004). Figure 10.3 depicts the arrangement of the Strange Situation and may characterize paradigmatically a central feature of the young child's attachment to mother, as described by Ainsworth. A young child, if alarmed, will go to her mother for reassurance and relaxation. This function of the mother is usually noted as a haven of safety.

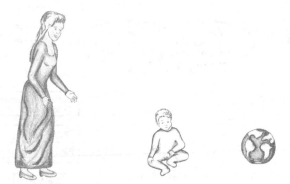

Figure 10.3 Characterization of the Strange Situation, as described by Ainsworth (by S. Kellinghaus).

However, by seeking proximity to the haven of safety, the child has to interrupt her exploration. If consolation is effective, the child will move off again to explore, demonstrating secure-base behavior. The Strange Situation procedure may certainly be a valid indicator of quality of infant attachment to mother but this method of assessment did not predict quality of attachment, friendship, and partnership representation beyond childhood in our two longitudinal studies. The second year of life may have been too early for the complex mental attachment organization assessed at 16 and 22 years (Grossmann, K. et al. 2005).

Figure 10.4 depicts how psychological security is acquired during exploration through having a trusted and protective companion nearby. In this image, the father monitors the child's intentions and supports her actions at the site of exploration or *Forschung*. This constellation is typical of fathers' interactions with their infants and children. In our longitudinal study, it turned out to be a valid and predictive indicator of the quality of the child–father relationship and the development in the child of later attachment (Grossmann, K. et al. 2005).

Both kinds of experiences with mother and with father were found to foster psychological security: a free, nonanxious access to others in case help,

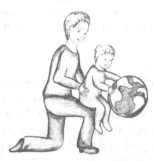

Figure 10.4 Characterization of the acquisition of psychological security during exploration in the presence of a trusted companion (the father) nearby (by S. Kellinghaus).

protection, and support is needed during challenging explorations. Conversely, children from our study, whose needs for secure proximity during distress and secure support during exploration were only insufficiently met by both parents, gave many indications of psychological insecurity, as evidenced, for example, by insecure representations of attachment and partnership (Grossmann, K. and Grossmann, K.E. 2004).

THE CHANGING THEORETICAL CONTEXT OF HUMAN SOCIAL ATTACHMENT

Attachment theory, as conceived by John Bowlby, and further developed through his interaction with Mary Ainsworth, has its roots in psychoanalysis and classical ethology. Ethology is the approach to animal behavior initiated by Lorenz and Tinbergen in the 1930s. Hinde recently said about ethology:

> It flowered between the fifties and seventies, and has now been largely assimilated into other disciplines. It is to be seen not as a theory about behavior, but in terms of three basic attitudes: 1. The description and classification of behavior is an essential preliminary to its understanding; 2. Behavior cannot be studied without some knowledge of the environment to which the species has become adapted in evolution; and [in referring to Tinbergen's four questions about causation, development, function, and evolution of behavioral characteristics (Tinbergen 1963), which are basic to the ethological approach, Hinde added] 3. Questions about the evolution and function of behavior are as important as those about its development and causation (Hinde 2005, p. 1).

Applying this approach to their work, Ainsworth and Bowlby regarded ethological observations as the *via regia* of attachment research and were convinced that the power of attachment theory owed much to its "ethological approach to personality development" (Ainsworth and Bowlby 1991). Recently, classical ethology has been assimilated by evolutionary psychology, sociobiology, physiology, and biological anthropology. Systematic observations of development and interactive behaviors, and its more or less adaptive functioning within and across various species, were its hallmark. Unfortunately, it has often given way to less detailed and less careful descriptions and documentation. For example, the extensive observational and descriptive work about maternal sensitivity, conducted by Ainsworth and her co-workers almost fifty years ago, have never been fully replicated in other cultures. Therefore, the full range of Ainsworth's observational implications could never be reliably compared, although there were many unwarranted assertions about inherent cultural differences regarding the relation between maternal sensitivity and infant attachment quality (e.g., Rothbaum et al. 2000).

For a new synthesis of attachment and bonding we feel that the following question must be addressed: How are causation, development, function, and evolution interrelated in humans as well as in animals? Below, we address briefly Tinbergen's four questions from our perspective, but the traditional orientation of attachment theory, which concentrates on the child's side of the attachment–caregiving relationship, must be integrated in a new synthesis of modern Darwinian life sciences. Otherwise it risks being left behind in scientific development. Our thoughts were greatly inspired by lively discussions with our colleagues from other disciplines, for instance by the sociobiologist, Eckart Voland, a fellow participant at this Dahlem Workshop.

Voland pointed us to the fact that the image of an "ideal" mother–child relationship as a *desideratum* of traditional attachment theory is not supported by neo-Darwinian concepts. Rather, sociobiologists recognize inherent structural conflicts between mothers and their offspring. In an ultimate sense, it may be adaptive for a mother to enhance her own reproductive fitness at the expense of any single particular child. This consideration can also provide a deeper understanding for proximate individual behavior, as it challenges some traditional assumptions of attachment theory. It came, for example, as a surprise to some attachment researchers that mothers could be differentially sensitive to their different infants, and that siblings' attachment classifications are largely unrelated (van IJzendoorn et al. 2000). Modern sociobiology may offer new insight as to whether variations in maternal sensitivity to different infants' signals are accidental (as we have implicitly assumed at the proximate level) or the result of variations in willingness to invest in children for ultimate strategic fitness reasons: consideration of present proximate living conditions in the culture (Rogoff 2003, pp. 111–116).

Next, we turn to the four concepts — causation, development, function and evolution (Tinbergen 1963) — basic to the ethological approach. Researchers often concentrate on these separately, but as Hinde (2005) points out, "all of these answers would be correct, but no one would be complete."

Causation

Much work has focused on the physiological mechanisms underlying social attachment and bonding (e.g., Keverne, this volume). The general assumption is that physiological structures of the central nervous system and hormonal processes "cause" human behavioral adaptation at the proximate level. These physiological mechanisms evolved because of fitness advantages of individuals thus endowed. Studies in many species show the interdependence between behavior and causation. On one hand, physiological and neurological changes are frequently linked to social events such as distress, separation, social rejection, and inappropriate care (Kraemer 1992; Kraemer et al., this volume). On the other, hormones that play a crucial role in close bonds, and particularly in attachment relationships, such as oxytocin and vasopressin, have been shown to influence emotions profoundly. Among many other things they enhance the capacity to overcome anxiety and fear in animals (Carter, this volume).

In human one-year-olds, elevated cortisol levels were related to patterns of insecure attachments (Spangler and Grossmann 1993). We interpreted these findings as an indication of the inability of the organism to find an appropriate behavioral strategy to cope with separation distress, a set of behaviors that would result in proximity to the protective attachment figure. Insecurity about the availability and responsiveness of the attachment figure would imply negative consequences for development, as outlined above.

There are some unanswered questions about the significance of these processes from an evolutionary perspective. Comparison of previously experienced maternal sensitivity of the insecurely with the securely attached toddlers suggests that the differences in physiological stress may have been a consequence of suboptimal attachment experiences, which, in turn, may have influenced the toddler's physiological reactions to stress. Hypo- or hyperactivation of physiological systems might be a response to past inappropriate management of the infant's homeostasis by the mothering figure, as Polan and Hofer (1999) suggested. Only if development is disregarded could physiological processes qualify as a *cause* for behavioral responses to the aroused attachment system. A test for a pure causation assumption would be whether certain pathological behavior processes could be reversed by physiological or pharmacological interventions *together* with investigating how this would affect the quality of social, emotional, or attachment behavior that is associated with the changed behavior in question.

In sum, the causal answers per se may be correct; however, without parallel consideration of development, function, and evolution of the behavior in question, the answer would be incomplete, if not misleading.

Development

In attachment theory, the developmental processes are assumed to be basic and thus universal for human infants. All infants are born prepared to become social and "ready to learn the ways of those around them…for joining human life, to attract the care of adults and many other things" (Rogoff 2003, pp. 67f). Differences in the distribution of qualities of attachment between or within cultures are considered to be variations depending on the ontogenetically experienced circumstances in line with Waddington's genetic landscape (Waddington 1957). As an open genetic program, infants' attachment development accommodates a limited variety of caregiving practices and styles if they comply at least minimally with an infants' basic attachment needs to be protected and cared for by at least one reliably available individual. Experiments of raising infants by an interchangeable number of caregivers (e.g., those conducted in some former Communist countries or in Israeli kibbutzim) were abandoned when it either became evident that the children developed less competently than children raised in families (Matejcek 1989), or when the families were physically threatened, as was the case for Israel during the Gulf War in 1991 (Aviezer and Sagi 1999).

Provided the basic requirements of infant attachment formation are fulfilled, phenotypic attachment behaviors are bound to have specific characteristics. Attachment behaviors (e.g., actively seeking proximity or only passively crying when left alone, exuberant or subdued greeting behaviors upon reunion, more or less expressed separation anxiety) will differ in distinct cultures and in different epochs depending on differences in customs of child care, family or social structures, devastating or benign living conditions and similar environmental circumstances (Grossmann, K.E. 1995; Rogoff 2003). Social structures may allow or restrict the number of available attachment persons to a young child, and social customs may enforce separations, painful procedures inflicted to the child in the mother's presence, or other traumatic blows to the child's attachment needs. Still, even these cultures respect the biological, i.e., evolutionary constraints of attachment formation by assigning each infant to a mother figure, mostly the biological mother, who will be the primary person providing protection and care.

Over the years, longitudinal attachment research has maintained its focus on Ainsworth's and Bowlby's main assumption: Will early experiences with the attachment figures influence the quality of later psychological functioning in close relationships, and on the development of IWMs of self and others? IWMs are hypothetical constructs about individual expectations. Expectations about how others will react to one's attachment needs and the need to explore influence a person's perceptions of social interactions, especially the organization of behavior strategies when distressed. Incoherent IWMs about self and others appear to be the central and essential issue in deviant development (Hennighausen and Lyons-Ruth, this volume).

Other developmental issues worth more investigations are: what will uphold and what will break an intergenerational transmission of quality of attachment, of unhealthy and unkind childcare practices, of child abuse, or of "inheriting" mental health or ill health. Bowlby (1973) posited that these processes are much more likely to be socially than genetically inherited.

Function

Bowlby's original idea about the evolutionary function of attachment was protection from wild animals or other dangers. Sociobiology today would also suggest that nonkin humans may have posed a much greater danger. For parents, the important issues are still protection from environmental dangers (e.g., getting hurt, burned, or poisoned) as well as protection from nonkin (e.g., prevention from abduction, abuse, or being lured into drug dependency).

As a clinician, Bowlby (1988) experienced that non-attachment or severe attachment trauma through separation, rejection, loss, etc. led to deviating developmental pathways in ontogeny that differed widely from the range of normal development. However, attachment theory provided for the discovery of secure and insecure patterns of attachment within nonclinical samples and their function within a specific parent–child relation (Main 1981), the discovery of incomplete attachment strategies because of internal motivational conflict leading to disorientation and disorganization, and the discovery of different rules behind secure and insecure IWMs and their functioning.

An "ideal" model of a secure human attachment developmental trajectory requires that it should function adaptively at different age periods and under a variety of psychological challenges. Optimal functioning, according to attachment theory, is evidenced by the ability to seek and accept help from trusted others and by undistorted perceptions, interpretations, and descriptions of complex social and emotional experiences, as well as motives and intentions of self and others. Variations between cultures are analogous to variations between different species as long as they remain functionally adaptive but originate from homologous origins (Lorenz 1974, 1977). "Similarities and differences across communities do not divide phenomena into biological and cultural," and "cultural differences are generally variations of themes of universal import with differing emphasis or value placed on particular practices rather than all-or-none differences" (Rogoff 2003, p. 64). This certainly is true for the function of attachment.

Why do some (insecure and/or disorganized) IWMs malfunction? One of the old psychoanalytic hypothesis summoned so-called defense mechanisms (A. Freud 1946). The term defense mechanism refers to a set of assumed mental rules in the service of protecting the person from emotional pain (purposefully? unconsciously?) by distorting perception and interpretation of situations, feelings, and intentions of others. However well they may function ad hoc, some defenses do not function well for long-term psychological adjustment. George Vaillant (1977, 1992; Vaillant et al. 1986) devised measurement procedures for maladaptive or "immature" as well as adaptive or "mature" psychological defenses. In one of our longitudinal studies, an analysis of defense mechanisms used by young adults with secure versus insecure attachment representations revealed a predominance of adaptive defenses in the secure interviews as compared to a predominance of maladaptive defenses in the insecure interviews (Hetterich 2004). This finding is another indication of variation in function as well as in development of attachment thoughts and behaviors which is "caused" by different attachment experiences.

Future research might find corresponding physiological processes of different defense mechanisms when a person confronts negative or positive attachment experiences such as separation and loss, or supportive helpful others, and the role culture plays during these experiences.

Evolution

Evolution, as a framework for understanding human development, has often been neglected in psychology (for a laudable exception, see Gray 2002) and attachment research (Ainsworth 1990). Our position in this chapter is rooted, but not limited, in the tradition of classical ethology. Ainsworth (pers. comm.) adopted the evolutionary concept of adaptation as a theoretical frame for psychological adaptation, that is, individual mental health when adjusting to complex social environments. Lorenz (1967, p. 379) asserted that any organismic adaptation to given qualities of its ecological space results in a change in the living system itself. It incorporates that environmental quality and thereby becomes part of it. The fin of a fish, in Lorenz's way of thinking, reflects the physical properties of water; the hoof of a horse the physical properties of the steppe.

What are the basic realities of human life? Bronislaw Malinowski (1949) and Sir James George Frazer — both eminent founders of cultural and social anthropology — offered the following answer derived from an observation of nature known across the ages: "to live and to create life, to eat and to generate children, these are the primary wish of man in all past times, and these will remain to be the primary wishes as long as the world will exist." Here, Malinowski (1949, freely translated from a German translation of an original manuscript written in 1942) asserts, "Frazer tells us that human culture constructs itself deeply from the biological needs of man."

Using the ethological approach to personality development, future research in attachment should pursue the phenotypic fate of the pre-programmed biological necessities in a given culture, and compare the psychological consequences of secure or insecure attachment experiences for the individuals concerned within "close similarities in the sequence and timing of some infant developmental milestones as the onset of smiling and distress over separation from an attachment figure" (Rogoff 2003, p. 68).

CONCLUSION

For us, the core interest of attachment research in individual children's optimal adaptive developmental outcomes, as stated by Ainsworth (1979, p. 14), is still an important issue from a developmental and mental health point of view, but not necessarily from a sociobiological perspective. It would be shortsighted, however, to ignore coherent and more integrative explanations suggested by modern evolutionary theory. In an attempt to incorporate these evolutionary hypotheses, future attachment research needs to go beyond the first generation of offspring to the fate of grandchildren (see Belsky et al. 1991; Belsky, this volume; Draper, this volume). Only by taking a long-term perspective will it be possible to differentiate between evolutionary conditional strategies and functional versus nonfunctional variation in attachment.

From a sociobiological perspective, Voland (pers. comm.) points out that biological normativity is nearly always expressed in all individuals of a species. In humans, the fact that insecure patterns of attachment occur relatively often in infants would speak against a genetically pre-programmed biological normativity of the secure pattern (Voland 1998), as would research results showing that attachment patterns are individually acquired, may underlie change, and may develop differently to different caregivers. Hinde and Stevenson-Hinde (1990) also argue in favor of conditional ontogenetic adaptivity of all attachment patterns — be they secure or insecure — implying that there may be ecological reasons for the development of secure as well as insecure patterns. This is granted. Nevertheless, it seems that the psychological consequences of security versus insecurity for each individual result in more or less psychological adaptivity in mental health terms. More research is needed to determine whether under some living conditions avoidance, enmeshment, or even disorganization and disorientation — rather than security of attachment — would indeed be more successful reproductively across generations. Attachment theory presently assumes that conditional adaptation through insecure patterns of attachment to adverse circumstances (e.g., war or epidemics which imply many losses) is advantageous only at the expense of psychological security of the individual human being. Similarly, using defenses that mentally distort or exclude decisive aspects of how the self and others are perceived will eventually not serve mental health.

In contrast to attachment theory, sociobiology has paid much less attention to the infant's part in the parent–offspring conflict. Hrdy (1999, this volume), however, does address an infant's self interest. She argues that infants, from the very beginning, demonstrate vitality as strategic players by, for example, crying, cuteness, cooing, and their appearance, the *Kindchen-Schema*. (Cuteness and cooing, however, are not yet necessarily present immediately after delivery.) These features, she believes, entice the mother to invest in the offspring. Hrdy's and Ainsworth's view on infant crying augment each other by adding cultural learning to the initial demonstration of vitality if life circumstances are not as harsh, as related by Rogoff (2003). An infant's cry surely alerts the mother, and when she responds sensitively, the infant will eventually replace crying by more differentiated preverbal means of communication. Still, attachment theory needs to address the correspondence between societal desiderata, parental investment interests, life circumstances, infant "genetic selfishness," and the psychologically healthy development of the individual child to keep pace with the continuing development of evolutionary theory.

In a future synthesis of attachment and bonding, a combined view of causation, development, function, and evolution will certainly constitute a new vital natural developmental science. It will enable us to analyze more broadly and with greater validity the various functions of attachment and bonding, pre-programmed by evolution and performed by individuals under various specific living conditions, and how they account for the development of individual's psychological security and adaptability across various cultures and in different natural and historical epochs in various kinds of bonds as well as in attachment development.

ACKNOWLEDGMENT

We thank Heidi Keller for her thoughtful and constructive comments on an earlier version of this paper.

224   K. E. Grossmann and K. Grossmann

REFERENCES

Abe, R. 2003. Lebensborn e.V. http://www.shoa.de/lebensborn.html.
Ainsworth, M.D.S. 1979. Attachment as related to mother–child interaction. In: Advances in the Study of Behavior, ed. J. Rosenblatt, R.A. Hinde, C. Beer, and M. Busnel, vol. 9, pp. 1–51. San Diego: Academic.
Ainsworth, M.D.S. 1985. Attachment across the life span. Bull. NY Acad. Med. 61:792–812.
Ainsworth, M.D.S. 1990. Some considerations regarding theory and assessment relevant to attachments beyond infancy. In: Attachment in the Preschool Years, ed. M.T. Greenberg, D. Chicchetti, and E.M. Cummings, pp. 463–488. Chicago/London: Univ. of Chicago Press.
Ainsworth, M.D.S. 1991. Attachments and other affectional bonds across the life cycle. In: Attachment across the Life Cycle, ed. C.M. Parkes, J. Stevenson-Hinde, and P. Marris, pp. 33–51. New York: Routledge.
Ainsworth, M.D.S., and S.M. Bell. 1974. Mother–infant interaction and the development of competence. In: The Growth of Competence, ed. K.J. Connolly and J. Bruner, pp. 97–118. London and New York: Academic.
Ainsworth, M.D.S., and S.M. Bell. 1977. Infant crying and maternal responsiveness: A rejoinder to Gewirtz and Boyd. Child Dev. 48:1208–1216.
Ainsworth, M.D.S., S.M. Bell, and D.J. Stayton. 1974. Infant–mother attachment and social development: "Socialization" as a product of reciprocal responsiveness to signals. In: The Integration of a Child into a Social World, ed. P.M. Richards, pp. 99–135. Cambridge: Cambridge Univ. Press.
Ainsworth, M.D.S., M.C. Blehar, E. Waters, and S. Wall. 1978. Patterns of Attachment: A Psychological Study of the Strange Situation. Hillsdale, NJ: Erlbaum.
Ainsworth, M.D.S., and J. Bowlby. 1991. 1989 APA award recipient address: An ethological approach to personality development. Am. Psychol. 46:333–341.
Ainsworth, M.D.S., and B.A. Wittig. 1969. Attachment and the exploratory behavior of one-year-olds in a strange situation. In: Determinants of Infant Behavior, ed. B.M. Foss, vol. 4, pp. 111–136. London: Methuen.
Aviezer, O., and A. Sagi. 1999. The rise and fall of collective sleeping and its impact on the relationships of kibbutz children and parents. In: The Transformation of Collective Education in the Kibbutz: The End of Utopia?, ed. W. Fölling and M. Fölling-Albers, pp. 192–211. Frankfurt: Peter Lang.
Barry, H., and L. Paxson. 1971. Infancy and early childhood: Cross-cultural codes. Ethology 10:466–508.
Belsky, J., L. Steinberg, and P. Draper. 1991. Childhood experience, interpersonal development, and reproductive strategy: An evolutionary theory of socialization. Child Dev. 62:647–670.
Bowlby, J. 1951. Maternal care and mental health. Bull. WHO 3:355–534.
Bowlby, J. 1960. Comment on Professor Piaget's paper. In: Discussions on Child Development, ed. J.M. Tanner and B. Inhelder, vol. 4, pp. 35–47. London: Tavistock.
Bowlby, J. 1973. Separation: Anxiety and Anger. Attachment and Loss, vol. 2. New York: Basic.
Bowlby, J. 1979. The Making and Breaking of Affectional Bonds. London: Tavistock.
Bowlby, J. 1980. Loss: Sadness and Depression. Attachment and Loss, vol. 3. New York: Basic.
Bowlby, J. 1982. Attachment. 2nd rev. ed. Attachment and Loss, vol. 1. New York: Basic.

Bowlby, J. 1987. Attachment. In: The Oxford Companion to the Mind, ed. R.L. Gregory, pp. 57–58. Oxford: Oxford Univ. Press.

Bowlby, J. 1988. Developmental psychiatry comes of age. *Am. J. Psych.* **145**:1–10.

Bowlby, J. 1991. Postscript. In: Attachment across the Life Cycle, ed. C.M. Parkes, J. Stevenson-Hinde, and P. Marris, pp. 293–297. New York: Routledge.

Bruner, J.S. 1982. The organization of action and the nature of adult–infant transaction. In: Analysis of Action, ed. M. von Cranach and R. Harre, pp. 313–327. Cambridge: Cambridge Univ. Press.

Bruner, J.S. 1983. In Search of Mind: Essays in Autobiography. New York: Harper and Row.

Bruner, J.S. 1990. Acts of Meaning. Cambridge, MA: Harvard Univ. Press.

Cairns, R.B. 1979. Social Development: The Origins and Plasticity of Interchanges. San Francisco: Freeman.

Cassidy, J. 1988. Child–mother attachment and the self in six-year-olds. *Child Dev.* **59**:121–134.

Cassidy, J., and P.R. Shaver, eds. 1999. Handbook of Attachment: Theory, Research, and Clinical Applications. New York: Guilford.

Cole, M. 1996. Cultural Psychology: A Once and Future Discipline. Cambridge, MA: Harvard Univ. Press.

Cosmides, L., and J. Tooby. 2000. Evolutionary psychology and the emotions. In: Handbook of Emotions, ed. M. Lewis and J.M. Haviland-Jones, 2nd ed., pp. 91–115. New York: Guilford.

Crowell, J., and E. Waters. 2005. Attachment representations, secure behaviour, and the evolution of adult relationship. In: Attachment from Infancy to Adulthood: The Major Longitudinal Studies, ed. K.E. Grossmann, K. Grossmann, and E. Waters, pp. 223–244. New York: Guilford.

Darwin, C. 1872/1998. The Expression of the Emotions in Man and Animals, 3rd ed. New York: Oxford Univ. Press.

De Wolff, M.S., and M.H. van IJzendoorn. 1997. Sensitivity and attachment: A meta-analysis on parental antecedents of infant attachment. *Child Dev.* **68**:571–746.

Dunn, J. 1993. Young Children's Close Relationships: Beyond Attachment. Newbury Park, CA: Sage.

Freud, A. 1946. The Ego and the Mechanisms of Defense. New York: Intl. Univ. Press.

Gray, P. 2002. Psychology. 4th ed. New York: Worth.

Grossmann, K., and K.E. Grossmann. 2004. Bindung: Das Gefüge psychischer Sicherheit. Stuttgart: Klett-Cotta.

Grossmann, K., K.E. Grossmann, E. Fremmer-Bombik et al. 2002. The uniqueness of the child–father attachment relationship: Fathers' sensitive and challenging play as the pivotal variable in a 16-year longitudinal study. *Soc. Dev.* **11**:307–331.

Grossmann, K., K.E. Grossmann, and H. Kindler. 2005. Early care and the roots of attachment and partnership representation. The Bielefeld and Regensburg Longitudinal studies. In: Attachment from Infancy to Adulthood: The Major Longitudinal Studies, ed. K.E. Grossmann, K. Grossmann, and E. Waters, pp. 98–136. New York: Guilford.

Grossmann, K., K.E. Grossmann, G. Spangler, G. Suess, and L. Unzner. 1985. Maternal sensitivity and newborns' orientation responses as related to quality of attachment in northern Germany. *Mono. Soc. Res. Child Dev.* **50**:233–256.

Grossmann, K., K. Thane, and K.E. Grossmann. 1981. Maternal tactual contact of the newborn after various postpartum conditions of mother–infant contact. *Dev. Psychol.* **17**:158–169.

Grossmann, K.E. 1995. The evolution and history of attachment research and theory. In: Attachment Theory: Social, Developmental and Clinical Perspectives, ed. S. Goldberg, R. Muir, and J. Kerr, pp. 85–102. Hillsdale, NJ: Analytic Press.

Grossmann, K.E. 1999. Old and new internal working models of attachment: The organization of feelings and language. *Attach. Hum. Dev.* **1**:253–269.

Grossmann, K.E., K. Grossmann, and A. Keppler. 2005. Universal and culturally specific aspects of human behavior: The case of attachment. In: Culture and Human Development: The Importance of Cross-cultural Research to the Social Sciences, ed. W. Friedlmeier, P. Chakkarath, and B. Schwarz. Amsterdam: Swetz and Zeitlinger.

Grossmann, K.E., K. Grossmann, M. Winter, and P. Zimmermann. 2002. Attachment relationships and appraisal of partnership: From early experience of sensitive support to later relationship representation. In: Paths to Successful Development, ed. L. Pulkkinen and A. Caspi, pp. 73–105. Cambridge: Cambridge Univ. Press.

Grossmann, K.E., K. Grossmann, and P. Zimmermann. 1999. A wider view of attachment and exploration: Stability and change during the years of immaturity. In: Handbook of Attachment: Theory, Research, and Clinical Applications, ed. J. Cassidy and P.R. Shaver, pp. 760–786. New York: Guilford.

Harlow, H.F. 1961. The development of affectional patterns in infant monkeys. In: Determinants of Infant Behavior, ed. B.M. Foss, vol. 1, pp. 75–97. New York: Wiley.

Harlow, H.F. 1971. Learning to Love. San Francisco: Albion.

Hesse, E. 1999. The Adult Attachment Interview: Historical and current perspectives. In: Handbook of Attachment: Theory, Research, and Clinical Applications, ed. J. Cassidy and P.R. Shaver, pp. 395–433. New York: Guilford.

Hetterich, S. 2004. Unterschiede in der Verwendung adaptiver und maladaptiver Abwehrmechanismen in narrativen Darstellungen früher Bindungserinnerungen. Diplom-Thesis. Universität Regensburg, Germany.

Hinde, R.A. 1976. On describing relationships. *J. Child Psychol. Psychiat.* **17**:1–19.

Hinde, R.A. 2005. Ethology and attachment theory. In: Attachment from Infancy to Adulthood: The Major Longitudinal Studies, ed. K.E. Grossmann, K. Grossmann, and E. Waters, pp. 1–12. New York: Guilford.

Hinde, R.A., and J. Stevenson-Hinde. 1990. Attachment: Biological, cultural, and individual desiderata. *Hum. Dev.* **33**:62–72.

Hrdy, S.B. 1977. The Langurs of Abu: Female and Male Strategies of Reproduction. Cambridge, MA: Harvard Univ. Press.

Hrdy, S.B. 1999. Mother Nature: A History of Mothers, Infants, and Natural Selection. New York: Pantheon.

Klaus, M.H., and J.H. Kennell. 1976. Maternal–infant Bonding. Saint Louis: Mosby.

Kliegl, R., J. Smith, and P.B. Baltes. 1989. Testing-the-limits and the study of adult age differences in cognitive plasticity of a mnemonic skill. *Dev. Psychol.* **25**:247–256.

Kraemer, G.W. 1992. A psychological theory of attachment. *Behav. Brain Sci.* **15**:493–541.

Lilienthal, G. 1993. Der Lebensborn e.V.: Ein Instrument nationalsozialistischer Rassenpolitik. Frankfurt: Fischer.

Lorenz, K. 1960. Various contributions to general discussions. In: Discussions on Child Development, ed. J.M. Tanner and B. Inhelder, vols. 1–4. (vols. 1 and 2: 1956; vol. 3: 1958; vol. 4: 1960.) London: Tavistock.

Lorenz, K. 1967. Die instinktiven Grundlagen menschlicher Kultur. *Naturwiss.* **54**:377–388.

Lorenz, K. 1974. Analogy as a source of knowledge. *Science* **185**:229–234.

Lorenz, K. 1977. Behind the Mirror: A Search for a Natural History of Human Knowledge. New York: Harcourt.

Main, M. 1981. Avoidance in the service of attachment: A working paper. In Behavioral Development: The Bielefeld Interdisciplinary Project, ed. K. Immelmann, G. Barlow, L. Petrinovich, and M. Main, pp. 651–693. New York: Cambridge Univ. Press.

Main, M., and N. Kaplan. 2005. Predictability of attachment behavior and representational processes at 1, 6, and 19 years of age. The Berkeley longitudinal study. In: Attachment from Infancy to Adulthood: The Major Longitudinal Studies, ed. K.E. Grossmann, K. Grossmann, and E. Waters, pp. 245–304. New York: Guilford.

Main, M., and J. Solomon. 1986. Discovery of an insecure disorganized/disoriented attachment pattern: Procedures, findings and implications for the classification of behavior. In: Affective Development in Infancy, ed. T.B. Brazelton and M. Yogman, pp. 95–124. Norwood, NJ: Ablex.

Malinowski, B. 1949. Sir James Frazer: Eine biographische Würdigung (1942). In: Bronislaw Malinowski: Eine wissenschaftliche Theorie der Kultur, pp. 171–208. Zurich: Pan.

Matejcek, Z. 1989. Krippen und die Prinzipien des Familienlebens [Crèches and the principles of family life]. *Der Kinderarzt* **20**:1091–1095.

Meins, E. 1999. Sensitivity, security, and internal working models: Bridging the transmission gap. *Attach. Hum. Dev.* **3**:325–342.

Minsky, M. 1987. The Society of Mind. London: Heinemann.

Miyake, K., S.-J. Chen, and J. Campos. 1985. Infant temperament, mother's mode of interaction, and attachment in Japan: An interim report. *Mono. Soc. Res. Child Dev.* **50**:276–297.

Nelson, K. 1996. Language in Cognitive Development. Cambridge: Cambridge Univ. Press.

Nelson, K. 1999. Event representations, narrative development, and internal working models. *Attach. Hum. Dev.* **1**:239–251.

Parke, R.D. 1996. Fatherhood. Cambridge, MA: Harvard Univ. Press.

Polan, H.J., and M.A. Hofer. 1999. Psychobiological origins of infant attachment and separation responses. In: Handbook of Attachment: Theory, Research, and Clinical Applications, ed. J. Cassidy and P.R. Shaver, pp. 162–180. New York: Guilford.

Rogoff, B. 2003. The Cultural Nature of Human Development. New York: Oxford Univ. Press.

Rothbaum, F., J. Weisz, M. Pott, K. Miyake, and G. Morelli. 2000. Attachment and culture: Security in the United States and Japan. *Am. Psychol.* **55**:1092–1104.

Sagi, A., M.H. van IJzendoorn, O. Aviezer, F. Donnell, and O. Mayseless. 1994. Sleeping out of home in a kibbutz communal arrangement: It makes a difference for infant–mother attachment. *Child Dev.* **65**:902–1004.

Sagi, A., M.H. van IJzendoorn, O. Aviezer et al. 1995. Attachments in a multiple-caregiver and multiple-infant environment: The case of the Israeli kibbutzim. *Mono. Soc. Res. Child Dev.* **60**:71–91.

Schaffer, H.R., and P.E. Emerson. 1964. The development of social attachments in infancy. *Mono. Soc. Res. Child Dev.* **29**.

Solomon, J., and C. George. 1999. The development of attachment in separated and divorced families. *Attach. Hum. Dev.* **1**:2–33.

Spangler, G., and K.E. Grossmann. 1993. Biobehavioral organization in securely and insecurely attached infants. *Child Dev.* **64**:1439–1450.

Spitz, R.A. 1945. Hospitalism. *Psychoan. Stud. Child* **1**:53–74.

Sroufe, L.A. 2000. Early relationships and the development of children. *Infant Mental Hlth. J.* **21**:67–74.

Sroufe, L.A., B. Egeland, E. Carlson, and W.A. Collins. 2005. Placing early attachment experiences in developmental context. In: Attachment from Infancy to Adulthood: The Major Longitudinal Studies, ed. K.E. Grossmann, K. Grossmann, and E. Waters, pp. 48–70. New York: Guilford.

Sternberg, R.J. 1997. The concept of intelligence and its role in lifelong learning and success. *Am. Psychol.* **52**:1030–1037.

Suess, G., K.E. Grossmann, and L.A. Sroufe. 1992. Effects of infant attachment to mother and father on quality of adaptation in preschool: From dyadic to individual organization of self. *Intl. J. Behav. Dev.* **15**:43–65.

Tanner, J.M., and B. Inhelder, eds. 1960. Discussions on Child Development. vols. 1–4. London: Tavistock. (vol. 1 and 2: 1956; vol. 3: 1958; vol. 4: 1960).

Thompson, R.A. 2000. The legacy of early attachments. *Child Dev.* **71**:145–152.

Tinbergen, N. 1951. The Study of Instinct. London: Oxford Univ. Press.

Tinbergen, N. 1963. On aims and methods in Ethology. *Z. Tierpsychologie* **20**:410–433.

Tomasello, M. 1999. The Cultural Origins of Human Cognition. Cambridge, MA: Harvard Univ. Press.

Trivers, R.L. 1974. Parent offspring conflict. *Am. Zoologist* **14**:249–264.

Vaillant, G.E. 1977. Adaptation to Life. Boston: Little Brown.

Vaillant, G.E. 1992. Ego Mechanisms of Defense. Washington: Am. Psychiatric Press.

Vaillant, G.E., M. Bond, and C.O. Vaillant. 1986. An empirically validated hierarchy of defense mechanisms. *Arch. Gen. Psychiatry* **43**:786–794.

Valenzuela, M. 1997. Maternal sensitivity in a developing society: The context of urban poverty and infant chronic undernutrition. *Dev. Psychol.* **33**:845–855.

van IJzendoorn, M.H., and P.M. Kroonenberg. 1988. Cross-cultural patterns of attachment: A meta-analysis of the strange situation. *Child Dev.* **59**:147–156.

van IJzendoorn, M., G. Moran, J. Belsky et al. 2000. The similarity of siblings' attachments to their mother. *Child Dev.* **71**:1086–1098.

van IJzendoorn, M.H., and A. Sagi. 1999. Cross-cultural patterns of attachment: Universal and contextual determinants. In: Handbook of Attachment: Theory, Research, and Clinical Applications, ed. J. Cassidy and P.R. Shaver, pp. 713–734. New York: Guilford.

van IJzendoorn, M., A. Sagi, and M.W.E. Lambermon. 1992. The multiple caretaker paradox: Some data from Holland and Israel. In: Relationships between Children and Non-parental Adults, ed. R.C. Pianta, pp. 5–24. New Directions in Child Development 57. San Francisco: Jossey-Bass.

Voland, E. 1998. Evolutionary ecology of human reproduction. *Ann. Rev. Anthropology* **27**:347–374.

Waddington, C.H. 1957. The Strategy of Genes. London: Allen and Unwin.

Waters, E., and E.M. Cummings. 2000. A secure base from which to explore close relationships. *Child Dev.* **71**:164–172.

Wensauer, M., and K.E. Grossmann. 1998. Bindungstheoretische Grundlagen subjektiver Lebenszufriedenheit und individueller Zukunftsorientierung im höheren Erwachsenenalter. *Z. Geront. Geriatrie* **31**:362–370.

11

Parenting and Alloparenting

The Impact on Attachment in Humans

L. AHNERT

Department of Education and Psychology, Freie Universität Berlin,
14195 Berlin, Germany

ABSTRACT

During the first months, child–mother attachment relationships are shaped by sensitive parenting, as evidenced by prompt reactions to the child's distress followed by positive affectional interactions. In contrast to a trait-like attribute, which remains stable in an individual throughout life, it is proposed that attachment is dynamic in nature, influenced by the necessary adjustment of sensitivity in response to the child's growing competence as well as age-appropriate changes in care contexts during infancy and beyond. A broad range of caregiving characteristics might explain how child–mother attachments are maintained, thereby revealing multidetermined aspects of attachment relationships. With increased heterogeneity of parenting, various forms of attachments develop based on different care practices, including alloparenting (being cared for by adults other than the biological parents). Alloparenting leads children to form relationships in addition to attachments to their mothers. To explain how children handle multiple attachment relationships and why attachments to different adults sometimes diverge but are still adaptive, the narrow optimum theorem of classical attachment theory is set aside and variations in attachments are evaluated according to how these relationships function in particular care environments.

VARIATIONS IN ATTACHMENT: AN INTRODUCTION

Bowlby (1969) and Ainsworth (1967) focused on the mother–child bond as a complementary but asymmetrical attachment relationship that is challenged by the child's responses to threat and by the mother's function as an attachment figure providing protection. In both animals and humans, it has been continually observed that young under threat do not flee but rather approach the mother as a secure base; this appears to be the result of an evolutionary adaptation. Foremost in humans, however, is secure-base behavior — the hallmark of "secure attachment" (Ainsworth et al. 1978). It has been proven to be strongly shaped by the child's experiences with an attachment figure who dominates the relationship.

In addition to secure-base behaviors, other attachment behaviors have also been observed in humans. Surprisingly, there are behaviors present in human mother–child relationships that run contrary to the expected secure base: infants avoid or resist their mothers when under threat. These insecure-avoidant or insecure-ambivalent attachments (Ainsworth et al. 1978) have been viewed as variations of attachment relationships because avoidance/resistance might be considered to serve attachment (Main 1981).

Main's analyses on communication patterns in animals and humans have revealed that certain behaviors (e.g., gaze aversion, movements away of the head or upper body, turning back and moving out of contact or immediate proximity) might help to *maintain* social contacts. In particular, if the attachment figure is difficult to approach or unpredictably available, interactions might be facilitated if a child shifts the focus of attention away and times behaviors stepwise. Furthermore, the three-part attachment classification system — insecure-avoidant (A), secure (B), and insecure-ambivalent (C) — was refined when Main and Solomon (1990) discovered disorganized features, which indicated troubled relationships in 15% of the A–B–C patterns in normal middle-class samples (van IJzendoorn et al. 1999).

In this chapter, I present variations of attachments in infancy and childhood and discuss their characteristics and functions. Because primary attachments develop through mother–child interaction, we investigate how parenting affects variations in child–mother attachments, whether and how alloparenting leads to attachment relationships, and children's experiences with multiple care providers. Finally, I discuss whether and how primary attachments influence and are influenced by alloparenting.

FORMATION OF ATTACHMENTS AND THE ROLE OF PARENTING

Attachment as a Dynamic Construct

As one of the first behavioral scientists to draw from biology, medicine, and the social sciences, Bowlby (1969) used features of circuit models in cybernetics to conceptualize his perspective on child–mother attachment relationships. This approach allowed him to think of child–mother attachments in terms of a dynamic, goal-corrected feedback process that regulates the child's attachment behaviors toward the mother, in an attempt to maintain a desired level of felt emotional security. In this model, threat activates the child's attachment behaviors and concurrently sets the goal that the behaviors are supposed to achieve, such as felt security. A feedback process compares current behaviors to the goal state as long as the set goal is not reached (Bretherton 1985). These processes lead to mental representations (internal working model or IWM), which serve as a selection mechanism for insuring emotional security by preferring contacts with the attachment figure over contacts with other adults (see Figure 11.1). In

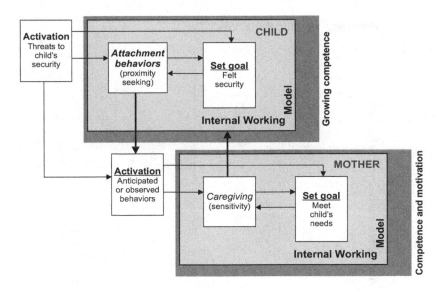

Figure 11.1 Dynamics of child–mother attachment relationships (adapted from Bell and Richard 2000, p. 71).

addition, the child's attachment behaviors have been described by two dimensions (*proximity-seeking* and *avoidance-resistance*), which have been hierarchically linked to form a behavioral matrix in which individual patterns can be classified along the A–B–C attachment system (Figure 11.2).

In his evolutionary approach to child–mother attachment relationships, in which maternal behaviors complement child behaviors, Bowlby (1969) explicitly stated that these nurturant caregiving behaviors are central to the child's IWM. Parenting experienced by the child is encoded as an essential part of the child's IWM, and sensitivity represents the most relevant characteristic. Moreover, parenting might be considered a cybernetic process of its own (Bell and Richard 2000; Solomon and George 1996), one closely linked to the child's attachment behaviors (Figure 11.1). Thus, the concept of child–mother attachment necessarily suggests a dynamic nature (Sroufe and Waters 1977; Waters et al. 1991) that is subject to change, just as other active and intrinsic concepts are, in contrast to a trait-like attribute, which remains stable in an individual throughout life. Child–mother attachments are therefore much more unstable, take much longer to become organized, and are much more dependent on supportive parental behavior (Lamb et al. 1985; Lamb et al. 1984; Sroufe and Jacobvitz 1989) than may have been originally assumed.

Modern neurobiological models describe how these bonds develop immediately after birth, linking emotional processes from the limbic system to the cortex of the child's maturing brain, where the mother's responses to the child's distress are processed and balance negative emotions (Buck 1994; Schore

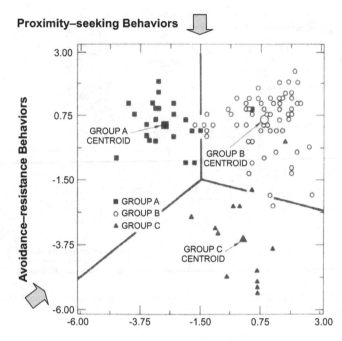

Figure 11.2   Behavioral matrix underlying the A–B–C attachment classification system (adapted from Ainsworth et al. 1978, p. 102).

2001). The early mother–child interaction that coincides with the early rapid brain development might thus make those primary attachments easier to establish and more influential on child's development than later attachments. That researchers regularly examine individual IWMs at the end of the child's first year of life only means that alternative measures for earlier processes are still under preparation (see Belsky et al. 1984; Leyendecker et al. 1997). Furthermore, this dynamic change in attachment is triggered by both mother and child. In accommodating new attachment experiences to the child's past experience and his/her growing competence, levels of sensitivity have to be adjusted in response to this growing experience and competence, which in turn depends on the mother's competence and motivation (Bell and Richard 2000; Bretherton et al. 1989; Solomon and George 1996). Consequently, enduring characteristics of attachment can be captured only if the characteristics of parenting adequately endure in accordance to the child's growing experience and competence.

Attachment as a Multidetermined Construct

The most important characteristic in parenting relevant to child–mother attachments has been described as *sensitivity.* Sensitivity captures the mother's ability to respond appropriately and promptly to the signals implicit in her child's behavior (especially distress cues) and to maintain positive affectional interactions (Ainsworth et al. 1974; Belsky and Fearon 2002). In Isabella's (1993, 1998) intensive observation studies, it became clear that sensitivity in parenting throughout the first three months was a much better predictor of attachment security than sensitivity in later parenting (see also, e.g., Grossmann et al. 1985). Consequently, convincing associations between sensitive parenting and secure child–mother attachments and, likewise, associations between insensitive parenting and insecure attachments, have only been demonstrated during the first months of a child's life. In addition, van IJzendoorn et al. (1995) reported that interventions on maternal sensitivity and infant attachment security, of which two-thirds started beyond the first three months, were more effective in changing mothers' insensitivity than in changing children's attachment security. In a meta-analysis of over 1,000 cases, De Wolff and van IJzendoorn (1997) discovered only moderate associations between types of sensitivity (which were sorted into various concepts of parenting) and attachment security, suggesting that sequelae of attachment might be reconsidered and not be limited to the classical concept of *sensitivity*.

The ways in which sensitivity diverges from other changing aspects of parenting throughout childhood might influence which other factors also help to maintain attachments, particularly when the child's behaviors become complex and increasingly independent from the attachment figure with growing age. Little is known, however, about how various attachments then intersect with age-appropriate features of child–mother relationships (see also Thompson 1999). For example, a mother's prompt and appropriate response to her infant's crying may be central to her parenting early in the first year, whereas positive affectional exchanges at sharing experiences during interactions (Mannle et al. 1992; Carpenter et al. 1998) and social referencing might be crucial in parenting later in child's life. In the first months, infants may attend to how well parents help them in coping with negative emotions; in later months, infants might attend more to the quality of the interactions that introduce them to a wider view into the social environment. Such a chronological shift from prioritizing emotional regulation to prioritizing shared social experiences would correspond to the rapid brain development and the activity of neural circuitry in the cortex (Siegel 1999).

The multidimensional character of parenting led Keller et al. (in prep.) to suggest a component model of parenting, which has some origin in MacDonald's (1992) relationship model. MacDonald proposed two discrete, evolutionarily independent affective systems, the *positive-social-reward* system and the *security-separation-distress* system, to distinguish warmth from security management in parenting. Whereas the *security-separation-distress* system focuses on the child's fear and how the parent's actions serve to reduce the child's negative affect, the *positive-social-reward* system addresses positive affect through the warm and nurturing contacts typical in mother–child interactions. Both systems might influence attachment relationships through combined high ratings, as is true for the traditional concept of *sensitivity*. However, various attachments might also emerge and be maintained by new combinations of high and low levels of both systems, and this can only be possible if these systems work separately. MacDonald's model helps to explain why a child might be able to develop different relationships with different adults in the same environment, and why he/she is able to maintain a relationship even when environments dramatically change.

Attachments as Variable Adaptations

Framing attachment relationships within human evolution has led to the portrayal of secure child–mother attachments as behaviorally adaptive, whereas insecure attachments have been viewed as maladaptive or as a second-best strategy for behavioral functioning (Main 1990). Classical attachment theory has thus provided a definite topology of attachment relationships in humans that designates an optimal pattern, that is, secure attachment. Evolutionary theories, however, do not define ad hoc criteria for optimal behavioral adaptation (e.g., Hinde 1982). Instead, different behaviors and perhaps different relationship types are better in different environments, and natural selection acts to favor individuals with a range of potential behaviors from which they select appropriately. Such reasoning leads to the proposal that children and their care providers would be programmed by evolution not simply to form one sort of relationship but to form a range of possible relationships according to the specific environment. In the course of evolution (and in habitats that are much more varied than "environment of evolutionary adaptedness," which Bowlby [1969] describes), human communities have created social structures for the care of young in which other adults have provided care in the mother's absence or have shared the care with the mother. To describe how children form multiple relationships with adults who fill diverse caregiving functions, the narrow optimum theorem must be relinquished, and the various attachments that are observed must be evaluated according to how these relationships function in particular care environments.

Even though we might currently observe only a subset of the attachment variations that might have once been active during evolution (Belsky 1999), the attachment patterns known today represent systematic variations on a behavioral matrix derived from two connected dimensions (*proximity-seeking* and *avoidance-resistance*), and these variations comprise species-specific social patterns. If psychological mechanisms have evolved through evocation of species-specific patterns based on environmental cues (Tooby and Cosmides 1992), then A–B–C attachments must be seen as variable but equivalent adaptations to different environments (Belsky 1999; Hinde 1982; Lamb et al. 1984). Because variability is limited by the defined structure of the behavioral matrix (Figure

11.2), disorganized attachment patterns, for example, can be excluded from adaptive variations of attachments. In this way, the current subset of attachment types might both represent flexible adaptations to different environments and distinguish adaptive from maladaptive patterns.

ALLOPARENTING AND CHILDREN'S RELATIONSHIPS TO NONMATERNAL CARE PROVIDERS

The Role of Alloparenting

The fact that humans evolved in social groups and show extensive psychological adaptations to social life raises questions about whether early human infants were carried and cared for exclusively by their mothers or, in contrast, with significant help from group members other than the parents (known as alloparenting). Both the exclusive caretaker model and the multiple caretaker model existed in hunter–gatherer (e.g., Hewlett 1989; Lee 1979; Tronick et al. 1992) as well as in modern societies. However, Hrdy (1999) argued that the cooperative provision of care (like collective breeding in avian and mammalian species) most likely allowed our ancestors to successfully rear the young (who mature very slowly and otherwise might not survive) and, at the same time, take advantage of new habitats. That mothers come to rely on assistance from other group members can be grounded in humans' high degree of sociability as well as the flexibility allowed by shifting roles, e.g., between care for their own and for other children, including the capability to understand and respond to children's signals. Availability of additional care providers clearly reduces the cost of parenting. Furthermore, a mother might give birth to another child while alloparents continue with caregiving, often employing different care practices. Not surprisingly, there is evidence that with the help of additional care providers, birthrates increase. Growing birthrates in many European countries today can be traced back to increased provision of public child care (especially for children under three) over the last two decades (Lamb and Ahnert 2004).

Whereas classical attachment theory has favored the exclusive-caretaker model over the multiple-caretaker model, which is seen as a modern deviation of "natural" care practices, Hrdy (1999) characterizes alloparenting as an ancient way of child rearing that might not even necessarily be based on kin grouping and degrees of relatedness. In chimpanzees, where mother–child bonds are strong and enduring, for example, mothers do selectively allow access for nonkin once these allomothers are highly motivated to take and carry infants (Nishida 1983). However, in many primates (such as Macaca, Papio, Presbytis) shared care almost certainly evolved within the context of matrilineal kin groups. Thus, kinship was probably essential in the evolutionary origin of allomothering (see review in Todt and Riechelmann 1998; Hrdy, pers. comm.).

Modern mothers often do not rely on relatives but instead use paid care providers outside of the private family networks, where children are normally cared for in groups. However, these evolutionarily novel institutions, which are based on civil order with a high degree of personal security, low child mortality and central control of child care services, make entrusting children to nonfamily members relatively risk free (Lamb et al. 1992; Melhuish and Moss 1991; Spiro 1965). The fact that care providers earn money by taking care of children, however, can raise questions about their motivation (Sonenstein and Wolf 1991); but even parents may need to provide services in return for the minding of children within extended family units (e.g., Tietze and Rossbach 1991). The long-lasting European traditions of kindergarten, nanny, and au-pair service indicate that young women can obtain experience taking care of other children before they have their own (Rauschenbach et al. 1995), suggesting that those care providers can be motivated to invest even emotionally in other's children, at least for a limited time. Bowlby (1951), however, was convinced that group care arrangements supervised by professional care providers cannot provide satisfactory environments for infants and young children. Most of his concerns focused on the question of how care providers manage to form and maintain attachment relationships, and how children develop and maintain attachment relationships under care practices that are consistently changing.

Children's Relationships to Nonmaternal Care Providers

Young children seek proximity and reassurance from nonmaternal providers when stressful mishaps occur under the conditions of group care. Obvious similarities between those secure-base behaviors and behaviors in child–mother attachments lead researchers to examine child–care provider relationships in the framework of attachment theory, but also to differentiate those relationships from non-attached patterns. A meta-analysis of nearly 3,000 cases (Ahnert et al., in prep.) revealed that insecure (A and C) types of attachments often dominate child–care provider attachment relationships, and that child–care provider attachments are both functionally and ontogenetically different.

In this analysis, there was controversy, for example, about the antecedents of child–care provider attachments. Some researchers argued that secure attachments to care providers (as with mother–child dyads) depend on sensitive caregiving toward individual children. Other researchers found no association between care providers' sensitivity and secure attachments. Moreover, children of the same group tended to develop attachments with their shared care providers that were of similar quality. In some groups, child–care provider attachments remained the same even when the particular care provider changed. These findings suggest that attachments to care providers might not be shaped primarily by individual-focused behaviors. Since some research evaluated care providers on the promptness and adequacy of their responses to individual children (using the classical *sensitivity* measure) whereas others used group-focused measures of responsiveness (using a group-related empathy measure), the meta-analysis

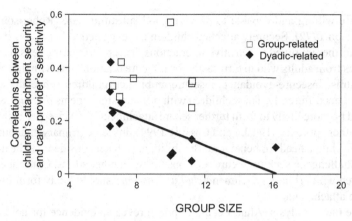

Figure 11.3 Correlations between security of child–care provider attachment and measures of care provider behaviors as related to group size (Ahnert et al., in prep.).

examined the differential impact of these two types of caregiving on emerging child–care provider relationships. As a result, child–care provider attachments, especially in centers, were predominantly shaped by care providers' empathetic behaviors toward the group as a whole reflecting selective problem-oriented sensitivity to the right signals at the right time in order to address the children's most important needs. Only in small groups were secure child–care provider attachments associated with measures of dyadic sensitivity similar to those that predict children's primary attachments in early infancy (see Figure 11.3).

Because groups of children segregate in gender-based groupings (e.g., Howes 1988), especially when children favor same-sex over cross-sex interactions particularly at formation of gender-based social identity (Leaper 2002; Maccoby 1998) care providers' group-oriented behaviors are linked to child gender. Not surprisingly, the formation of child–care provider attachments appeared to vary depending on child gender, which is not something typical discovered in studies of attachment. Girls tended to develop secure attachments in child care more often than did boys, which suggests that care providers' (gender biased) behaviors might be enforced by these groupings, might lead to more frequent care provider–girl than provider–boy interaction and to a better match between girls' social identity and care providers educational goals. Consistent with this, secure child–care provider attachments were more common when children had experience of continued child care histories, and were exposed to the care provider whom they become attached to, longer after enrollment.

Multiple Adult–Child Attachments

In the framework of classical attachment theory, the child's main attachment to the primary caregiver provides the basis for his/her expectations of other adults who are willing and capable to provide good substitute care (Robertson and Robertson 1972). Securely attached children are expected to behave as if they were further involved in sensitive interactions, thereby triggering sensitive behaviors from adults who in turn easily form secure relationships with that child. In contrast, insecure-avoidant or insecure-ambivalent children impact the social encounters differently. Thus, children with primary attachments *that are secure* should be more likely to form further secure attachments than insecure children. In another approach (Belsky and Cassidy 1994), insecure primary attachments and the child's need for behavioral flexibility have been considered to be a specific challenge in seeking secure relationships with other adults. Consequently, children with primary attachments *that are insecure* should likely form further secure attachments.

The meta-analysis (Ahnert et al., in prep.) revealed evidence for neither of these assumptions. Instead, nondirectional discordance between the security of child–parent and child–care provider attachments was common (i.e., these attachments represented specific adaptations to care environments with different qualities). However, security of the children's relationships with their parents (both mothers and fathers) and with their care providers were minimally but significantly intercorrelated. This suggests that children construct complex internal working models of significant relationships to adults. Not surprisingly, child–mother attachments developed independently of out-of-home care, and the security of child–mother attachment was associated with maternal sensitivity, regardless of types of the out-of-home care arrangements (NICHD Early Child Care Research Network 1997). Since, as a rule, children develop different attachment relationships to different caretakers and because discordance between child–parent and child–care provider attachments were common, child–parent and child–care provider attachments seem to be equally important in the respective environments in which they develop. Normally, parents and care providers are not simultaneously available. Thus, it is unclear whether the primary IWMs always exert the strongest influence on children's behavioral organization in situations of uncertainty (cf. Farran and Ramey 1977) or how important secondary IWMs are in children's later lives (e.g., Oppenheim et al. 1988).

SHARED CARE AND MAINTENANCE OF ATTACHMENT

Discontinuity in Parenting

According to Ainsworth et al.'s (1974) and Bowlby's (1973) *Security–Attachment* concept, the more stable and predictably sensitive mother–child interactions are, the more likely it is that secure attachments will be formed. This proposition is challenged by the fact that secure child–mother attachments are developed and maintained even when children spend a substantial part of the day away from their mothers. Based on the understanding of cognitive development at the time, Bowlby (1973) was convinced that infants under one year do not acquire person permanence and thus are unable to form IWMs under discontinuous parenting. Accordingly, periods of mother–child separations must thus be minimized as they work against the formation of relationships. Claims of strict continuity in parenting, however, refer to good parenting in terms of *monotropy*. This concept is closely related to the psychoanalytic concept of *symbiosis*, which means "reared by only one person" [Greek]. In today's developmental pediatrics, however, symbiotic aspects of child–mother relationships pose a potential barrier to the child's social competence, and are thus more likely to be related to pathological aspects of social development than to healthy mother–child bonds. Research on parenting has further shown that infants enjoy interacting with more than one person and do not get overwhelmed very easily. Moreover, modern cognitive science and neuroscience reveal that an infant's social memory is capable of bridging even sustained separations (e.g., Bauer 1996). Yet there are substantial contributions on the mother's (parents') side to the maintenance of the attachment relationship, particularly when care by other adults is considered. Parents might then be influential, specifically in the ways they perceive and select out-of-home care arrangements, and adjust their parenting to shared care (see also Ahnert and Lamb 2003).

Selection of Out-of-home Care Arrangements

Parents' educational histories, occupations, and incomes, like their attitudes and beliefs about parenting, family life, and maternal employment, certainly influence children's care environments. For example, parents with higher education and income levels tend to select out-of-home care of higher quality, and tend to prefer center-based care rather than home-based care because they value the enhanced opportunities for cognitive stimulation and education. Some parents also consider aspects of care that directly complement their own daily lives (such as a convenient location which allows them more time with the child) over educational features that might promote their child's development. These associations are moderated by child age, however. More specifically, regardless of their educational backgrounds, parents of infants and toddlers (as opposed to parents of preschoolers) emphasize concerns about health and well-being and seek care environments likely to encourage warm childcare provider relationships. In other words, parents of infants expect care providers to provide care similar to home and encourage caretakers to form secure attachments with their children, whereas parents of older children often do not want to "compete" over the affection of their child. Unlike parents for whom quality care matters, parents who do not prioritize quality of out-of-home care have more stressful lives, more restrictive parenting attitudes, and seem to be less invested in their children. Summarizing those studies (see Ahnert et al. 2000), parents' careful choices for types of out-of-home care which they trust are much better predictors of sensitivity in parenting than whether they do or do not use out-of-home care (see also Ahnert and Lamb 2003).

Adjustment of Parenting to Shared Care

Sensitive parenting and child–mother attachments seem to be well predicted by how parents adjust family life to shared care. Research has shown that mothers whose children are in high-quality daycare compensate for their time away from their children by interacting with increased intensity when they are together (e.g., during the early morning and evening) (Ahnert et al. 2000). This time is characterized by increased attention, stimulation, affective exchange, emotional display, and other forms of social interaction (Figure 11.4). Children, in turn, show heightened levels of distress when they are picked up from the daycare center, but not during the time when they are at the center. After retrieving their children, mothers tend to respond less promptly to a child's stress signals (Figure 11.5). This may reflect their low energy level, as a result of work commitments. Nonetheless, positive child–mother relationships could be maintained.

From the perspective of MacDonald's (1992) models, secure child–mother attachment might not have been maintained by the *security-separation-distress* system, even though it may have been maintained by intensifying the *positive-social-reward* system. This suggests that assumptions of the multidetermination of attachment are particularly useful in changing care environments.

CONCLUSION

In contrast to the narrow optimum theorem, which is articulated in classical attachment theory, the studies described here suggest that attachment is regulated by a multitude of factors. These may be especially apparent under the variable conditions present in changing care arrangements, in particular when individuals other than the parents or familiar relatives are involved.

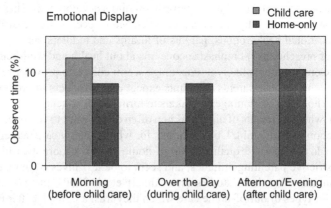

Figure 11.4 Emotional display between children and adults at home and in child care over the course of the day (adapted from Ahnert et al. 2000).

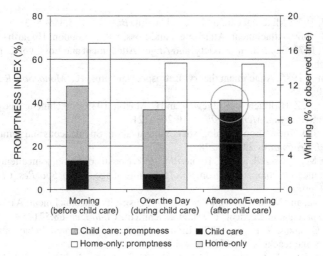

Figure 11.5   Children's whining and adults' responses at home and in child care over the course of the day (adapted from Ahnert et al. 2000).

REFERENCES

Ahnert, L., and M.E. Lamb. 2003. Shared care: Establishing a balance between home and child care. *Child Dev.* **74**:1–6.

Ahnert, L., H. Rickert, and M.E. Lamb. 2000. Shared caregiving: Comparison between home and child care. *Dev. Psychol.* **36**:339–351.

Ainsworth, M.D.S. 1967. Infancy in Uganda: Infant Care and the Growth of Love. Baltimore: Johns Hopkins Univ. Press.

Ainsworth, M.D.S., S.M. Bell, and D.J. Stayton. 1974. Infant–mother attachment and social development: "Socialization" as a product of reciprocal responsiveness to signals. In: The Integration of a Child into a Social World, ed. M.P.M. Richards, pp. 99–135. New York: Cambridge Univ. Press.

Ainsworth, M.D.S., M.C. Blehar, E. Waters, and S. Wall. 1978. Patterns of Attachment: A Psychological Study of the Strange Situation. Hillsdale, NJ: Erlbaum.

Bauer, P.J. 1996. What do infants recall of their lives? Memory for specific events by one- to two-year-olds. *Am. Psychol.* **51**:29–41.

Bell, D.C., and A.J. Richard. 2000. Caregiving: The forgotten element in attachment. *Psychol. Inq.* **11**:69–83.

Belsky, J. 1999. Modern evolutionary theory and patterns of attachment. In: Handbook of Attachment: Theory, Research, and Clinical Applications, ed. J. Cassidy and P.R. Shaver, pp. 141–161. New York: Guilford.

Belsky, J., and J. Cassidy. 1994. Attachment: Theory and evidence. In: Development through Life: A Handbook for Clinicians, ed. M. Rutter and D. Hay, pp. 373–402. Oxford: Blackwell.

Belsky, J., and R.M.P. Fearon. 2002. Early attachment security, subsequent maternal sensitivity, and later child development: Does continuity in development depend upon continuity of caregiving? *Attach. Hum. Dev.* **3**:361–387.

Belsky, J., M. Rovine, and D.G. Taylor. 1984. The Pennsylvania Infant and Family Development Project. III. The origins of individual differences in infant–mother attachment: Maternal and infant contributions. *Child Dev.* **55**:718–728.

Bowlby, J. 1951. Maternal care and mental health. *Bull. WHO* **3**:355–533.

Bowlby, J. 1969. Attachment. Attachment and Loss, vol. 1. London: Hogarth.

Bowlby, J. 1973. Separation: Anxiety, and Anger. Attachment and Loss, vol. 2. London: Hogarth.

Bretherton, I. 1985. Attachment theory: Retrospect and prospect. *Mono. Soc. Res. Child Dev.* **50**:3–35.

Bretherton, I., Z. Biringen, D. Ridgeway, and C. Maslin. 1989. Attachment: The parental perspective. *Infant Mental Hlth. J.* **10**:203–221.

Buck, R. 1994. The neuropsychology of communication: Spontaneous and symbolic aspects. *J. Pragmatics* **22**:265–278.

Carpenter, M., K. Nagell, and M. Tomasello. 1998. Social cognition, joint attention, and communicative competence from 9 to 15 months of age. *Mono. Soc. Res. Child Dev.* **63**, 176 pp.

De Wolff, M., and M.H. van IJzendoorn. 1997. Sensitivity and attachment: A meta-analysis on parental antecedents of infant attachment. *Child Dev.* **68**:571–591.

Farran, D.C., and C.T. Ramey. 1977. Infant day care and attachment behaviors toward mothers and teachers. *Child Dev.* **48**:1112–1116.

Grossmann, K., K.E. Grossmann, G. Spangler, G. Suess, and L. Uzner. 1985. Maternal sensitivity and newborns' orientation responses as related to quality of attachment in Northern Germany. *Mono. Soc. Res. Child Dev.* **50**:233–256.

Hewlett, B.S. 1989. Multiple caretaking among African Pygmies. *Am. Anthropologist* **91**:186–191.

Hinde, R.A. 1982. Attachment: Some conceptual and biological issues. In: The Place of Attachment in Human Behavior, ed. C.M. Parkes and J. Stevenson-Hinde, pp. 60–76. New York: Basic.

Howes, C. 1988. Same- and cross-sex friends: Implications for interaction and social skills. *Early Childh. Res. Qtly.* **3**:21–37.

Hrdy, S.B. 1999. Mother Nature: A History of Mothers, Infants, and Natural Selection. New York: Pantheon.

Isabella, R.A. 1993. Origins of attachment: Maternal interactive behavior across the first year. *Child Dev.* **64**:605–621.

Isabella, R.A. 1998. Origins of attachment: The role of context, duration, frequency of observation, and infant age in measuring maternal behavior. *J. Soc. Pers. Rel.* **15**: 538–554.

Lamb, M.E., and L. Ahnert. 2004. Nonparental child care: Context, concepts, and consequences. In: Handbook of Child Psychology, ed. W. Damon, I. E. Sigel, and K.A. Renninger. (vol. 4: Child Psychology in Practice). New York: Wiley.

Lamb, M.E., K.J. Sternberg, C.P. Hwang, and A.G. Broberg. 1992. Child Care in Context: Cross-cultural Perspectives. Hillsdale, NJ: Erlbaum.

Lamb, M.E., R.A. Thompson, W.P. Gardner, and E.L. Charnov. 1985. Infant–mother Attachment: The Origins and Developmental Significance of Individual Differences in Strange Situation Behavior. Hillsdale, NJ: Erlbaum.

Lamb, M.E., R.A. Thompson, W.P. Gardner, E.L. Charnov, and D. Estes. 1984. Security of infantile attachment as assessed in the Strange Situation: Its study and biological interpretation. *Behav. Brain Sci.* **7**:127–171.

Leaper, C. 2002. Parenting girls and boys. In: Handbook of Parenting: Children and Parenting, ed. M. Bornstein, 2nd ed., vol. 1, pp. 189–225. Mahwah, NJ: Erlbaum.

Lee, R.B. 1979. The !Kung San: Men, Women, and Work in a Foraging Society. New York: Cambridge Univ. Press.

Leyendecker, B., M.E. Lamb, M.P. Fracasso, A. Schölmerich, and C. Larson. 1997. Playful interaction and the antecedents of attachment: A longitudinal study of Central American and Euro-American mothers and infants. *Merrill-Palmer Qtly.* **43**:24–47.

Maccoby, E.E. 1998. The Two Sexes: Growing Up Apart, Coming Together. Cambridge, MA: Harvard Univ. Press.

MacDonald, K. 1992. Warmth as a developmental construct: An evolutionary analysis. *Child Dev.* **63**:753–773.

Main, M. 1981. Avoidance in the service of attachment: A working paper. In: Behavioral Development: The Bielefeld Interdisciplinary Project, ed. K. Immelmann, G. Barlow, L. Petrinovich, and M. Main, pp. 651–693. New York: Cambridge Univ. Press.

Main, M. 1990. Cross-cultural studies of attachment organization: Recent studies, changing methodologies, and the concept of conditional strategies. *Hum. Dev.* **33**:48–61.

Main, M., and J. Solomon. 1990. Procedures for identifying infants as disorganized/disoriented during the Ainsworth Strange Situation. In: Attachment in the Preschool Years: Theory, Research and Intervention, ed. M.T. Greenberg, D. Cicchetti, and E.M. Cummings, pp. 121–160. Chicago: Univ. of Chicago Press.

Mannle, S., M. Barton, and M. Tomasello. 1992. Two-year-olds' conversations with their mothers and preschool-aged siblings. *First Lang.* **12**:57–71.

Melhuish, E.C., and P. Moss. 1991. Day Care for Young Children: International Perspectives. New York: Routledge.

NICHD Early Child Care Research Network. 1997. The effects of infant child care on infant–mother attachment security: Results of the NICHD study of early child care. *Child Dev.* **68**:860–879.

Nishida, T. 1983. Alloparental behavior in wild chimpanzees of the Mahale Mountains, Tanzania. *Folia Primatol.* **41**:318–336.

Oppenheim, D., A. Sagi, and M.E. Lamb. 1988. Infant–adult attachments on the kibbutz and their relation to socio-emotional development four years later. *Dev. Psychol.* **24**:427–433.

Rauschenbach, T., K. Beher, and D. Knauer. 1995. Die Erzieherin: Ausbildung und Arbeitsmarkt [The Care Provider: Education and Job Market]. Weinheim: Juventa.

Robertson, J., and J. Robertson. 1972. Quality of substitute care as an influence on separation responses. *J. Psychosom. Res.* **16**:261–265.

Schore, A.N. 2001. Effects of a secure attachment relationship on right brain development, affect regulation, infant mental health. *Infant Mental Hlth J.* **22**:7–66.

Siegel, D.J. 1999. The Developing Mind: Toward a Neurobiology of Interpersonal Experience. New York: Guilford.

Solomon, J., and C. George. 1996. Defining the caregiving system: Toward a theory of caregiving. *Infant Mental Hlth. J.* **17**:183–197.

Sonenstein, F.L., and D.A. Wolf. 1991. Satisfaction with child care: Perspectives of welfare mothers. *J. Soc. Iss.* **47**:15–31.

Spiro, M.E. 1965. Children of the Kibbutz. New York: Schocken.

Sroufe, L.A., and D. Jacobvitz. 1989. Diverging pathways, developmental transformations, multiple etiologies and the problem of continuity in development. *Hum. Dev.* **32**:196–203.

Sroufe, L.A., and E. Waters. 1977. Attachment as an organizational construct. *Child Dev.* **48**:1184–1199.

Thompson, R.A. 1999. Early attachment and later development. In: Handbook of Attachment: Theory, Research, and Clinical Applications, ed. J. Cassidy and P.R. Shaver, pp. 265–286. New York: Guilford.

Tietze, W., and H.-G. Rossbach. 1991. Die Betreuung von Kindern im vorschulischen Alter [Minding pre-schoolers]. *Z. Pädagogik* **37**:555–579.

Todt, D., and C. Riechelmann. 1998. Formen der frühen Sozialisierung bei nicht-menschlichen Primaten [Types of early sozialization in nonhuman primates]. In: Tagesbetreuung für Kinder unter 3 Jahren: Theorien und Tatsachen [Child Care for Children under Three Years of Age: Theories and Facts], ed. L. Ahnert, pp. 173–192. Bern: Huber.

Tooby, J., and L. Cosmides. 1992. The psychological foundations of culture. In: The Adapted Mind: Evolutionary Psychology and the Generation of Culture, ed. J.H. Barkow, L. Cosmides, and J. Tooby, pp. 19–136. New York: Oxford Univ. Press.

Tronick, E.Z., G.A. Morelli, and P.K. Ivey. 1992. The Efe forager infant and toddler's pattern of social relationships: Multiple and simultaneous. *Dev. Psychol.* **28**:568–577.

van IJzendoorn, M.H., F. Juffer, and M.G.C. Duyvesteyn. 1995. Breaking the intergenerational cycle of insecure attachment: A review of the effects of attachment-based interventions on maternal sensitivity and infant security. *J. Child Psychol. Psychiat.* **36**:225–248.

van IJzendoorn, M.H., C. Schuengel, and M.J. Bakermans-Kranenburg. 1999. Disorganized attachment in early childhood: Meta-analysis of precursors, concomitants, and sequelae. *Dev. Psychopathol.* **2**:225–249.

Waters, E., K. Kondo Ikemura, G. Posada, and J.E. Richters. 1991. Learning to love: Mechanisms and milestones. In: Self Processes and Development: The Minnesota Symposia on Child Psychology, ed. M.R. Gunnar and L.A. Sroufe, vol. 23, pp. 217–255. Hillsdale, NJ: Erlbaum.

12

Attachment and Stress in Early Development

Does Attachment Add to the Potency of Social Regulators of Infant Stress?

M. R. GUNNAR

Institute of Child Development, University of Minnesota,
Minneapolis, MN 55455, U.S.A.

ABSTRACT

For the last forty some years, studies of stress and attachment have been mainstays of primate psychoendocrine research. These studies have focused on the limbic–hypothalamic–pituitary–adrenal (LHPA) system, a system critical to adaptation and survival. They have shown that activity of this neuroendocrine system is sensitive to the availability and responsiveness of the attachment figure. Separation produces elevations in cortisol, the primary hormone of this system, in both monkey and human infants. In the presence of the attachment figure, elevations in cortisol to a range of stressors are reduced or prevented altogether. Finally, within the attachment relationship, insensitive, intrusive, or, in the extreme, abusive care stimulates increases in this stress hormone. These findings fit well with arguments that attachment provides primate infants with a secure base for exploration and that separation or loss is stressful or traumatic. In addition, because stress influences immune competence and brain development, these findings suggest one mechanism by which attachment protects the developing primate's physical and mental health. We need, however, to ask whether the significance of attachment–stress findings have been overplayed. Are any of these findings unique to attachment relationships? It will be argued that evidence, to date, fails to show that attachment plays a unique role in stress regulation in developing primates. In part, this conclusion is necessary because certain critical studies have not been done. In the absence of definitive studies, we may be wise to limit conclusions to more general statements about sensitive and responsive social relationships as powerful regulators of stress in early development.

INTRODUCTION

Among John Bowlby's seminal insights was the idea that in the primate central nervous system a motivational system evolved to insure that an infant will attempt to maintain proximity and contact with the conspecifics who are the most likely to provide it with nurturance and protection (Bowlby 1969). He termed this system *attachment*. Protection from dangerous elements of the environment and regulation of the infant's internal state are two of the principal functions of caregiving. Thus, the ultimate function of attachment is achieved through the attachment system that operates to maintain proximity between caregivers and infants. Protection of the infant's internal state from internal and external threats to homeostasis is not solely the responsibility of the caregivers. Evolution has also conferred on mammals and their young stress-sensitive neurobiological systems that operate in the face of threat to shift and liberate metabolic resources and orchestrate behavior and physiology to increase survival. Activating these stress-sensitive systems, however, also brings costs to the organism, which in early development may include impairments in physical growth and shaping of the nervous system in ways that increase vulnerability to stress during throughout the lifespan (McEwen 1998).

In another of Bowlby's insights he argued that when the caregiving system is up to the task of providing protection and external regulation of the infant's internal milieu, the infant will be able to direct its resources to other activities (Bowlby 1969). Bowlby, thus, provided a framework that anticipated an inverse relationship between the availability and responsiveness of the attachment figure(s) and activity of stress-sensitive neurobiological systems. In this chapter, I outline the neurobiology of one of the principal components of the mammalian stress system: the limbic–hypothalamic–pituitary–adrenocortical (LHPA) system. This system has most often been the focus of research on stress and attachment in monkeys and humans. I summarize some of the key studies supporting the argument that in primates the caregiver–infant attachment system functions to regulate this stress-sensitive neurobiological system. I address studies currently available to examine whether the attachment relationship plays a unique role in stress regulation during primate development, or, alternatively, is merely a reflection of the importance of social processes in stress regulation throughout the lifespan. Finally, I discuss implications of this work for our understanding of the roles of both attachment and stress in primate development.

THE LHPA SYSTEM: A BRIEF OVERVIEW

Current views of stress neurobiology describe a loosely integrated system consisting of neuroanatomically and functionally related subsystems. In the periphery, stress biology centers on the regulation of glucocorticoids or CORT (cortisol in primates, corticosterone in rodents) and catecholamines (norepinephrine [NE] and epinephrine [EPI]; Johnson et al. 1992). CORT and catecholamines operate to increase metabolism and stimulate cardiovascular and pulmonary function. In concert with central components of the stress system, they inhibit the biology of growth and repair, including digestion, physical growth, immune function, and reproduction. In the brain, the stress system is orchestrated through reciprocal interactions among NE and hypothalamic and extra-hypothalamic corticotropin-releasing hormone (CRH).

CRH is a neuroactive peptide produced in the hypothalamus and in extra-hypothalamic sites (Strand 1999). Its production in the hypothalamus initiates the cascade of events that culminate in increased production of CORT by the adrenal glands (see Figure 12.1). CRH and other peptides, principally, arginine vasopressin (AVP), regulate the production of adrenocorticotropic hormone (ACTH) by cells in the anterior pituitary. ACTH binds to receptors in the cortex of the adrenal glands and causes the biosynthesis and release of CORT into general circulation. CORT primarily acts by binding to receptors in the cytoplasm of cells, including nerve cells. The activated hormone-receptor complex then enters the nucleus of the cell where it regulates gene transcription on genes with glucocorticoid receptive elements (GREs). Negative feedback loops operating at the levels of the pituitary, hypothalamus, hippocampus, and possibly frontal cortex (Sullivan and Gratton 2002) terminate and contain the stress response.

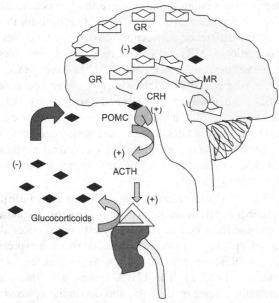

Figure 12.1 The limbic–hypothalamic–pituitary–adrenal (LHPA) axis and corticoid receptor distribution and function in brain. The corticotropin-releasing hormone (CRH) molecule originating in the hypothalamus is at the center of the activation of the system. CRH acts on the release of adrenocorticotropic hormone (ACTH) from the pituitary, which in turn acts on the adrenal to release glucocorticoids. Glucocorticoids act on tissues peripherally from the brain and are also "key" for LHPA axis "brake." Two receptors are the "locks": glucocorticoid (GR) and mineralocorticoid (MR) receptors, with GR widely distributed throughout the brain and MR localized exclusively in "the emotional brain" or limbic structures. POMC = proopiomelanocortin. Adapted from Muller et al. (2002).

Hypothalamic CRH-producing neurons receive input from other hypothalamic and brainstem nuclei, with NE being a major stimulus of increased hypothalamic CRH activity. However, there are multiple neurotransmitter and
neuropeptide systems, beyond the NE system, that are involved in regulating
hypothalamic CRH activity (Herman and Cullinan 1997). Activation and regulation of CRH in the hypothalamus is, thus, multifactorial, reflecting the current
and previous state of the organism in conjunction with current, previous, and anticipated demands. The balancing of internal and external demands is also reflected in the regulation of what has been called extra-hypothalamic CRH. CRH
is produced in many limbic structures, brainstem nuclei, and neocortical areas
involved in stress reactivity and regulation. One subtype of the CRH receptor,
CRH1, appears to mediate many stress and anxiety related functions; while the
other subtype, CRH2, appears to mediate functions (e.g., eating, sleeping) that
are often inhibited during stressful periods (Steckler and Holsboer 1999).

One common fallacy about the LHPA system is that CORT and CRH are necessarily detrimental to health and well-being. In fact, the relationship between
CORT and adaptive functioning is often an inverted-U function. Both too little
and too much can be detrimental (McEwen 1998). One basis for the inverted-U
function may be the difference between the two major receptors for CORT,
termed mineralocorticoid (MR) and glucocorticoid (GR) receptors (De Kloet
1991). In the central nervous system, MRs tend to have growth and health
promotive effects, whereas GRs tend to have catabolic and potentially damaging effects. CORT has high affinity for MRs and lower affinity for GRs. Thus at
low levels of the hormone, MRs in the central nervous system are primarily occupied, while at higher levels, GRs become increasingly occupied. MRs are believed to be critically involved in regulating the diurnal rhythm of CORT,
whereas GRs serve in negative feedback of the system to terminate and contain
stress elevations of the hormone.

In rodents, vigorous maternal care during the first weeks of life permanently
increases the number of GR available to contain the stress response (Liu et al.
1997). In rodents and monkeys, negative early care experiences also increase
CRH production (Coplan et al. 1996) and alter CRH receptor expression, resulting in increases in CRH1 receptors in regions involved in fearful/anxious behavior (Sanchez et al. 2001). The LHPA system also interacts with the
developing serotonin (Lopez et al. 1998) and dopamine systems (Pani et al.
2000) in complex ways that may affect vulnerability to anxiety, depression, and
substance abuse disorders. Cortisol and CRH also influence neural systems involved in learning and memory, including circuits in the hippocampus
(McEwen 1998) and prefrontal cortex (Sullivan and Gratton 2002). With regard
to the former, the same dimensions of maternal care associated with changes in
LHPA activity in the rodent influence synaptogenesis and memory function (Liu
et al. 2000). With regard to the latter, there is some evidence that side matters,
with right prefrontal activity being more closely associated with elevated CORT

in animals and humans, consistent with evidence that right frontal EEG asymmetry is associated with depression and withdrawal behavior (Buss et al. 2003; Sullivan and Gratton 2002). The impact of early care experiences on neural systems regulating stress, emotion, and cognition provides a strong impetus for understanding how and whether experiences within the caregiver–infant attachment relationship have a unique role to play in stress regulation in primate development.

ATTACHMENT AND LHPA ACTIVITY IN DEVELOPING PRIMATES

Basic Findings

Borrowing from the human literature on stress and coping, in monkeys the mother has been conceptualized as providing a social buffer against stress. Maternal buffering describes situations in which the infant exhibits behavioral distress; nonetheless in the mother's presence, LHPA and autonomic reactions to the stressor are attenuated. A classic example is capture and handling in naïve infant monkey. Typically, this provokes marked increases in infant cortisol levels; however, when the infant is put back with the mother immediately, having never lost sight of her, the cortisol response is greatly reduced (for a review, see Levine and Wiener 1988). Physical contact with the mother does not appear to be necessary in monkey infants in order for maternal buffering to reduce cortisol increases. Infants separated and placed in cages adjacent to their mothers show markedly more distress vocalizations and behavioral agitation, but they exhibit lower cortisol increases compared to infants who cannot hear, smell, or see their mothers. In human infants it becomes difficult to elevate cortisol to a range of stressors (e.g., doctor's exams and inoculations, the approach of strangers and/or exposure to odd, anxiety-eliciting stimuli) by the end of the first year, as long as the child is in a secure attachment relationship with the parent who accompanies the child (Gunnar and Donzella 2002).

Separation from the attachment figure provokes marked elevations in cortisol in monkey infants that does not habituate over repeated trials (Levine and Wiener 1988). In human infants, brief separations such as those in the Ainsworth and Wittag Strange Situation produce increases in cortisol for infants in insecure attachment relationships (Spangler and Schieche 1998). More striking, regardless of attachment security, toddlers show marked elevations in cortisol over home baseline levels during the first several weeks after entering center-based child care (Ahnert et al. 2004). In monkey infants, separations induce long-term effects on the LHPA system. Unlike in rodents, however, where increases in LHPA axis reactivity is stimulated by single or repeated bouts of prolonged (3 to 24 hr) removal of the pup from maternal care, in monkey infants, separations of similar duration may result in blunted or suppressed activity of the LHPA system, sometimes but not always in the context of increased fearful, anxious behavior (Dettling et al. 2002; Levine et al. 1997).

If the attachment figure provides stress regulation and if separation elevates stress hormones, does rearing in the absence of an attachment figure produce marked dysregulation of the stress system? There is little evidence that such abnormal rearing environments affect the development of the HPA components of the axis, perhaps because these are well developed prior to birth in monkeys and humans (Sanchez et al. 2001). However, later developing limbic and cortical regions, which are important in the regulation of fear and stress, do show alterations. These changes include increased density of CRH1 receptors in the prefrontal cortex and down regulation of CRF2 receptors in the amygdala. Several studies of orphanage-reared children conducted several years after their adoption into families have indicated slight alterations in basal cortisol levels, particularly near the peak of the circadian cycle (for a review, see Gunnar and Donzella 2002).

In human infants, a number of studies indicate that attachment figures who are insensitive and/or intrusive provoke increases in cortisol. More intrusive, insensitive caregiving has been associated with increases in cortisol during mother–infant play bouts for infants between three and nine months of age (Spangler et al. 1994). Similarly, insensitive, intrusive mothers observed during well-child visits at two, four, and six months had infants who at those visits had higher pre-stressor levels of cortisol (Gunnar and Donzella 2002). With toddlers, mothers who were overly solicitous and who intrusively attempted to get their toddlers to approach arousing stimuli have toddlers who exhibit greater cortisol responses (Nachmias et al. 1996). In preschoolers, mothers who are less involved and responsive have children whose basal cortisol levels remain higher over the day (P. Pendry and E.K. Adam, pers. comm.). Severe failures in the caregiving system, such as those associated with abuse, produce long-term alterations in the LHPA system, perhaps especially in genetically vulnerable individuals (Heim et al. 1997). There is also evidence that manipulations which lead mother monkeys to be rejecting and unresponsive to their infants result in elevated central CRH levels measured in adulthood (Coplan et al. 1996). Noradrenergic and serotonergic systems are also affected in the same animals.

Does the Attachment Relationship Play a Unique Role in Infant Stress Regulation?

Here we explore whether the attachment relationship is unique in its stress regulatory function in primate development. I provide evidence to answer each of the following questions:

- Does the infant need to be attached to the caregiver before that individual can serve a stress regulatory function for the infant?
- Is the increase in cortisol during separation a response to separation from the attachment figure, or is it due to other changes in the environment that often co-occur with separation?

Is the Stress-buffering Effect Specific to the Attachment Relationship?

Predictability and control are two of the core psychological variables that regulate activity of the LHPA system throughout the lifespan (Levine and Ursin 1979). When we are reliant on others to exercise reliable control over threat, their sensitivity and responsiveness to our signals become principal determinants of our coping resources (Glass and Singer 1972). Caregiver sensitivity and responsivity form the basis for the development of secure attachment relationships (Ainsworth et al. 1978). However, is it necessary for the infant to be attached to a caregiver in order for their sensitivity and responsiveness to the infant's signals to regulate reactivity of the LHPA system? In some monkeys, infants receive caregiving from many female members of the troupe, whereas in others, a separated infant is less likely to direct and receive comfort from other troupe members. Studying monkeys where *aunting* or *alloparenting* is common, researchers have found that increases in cortisol upon separation return to baseline by 60–90 minutes as the infant receives care from other adult females (Levine and Wiener 1988). Because these females are familiar to the infant, one could argue that the infants might have already formed some attachment to them. More striking evidence that an attachment bond may not be necessary comes from a study of 9-month-old human infants (Gunnar and Donzella 2002). In this study, the infants were given a babysitter during a 30-minute maternal separation. The babysitter was either programmed to be sensitive and responsive or relatively cold and aloof. In the presence of the sensitive and responsive babysitter no increase in cortisol was observed, whereas elevations were observed with the colder and more distant babysitter. Certainly, the infants could not have been attached to the sensitive and responsive babysitter as they had never seen her before the moment of separation. While this study is provocative, it is important to note that we do not know whether the responsive babysitter would have been able to maintain low cortisol levels in the infant if the separation period had been extended into hours or days. Nor do we know whether infants older than nine months would have shown the same propensity to maintain baseline levels of cortisol with a high-responsive as compared to low-responsive babysitter.

Does attachment confer any added benefit to sensitive and responsive caregiving in stress regulation? Unfortunately, the aunting and babysitting studies described above do not tell us. What we need are studies that pit secure and insecure attachment against sensitive versus insensitive caregiving by individuals for whom there is no attachment bond with the child. As discussed, there is already evidence that the presence of the attachment figure in an insecure relationship results in greater cortisol responses to threatening events than it does in a secure relationship. However, it is difficult in these studies to determine whether it is the insecure relationship history or the behavior of the attachment figure during the stressor that affects the cortisol response. If it is the concurrent behavior, then we might well find that for insecurely attached infants, cortisol reactions to potentially threatening events might be lower when they are with a sensitive and responsive stranger than when they are with their attachment figure. This would certainly argue that it is the caregiving style and not the attachment relationship that regulates the LHPA axis. Although such studies would be difficult to construct, they would be the kind of studies we need to know whether the attachment relationship confers special potency in stress regulation.

There is actually a naturally occurring situation that might be used to address this question. Dozier and colleagues (Stovall and Dozier 2000) have studied infants and toddlers in the U.S. foster care system during the first days and weeks of their transition into the care of the foster parent. Using a daily diary method, the foster mothers record the secure base behavior of the children in response to mild stressors (e.g., falling down, brief separations from the foster mother). Dozier and colleagues then classify these behaviors as secure, avoidant, or resistant and examine over days the emergence, or not, of secure attachment behaviors in the children. Some of these foster mothers are very sensitive and responsive to children in their care, others are less. One could ask, then, whether cortisol levels and reactivity in the infant during the infant's transition into the foster home track the sensitivity and responsiveness of the foster parent and whether changes in cortisol activity are noted before or after the infant begins to exhibit consistent patterns of attachment behavior towards the foster parents.

Is the LHPA Response to Separation a Response to Loss of the Attachment Figure?

Separation induces attachment behaviors (proximity/contact seeking, separation distress vocalizations), as well as other behaviors that may reflect fear and anxiety (freezing and inhibition of exploration). Separation reactions, thus, are not unitary phenomena (Kraemer et al. 1991). This may explain one of the more persistent and perplexing findings in the psychoneuroendocrine literature. Specifically, protest behaviors (crying, searching) at times are inversely related to separation-induced activity of the LHPA system. Levine and Wiener (1988) argue that protest behaviors reflect the infant's active attempt to cope with separation, whereas activation of the LHPA system reflects failed coping. An alternative explanation is that protest behaviors reflect the operation of the attachment system, and that LHPA responses reflect the operation of fear/anxiety systems in the central nervous system.

Kalin and colleagues (e.g., Kalin et al. 1988) provide support for this latter hypothesis. They have shown that calling and searching for the mother is regulated by central opioid activity. Exogenous opiates affect this type of protest behavior in infant monkeys, but they do not affect fear and defensive behaviors (e.g., freezing and threatening experimenters). Exogenous opiates also do not affect cortisol increases to maternal separation. In contrast, freezing, barking and other defensive behaviors during separation are regulated by central fear/anxiety systems orchestrated, in part, by extra-hypothalamic CRH. Central administration of CRH mediates the intensity of defensive behaviors but does not affect protest vocalizations. Indeed, in monkey infants there seems to be a close correspondence between freezing and other defensive behaviors and measures of ACTH and cortisol in response to separation.

In human infants, separation distress (fussing, crying) varies as a function of the infant's attachment classification. Insecure avoidant attachment is associated with less protest than is insecure resistant attachment. Indeed, it has been noted that the security dimension of attachment is orthogonal to the protest dimension of reaction to separation (Belsky and Rovine 1987). Cortisol increases are noted for both low-protest, avoidant babies and high-protest, resistant babies. Among securely attached infants, protest and cortisol responses in the Strange Situation are uncorrelated, while in insecurely attached infants, significant associations are observed, consistent with evidence that resistant infants tend to be more anxious and fearful (Spangler and Schieche 1998). Similarly, there is evidence that freezing/withdrawal during separation is associated with large increases in cortisol among year-old infants (Gunnar and Donzella 2002).

Separation may stimulate fear in infants and young children, but how much fear the infant experiences likely depends on the infant's temperament and the nature of the separation environment. As already discussed above, when the infant is provided with a sensitive and responsive caregiver, this blocks increases in cortisol and likely reduces the threat the infant experiences in the separation context. However, when the infant is fearful of strangers, this may make it difficult for her to use the comfort of a strange adult to regulate stress in the separation environment. Thus, not only the quality of care provided the infant, but the child's temperament may be expected to influence increases in cortisol during periods spent away from primary attachment figures. Recent studies of cortisol activity in infants, toddlers, and preschoolers studied in out-of-home childcare arrangements confirm these predictions. Quality of care and fearful temperament are both associated with rising levels of cortisol over the childcare day (Gunnar and Donzella 2002).

Continuity with Rodent Studies

Maternal care in rodents is critical to shaping the developing nervous system and in providing protection and nurturance. Distress vocalizations and LHPA activity in response to separation, however, appear to be mediated by opiate and CRH system, as described for the monkey infant. Similarly, LHPA activity during separation does not seem to reflect loss of the mother, but rather loss of certain stimuli correlated with maternal care (Suchecki et al. 1993). Although it can be argued that pups do not form primate-like attachment bonds to their mothers, it appears from the above review that there may be considerable continuity in the social mechanisms regulating stress from rodents to monkeys to humans. The attachment motivational system may help insure that the primate infant maintains proximity to the adult who is the most likely to provide adequate social regulation of the axis. However, there is as yet no evidence that having formed an attachment relationship, the infant loses the capacity to regulate stress physiology through interaction with other sensitive and responsive caregivers. Evidence is also lacking to indicate that separation from the attachment figure, per se, is a potent stimulator of the primate infant's LHPA system, as opposed to behavioral systems orchestrated around regaining contact (e.g., calling, searching).

ACKNOWLEDGMENTS

Preparation of this manuscript was supported by a K05 award (MH 66208) and network grant (MH 65046) to the author.

REFERENCES

Ahnert, L., M.R. Gunnar, M.E. Lamb, and M. Barthel. 2004. Transition to child care: Association of infant–mother attachment, infant negative emotion and cortisol elevations. *Child Dev.* **75**:629–650.

Ainsworth, M.D.S., M.C. Blehar, E. Waters, and S. Wall. 1978. Patterns of Attachment: A Psychological Study of the Strange Situation. Hillsdale, NJ: Erlbaum.

Belsky, J., and M. Rovine. 1987. Temperament and attachment security in the strange situation: An empirical rapproachement. *Child Dev.* **58**:787–795.

Bowlby, J. 1969. Attachment. Attachment and Loss, vol. 1. New York: Basic.

Buss, K.A., J.R.M. Schumacher, I. Dolski et al. 2003. Right frontal brain activity, cortisol, and withdrawal behavior in 6-month-old infants. *Behav. Neurosci.* **117**:11–20.

Coplan, J.D., M.W. Andrews, M.H. Owens et al. 1996. Persistent elevations of cerebrospinal fluid concentrations of corticotropin-releasing factor in adult nonhuman primates exposed to early-life stressors: Implications for the pathophysiology of mood and anxiety disorders. *PNAS* **93**:1619–1623.

De Kloet, E.R. 1991. Brain corticosteroid receptor balance and homeostatic control. *Front. Neuroendocrin.* **12**:95–164.

Dettling, A., J. Feldon, and C.R. Pryce. 2002. Repeated parental deprivation in the infant common marmoset (*Callithrix jacchus*, primates) and analysis of its effects on early development. *Biol. Psych.* **52**:1037–1046.

Glass, D.C., and J.W. Singer. 1972. Urban Stress: Experiments on Noise and Social Stressors. New York: Academic.

Gunnar, M.R., and B. Donzella. 2002. Social regulation of the LHPA axis in early human development. *Psychoneuroendocrin.* **27**:199–220.

Heim, C., M.J. Owen, P.M. Plotsky, and C.B. Nemeroff. 1997. The role of early adverse life events in the etiology of depression and posttraumatic stress disorder: Focus on corticotropin-releasing factor. *Ann. NY Acad. Sci.* **821**:194–207.

Herman, J.P., and W.E. Cullinan. 1997. Neurocircuitry of stress: Central control of the hypothalamo–pituitary–adrenocortical axis. *Trends Neurosci.* **20**:78–84.

Johnson, E.O., T.C. Kamilaris, G.P. Chrousos, and P.W. Gold. 1992. Mechanisms of stress: A dynamic overview of hormonal and behavioral homeostasis. *Neurosci. Biobehav. Rev.* **16**:115–130.

Kalin, N.H., S.E. Shelton, and C.M. Barksdale. 1988. Opiate modulation of separation-induced distress in non-human primates. *Brain Res.* **440**:856–862.

Kraemer, G.W., M.H. Ebert, D.E. Schmidt, and W.T. McKinney. 1991. Strangers in a strange land: A psychobiological study of infant monkeys before and after separation from real or inanimate mothers. *Child Dev.* **62**:548–566.

Levine, S., D.M. Lyons, and A.F. Schatzberg. 1997. Psychobiological consequences of social relationships. *Ann. NY Acad. Sci.* **807**:210–218.

Levine, S., and H. Ursin, eds. 1979. Coping and Health. New York: Plenum.

Levine, S., and S.G. Wiener. 1988. Psychoendocrine aspects of mother–infant relationships in nonhuman primates. *Psychoneuorendocrin.* **13**:143–154.

Liu, D., J. Diorio, J.C. Day et al. 2000. Maternal care, hippocampal synaptogenesis and cognitive development in rats. *Nature Neurosci.* **3**:799–806.

Liu, D., J. Diorio, B. Tannenbaum et al. 1997. Maternal care, hippocampal glucocorticoid receptors, and hypothalamic–pituitary–adrenal responses to stress. *Science* **227**:1659–1662.

Lopez, J.F., D.T.Chalmers, K.Y. Little, and S.J. Watson. 1998. Regulation of serotonin 1A, glucocorticoid, and mineralocorticoid receptor in rat and human hippocampus: Implications for the neurobiology of depression. *Biol. Psych.* **43**:547–573.

McEwen, B. 1998. Stress, adaptation, and disease: Allostasis and allostatic load. *Ann. NY Acad. Sci.* **840**:33–44.

Muller, M.B., F. Holsboer, and M.E. Keck. 2002. Genetic modification of corticosteroid receptor signaling: Novel insights into pathophysiology and treatment strategies of human affective disorders. *Neuropeptide* **36**:117–135.

Nachmias, M., M.R. Gunnar, S. Mangelsdorf et al. 1996. Behavioral inhibition and stress reactivity: Moderating role of attachment security. *Child Dev.* **67**:508–522.

Pani, L., A. Porcella, and G.L. Gessa. 2000. The role of stress in the pathophysiology of the dopaminergic system. *Molec. Psychiatry* **5**:14–21.

Sanchez, M.M., C.O. Ladd, and P.M. Plotsky. 2001. Early adverse experience as a developmental risk factor for later psychopathology: Evidence from rodent and primate models. *Dev. Psychopathol.* **13**:419–450.

Spangler, G., and M. Schieche. 1998. Emotional and adrenocortical responses of infants to the strange situation: The differential function of emotional expression. *Intl. J. Behav. Dev.* **22**:681–706.

Spangler, G., M. Schieche, U. Ilg et al. 1994. Maternal sensitivity as an external organizer for biobehavioral regulation in infancy. *Dev. Psychobiol.* **27**:425–437.

Steckler, T., and F. Holsboer. 1999. Corticotropin-releasing hormone receptor subtypes and emotion. *Biol. Psych.* **46**:1480–1508.

Stovall, K.C., and M. Dozier. 2000. The development of attachment in new relationships: Single subject analyses for 10 foster infants. *Dev. Psychopathol.* **12**:133–156.

Strand, F.L. 1999. Neuropeptides: Regulators of Physiological Processes. Cambridge, MA: MIT Press.

Suchecki, D., P. Rosenfeld, and S. Levine. 1993. Maternal regulation of the hypothalamic–pituitary–adrenal axis in the rat: The roles of feeding and stroking. *Dev. Brain Res.* **75**:185–192.

Sullivan, R.M., and A. Gratton. 2002. Prefontal cortical regulation of hypothalamic–pituitary–adrenal function in the rat and implications for psychopathology: Side matters. *Psychoneuroendocrin.* **27**:99–114.

13

Attachment Disturbances Associated with Early Severe Deprivation

T. G. O'CONNOR

Department of Psychiatry, University of Rochester Medical Center,
Rochester, NY 14642, U.S.A.

ABSTRACT

Clinical and research findings dating back many years indicate that early institutional deprivation is associated with a range of social behavior and relationship disturbances that persist into middle childhood in a minority of children. These observations prompted extensive theorizing on the nature of the child's early experiences on long-term psychological development and the role of early caregiving in particular. Indeed, attachment theory was developed, in part, to account for what is particular about these early caregiving experiences for healthy development. A central aim in the earlier (e.g., 1960s) research work was to examine the developmental significance of the child's formation of a discriminating or selective attachment relationship (Bowlby 1982). That is, there was a strong emphasis on species-typical behavior and development. Subsequent research, stimulated by the descriptive and predictive research on individual differences in attachment security and insecurity (Ainsworth et al. 1978), focused instead on individual differences. Stimulated by the intriguing findings on attachment and social and relationship disturbances in children who did not have the opportunity for selective attachments in infancy, this chapter revisits the kinds of questions posed by the early research on species-typical development of attachment relationships formed in infancy and beyond.

Recent trends in international adoption and the greater clinical sensitivity to children in care provide an opportunity to reconsider basic yet largely unexamined questions concerning the formation of post-infancy attachment relationships and the link between early deprivation/neglectful caregiving and long-term development. Importantly, to a greater extent than previous research, this new set of studies combines perspectives on normative and species-typical development with a consideration for individual differences. Some of the findings from studies of children who experienced early caregiving deprivation and severe maltreatment have raised new questions and stirred considerable controversy in the clinical and research literatures. Contemporary debate concerning the nature of social and attachment relationship disturbances in this population of children are seen in the concept of "Reactive Attachment Disorder" and in the nontraditional interventions that have been proposed for these children. This chapter discusses the history and the current state of research in this area and identifies topics for further research.

INTRODUCTION

Observations of children who experienced poor, absent, or disrupted care in infancy provided a core building block in the history of attachment theory and set in motion an overhaul in how the state looked after vulnerable young people (Bowlby 1951, 1982). It is therefore ironic that, several decades later, the nature of attachment relationships in children who experienced the kind of severe early caregiving deprivation that was so formative for attachment theory is a topic of significant controversy.

The context for revisiting the nature of attachment disturbances in children who experienced severe early deprivation is a recent increase in international adoption, which often involves children who experience institutional rearing (Gunnar et al. 2000), and the greater attention directed toward children in the social care system from traditional attachment perspectives (e.g., Stovall and Dozier 2000). These studies provide a "natural experiment" to examine basic conceptual issues concerning the failure to develop attachments in early life and the processes by which new attachment relationships develop after infancy. The topics of species-typical behavior and normative development were central in the early writings on attachment but were subsequently given less attention, as empirical research focused instead on the predictors and sequelae of individual differences in attachment security and insecurity. One helpful side effect of recent research on ex-institutionalized and foster care samples is that it has rekindled interest in studying normative developmental and species-typical processes in the making of attachment relationships.

The goals of this chapter are to review the historical and contemporary accounts of disturbances in attachment and social behavior in children who experienced early caregiving deprivation and to highlight how the study of children who experienced early severe deprivation present some particular and unique challenges for theory and research.

HISTORICAL AND CONTEMPORARY APPROACHES TO THE STUDY OF ATTACHMENT DISTURBANCES ASSOCIATED WITH DEPRIVATION

It has been known for decades that children who experienced severe early caregiving deprivation show disturbances in social, emotional, and behavioral development. In fact, there is a surprising degree of correspondence in the description of the social and relationship disturbances in these children. Although different phrases were sometimes used, including "superficially affectionate," "excessive need for adult attention," and "indiscriminately friendly," the basic behavioral disturbance described was similar: a tendency for children to approach relative strangers openly and without apparent inhibition or wariness, sometimes involving physical contact; the nature of the approach seemed impersonal and superficial rather than reciprocal and truly "social" (reviewed in O'Connor 2002). This pattern is also found in contemporary reports of (ex-)institutionalized children, including those that followed up children post-adoption (Chisholm 1998; O'Connor et al. 2000) and those that tracked children's development while still in institutions (Smyke et al. 2002). Moreover, this pattern of disturbance has been reliably assessed using interview and observational methods (O'Connor et al. 2003; Zeanah et al. 2002), providing a much-needed methodological depth that was missing from the earlier reports. Consistent with the terminology used in the Diagnostic and Statistical Manual of the American Psychiatric Association (DSM-IV), this form of disturbance is hereafter referred to as a disinhibited disturbance.

Other severe disturbances in attachment behavior have been noted in deprived samples, such as severe withdrawal and reluctance to seek out attachment figures when it would be normative and expected (e.g., when distressed or fearful; this pattern is referred to as an "inhibited" in the DSM-IV). However, these disturbances are less consistently reported or, if they are common, seem more likely to dissipate after placement with a consistent caregiver. Given that the previously described "disinhibited" form of disturbance is much more clearly linked with lack of consistent care and has received much more research than the "inhibited" variety, it is the focus of the remainder of this chapter.

Severe disturbances in attachment behavior as described above (particularly the disinhibited variety) are most closely associated with institutional rearing; however, Howe (1995) has shown that parallel disturbances are found in children in foster care. Direct comparisons of children from institutional rearing and foster care settings are difficult to make, however, and important differences between institutionalized and foster care samples are consistently found in clinical research. For example, aggression is not consistently reported in ex-institutionalized samples (indeed, the lack of aggression is often noteworthy), but it is extremely common in foster care samples (most likely because of a history of exposure to abuse). A second distinction is that children who experienced institutional rearing most likely did not form a selective attachment because no consistent caregiver was available. In contrast, it is likely that most children in the foster care system had developed a selective attachment with an attachment figure, however insecure it may have been (evidence confirming this impression is lacking, but is consistent with a series of reports). In other words, these two groups are most often cited in the context of research on severe attachment disturbances, but there are important and perhaps critical differences in the childrearing histories of children who experienced institutionalization and maltreatment leading to the foster care system. The implication is that further research in this area needs to consider both populations of children.

It is noteworthy that extensive research on several high-risk groups of children has not found evidence of the kinds of severe attachment disturbance described above — at least not yet. Specifically, attachment research on maltreated children and children of psychiatrically ill parents has not reported signs of disinhibited behavior (whether there is some evidence of inhibited behavior is more difficult to judge). The implication is that it is not markedly insensitive care per se that is linked with severe attachment disturbances. Instead, a reasonable inference from existing data is that it is the *absence of a consistent caregiver* that is associated with disinhibited attachment disturbance described above. If that is so, then research assessing animal or human offspring who had the opportunity to form selective attachments may be irrelevant for understanding the particular nature of relationship and social impairments associated with caregiving deprivation. Similarly, the research instruments and paradigms used to study the effects of insensitive care (e.g., insecure attachment) may not necessarily be useful for studying the effects of caregiving deprivation. A distinction needs to be drawn between the developmental sequelae of insensitive care and that associated with an absence of care.

The Notion of an Attachment "Disorder"

Professional opinion about the assessment, care, and treatment of children who experienced severe caregiving deprivation is divergent and contradictory. A concept that encapsulates much of this debate is "Reactive Attachment Disorder," a nosological construct that first appeared in the Diagnostic and Statistical Manual of the American Psychiatric Association in 1980. An aim of the diagnosis was to identify the kinds of disturbances associated with very poor early (institutional) care because they were thought to describe a distinct set of disturbances and to require a particular treatment regiment. It might be expected that formulating a disorder would improve (e.g., systematize, coordinate) assessment and treatment of children with severe attachment disturbances. This has not happened. Moreover, despite the existence of attachment disorder in the psychiatric nomenclature for more than twenty years, it remains the subject of little systematic study.

The absence of a sound empirical foundation for the attachment disorder concept has promoted a range of views about its usefulness. First, there are those who suggest that the notion of attachment disorder is hopelessly vague and should be dismissed. Then there are those who reject the linking of "disorder" with "attachment" and develop alternative epistemologies to settle (or avoid) problems in translating attachment classifications to attachment disorders (e.g., there are "relationship disorders"). Others have accepted the idea underlying the disorder, but nevertheless offer alternative definitions to those provided by DSM-IV and ICD-10 (International Statistical Classification of Diseases, 10th rev.). There are others still whose investment in the validity of the diagnosis is so well-developed that they have invented specialty "Reactive Attachment Disorder" interventions.

Notwithstanding the problems associated with the current diagnosis, it is a useful focus for discussion on the effects of early caregiving deprivation on attachment behavior for at least two reasons. First, although widely criticized, the DSM-IV and ICD-10 provide the clearest attempt thus far to codify the kinds of severe behavioral disturbances in children who experienced severe caregiving deprivation. Alternative definitions have not yet garnered significant clinical or research attention and, in addition, formulations from mainstream attachment research (e.g., Avoidant, Disorganized forms of insecure attachment) are of very limited usefulness for describing the behavioral phenomena. Second, current diagnostic criteria are increasingly applied to children in the foster care system and the growing number of children adopted from very poor circumstances, notably institutions from abroad. That is, the disorder has not only entered the clinical lexicon, but also influenced clinical practice (to varying degrees). In sum, more systematic research is needed to consider whether current diagnostic criteria adequately define the phenomena, but there is little doubt that the disturbance to which "Reactive Attachment Disorder" refers is a real phenomena that is linked with severe early caregiving deprivation.

Insofar as the diagnostic descriptions of disturbances associated with institutionalization provide a natural starting point for discussion, a brief review is provided. First, the behavioral descriptions in DSM-IV and ICD-10 have much in common with one another and with the early reports of ex-institutionalized children. According to DSM-IV, two forms of disturbance are identified: (a) an *inhibited* form of disturbance is characterized by a "persistent failure to respond ... to social interactions, as manifest by excessively inhibited" behavior; (b) a *disinhibited* form of disturbance is defined as "diffuse attachments as manifest by indiscriminate sociability."

In addition to describing briefly the behavioral markers of the disturbance, several conditions are also set by the diagnosis. The first is that there is a history of "grossly pathogenic care." What is implied by grossly pathogenic is not obvious, but this condition is specified to make clear that the disturbance is associated with environmental deprivation. Defining pathogenic care is not straightforward, partly because it is not yet certain what it is about the caregiving environment that is causally linked with the disturbance. Moreover, "grossly pathogenic care" would hardly be the term that caregivers (or the researchers) might have used to describe the care received by children reared in English residential units who were studied by Tizard and colleagues (Tizard and Rees 1975). Nonetheless, a sizable number of children in that study exhibited markedly disinhibited attachment disorder behavior. Therefore, as currently conceived, "pathogenic care" is clearly more than maltreatment and may be best operationalized as the absence of normally expected opportunities to form selective or discriminating attachment relationships.

Additional diagnostic criteria specify that the disturbance is not solely accounted for by developmental delay or pervasive developmental disorder. This criterion helps to establish the caregiving environment as having a causal influence. Also, it is specified that the disturbance has an early onset, defined as before five years of age. Finally, consistent with the notion of a disorder, it is required that the behavioral disturbances be evidence across situations and relationships, that is, not confined to a particular relationship. In that way, the diagnosis is clearly not to be seen as a *relationship-specific* disturbance.

Remarkably few studies are available that specifically examined children diagnosed with an attachment disorder. Nonetheless, there are many studies that assess children who show the kinds of disturbance implied by the disorder and noted in the early reports of institutionalized children. Findings from these studies, almost all of which assess the disinhibited form of disturbance, offer several important lessons for further research (see Chisholm 1998; Goldfarb 1943; Howe 1995; Hughes 1999; O'Connor et al. 2000, 2003; Provence and Lipton 1962; Rushton et al. 1995; Rutter 1981; Smyke et al. 2002; Tizard and Rees 1975; Zeanah et al. 2002).

First, the disinhibited disturbance is associated with caregiving deprivation even in the absence of nutritional, social, and cognitive deprivation. Thus, for example, in their study of young children who were reared since infancy in residential settings in England, Tizard and colleagues reported that several children showed "indiscriminate friendly" behavior toward strangers. That study is especially noteworthy because the children were cared for adequately in many respects, including adequate nutrition, cognitive stimulation, and opportunities for social play with adults and peers; they also exhibited normal intelligence. What they did lack was a consistent caregiver, and this likely explains the particular form of disturbance that was reported. In this regard it is noteworthy that Smyke et al. (2002) found that improving the child:caregiver ratio and decreasing the number of caregivers in institutions in Romania was associated with a decrease in disinhibited disturbance. The implication is that the disinhibited disturbance is not an "institutional syndrome," but is instead more closely linked with caregiver deprivation.

A second lesson from research is that the disinhibited disturbance appears to be persistent in at least a sizable minority of children, even in the absence of risk in the *current* caregiving environment. This is most clearly seen in the studies of children who were "rescued" from institutions and reared in normal-low risk families in the U.S., Canada, the U.K., and elsewhere. Two of these studies that assessed children from early to middle childhood (Chisholm 1998; O'Connor et al. 2000) found that duration of deprivation continued to be associated with disinhibited attachment disturbance several years after the children were placed in low- to normal-risk families. What is not yet known is how persistent the disturbance is and if it takes a different form in older children (e.g., are older children still showing "indiscriminate friendliness" and inappropriate social approach to strangers?). Recent findings from the 11-year-old follow-up of children adopted into the U.K. from Romania show that there are persisting disturbances in approximately one-quarter of the children adopted after two years of age; furthermore, the effect of duration of deprivation remained a robust predictor of disturbance at age 11 years, despite the fact that the children had been living in a sensitive, low-risk home for a minimum of 7.5 years (O'Connor, unpublished paper, Society for Research in Child Development 2003).

Third, the type of disturbances found in children who experienced early caregiver deprivation do not resemble insecure attachment found in high-risk samples, such as those children who experience maltreatment or parental mental illness (O'Connor et al. 2003). The implications of this are substantial. Most importantly, this implies that disturbances (where they exist) in children who experienced caregiver deprivation may be different in kind from those found in children who had the opportunity to form a selective attachment in infancy, however insensitive the care received. As noted above, it is striking that reports of "indiscriminate friendliness" are confined to reports of institutionally reared children and children in the foster care system. Children whose experiences lay outside the range of evolutionary adaptation — such as those who experience institutionalization — may show disturbances in species-typical development that are difficult to reconcile with those found in children who had the opportunity to develop selective attachments in infancy.

Fourth, disturbances defined by attachment disorder are readily distinguishable from other forms of psychopathology, although co-occurring problems of inattention, conduct disturbance, and emotional problems as well as cognitive and language problems are widely reported. A clear distinction between disinhibited attachment disorder behavior and other forms of psychopathology is noteworthy, given the multitude of risks that impact these children.

Fifth, attachment disorder behavior is not secondary to cognitive delay, although children who show attachment disorder behavior often exhibit cognitive, linguistic, or broad developmental delay.

In summary, the specific definition of *attachment disorder* in the psychiatric nomenclature remains controversial and supported only indirectly by research findings. On the other hand, the broader concept underlying attachment disorder, that there is a particular disturbance associated with caregiving deprivation, is supported by a long history of research. Furthermore, a coherent set of findings is emerging on the form of disturbance associated with caregiving derivation. The implication is that more work is needed to construct the definition of *attachment disorder* so that it has greater application and significance in clinical settings. Toward that aim, one specific issue that needs attention is the question of how, and if, to bring together the concepts of attachment disorder with the research on individual differences in attachment (in)security.

CONCEPTUAL AND CLINICAL CHALLENGES ASSOCIATED WITH SEVERE ATTACHMENT DISTURBANCES

Careful study of the processes by which new attachment relationships are formed by children who experienced gross early deprivation has both practical and theoretical importance. Practically, research of this kind may lead to a better understanding of how to promote new attachments between children and foster/adoptive parents and reduce the rate of placement breakdown among late-placed or hard to place children. This is acknowledged as a substantial public health concern. Conceptually, research of this kind would fill an important gap in the human literature, which has largely ignored the question of how new attachment relationships form past infancy in those with a history of no or severely neglectful caregiving. That is, there is remarkably little human research that parallels the animal research on maternal deprivation (Kraemer 1992; Ramey and Sackett 2000), although that is changing in light of the recent studies in the U.S., U.K., and elsewhere cited above.

Links and Contrasts between Attachment Disorder and Research on Attachment (In)Security

Perhaps the most important issue to resolve to advance research in this area is to understand the links and contrasts between attachment disorder behavior and the wealth of research on individual differences in attachment. The notion of attachment disorder (e.g., as defined by DSM-IV), has at best a tenuous link with the extensive research based on individual differences in child–parent attachment (in)security associated with Ainsworth, Bowlby, and others.

Comparisons between the notion of attachment disorder and attachment security must take note of several distinctions. For example, whereas attachment disorder is focused on the existence (or not) of a current or past discriminating or selective attachment relationship, research on attachment (in)security is concerned with individual differences among those who definitely had and have a selective attachment relationship. Another way of defining this contrast is that attachment disorder is concerned with species-typical or species-expectant experiences and not individual differences in caregiver sensitivity. In addition, whereas attachment disorder is concerned with cross-relationship or cross-setting disturbances (e.g., lack of wariness of strangers), research on attachment (in)security proposes that security or insecurity is a function of the history of care between a child and a *particular* caregiver; a child may have a secure attachment with one figure but an insecure attachment with another, and so there is relationship-specificity to attachment (in)security.

In terms of assessment strategy, the key determination for attachment disorder is to assess whether there is a selective or discriminating attachment relationship; in contrast, research on attachment (in)security takes that as a given and instead assesses children's responses to separation–reunion and other stressful behavioral and cognitive paradigms. The rich array of assessment paradigms, so useful for assessing individual differences in attachment quality, will likely be of limited value for determining if an attachment relationship had formed. Specifically, the use of separation–reunion procedures to assess attachment (in) security was never meant to establish if an attachment relationship had formed. Unfortunately, there are no validated measures that assess presence/absence of an attachment relationship (largely because research has focused on samples in which there was no question that an attachment relationship did exist). New paradigms are needed.

Finally, in terms of treatment, the treatment goals for children with an attachment disorder cannot yet be discerned from available research; this contrasts with the very clear treatment goal derived from research on attachment security, which is to enhance the capability of the caregiver to be able to respond more sensitively to the child and thereby help the child to use the parent as a secure base for exploration.

The Impact of Findings on "Attachment Disorder" to Normative Research on Individual Differences

The ultimate goal of research on children showing attachment disorder is not only to inform the clinical management of the significant minority of children who show this form of disturbance, but also to feed back to a larger set of questions concerning the nature of attachment relationships more broadly. Evidence of this is found, for example, in the question of timing that is raised by the study of children rescued from institutions or placed into foster care following severe adverse care (e.g., is there a point in development by which recovery following deprivation is unlikely?). There is as yet no clear answer to this question, and data that do exist in humans suggest that there is nowhere near the strong timing effect that is found in the nonhuman primate data. On the other hand, given the persistence of the attachment disorder disturbance in a minority of children, we can reject the simple notion that complete "recovery" is possible, at least in some cases (what accounts for individual differences in vulnerability to persistence of disturbance or recovery is not known). Furthermore, follow-up naturalistic studies indicate that attachment disorder behavior persists following adoption into low-risk, caring families for a period of many years. If an intervention as intensive as adoption shows comparatively little evidence of improvement after several years, then basic questions need to be asked about the basis for expecting sizable clinical gains from treatment lasting weeks or months. This is a controversial area, and one that needs carefully designed and clinically relevant research. In any event, the study of children who experience severe early caregiving deprivation have raised issues of developmental timing, sensitive periods, and resilience far more dramatically than studies of children who received continuous care from infancy.

A second illustration of how research on children who show attachment disorder behavior may illuminate the broader field of research concerns the emerging findings on the biological basis of attachment and social behavior (e.g., Carter 1998; Insel 1997). Studies of children who experienced deprivation are beginning to tackle the question of how attachment relationships serve biological functions, such as stress regulation (Gunnar, this volume). That will allow investigators to consider how far the important findings from the animal literature generalize to humans.

CONCLUSION

Both animal and human research have long considered the extent to which, and by what mechanisms, early experiences in the child–caregiver relationship have lasting effects on social and behavioral/emotional development in the child. Research strategies tackling this question pose several different kinds of questions, propose several levels of analysis, and provide a rich set of findings. An important feature of this work on animal and human parent–offspring attachment — including most of the contributions to the current volume — is that it focuses on caregiving environments that Bowlby described as within the range of evolutionary adaptiveness. To put this more concretely, most studies describe normative development (ontogeny), the origins and consequences of individual differences in attachment (in)security, and the effects of disruptions or stressors to attachment relationships among those offspring who has the opportunity to form selective attachments from infancy. A central theme of this chapter is that the forms of behavioral (and possibly physiological) attachment-related disturbances found in children who had the opportunity to form selective attachments from infancy differ in important ways from the disturbances observed in children who did not have such opportunities. In fact, recent research findings from careful longitudinal studies of children who experienced early caregiving deprivation are important because they document how different developmental outcomes (e.g., attachment disorder versus attachment insecurity) may be linked with different caregiving experiences in early life (e.g., absence of consistent caregiver vs. insensitive care).

Further attachment research in children needs to address the specific questions that arise from reports of children who experience caregiving deprivation. Answers to these questions would not only fill conceptual gaps in the theory, but also provide directions for assessment and treatment for a significant number of children who present substantial levels of clinical need that often go unmet. Studies of children who experienced caregiving deprivation have opened up a broader set of concerns that extend well beyond the population of children who experienced deprivation, such as the formation of attachment relationships beyond infancy (following deprivation or not).

REFERENCES

Ainsworth, M.D.S., M.C. Blehar, E. Waters, and S. Wall. 1978. Patterns of Attachment: A Psychological Study of the Strange Situation. Hillsdale, NJ: Erlbaum.

Bowlby, J. 1951. Maternal Care and Mental Health. Geneva: WHO.

Bowlby, J. 1982. Attachment. 2nd ed. Attachment and Loss, vol. 1. New York: Basic.

Carter, C.S. 1998. Neuroendocrine perspectives on social attachment and love. *Psychoneuroendocrin.* **23**:779–818.

Chisholm, K. 1998. A three year follow-up of attachment and indiscriminate friendliness in children adopted from Romanian orphanages. *Child Dev.* **69**:1092–1106.

Goldfarb, W. 1943. The effects of early institutional care on adolescent personality. *J. Exp. Educ.* **12**:106–129.

Gunnar, M.R., J. Bruce, and H.D. Grotevant. 2000. International adoption of institutionally reared children: Research and policy. *Dev. Psychopathol.* **12**:677–697.

Howe, D. 1995. Adoption and attachment. *Adoption Fostering* **19**:7–15.

Hughes, D.A. 1999. Adopting children with attachment problems. *Child Welfare* **78**:541–560.

Insel, T.R. 1997. A neurobiological basis of social attachment. *Am. J. Psych.* **154**:726–735.

Kraemer, G. 1992. A psychobiological theory of attachment. *Behav. Brain Sci.* **15**:494–551.

O'Connor, T.G. 2002. Attachment disorders in infancy and childhood. In: Child and Adolescent Psychiatry: Modern Approaches, ed. M. Rutter and E. Taylor, pp. 776–792. 4th ed. Oxford: Blackwell.

O'Connor, T.G., R.S. Marvin, M. Rutter et al. 2003. Child–parent attachment following early institutional deprivation. *Dev. Psychopathol.* **15**:19–38.

O'Connor, T.G., M. Rutter, and the English and Romanian Adoptees Study Team. 2000. Attachment disorder behavior following early severe deprivation: Extension and longitudinal follow-up. *J. Am. Acad. Child and Adoles. Psychiatry* **39**:703–712.

Provence, S, and R.C. Lipton. 1962. Infants Reared in Institutions. New York: Intl. Univ. Press.

Ramey, S.L., and G.P. Sackett. 2000. The early caregiving environment: Expanding views on nonparental care and cumulative life experiences. In: Handbook of Developmental Psychopathology, ed. A.J. Sameroff, M. Lewis, and S.M. Miller, pp. 365–380. 2nd ed. New York: Kluwer.

Rushton, A., J. Treseder, and D. Quinton. 1995. An eight-year prospective study of older boys placed in permanent substitute families: A research note. *J. Child Psychol. Psychiat.* **36**:687–695.

Rutter, M. 1981. Maternal Deprivation Reassessed. 2nd ed. Harmondsworth: Penguin.

Smyke, A.T., A. Dumitrescu, and C.H. Zeanah. 2002. Attachment disturbances in young children. I. The continuum of caretaking casualty. *J. Am. Acad. Child Adoles. Psych.* **41**:972–982.

Stovall, K.C., and M. Dozier. 2000. The development of attachment in new relationships: Single subject analyses for 10 foster infants. *Dev. Psychopathol.* **12**:133–156.

Tizard, B., and J. Rees. 1975. The effect of early institutional rearing on the behavioral problems and affectional relationships of four-year-old children. *J. Child Psychol. Psychiat.* **16**:61–73.

Zeanah, C.H., A.T. Smyke, and A. Dumitrescu. 2002. Attachment disturbances in young children. II. Indiscriminate behavior and institutional care. *J. Am. Acad. Child Adoles. Psych.* **41**:983–989.

14

Disorganization of Behavioral and Attentional Strategies toward Primary Attachment Figures

From Biologic to Dialogic Processes

K. H. HENNIGHAUSEN and K. LYONS-RUTH

Harvard Medical School, Cambridge, MA 02139, U.S.A.

ABSTRACT

This chapter reviews disorganized behavioral and attentional strategies used by the child to seek comfort and care from the parent in the face of fearful arousal, and how these disorganized strategies relate to maladaptive outcomes. Relational and biological mechanisms related to disorganized attachment during the first years of life are reviewed, emphasizing the importance of developmental changes in the capacity for intersubjective sharing. The early childhood shift from disorganized to controlling strategies is described and related to current and future psychopathology. Finally, an expanded etiological model is proposed for intergenerational transmission of disorganized attachment strategies. Three theoretical issues requring further attention are highlighted: (a) the need to reconsider the evolutionary base of human attachment to include the specifically human capacity for intersubjective sharing; (b) the need to consider mechanisms embedded in positive interactions with others that may regulate fearful arousal; and (c) the need to reconcile the existing competing models of the etiology of attachment disorganization in the parent and in the infant.

INTRODUCTION

The parent–infant attachment relationship is the relational system most fundamentally involved in the regulation of the child's fearful arousal from the beginning of life. Although recent animal models have focused most systematically on neurobiological and neurobehavioral systems underlying the attachment bond from mother to infant, human attachment studies have focused most intensively on the bond from infant to parent (Cassidy and Shaver 1999).

This difference in focus does not occur by chance. In most other mammalian species, maternal behavior is strongly prepared by physiological mechanisms, and it is the mother, more than the infant, who exhibits specific biologically prepared behaviors to insure the infant's survival, including selective caregiving, selective recognition and attention, and selective protective actions in favor of her own offspring (e.g., Carter, this volume; Keverne; this volume). In the human species, however, the role of the infant's expressive repertoire for attracting and maintaining parental investment is heightened (Hrdy, this volume). Parallel to this expanded role for infant behavior is the decreased uniformity of human maternal behavior from parturition onwards, with an associated decrease in the role of specific biological mechanisms in the onset and maintenance of maternal care. This increased variability in human maternal care allows, in turn, for increased variability in the quality of arousal regulation for the offspring.

In this chapter we review the relation between maladaptive developmental pathways and the infant's strategies for seeking comfort and care in the face of fearful arousal, with a focus on the disorganized strategies that have been most clearly associated with later negative outcomes. Disorganized behavioral and attentional processes in relation to a primary attachment figure subsume one set of indicators of dysregulation in the infant–parent attachment relationship. Because the attachment system is active from the beginning of life and regulates key homeostatic functions related to safety and survival, such dysregulation has potentially far-reaching consequences for the further development of both behavioral and physiological systems related to psychopathology.

Our understanding of the family contexts and developmental transformations associated with disorganization of infant attachment strategies still contains many areas of controversy. Here we highlight the significant gaps and questions that need to be addressed to advance understanding of the role that disorganized attachment relationships play in development and psychopathology. Because some of the most significant, interesting gaps and controversies concern the ability to envision developmental pathways associated with attachment disorganization over time, we focus discussion developmentally as of infancy.

VARIABILITY IN MATERNAL CARE FROM AN EVOLUTIONARY PERSPECTIVE

Immediately after birth, primate mothers do not engage in many of the highly specific behaviors seen in small-brained mammals, such as nest-building prior to birth, eating the placenta, licking themselves to spread the odor of the placenta, or needing to see or smell the infant within a specified period after birth to recognize and care for the infant (e.g., Keverne, this volume; Carter, this volume). Maternal behavior among primates is notable for its absence of fixed action patterns associated with birth and bonding.

Maternal behavior among humans is even more notable for its variability and absence of fixed action patterns around birth and bonding (Hrdy, this volume).

For many of its specifics on cultural practices, human mothering depends on conditions surrounding childbirth, sleeping arrangements, nursing, and weaning. This variability across cultures in the patterns characterizing birth and early care indicate a lack of strong biological control of early patterns of mothering. This absence of strong biological control can be seen in the case of the attachments that are made between adoptive parents and their children, where biological processes associated with pregnancy and parturition play no role in the development of adequate parental care and affectionate attachment. Equally striking is the relatively high rate of infanticide among human mothers who *have* given birth (Hrdy, this volume). It appears, therefore, that maternal behavior in humans is mediated more strongly by the neocortex than is maternal behavior in all other mammals.

Given the necessity of adequate care for the survival of the infant, why would such extensive variability in maternal behavior have evolved? First, even in small-brained mammals where specific biological mechanisms channel maternal behavior, maternal behavior also benefits from experience in that first litters receive less skilled mothering than subsequent litters (Fleming, this volume). The effect of prior maternal experience, seen almost universally among mammals, is likely to be even more potent among human mothers, given the greater variation in parenting behavior in general and the complexity of care needed to adjust to the rapidly changing needs of the human child. Consistent with the well-documented positive effect of prior maternal experience in other mammals, disorganized human infant attachment behaviors have been found to be less frequent among later-borns than among first-borns (Lyons-Ruth, Bronfman, and Parsons 1999).

Second, Hrdy (this volume) points out that human children take a long time to mature, and rearing them is more costly than a mother fending for herself could have managed in the Pleistocene environments in which our ancestors evolved. Assistance from fathers is important, but fathers are not always a sufficient or reliable source of help. Hence, mothers often rely on assistance from other group members, including siblings, aunts, uncles, and grandmothers. Hrdy argues that because of the cost of parenting to human mothers, it may not be adaptive to have unconditional commitment to the care of every offspring. Instead, a human mother may need to make decisions about when and how much care is needed to devote to a given offspring to maximize both her own reproductive potential and the reproductive potential of older offspring to whom a large amount of resources may already have been devoted. In support of this argument, Hrdy points out that there is a high rate of infanticide among humans compared to other species. Given the very large resource allocation that must be devoted to the care of human children, Hrdy also argues that the availability of allomaternal care, or care of the infant by adults and subadults other than the mother, will be an important factor in a mother's implicit decision making regarding how vigorously to commit herself to the care of a given infant. Hrdy reasons that low social support may lead to less maternal resource allocation to a given infant and more resource allocation to maintaining her own and her other offspring's survival and reproductive potential. Thus, maternal behavior may show variability in relation to available parenting support from other adults and the larger society.

Hrdy's discussion of the conditional nature of human maternal care offers a framework for considering disorganized infant attachment behaviors within evolutionary and cultural perspectives. Whereas evolutionary theory has been extended to the understanding of variations in organized forms of infant attachment strategies (Belsky, this volume), disorganized forms of infant attachment have been viewed primarily through the lens of developmental psychopathology. This view has emerged from a variety of evidence that both psychological regulation and neurobiological functioning are less optimal among disorganized infants than among infants with organized attachment behaviors, as reviewed below. However, to extend Hrdy's reasoning, every family and culture makes a variety of implicit and explicit decisions about how to value the infant's biological and psychological regulation in relation to the demands of the larger collective units that provide life support for the infant. The parent–infant attachment patterns observed in human societies represent one set of decisions about how the infant's growth, development, and regulation of fearful arousal should be prioritized relative to the reproductive advantages accruing to other allocations of caregiver and family resources.

Variability in parenting behavior may be important to allow the human species as a whole to engage in and transmit the wide range of cultural experiments that are associated with a rapid rate of cultural change and ever-new patterns of culturally transmitted learning. Our current massive cultural experiment with out-of-home care for infants is one example of how a lack of fixed patterns of maternal care allows radically different forms of family organization to emerge and be transmitted culturally. The impact of such innovations on the reproductive fitness of the individual infant, the mother, and the kinship group as a whole is currently a topic of intense debate (Ahnert, this volume). Conflict behaviors, increased fearful arousal, and role-reversed behaviors seen among disorganized infants are associated with low resource environments and with deviations in parental responsiveness to infants' cues (Lyons-Ruth and Jacobvitz 1999). Although costly to the infant, this decrease in maternal commitment may maximize reproductive outcomes for the family unit as a whole. In addition, if the parent is psychologically vulnerable, decreased involvement in the parenting role may also be important to maintain the functioning of the parent.

A third contributor to variability in human maternal behavior may be the shift in the human species to the transmission of experience from one generation to the next through processes of intersubjective sharing (e.g., Tomasello 1999). Hrdy (this volume) has speculated that the enhanced capacity of the human infant to engage the caregiver very early through the exchange of modulated emotional and intentional signals may be one evolutionary consequence of the conditional maternal commitment seen in the human species. The ability of the infant to engage the mother in an emotional dialog may have important survival value for the infant if the mother's commitment to the infant's care is not strongly biologically channeled. Whatever its origins, however, the enhanced human capacity for intersubjective sharing allows a shift in the regulation of attachment relationships from more strongly channeled biologic mechanisms to more finely modulated but also more variable communication processes.

Much has been written recently about the shift in the basis of evolutionary change from biologic to what we will call dialogic mechanisms, or from "genes to memes." For example, Tomasello (1999) pointed out that sometime after 200,000 years ago, with the emergence of *Homo sapiens*, more complex cultural innovations were introduced into human life than in the previous six million years. He theorizes that a biological change occurred to shift the basis for innovation in human life from biological evolutionary mechanisms to mechanisms of cultural transmission, which are many orders of magnitude faster than those of organic evolution. He assigns this shift to the increased ability of humans, relative to other primates, to imagine the thoughts and feelings of others and to share those thoughts and feelings intentionally in the form of explicit teaching and learning. In contrast to other primates, the human infant does not have to acquire all knowledge and experiences necessary to survival first-hand. Instead, the infant needs to acquire skills for sharing affective valences and intentional states with others to participate in the cultural learning processes of human society. The early parent–infant attachment relationship, then, must insure the infant's immediate biological survival and also contribute to later reproductive fitness by equipping the infant to participate in the learning processes and extensive social exchanges of a particular kin or community network. Thus, in contrast to primate attachment behaviors, the human attachment system is filtered through and mediated by the increasingly complex intersubjective processes that emerge as of birth. (Evolutionary recontextualization of the human attachment system is considered further below.) Thus, the more molar infant attachment behaviors seen in other species (e.g., crying, clinging, following) became more recontextualized from the beginning of human life within a much more finely modulated intersubjective regulatory system involving the exchange of a wider array of subtle facial and vocal cues as to one's intentional states.

Intersubjective communication as part of a species-wide attachment regulatory system is further contextualized by the function of intersubjective communication as a culturally specific set of procedures for insuring integration of the individual into a specific cultural group and adaptation of the group as a whole. Human cultural groups develop different ways of managing social communications and the exchange of potent affect cues in the service of group adaptation and survival. The infant's signaling of attachment needs and a caregiver's affective responses are thus shaped by the larger cultural regulations that are imposed on the attachment system by the cultural group. This more complex system creates the potential for tensions to exist between optimal regulation of the individual infant and the need to socialize the infant to participate in the patterns of affect expression and intersubjective exchange adopted by the group as a whole.

In summary, when considering the caregiving contexts associated with disorganized infant attachment behaviors, it is important to recognize the extensive variability in patterns of human mothering and the potential relation of such variability to evolutionary mechanisms governing maternal investment and overall reproductive fitness. In addition, variability in human mothering is further contextualized by the variability inherent in the greater specificity of the exchange and calibration of affect and intention signals between human parents and their infants, which provides a foundation for the further development of shared mental states between the infant and its cultural surround. In addition to adaptive variability, the shift to an intersubjective basis for attachment also opens the way for a wider variety of nonlethal dysfunctions in the parent–infant relationship.

RETHINKING MECHANISMS OF ATTACHMENT DURING THE FIRST YEAR: EVOLUTION AND INTERSUBJECTIVE AWARENESS

John Bowlby thoroughly documented the similarities in attachment behaviors across primate species and human cultures. At the time Bowlby (1969) was writing, however, little was known about the capacities of the very young human infant for establishing intersubjective communication with a caregiver. Therefore, in discussing the attachment behavioral system during the first year of life, Bowlby located the human attachment system within the context of primate evolution and identified the more molar and visible human attachment behaviors shared with other primates, such as clinging, following, and crying, as the infant's contribution to the attachment relationship during the first year. However, not until the end of the first year of human life do these more molar behaviors take on the characteristic pattern described by Bowlby of maintaining proximity to the caregiver and protesting separation. Therefore, these studies of the infant attachment system focused on behaviors as of 12 months.

In following up Bowlby's central insights, Ainsworth et al. (1978) elaborated in much more detail the role of the mother's sensitivity to infant cues over the first year in fostering the infant's open emotional communication and associated sense of security in the face of mild threat. She began to document the variation among human mothers in their responses to infant cues. We would argue that the full implications of Ainsworth's focus on maternal sensitivity, as the critical variable mediating attachment security, have yet to be fully integrated with Bowlby's more separation-related version of attachment theory. Essentially, Ainsworth's focus on maternal sensitive responsiveness shifted the focus of attachment theory from separation and protection to the moment-to-moment negotiation of the balance between fearful arousal and engaged exploration of the social environment, with such negotiations occurring through finely modulated, intersubjective affective communication between parent and infant.

Over time, these caregiver–infant negotiations lead to increasingly complex internal working models of how to approach and engage others in ways that do not result in overwhelming fearful arousal. These models concern the degree to which others are perceived as a source of threat versus the degree to which they can be engaged around the affectively central concerns of early life, as well as the kinds of engagements that are possible around those concerns. The infant's security in exploring will then partly contextualize how complex and skilled the resulting internal models of how to engage with others will become.

Since Bowlby's early writing, numerous studies using diverse methodologies have demonstrated that human infants are equipped with much more elaborate capacities than other primates for sharing both affective signals and intersubjective states with others (e.g., Jaffe et al. 2001; Tomasello 1999). This allows the infant to participate in the human capacity for sharing another's emotional states from very early in life and also equips the infant to draw the caregiver into sharing the infant's emotional states. Tomasello argues that only humans develop the capacity to attribute to others a mental life similar to one's own. The rudiments of such a theory of mind are evident by the end of the first year of life (e.g., Lyons-Ruth and Zeanah 1993). Further, Tomasello reasons that humans use this awareness to learn from and transmit knowledge to others, and that this capacity for conceiving of other minds accounts for the explosive rate of cultural evolution over the past 200,000 years. We would argue that the greatly enhanced intersubjective capacity of the human infant compared to other primates partially displaces the human attachment system from its primate base and recontextualizes it within particularly human forms of intersubjective relatedness from the beginning of life.

As the explicit sharing of intentional states became a more powerful force in human evolution, we would argue that this shift also affected the infant–parent attachment system, moving the center of the attachment relationship to primarily intersubjective processes, as implicitly recognized in Ainsworth et al.'s (1978) work and in much of Bowlby's later work. The primate attachment behaviors of clinging, following, and close bodily contact as means of soothing the infant and maintaining a positive state are partially displaced by the sharing of emotional cues. The capacity for emotional sharing and signaling becomes a primary way of regulating fear states or security of attachment in the infant from very early in life. The infant's tendency to seek out a caregiver for comfort is based on a hierarchy of preference related to which caregiver best knows the infant's mind and can interpret the infant's intentional signals. The release of neurotransmitters, neuropeptides, and neurohormones that may partially mediate the feeling components of attachment relationships, including, for example, dopamine, serotonin, oxytocin, prolactin, vasopressin, and cortisol, would then become mediated through the exchange of affective and intentional cues, rather than primarily through close holding or simple visual proximity.

This shift to an intersubjective basis for regulating the underlying physiology of attachment also introduces the possibility that in the human species a greater variety of caregivers, other than biological mothers alone, can be involved with the infant. All human adults have a capacity to relate intersubjectively and this mechanism is not dependent on particular hormonal events of pregnancy and parturition, as in many other mammalian species. However, the specificity of intersubjective processes requires that a caregiver come to know the mind of the infant well if adequate regulation is to be achieved.

This proposed evolutionary shift to an intersubjective basis for attachment allows much more subtlety and variation in the quality of relatedness and in the adaptiveness of the parent–infant interactions, simply because the intersubjective mechanisms involved are so variable and less canalized by more molecular biological mechanisms. In addition to adaptive variations, the shift to an intersubjective basis for attachment also opens the way for a wider variety of nonlethal dysfunctions in the parent–infant relationship. If stress regulation is based less directly on aspects of physical care than in smaller-brained mammals and more directly on complex and variable subjective sharing mechanisms, there is the opportunity for very wide variation in felt security, or in the quality of regulation of stressful arousal available to the infant.

These early patterns of sharing intentional states with caregivers occur as the neocortex is forming synaptic connections during the early years, so that the patterning of social exchanges with primary family members are literally being wired into the neocortical areas of the brain of the infant. This wiring of the brain to incorporate early patterns of social interaction provides one potential mechanism for adapting the child to survive and reproduce within a particular family and social group. Although we assume that such early structuring is plastic to some extent, further brain structures and learning processes build on these early patternings, so that restructuring of early patterns of attachment-related social communication in later life would be expected to be difficult. Many of the phenomena studied under the topic of disorganization of attachment, as reviewed below, are an attempt to map the less adequate varieties of intentional sharing that occur among parents and infants and their relation to the infant's felt security and biological regulation of fearful arousal.

Such a view of specifically human attachment requires greater elaboration of how attachment processes during the first year are embedded within a matrix of shared communication of experiences with the caregiver. This greater elaboration is particularly critical to understanding the relations among the attachment system, regulation of fearful arousal, and the development of the hypothalamic–pituitary–adrenal (HPA) axis during the first year. Drawing on the body of infancy research, Schuder and Lyons-Ruth (2004) have elaborated a dual-level model of attachment processes during the first year, with regulatory mechanisms both at the behavioral/physiological level and at the level of intersubjective affective communication. References for the developmental work referred to below are available in Lyons-Ruth and Zeanah (1993) and Schuder and Lyons-Ruth (2004).

Primary Intersubjective Communication

Contemporary biologists have reconceptualized the capacity to regulate states of emotional security as a developmental process that begins with the dyadic regulation of the infant's earliest physiological homeostasis (Hofer 1996). The caregiver facilitates the infant's capacity to maintain internal homeostasis by adjusting the mode, amount, timing, and variability of relational stimulation to the infant's signals. The human infant appears uniquely well-equipped at birth to exchange affective signals with a caregiver. Emotions such as sadness, anger, disgust, fear, joy, and interest can be identified reliably from the facial displays of infants aged 1–9 months. The resulting subtlety of this capacity for exchanging affective signals in face-to-face communication by 2–3 months of age, as well as the statistical dependency of maternal and infant cues, has been described in detail in time-series analyses (e.g., Jaffe et al. 2001).

A number of researchers have concluded that there is a preadapted intention toward cooperative communication in the human infant as well as a preadapted capacity for coordination of subjectivities. According to Murray and Trevarthen (1985, p. 194), "the forms and communicative values of human emotions are innately formulated." We would add that in this earliest expression of intersubjective communication, the "topic" or referent of the shared affective "comment" is simply the hedonic quality of the relationship itself. There is a primary affective communication of "We make pleasure or displeasure together," with no reference to outside objects or events. Therefore, the earliest phase of intentional sharing involves calibrating the infant–caregiver relationship itself in regard to maintaining a positive state for the infant. The parent's role in regulating negative arousal during the first year is not simply to respond with comfort when the infant is disturbed, but to avert distress by maintaining the infant's interest and engagement in a positively toned dialog with the social and physical environment. We would argue that, during the first year in particular, the infant attachment relationship cannot be defined primarily in terms of caregiver responses to infant distress. Instead, maintenance of a positively toned state is critical to the infant's felt security and stress modulation, and this requires a responsive intersubjective dialog between caregiver and infant.

Parental responsiveness is perhaps best viewed as parental sensitivity and flexibility in continually adjusting interaction to respond to infant signals. The most obvious examples of this process occur when the interaction is ruptured by a negative state of the infant and "repaired" by sensitive parental response. However, much parent–child interaction involves more continual and subtle mutual modifications in behavior such that obvious ruptures do not occur.

Recent animal models of attachment processes support the idea that biological mechanisms for the enhancement of positive feeling states may play a role in establishing selective attachments and reducing fearful arousal. As described elsewhere in this volume, (e.g., Keverne, this volume; Carter, this volume), oxytocin is a neuropeptide that is related to pair bonding, parturition, and lactation in many mammalian species. In animal models, oxytocin is also related to decreases in the stress hormone cortisol in cerebrospinal fluid. Therefore, oxytocin provides one evolutionarily prepared biological mechanism that may mediate the role of positive parent–infant interactions in facilitating secure attachments and buffering the infant's potential for fearful arousal. Unfortunately, animal models have concentrated on the role of oxytocin in maternal behavior and bonding, so that relatively little is known about the role of oxytocin in mediating infant behavior and stressful arousal, even among other mammals. In addition, oxytocin does not readily pass the blood–brain barrier, so assessments of oxytocin function in humans are hampered by the need to sample cerebrospinal fluid. Nevertheless, the accumulated research findings regarding the stress-reducing properties of social affiliation are clear (e.g., Taylor et al. 2000); biological effects of positive engagement with the attachment figure are likely to play a role in reducing fearful arousal in infancy. Porges (this volume) proposes a model of how positive social engagement may decrease sympathetic arousal, mediated through the ventral vagal components of the parasympathetic nervous system. Thus, there is now a convergence of developmental/behavioral, biological, and evolutionary arguments for enlarging our model of the attachment behavioral system to include positive components of the infant–caregiver relationship that also serve the function of regulating fearful arousal.

Recent work on the early functioning of the HPA axis has already documented the importance of infant–caregiver affective communication in setting parameters of the early functioning of stress response systems in other mammals (e.g., Francis et al. 1999). Although much of this work has come from animal models where experimental controls can be instituted, related findings are also being reported for human infants. For example, Thompson et al. (unpublished paper, Society for Research in Child Development 2003) have reported that cortisol change to a mildly stressful event occurs in the same direction for mother and baby by six months of age, and Ashman et al. (2002) have found cortisol elevations among infants of depressed mothers. The literature also indicates that by the end of the first year, intersubjective communication with the caregiver has become the primary regulator of fearful arousal, in that caregiver regulation can override inhibited temperamental predisposition (Schuder and Lyons-Ruth 2004).

Unfortunately, very little work has directly examined the relations between disorganized attachment strategies at one year and the characteristics of infant and maternal affective communication in the first 8 months of life. In one exception, Jaffe et al. (2001) found that "hypervigilant" tight vocal rhythm tracking by both mother and baby at four months of age, combined with the baby's postural and visual avoidance, was a predictor of disorganization of attachment strategies at 12 months. They postulated that hypervigilance was an indicator of maternal stress or anxiety and also found that babies who became disorganized showed more vocal and facial distress at four months. In addition, Kelly, Ueng-Hale, Grienberger, and Slade (unpublished paper, Society for Research in Child Development 2003) found that maternal disrupted communication with the infant at four months of age, assessed by the AMBIANCE scales, predicted disorganized attachment behavior at one year. It will be critical to understand the early parent–infant interactive processes that affect the infant's stress physiology and to explore the early physiological adaptations that precede and predict the emergence of behavioral disorganization in relation to the caregiver by the end of the first year.

While available data point to the likelihood that parent–infant affective interactions are disrupted from early in the first year, it is more difficult to tease apart whether the infant is difficult to engage or whether the parent is unskilled at engaging the infant. Videotaped observations clearly reveal that parents override or ignore clear and appropriate infant cues in many cases, and that infants may respond with more positive engagement to strangers than to the parent. However, from very early on, a number of infants also begin to display more avoidance and more conflict behavior toward the parent, and an increasingly problematic interaction pattern results that involves difficult behaviors from both partners. Pairing both the parent and the infant with other interactive partners would be one way of examining the relative contributions of each. Randomized interventions with parents would also help chart the extent to which changes in parental behavior influence changes in infant behavior.

Secondary Intersubjective Communication

As infants approach nine months of age, they increasingly look to their familiar social partners for affective cues to guide responses to objects and events outside the relationship itself, a process referred to as "social referencing." This capacity has been related to other indicators of a broad capacity for mutual sharing of subjective states, or affective comments, toward other objects and events that emerge during the last quarter of the first year (for a review, see Lyons-Ruth and Zeanah 1993). As an infant becomes more mobile, social referencing of the parent serves as an anticipatory affective guide to inform the infant about sources of danger or pleasure and serves to regulate the infant's affect and behavior from a distance. The sense of shared emotional states and mutually regulated affective displays underlying this behavior is likely to have been constructed, at least in part, upon the earlier processes of affective communication observed during the first six months of life.

The literature on social referencing and secondary intersubjectivity has not yet been extended to infants at social risk nor has it been related theoretically to attachment processes. However, we hypothesize that this emergent capacity for using parental affective signals as cues to safety and pleasure in the larger environment promotes the increasingly selective preference for particular attachment figures observed by 12 months of age. The wariness to strangers at 9 months may also stem from the increased intersubjective sharing capacity of the 9- to 12-month-old, a capacity that makes a stranger's unknown affective communicative repertoire a source of uncertainty and therefore potentially unsafe. Therefore, embedding attachment processes more fully in a theory of the development of intersubjective sharing could offer a host of new insights.

Potential disruptions in the development of normal social referencing behavior among high-risk infants and toddlers are strongly implied in the clinical descriptions of the absence of stranger wariness and cautious behavior among children who have experienced early deprivation and neglect. This absence of wariness is a criterion for the diagnosis of "Reactive Attachment Disorder." Indiscriminate friendliness toward strangers is often displayed by international adoptees from severely deprived institutional settings (O'Connor, this volume). Such indiscriminate friendliness may rest on very early disruptions in the development of normative forms of affective sharing, with subsequent impact on social referencing behaviors. Potential links between developing forms of intersubjective communication and risk-related deviations in attachment behaviors speak to the importance of embedding attachment processes more fully within a view of the development of intersubjective sharing over the first year. More research on this interface is greatly needed.

Infant Attachment and Disorganization of Attachment by Twelve Months of Age

As noted earlier, organized strategies for maintaining proximity to the caregiver are first evident at around 12 months of age (see Grossmann and Grossmann, this volume; Belsky, this volume). Similarly, disorganized attachment strategies, or contradictory and unintegrated behaviors toward the caregiver when comfort is needed, can first be identified at 12 months of age. A large body of research on fearful arousal has documented the range of coping responses to pain or fear displayed by individuals when exposed to severe stressors. These have been captured by the summary label "fight or flight." In addition, Seligman (1975) and others have described "freezing" and "learned helplessness" as responses occurring when more active coping responses are unavailable or ineffective. More recently, Shelly Taylor and colleagues (2000) have advanced a "tend or befriend" hypothesis regarding primary responses to threat among social primates, arguing that "fight or flight" may be more relevant to the stress responses of males, whereas various forms of affiliative responses may be more common stress responses of females.

This entire array of coping or defensive responses appears in some form in the behaviors that are part of the disorganized/controlling spectrum, as shown in

Table 14.1 Indices of infant disorganization and disorientation in the presence of the parent. For complete descriptions, see Main and Solomon (1990).

1. Sequential display of contradictory behavior patterns, such as strong attachment behavior followed by avoidance or disorientation.
2. Simultaneous display of contradictory behavior patterns, such as strong avoidance with strong contact seeking, distress, or anger.
3. Undirected, misdirected, incomplete, and interrupted movements and expressions.
4. Stereotypies, asymmetrical movements, mistimed movements, and anomalous postures.
5. Freezing, stilling, or "slow-motion" movements and expressions.
6. Direct indices of apprehension regarding the parent.
7. Direct indices of disorganization or disorientation in presence of parent, such as disoriented wandering, confused or dazed expressions, or multiple, rapid changes.

Table 14.1. For example, freezing, huddling on the floor, and other depressed behaviors are part of the coding criteria for disorganized behaviors, as are contradictory approach–avoidance behaviors that often mix angry resistance with avoidant behaviors such as running away or hiding under a chair. In addition, a majority of disorganized infants continue to approach and seek contact with the caregiver while also displaying conflict behaviors.

Etiological Models of Infant Disorganization

The etiological model of the genesis of disorganized attachment strategies in infancy, initially proposed by Main and Hesse (1990), is presented in Figure 14.1. According to this model, parental experiences of loss or abuse may lead to unintegrated states of mind in the parent, states of mind that generate lapses in reasoning or discourse when interviewed on the Adult Attachment Interview (AAI). This is termed an "Unresolved" state of mind and is the adult representational measure of a disorganized working model of attachment. This "Unresolved" adult state of mind, in turn, is predicted to be associated with frightened or frightening (FR) parental behavior toward the infant, due to the lack of mental and behavioral integration of the fearful affect associated with the loss or abuse experience. The parent's FR behavior, in turn, is seen as placing the infant in an irresolvable conflict because the parent becomes a source of fear for the infant as well as the primary source of comfort. This conflict is viewed as leading to the contradictory and unintegrated behaviors toward the caregiver that are the hallmark of attachment disorganization (Main and Solomon 1990).

Of the proposed relations in this model, there is meta-analytic confirmation that unresolved parental states of mind are associated with infant disorganization, $r = 0.31$ (van IJzendoorn et al. 1999), mixed support for the mediating role of FR parental behaviors, and surprisingly little support for an etiological connection between severity of maternal experiences of loss or trauma in childhood and maternal "Unresolved" states of mind on the AAI (Ainsworth and Eichberg

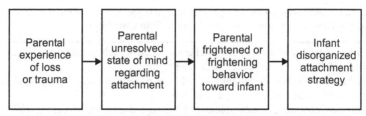

Figure 14.1 Etiological model of the transmission of disorganized attachment from parent to infant.

1991; Lyons-Ruth et al. 2005; Schuengel et al. 1999). The relations between severity of experiences of loss or trauma and "Unresolved" status on the AAI have received less attention, however. Thus, additional work is needed to explore their etiological contribution.

The etiological model focuses on active parental stimulation of infant fear as key to the etiology of disorganization. However, the primate literature has been unequivocal in demonstrating that parental lack of response, or at the extreme, parental absence, is associated with highly fearful infant behavior and associated hyper-responsiveness of the HPA stress response system (Coplan et al. 1996). An alternative account is that disorganized infant behaviors are related to a broader spectrum of disturbed caregiving interactions, including parental withdrawal, that are unresponsive to the infant's attachment needs and that leave the infant subject to unregulated fearful arousal. Recent research has generated support for such a broader etiological model of infant disorganization that includes parental nonresponse or withdrawal in the face of infant attachment initiatives (e.g., Goldberg et al. 2003; Lyons-Ruth, Bronfman, and Parsons 1999; Madigan, Pederson, and Moran, unpublished paper, Society for Research in Child Development 2003; Kelly, Ueng-Hale, Grienberger, and Slade, unpublished paper, Society for Research in Child Development 2003). This view of disrupted affective communication processes between caregiver and infant early in the first year as leading to disorganized and unintegrated attachment behaviors is consonant with the need to embed attachment processes more fully in a context of intersubjective sharing in the parent–infant relationship.

Subtypes of Infant and Parent Behavior within the Disorganized Group

Within the broad array of disorganized infant behaviors, there are at least two distinct subgroups. Disorganized attachment behaviors may occur in concert with other insecure behaviors that are part of an avoidant or ambivalent attachment strategy, resulting in a primary classification of disorganized attachment and a secondary classification of avoidant or ambivalent (hereafter referred to as D-insecure). Disorganized behaviors, however, are also displayed in the context of behaviors that are usually part of a secure strategy, such as protesting separation, seeking contact with mother at reunion, and ceasing distress after being

Table 14.2 Disorganized attachment in infancy: subgroups.

INFANT BEHAVIORS

Disorganized–Secure: "Pseudo–Secure"	*Disorganized–Insecure: "Avoidant–Resistant"*
• Disorganized behaviors	• Disorganized behaviors
• Little avoidance or resistance	• Avoidance, resistance, or both
• Distress to separation	• Often appears quite conflicted
• May appear passive, depressed, aimless, hesitant, or apprehensive	• May combine marked separation distress with marked avoidance at reunion
• Some proximity-seeking	
• Calm in parent's presence	

PARENTAL BEHAVIORS

Helpless–Fearful	*Hostile–Self-Referential*
• Contradictory affective cues	• Contradictory affective cues
• Lack of parental structuring	• Hostile or threatening behaviors
• Subtle withdrawal from contact	• Seeking contact/attention from infant
• Hesitant, fearful, or deferential behaviors	• Intrusive parental control

picked up (Table 14.2). This disorganized subgroup is given a secondary classification of secure (referred to hereafter as D-secure). The D-secure group constitutes the majority (52%) of infants classified disorganized (unpublished data, NICHD Early Child Care Research Network 2001).

There are parallel differences in the maternal behaviors associated with infant disorganization, as shown in Table 14.2. Mothers of D-insecure infants display significantly higher rates of role confusion, negative-intrusive behavior, and frightening behavior than mothers of D-secure infants. In contrast, mothers of D-secure infants exhibit significantly higher rates of withdrawal than mothers of D-insecure infants (Lyons-Ruth, Bronfman, and Atwood 1999). These two profiles of maternal behavior will be referred to here as "hostile–self-referential" and "helpless–fearful." The behaviors contributing to these profiles are described in more detail in Lyons-Ruth, Bronfman, and Atwood (1999).

The subtle nature of the helpless–fearful profile of maternal behavior is important to note, as is the subtlety of many of the disorganized behaviors of D-secure infants. The more hostile–self referential maternal behaviors and the more flagrantly contradictory infant behaviors of the D-insecure group are much easier to identify as maladaptive, yet recent data indicate that these behaviors characterize slightly less than half of the mothers and infants who experience disorganized attachment relationships.

Both of these maternal profiles, however, can be viewed as stances that conserve maternal resources. In both profiles of behavior, clear attachment cues of the infant are ignored or overridden in favor of the preferred directions of the parent. In both profiles of interaction, then, the parent imposes a more unilateral agenda and fails to engage in a more mutual process of attention to and negotiation with the infant's needs and directions. In some cases, this more unilateral stance takes the form of lack of response; in others it takes the form of more intrusive insistence that the infant conform to the parent's agenda. These more intrusive behaviors are also highly correlated with self-referential behaviors on the part of the parent (e.g., "Did you miss me?" "He doesn't like me."), providing further indication that the parent is looking to the infant to conform to the needs of the parent. We would argue that maintaining a more mutually negotiated dialog with the infant requires more sustained and skilled attention and more available parental resources to allocate to the task than a focus that remains more consistently on the parent's own needs.

Socially Indiscriminate Behavior

Another form of atypical attachment behavior that is likely to be the most deviant and the most predictive of long-term impairment is the indiscriminate attachment behavior referred to earlier, in which infants seek close contact or comfort from strangers. Such behavior is seen among infants reared in institutional settings with very poor care and with no selective attachment figure available (O'Connor et al. 2000). Such indiscriminate attachment behavior is atypical not only in modern societies but in non-Western cultures as well (Ainsworth 1967; True 2001). It remains unclear how this form of deviant attachment behavior is related to the disorganized forms of attachment behavior described among home-reared infants. However, a lack of selectivity in attachment behavior is also noted clinically among high-risk, home-reared infants and can be observed in the standard Strange Situation assessment in the infant's tendency to accept comfort from the stranger even though actively distressed. Even more dramatically, the infant may display an active preference for the stranger over the mother, where close physical contact is accepted from the stranger but not the mother, or where the infant becomes distressed at the stranger's departure in the presence of the mother. These observations have not yet been documented systematically in the literature. Further work is needed to develop a reliable assessment procedure that can encompass the varieties of indiscriminate attachment behavior observed across the spectrum of institutionalized and home-reared children.

In addition, evidence now suggests that when caregivers are not hostile, but are withdrawn or emotionally unavailable, infants' approach behaviors to attachment figures are heightened and angry or avoidant behavior is inhibited (Lyons-Ruth, Bronfman, and Parsons 1999). This nonhostile but emotionally withdrawn caregiving may also characterize the behavior of childcare personnel in substandard orphanages and may be related to the increases in indiscriminate approach behavior seen among orphanage-reared children. More work is needed to assess whether care by nonhostile but withdrawing, neglecting, or emotionally unavailable caregivers could account for the heightened indiscriminate approach behaviors of infants from both home and orphanage settings.

TODDLERHOOD: SELF-AWARE INTERSUBJECTIVITY AND THE EMERGENCE OF CONTROLLING ATTACHMENT PATTERNS

Self-aware Intersubjectivity

As infants become toddlers and move into the second half of the second year, the emergence of symbolic representational capacity and the associated emergence of self-awareness, empathy, evaluative standards, and the "early moral emotions" brings a new level of intersubjective capacity (for a review, see Lyons-Ruth and Zeanah 1993). The rapid development of language after 18 months of age is one of the most striking signs of this advance. Other signs of new capacities that can be seen toward the end of the second year include the child's recognition of the self in mirrors and video images, the emergence of "no" as an indicator of a new level of self-aware autonomy, and the appearance of self-conscious emotions such as embarrassment.

By 18 months of age, normative developmental studies also indicate that the toddler has the capacity to represent, at a symbolic level, simple perceptual, intentional, and emotional states of another person. A central task of the toddler from 18 months to 3–4 years of age is to create and coordinate these symbolic representations of the perceptual, affective, and evaluative qualities assigned to objects and events by others, qualities such as "red," "bad," "pretty," and "sad." This includes assigning evaluative dimensions to the self and the self's actions and developing responsive and empathic behaviors to parents' and peers' affective states. From 4–6 years of age, preschoolers begin to develop a true "theory of mind," with the capacity to represent more complex mental processes and to mentally differentiate and coordinate the complex thought processes of others and of the self. Although these constitute striking new capacities that the child brings to interactions, relatively little research has focused directly on whether and how these new capacities develop within disorganized attachment relationships.

From 18 months to 3 years, the child is also increasingly able to hold his or her own goals in mind in opposition to the parent's wishes, represent the parent's evaluative responses to the child's behavior, and test the flexibility of the parents' limits. The child's increasingly sophisticated capacity to represent states of mind of others contributes to the development of the "goal corrected partnership" that emerges between parent and child during the preschool years (Bowlby 1969), in which parent and child express their respective intentions and negotiate for their inclusion in joint plans. The parent–toddler system must encompass a variety of new capacities and behaviors. Indeed, research suggests that the parent–child capacity to negotiate successfully a balance between the goals of the parent and the goals of the child provides the underpinnings for effective social behavior at later ages. It is within this context of sharing increasingly complex states of mind and negotiating shared intentional directions with the parent that the toddler's attachment strategies and HPA axis functioning develop further. When parent–child interactions are very unbalanced and the parent's needs continually override those of the child, disorganized behaviors may develop into controlling attachment strategies.

The Emergence of Controlling Attachment Strategies

Sometime between 18 months of age and 6 years, with the cognitive developments of the preschool period, the disorganized attachment behaviors of many infants become organized around the apparent goal of controlling the interaction with the attachment figure (Main et al. 1985; Wartner et al. 1994). The best stability and validity data in relation to the disorganized/controlling behaviors seen in the preschool period come from the NICHD Early Childcare Research Study (2001), a large-scale longitudinal investigation ($N = 1,364$) that found stability between disorganized classifications at 15 months using the Strange Situation and disorganized/controlling classifications at 36 months using the Preschool Attachment Classification System (PACS; Cassidy et al. 1992, unpublished).

Controlling strategies are likely to be discontinuous with responses seen in other primates because they may require the increasingly sophisticated subjective perspective-taking capacities that emerge in human children over the preschool years. Such parent–offspring role reversal is virtually unknown in primate groups (Hrdy, pers. comm.). Among chimps or baboons, offspring may serve as allies to the mother in alliances, groom the mother, or huddle to keep warm, but these behaviors tend to be reciprocal and mutually beneficial to both. The juveniles in these species do not take responsibility for organizing or directing the behavior of the parent and do not become involved in initiating cycles of provocative behavior to maintain the parent's attention and involvement.

As noted earlier, Hrdy (this volume) has argued that the capacity of the human infant to engage the caregiver through the exchange of emotional signals may be one evolutionary consequence of the conditional maternal commitment among human parents. The ability of the infant to engage the mother may have important survival value for the infant if the mother's commitment to the infant's care is not strongly biologically channeled. Attachment studies of infants of mothers with limited social resources further this argument. A significant subgroup of young children display role-reversed patterns of behavior in relation to the caregiver as early as two years of age. Caregivers of these infants are more likely to be depressed or have low social resources so that the child's behavior in taking over some basic relationship-maintaining functions from the parent can be viewed as adaptive. The capacity for sharing emotional states with the caregiver not only functions to engage the caregiver, but also allows the child to participate actively in the care of the caregiver as it matures. For a deprived and isolated caregiver, the empathy and comforting behaviors of a two-year-old or the organizing and entertaining behaviors of an older child may significantly influence the mother's functioning.

There is striking phenotypic discontinuity in the shift from disorganized behavior to a controlling strategy in that the surface behaviors and the apparent emotional tone of the attachment-related interactions become quite different from the hesitant, apprehensive, or conflicted behaviors observed in infancy. Extensive longitudinal data have not been available to chart this process of reorganization over time, however, so that little is understood about when these changes typically occur, what proportion of disorganized infants are able to make this developmental shift, what strengths or vulnerabilities are associated with the shift, and whether similar controlling strategies are shown in relation to peers, teachers, or other adults.

Two Forms of Controlling Attachment Behavior

The developmental shift to controlling strategies is made more complex by the bifurcation that becomes prominent in the controlling group by 5–6 years of age. Controlling attachment behaviors have been found to take two very different forms: Controlling-punitive behavior involves the child's attempts to take control of the relationship with the parent through hostile, coercive, or more subtly humiliating behaviors when attachment concerns are aroused. Controlling-caregiving behavior involves the child's attempts to control by entertaining, organizing, directing, or giving approval to the parent.

This bifurcation is foreshadowed by the large differences noted earlier in the organization of mother–infant interaction within the disorganized group in infancy. We speculate that the two disorganized infant subgroups mentioned earlier, D-secure and D-insecure, are early anlagen of the caregiving and punitive stances observed among controlling children at age 6. However, longitudinal data are not yet available to evaluate these postulated links between the two D subgroups in infancy and the two controlling subgroups during the preschool period. Given the sharp behavioral differences between the two forms of controlling attachment behavior and the likelihood that these two forms continue on separate developmental pathways, we briefly discuss each in turn.

Controlling-Caregiving Strategies

Zahn-Waxler and Kochanska (1990) describe both the depressed parent's tendency to resort to role-reversing and guilt-inducing disciplinary tactics and the tendency of some young preschoolers to become quite anxious in response to these parental techniques of discipline and to develop inhibition of aggression and more elaborate expressions of concern and empathy for the parent. The exaggerated anxiety and sense of responsibility or guilt described by Zahn-Waxler and Kochanska among two- to three-year-olds may constitute early signs of an emerging controlling/caregiving stance.

Caregiving behaviors, in particular, seem to depend on the capacity to think about the states of mind of others and we would speculate that more elaborate, sophisticated, and integrated forms of caregiving behavior would emerge with each succeeding developmental elaboration of the child's intersubjective capacities. Teti (1999) observed mothers with their controlling preschoolers during play interactions and found no reliable differences between the secure and caregiving groups, while punitive children were significantly more negative than both secure and caregiving children in emotional tone.

Although it would be tempting to conclude from the above findings that D-secure infants or controlling-caregiving children may be less at risk for negative outcomes, this conclusion is at odds with a large body of data. Compared to D-insecure infants, D-secure infants are at equal risk for a variety of negative outcomes, including elevated cortisol secretion to mild stressors in infancy, elevated distress during interactions with mother at home, elevated hostile-aggressive behaviors towards peers in kindergarten and second grade, and elevated rates of controlling attachment patterns towards parents by age 6 (see Lyons-Ruth and Jacobvitz 1999). Controlling-caregiving children assessed at age 6 are also at elevated risk for behavior problems reported by both mothers and teachers (Solomon et al. 1995). The behaviors of controlling-caregiving children may look better than average when interacting with their parents, but worse than average in other assessment settings, including interactions with peers and teachers at school (see Lyons-Ruth and Jacobvitz 1999).

Controlling-Punitive Strategies

In addition to an increased capacity for empathy and guilt, the emergence of self-aware intersubjectivity may also allow the toddler to represent mentally the parent's hostile affect, as related to the self, and to respond with more directed anger and avoidance toward the parent. This may contribute to the emergence of punitive strategies during preschool (Lyons-Ruth and Jacobvitz 1999).

It is also likely that among parents with histories of emotional or physical abuse, the toddler's increased willfulness and resistant behavior activates the parent's representations of prior unbalanced and abusive relational patterns and increases parental tendencies toward hostile attributions and coercive cycles of interaction. By 4 to 6 years of age, the association between infant disorganized behaviors or preschool controlling behaviors and teacher-reported aggressive behaviors toward peers is well replicated. In addition, controlling behaviors toward the parent are associated with clinically diagnosed oppositional defiant disorder. The developmental pathways associated with coercive cycles and early oppositional defiant disorder have been well characterized in the literature and will not be described further here (see Lyons-Ruth and Jacobvitz 1999).

Given the large gender differences found in internalizing and externalizing symptomatology, it is plausible to speculate that female gender may be differentially related to internalization of dysphoric affect and caregiving forms of control, whereas male gender may predispose to externalization of anger and punitive forms of control. However, the small cell sizes that occur when controlling or disorganized groups are subdivided by gender have precluded any definitive test of this hypothesis.

The capacity for intersubjective sharing among controlling children also needs more investigation. Given the disruptions in maternal affective communication with the infant documented over the first 18 months, as well as the dysfluency in parent–child discourse reported at age 6 (Main et al. 1985), one would expect that disturbances in intersubjective sharing would be transmitted from parent to child. However, as noted, some disorganized children attempt to organize, entertain, and care for the parent, which entails heightened attention to the parent's states of mind. In addition, the parent's frightening and unpredictable behavior could lead the child to be hypervigilant of the parent's states of mind. Whether such demands on the child contribute, in some cases, to the precocious ability to represent the viewpoint of others remains relatively unstudied. Given the dysfluencies in both affective and verbal forms of parent–child dialog, however, it is more likely that disorganized children will show hyper-alertness to subtle affective cues from the parent but will lack the background of rich exchanges with others that would allow them to place those cues into a more complex theory of mind.

CONTROLLING STRATEGIES AND FUNCTIONING BEYOND EARLY CHILDHOOD

Additional work is needed to track the developmental pathways associated with controlling forms of attachment behavior beyond early school entry. Almost nothing is currently known about the forms these behaviors will take across the transitions from middle childhood to adolescence and from adolescence to adulthood. It is also of particular interest to explore whether controlling strategies may allow more advantageous behavioral and HPA axis functioning than occurs among children who are not able to organize a controlling strategy.

In middle childhood, caregiving children may adopt an increasingly role-reversed relationship with caregivers as they become more adept at regulating both their own behavior and their parent's negative affective states. Parents who have difficulty regulating their own emotional experiences due to trauma or psychopathology may derive greater comfort within role-reversed than veridical parent–child relationships. Moss (unpublished paper, Society for

Research in Child Development 2001) found that decreases in maternal self-reports of depression were associated with increases in teacher reports of child depression between ages 4 to 8 years among controlling children; this was not the case in noncontrolling children. Furthermore, within the controlling group, higher levels of role reversal were related to decreases in maternal depression. Moss concluded that controlling children were effective in their efforts "to orient, contain, or cheer up" their mothers, but they could not use the caregiver to regulate their own emotions and therefore needed to manage this burden themselves. Consistent with the evolutionary perspective advanced earlier, these behaviors may be quite adaptive in stabilizing parental mental health and parental investment in the parent–child relationship. Moss speculates further that controlling children may develop split, segregated, or confused models of the self because of the conflicting demands of appearing competent with the caregiver while feeling worried or fearful.

Dissociative symptomatology has been one of the most striking longitudinal outcomes of early disorganization beyond middle childhood. Carlson (1998) found that disorganization in infancy was related to teacher reports of dissociation, internalizing behavior, and poorer overall emotional health in Grades 1, 2, 3, and 6, as well as elevated levels of dissociative symptoms and overall psychopathology in late adolescence (age 19). Working with the same sample, Ogawa et al. (1997) found that an emotionally unavailable caregiver in early childhood and a disorganized classification during infancy were independent predictors of dissociative symptoms in adolescence, whereas a wide array of other variables, including trauma and abuse, were less predictive. These data support the hypothesis that dissociative processes emerge from disorganized forms of relational dialog rather than from abusive experiences alone.

DISORGANIZED ATTACHMENT IN ADOLESCENCE AND ADULTHOOD

Whereas attachment assessments in infancy and childhood have primarily focused on direct observation of parent–child interaction, attachment assessments in adolescence and adulthood have relied on the AAI. Through this semi-structured interview format, participants are asked about various aspects of their childhood attachment relationships. Disorganization in adolescence and adulthood is based on the presence of particular kinds of incoherence in discourse while discussing experiences of loss or abuse, which leads to a classification of "Unresolved" in relation to loss or trauma. Although some studies are beginning to explore attachment-related interaction patterns among romantic partners, few have included enough couples in the disorganized-unresolved spectrum to draw any conclusions from this work. Thus, we will discuss work using the AAI and indicate gaps or controversies in the model of intergenerational transmission of attachment disorganization that has emerged.

The model presented earlier in Figure 14.1 represents how disorganization is thought to be transmitted from parent to infant. However, a different and in some ways incompatible model has emerged of how disorganization develops from infancy to adulthood. In Figure 14.1, caregivers are viewed as developing unresolved states of mind in relation to specific experiences of loss or trauma that usually occur later than the first few years of life. In contrast, infants are viewed as developing disorganized attachment strategies in interaction with the caregiver, through exposure to the caregiver's unintegrated fear (Main and Hesse 1990). Thus, different etiological mechanisms are proposed for the parent and for the infant. This leads to the conundrum that if a disorganized infant grows up without specific experiences of additional loss or trauma, then methodologically he or she cannot be judged as "Disorganized/Unresolved" on the AAI. However, as already reviewed, infant disorganization has predicted controlling attachment strategies at least through age 6 in low-risk samples in which neither parental death nor abuse were observed to be associated with the infant's continued deviance. Lyons-Ruth et al. (2005) have termed this a "transmission block" in the conceptual model for how disorganized attachment is transmitted to the third generation (see Figure 14.2).

One critical theoretical issue that emerges, then, is how we should conceptualize the etiological mechanisms that contribute to the maintenance of disorganized attachment strategies into adolescence and adulthood in the absence of specific incidents of loss or trauma. The corresponding methodological issue that emerges is how we should assess disorganized sequelae in adolescence or adulthood when there has been no serious loss or abuse. In one approach to this dilemma, Hesse (1999) has developed criteria for designating an AAI as "Cannot Classify" if it contains contradictory or incompatible content over the entire interview. Due to the rarity of these protocols, however, reliability and validity

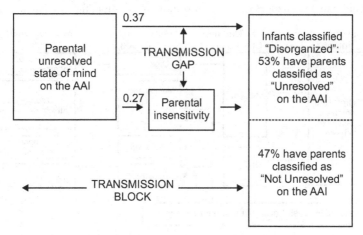

Figure 14.2   The transmission block in theory and research on disorganized attachments (AAI = Adult Assessment Interview).

data are not yet available to tie these adult characteristics to the developmental pathways involving disorganized attachments. A second approach to coding interview-wide indices of disorganization assesses what is termed a hostile-helpless state of mind. Hostile-helpless states of mind have recently been validated in relation to infant disorganization by Lyons-Ruth et al. (2005). More work is needed to identify indices of atypical states of mind on the AAI that can predict infant disorganization independent of indices of loss or trauma.

For some individuals, it is possible for the unintegrated fearful affect to be rooted solely in the relationship with the caregiver, generated, for example, by implacably hostile parental affect or parental childlike behavior. For others, fearful affect may be rooted in an experience of loss or trauma that is difficult to integrate due to its unusual and fear-inducing characteristics. Data, however, remain unclear whether the severity of loss or trauma in itself can be etiological or whether additional deviations in early caregiving and/or other individual temperamental vulnerabilities will be needed to predict unresolved lapses of reasoning or discourse when discussing emotion-laden topics on the AAI. Perhaps the most pressing need in the assessment of disorganized attachment is an observationally based measure of how disorganized parent–child interactions present in adolescence and early adulthood. Observations during these age periods might provide a more direct assessment of how disorganized/controlling behaviors continue over time.

An expanded model of the potential influences of a relational diathesis on the intergenerational transmission of disorganized attachment patterns is presented in Figure 14.3. In this model, unintegrated states of mind are proposed to result either from fear-inducing experiences or from deviant caregiving over time or from their joint effect.

Future work is needed to expand this model to include possible individual and contextual influences on disorganization. In addition, factors that attenuate

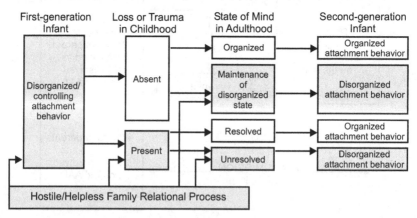

Figure 14.3   Relational diathesis model of the development of disorganized attachment from infancy to adulthood.

developmental or intergenerational continuity over time in disorganization need particular attention (Sagi-Schwartz et al. 2003). Individual factors, such as genetics, temperament or gender, have generally not been related to *organized* attachment classifications, but less is known about how these individual factors relate to disorganized classifications (Lyons-Ruth and Jacobvitz 1999; van IJzendoorn et al. 1999). Spangler and Grossmann (1999) found that newborn behavioral organization predicted later disorganized classifications, but this has not been a consistent finding (e.g., Carlson 1998). Within the family, maternal psychopathology, marital conflict, and child maltreatment have all been linked with infant disorganization, but the potential influence of paternal psychopathology on infant disorganization remains to be explored (Lyons-Ruth and Jacobvitz 1999). Outside the family, relationships with friends, teachers, and other significant figures develop throughout childhood and adolescence, and these relationships may play a role in perpetuating or ameliorating disorganized attachment patterns. Poverty is a broader contextual factor that increases the incidence of infant disorganization from 15–25%, but those increases are likely to be mediated by the rise in incidence of parental depression, trauma, withdrawal from interaction, and punitive discipline associated with poverty (Lyons-Ruth et al. 2002).

GENETIC CONTRIBUTIONS TO DISORGANIZED ATTACHMENT

Recent evidence suggests that genetic factors may also contribute to an individual's vulnerability to attachment disorganization. Investigators from the Budapest Infant–Parent Study found that 71% of the infants classified as disorganized had at least one 7-repeat allele of the DRD4 gene, in contrast to 29% of the nondisorganized group (Lakatos et al. 2000). Infants carrying the 7-repeat allele were four times more likely to be classified disorganized ($OR = 4.15$). However, only 36% of infants carrying this allele were classified disorganized, compared to 9% without the allele. Further analyses revealed that the association between disorganized attachment and the 7-repeat allele was observed only in the presence of the –521 T allele. In the presence of both risk alleles, incidence of disorganized attachment was 40% compared to 11% for the rest of the sample (Lakatos et al. 2002). A review by Swanson and colleagues (2000) confirmed the likely role of the 7-repeat allele of this gene in making the postsynaptic dopamine receptor subsensitive and suggests that dopamine underactivity compromises attentional systems.

Congruent with this data, a recent behavioral genetic comparison of the preschool attachment classifications of 110 same-sex monozygotic or dizygotic twin pairs (age 3 ½) found no genetic contribution to organized attachment patterns (O'Connor and Croft 2001). The degree of concordance at the level of secure/insecure attachment was equally high among monozygotic and dizygotic pairs (70% and 64%, respectively), suggesting little genetic influence on organized forms of attachment and substantial shared and nonshared environmental influence. However, the data were not analyzed for the organized/disorganized contrast, and the genetic effect was much stronger for the disorganized group. The odds ratio was 15.33 that if one monozygotic twin ($n = 11$) displayed disorganized attachment, the other would as well. Among dizygotic twins ($n = 6$), the OR was 0 (no concordance). Although provocative, the findings give no support for a specifically genetic interpretation because of the small n's in these cells. Disorganization was also twice as frequent among monozygotic twins, and environmental influences specific to monozygotic twins may account for their concordance. However, the high concordance in the disorganized group diverges from the findings of the study as a whole and makes these data potentially congruent with the molecular genetic findings cited above. We note that this study involved the preschool rather than infant attachment assessment, for which there is less extensive validity data.

A second behavioral genetic study by van IJzendoorn and Fonagy (unpublished paper, Society for Research in Child Development 2003) found that, over the entire spectrum of attachment classifications, nonshared environments accounted for more variance than genetics or shared environments. This led the authors to surmise that nonshared factors such as trauma, differential parental treatment, and/or measurement error due to the difficulty of coding disorganization may influence behavioral genetic models.

To date, no behavioral or molecular genetic study has included quality of caregiving in the model. Because gene–environment interactions have been the rule rather than the exception in studies that have examined such interaction effects, more complex designs are now needed for evaluating the interactions that are likely to occur between family interactive process and genetic endowment (e.g., Caspi et al. 2002). If caregiver behavior constitutes a strong influence on gene expression related to fearful arousal, as has been demonstrated in other species, the degree of overlap that occurs randomly between infant genotype and atypical caregiver behavior in a small cohort of disorganized infants will greatly influence the association obtained between genotype and the disorganized phenotype. Therefore, it will be critical to include the quality of caregiving in the model.

CONCLUSIONS

Disorganized attachment behaviors are one of the only behavioral predictors of later psychopathology that have been identified as early as infancy among biologically normal individuals. Although parental psychopathology, low socioeconomic status, and other indices of low resource family environments also predict elevated rates of psychopathology, those are distal processes that need more proximal mediating mechanisms to explain psychopathology in the child.

As we have discussed, the relation between attachment disorganization and psychopathology is complex. Summarizing across studies, disorganized attachment processes are early predictors of both internalizing and externalizing forms of psychopathology from the preschool period onward. Disorganized attachment processes are distinct from child temperament and appear to reside in child–caregiver relational processes rather than in one partner alone. As such, attachment disorganization is likely to index a broad relational contribution to psychopathology that cuts across conventional diagnostic categories and interacts with individual biological vulnerability to produce a range of psychiatric symptoms.

However, it is also likely that disorganized and controlling attachment behaviors, as well as many behaviors considered to represent psychiatric disorders, constitute adaptations to particular family and social circumstances. These adaptations may carry considerable biological and social costs to the individual while contributing to the survival of the kinship group as a whole. Consistent with the argument advanced by Hrdy (this volume), less commitment to a given child may be adaptive for a single mother with few social and emotional resources to invest. In turn, the child's taking over direction of the parent–child relationship through controlling attachment strategies may contribute to the care of the parent. In addition, the human child needs not only protection from predators and physical comfort, but also communicative interaction to survive and develop flexible and secure strategies for regulatory fearful arousal. Controlling attachment strategies insure that parental attention and interaction will occur, even if fear modulation or actual protection is seriously compromised. Thus, in very low resource environments, child-controlling strategies may be adaptive both for the individual and the family unit as a whole, from an evolutionary perspective, even though costly to the child in terms of physiological regulation of stressful arousal.

In this chapter, we have highlighted the most important gaps and controversies in theory and research regarding disorganized attachment. First, the need to reconceptualize the evolutionary basis of human attachment to include the specifically human capacities for shared intersubjective states was noted. There is now a convergence of developmental, behavioral, biological, and evolutionary arguments for enlarging the theoretical model of the components of the infant–caregiver relationship that serve the attachment (i.e., fear-regulating) behavioral system. Modulation of fearful arousal during the first year is dependent on the exchange of shared affect signals, and the maintenance of positive states is critically dependent on such fine-grained interactive processes. Consistent with this emphasis, an expanded model is needed of how the attachment relationship maintains positive infant states and regulates fearful arousal during the first year of life through intersubjective processes. In addition, a more integrated developmental account should be attempted of how attachment strategies evolve in relation to advances in the child's capacities for engaging with and representing other minds over subsequent periods of development.

Spanning all developmental periods, we need to understand the dynamic interplay between neurobiological and behavioral attachment processes. With the advent of neurobiological measurement, adequate assessments of attachment outcomes may need to include physiological measures as well as behavioral and representational assessments. In particular, etiological models of disorganized attachment may need to be expanded further to include the role of genetic vulnerability to disorganization. The role of genetic mechanisms is only beginning to be studied, and emerging evidence suggests that there may be genetic contributions to disorganized attachment processes. However, no studies to date have explored gene–environment interactions among disorganized children. Furthermore, variability in behavioral profiles within the disorganized group suggests that multiple etiological models may be needed. Differing biological vulnerabilities interacting with varying experiences of loss, abuse, and/or chronically hostile or neglecting relationships may lead to quite different biobehavioral developmental trajectories and adult outcomes.

Finally, a "transmission block" was described in the current model of what happens to disorganized/controlling attachment strategies as the child moves into adolescence and adulthood in the absence of particular experiences of loss or abuse. To address this block, an expanded model was proposed that allows unintegrated states of mind in adulthood to result either from fear-inducing experiences, from deviant caregiving over time, or from their joint effect.

In summary, with the current confluence of neurobiological, genetic, and relational assessments, there is now the potential to delineate many of the interactions between biological and relational processes that contribute to the emergence of child and adult psychopathology. Given current data, disorganized attachment processes are likely to play a prominent role in those developmental trajectories.

REFERENCES

Ainsworth, M.D.S. 1967. Infancy in Uganda: Infant Care and the Growth of Love. Baltimore: Johns Hopkins Univ. Press.
Ainsworth, M.D.S., M. Blehar, E. Waters, and S. Wall. 1978. Patterns of Attachment. Hillsdale, NJ: Erlbaum.
Ainsworth, M.D.S., and C.G. Eichberg. 1991. Effects on infant–mother attachment of mother's unresolved loss of an attachment figure or other traumatic experience. In: Attachment across the Life Cycle, ed. C. Parkes, J. Stevenson-Hinde, and P. Marris, pp. 160–186. New York: Routledge.
Ashman, S.B., G. Dawson, H. Panagiotides, E. Yamada, and C.W. Wilkinson. 2002. Stress hormone levels of children of depressed mothers. Dev. Psychopathol. 14: 333–349.
Bowlby, J. 1969. Attachment. Attachment and Loss, vol. 1. New York: Basic.
Carlson, E.A. 1998. A prospective longitudinal study of disorganized attachment. Child Dev. 69:1107–1128.
Caspi, A., J. McClay, T.E. Moffitt et al. 2002. Role of genotype in the cycle of violence in maltreated children. Science 297:851–854.

Cassidy, J., and P.R. Shaver, eds. 1999. Handbook of Attachment: Theory, Research, and Clinical Applications. New York: Guilford.

Coplan, J.D., M.W. Andrews, L.A. Rosenblum, et al. 1996. Persistent elevations of cerebrospinal fluid concentrations of corticotropin-releasing factor in adult nonhuman primates exposed to early-life stressors: Implications for the pathophysiology of mood and anxiety disorders. *Neuorobiology* **93**:1619–1623.

Francis, D., J. Diorio, D. Liu, and M. Meaney. 1999. Nongenomic transmission across generations of maternal behavior and stress responses in the rat. *Science* **286**: 1155–1158.

Goldberg, S., D. Benoit, K. Blokland, and S. Madigan. 2003. Atypical maternal behavior, maternal representations and infant disorganized attachment. *Dev. Psychopathol.* **15**:239–257.

Hesse, E. 1999. The Adult Attachment Interview: Historical and current perspectives. In: Handbook of Attachment: Theory, Research, and Clinical Applications, ed. J. Cassidy and P.R. Shaver, pp. 395–433. New York: Guilford.

Hofer, M.A. 1996. On the nature and consequences of early loss. *Psychosom. Med.* **58**: 570–581.

Jaffe, J., B. Beebe, S. Feldstein, C. Crown, and M. Jasnow. 2001. Rhythms of dialog in infancy. *Mono. Soc. Res. Child Dev.* **66**:1–132.

Lakatos, K., Z. Nemoda, I. Toth et al. 2002. Further evidence for the role of the dopamine D4 receptor (DRD4) gene in attachment disorganization: Interaction of the exon III 48 bp repeat and the –521 C/T promotor polymorphisms. *Molec. Psychiatry* **7**:27–31.

Lakatos, K., I. Toth, Z. Nemoda et al. 2000. Dopamine D4 receptor (DRD4) gene polymorphism as associated with attachment disorganization in infants. *Molec. Psychiatry* **5**:633–637.

Lyons-Ruth, K., E. Bronfman, and G. Atwood. 1999. A relational diathesis model of hostile-helpless states of mind: Expressions in mother–infant interaction. In: Attachment Disorganization, ed. J. Solomon and C. George, pp. 33–70. New York: Guilford.

Lyons-Ruth, K., E. Bronfman, and E. Parsons. 1999. Frightened, frightening, and atypical maternal behavior and disorganized infant attachment strategies. *Mono. Soc. Res. Child Dev.* **64**:67–96.

Lyons-Ruth, K., and D. Jacobvitz. 1999. Attachment disorganization: Unresolved loss, relational violence, and lapses in behavioral and attentional strategies. In: Handbook of Attachment: Theory, Research, and Clinical Applications, ed. J. Cassidy and P.R. Shaver, pp. 520–554. New York: Guilford.

Lyons-Ruth, K., R. Wolfe, A. Lyubchik, T. Grogan, and R. Steingard. 2002. Prevalence and correlates of depressive symptoms in parents of children under three: Results of the Commonwealth Survey. In: Child Rearing in America: Challenges Facing Parents with Young Children, ed. N. Halfon, K. McLearn, and M. Schuster, pp. 217–259. Cambridge: Cambridge Univ. Press.

Lyons-Ruth, K., C. Yellin, S.M. Melnick, and G. Atwood. 2005. Expanding the concept of unresolved mental states: Hostile/helpless states of mind on the Adult Attachment Interview are associated with disrupted mother–infant communication and infant disorganization. *Dev. Psychopathol.*, in press.

Lyons-Ruth, K., and C. Zeanah. 1993. The family context of infant mental health. I. Affective development in the primary caregiving relationship. In: Handbook of Infant Mental Health, ed. C. Zeanah, pp. 14–37. New York: Guilford.

Main, M., and E. Hesse. 1990. Parents' unresolved traumatic experiences are related to infant disorganized attachment status: Is frightened and/or frightening parental behavior the linking mechanism? In: Attachment in the Preschool Years: Theory,

Research and Intervention, ed. M. Greenberg, D. Cicchetti, and E.M. Cummings, pp. 161–184. Chicago: Univ. of Chicago Press.

Main, M., N. Kaplan, and J. Cassidy. 1985. Security in infancy, childhood and adulthood: A move to the level of representation. *Mono. Soc. Res. Child Dev.* **50**:66–104.

Main, M., and J. Solomon. 1990. Procedures for identifying infants as disorganized/disoriented during the Ainsworth Strange Situation. In: Attachment in the Preschool Years: Theory, Research and Intervention, ed. M. Greenberg, D. Cicchetti, and E.M. Cummings, pp. 121–160. Chicago: Univ. of Chicago Press.

Murray, L., and C. Trevarthen. 1985. Emotional regulation of interactions between two-month olds and their mothers. In: Social Perception in Infants, ed. T.M. Field and N.A. Fox, pp. 177–197. Norwood, NJ: Ablex.

NICHD Early Child Care Research Network. 2001. Child-care and family predictors of preschool attachment and stability from infancy. *Dev. Psychol.* **37**:847–862.

O'Connor, T.G., and C.M. Croft. 2001. A twin study in attachment in preschool children. *Child Dev.* **72**:1501–1511.

O'Connor, T.G., M. Rutter, and the English and Romanian Adoptees Study Team. 2000. Attachment disorder behavior following early severe deprivation: Extension and longitudinal follow-up. *J. Am. Acad. Child Adoles. Psych.* **39**:703–712.

Ogawa, J.R., L.A. Sroufe, N.S. Weinfield, E.A. Carlson, and B. Egeland. 1997. Development and the fragmented self: Longitudinal study of dissociative symptomatology in a nonclinical sample. *Dev. Psychopathol.* **9**:855–879.

Sagi-Schwartz, A. M.H. van IJzendoorn, K.E. Grossmann, et al. 2003. Attachment and traumatic stress in female Holocaust child survivors and their daughters. *Am. J. Psych.* **160**:1086–1092.

Schuder, M., and K. Lyons-Ruth. 2004. "Hidden trauma" in infancy: Attachment, fearful arousal, and early dysfunction of the stress response system. In: Trauma in Infancy and Toddlerhood, ed. J. Osofsky, pp. 69–104. New York: Guilford.

Schuengel, C., M. Bakermans-Kranenburg, and M. van IJzendoorn. 1999. Frightening maternal behavior linking unresolved loss and disorganized infant attachment. *J. Cons. Clin. Psychol.* **67**:54–63.

Seligman, M.E.D. 1975. Helplessness: On Depression, Development and Death. San Francisco: Freeman.

Solomon, J., C. George, and A. DeJong. 1995. Children classified as controlling at age six: Evidence of disorganized representational strategies and aggression at home and at school. *Dev. Psychopathol.* **7**:447–463.

Spangler, G., and K. Grossmann. 1999. Individual and physiological correlates of attachment disorganization in infancy. In: Attachment Disorganization, ed. J. Solomon and C. George, pp. 95–124. New York: Guilford.

Swanson, J.M., P. Flodman, J. Kennedy et al. 2000. Dopamine genes and ADHD. *Neurosci. Biobehav. Rev.* **24**:21–25.

Taylor, S.E., L.C. Klein, B.P. Lewis et al. 2000. Biobehavioral responses to stress in females: Tend-and-befriend, not fight-or-flight. *Psychol. Rev.* **107**:411–429.

Teti, D.M. 1999. Conceptualizations of disorganization in the preschool years: An integration. In: Attachment Disorganization, ed. J. Solomon and C. George, pp. 213–242. New York: Guilford.

Tomasello, M. 1999. The Cultural Origins of Human Cognition. Cambridge, MA: Harvard Univ. Press.

True, M.M. 2001. Relationships and interactions: Infant–mother attachment among the Dogon of Mali. *Child Dev.* **72**:1451–1466.

van IJzendoorn, M.H., C. Schuengel, and M.J. Bakermans-Kranenburg 1999. Disorganized attachment in early childhood: Meta-analysis of precursors, concomitants, and sequelae. *Dev. Psychopathol.* **11**:225–249.

Wartner, U.G., K. Grossmann, E. Fremmer-Bombik, and G. Suess. 1994. Attachment patterns at age six in south Germany: Predictability from infancy and implications for preschool behavior. *Child Dev.* **65**:1014–1027.

Zahn-Waxler, C., and G. Kochanska. 1990. The origins of guilt. In: Socio-emotional Development, ed. R. Thompson, pp. 183–258. Nebraska Symposium on Motivation 26. Lincoln: Univ. of Nebraska Press.

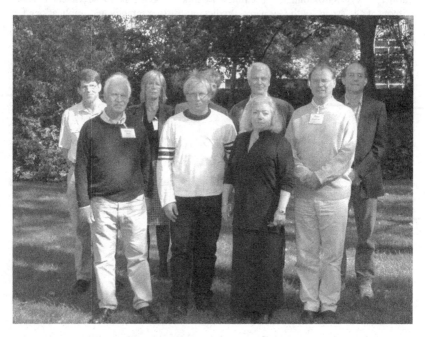

Back, left to right: Mike Hennessy, Gisela Klann-Delius, Sarah Hrdy,
    Dietrich von Holst, Jim Leckman
Front, left to right: Dietmar Todt, Carsten Schradin, Sue Carter, Barry Keverne

15

Group Report: Biobehavioral Processes in Attachment and Bonding

J. F. LECKMAN, Rapporteur

C. S. CARTER, M. B. HENNESSY, S. B. HRDY, E. B. KEVERNE,
G. KLANN-DELIUS, C. SCHRADIN, D. TODT, and D. VON HOLST

> Every variety of love...is born, lives, dies, or attains immortality in accordance with the same laws.
> — Henri Marie Beyle (Stendhal), 1822

> It may in fact be that not only do attachment and sexual behavior share certain components and causal mechanisms but that parental behavior shares some of them as well.
> — John Bowlby, 1969

INTRODUCTION

The goal of our group was to identify common biobehavioral processes in attachment and bonding in an effort to advance our understanding of our place in the world, the nature of human relationships, the origins of some forms of psychopathology and, where possible, to inform social policy. Before reviewing specific findings, we articulate our evolutionary point-of-view concerning the likely existence of common biobehavioral processes in attachment and bonding among mammals.

Point-of-view and Initial Caveats

The human brain is a remarkable product of evolution. While the basic machinery of the vertebrate brain has been in place for more than 450 million years, the appearance of our subspecies (*Homo sapiens sapiens*) emerged between 100,000 and 200,000 years ago. In the struggle for life, certain traits have come to predominate. We might surmise that elements in our mental and behavioral repertoire related to successful mammalian reproduction have been the focus of intense selective pressures ever since the first lactating proto-mammals emerged some 300 million years ago. The selection of a mate, bearing of viable offspring, and the formation of parental commitments that will sustain an infant through varying periods of dependency (especially lengthy for humans) are just a few of the crucial complex, interdependent processes needed for individual survival and, hence, species viability. Although most of our biological and behavioral potentialities are likely called upon at one point or another in the service of these goals, there must be highly conserved brain-based systems that are specifically activated at developmentally appropriate moments to achieve and sustain these processes. We hypothesize that a thorough understanding of these "normal" processes will also lead to deeper insights into our vulnerability to develop a range of psychopathological outcomes.

Definitions

In this chapter, we use the term *bond* to refer to the study of biological processes that mediate parental behaviors and infant responsiveness, whereas the term *attachment* has a stronger psychological and consequently human connotation; some overlap in the use of these terms is inevitable. Initial bond formation in mammals is marked by the selective recognition of an individual or individuals associated with proximity seeking, separation distress, and altered autonomic and behavioral responsivity conditioned by the absence, presence, or merely cues of the other(s). Affiliative bond formation alters in a fundamental and profound fashion what is important in the world. Attachments embellish bonds and refer to a complex developmental process between human beings that is dependent on learning and memory and based on specific histories of emotionally charged interactions, including caretaking, care receiving, communication, negotiation of affection, protection, and commitment, and the creation of metacognitive domains. These attachments and bonds often serve to enhance security and a sense of well-being as well as to reduce the impact of potentially stressful future events. Indeed, bonds may be seen as a means by which the individual is prepared for an uncertain future. However, the loss or threatened loss of such bonds and attachments can have catastrophic consequences.

An Emerging Model

We offer a tentative biobehavioral model of bonding and attachment that focuses on the interface of several highly conserved neural systems involved in perception, arousal, maintenance of physiological homeostasis, as well as reward and threat detection and response pathways. We propose that in the course of evolution, natural selection led to a species-specific integration of these systems producing the diversity of affiliative behaviors observable today. In our estimation, the utility of this integrative model comes in the identification of which of these biobehavioral components are active in any one of a range of adaptive and maladaptive outcomes. We encourage investigators to explore how these systems interact with each other at each level of analysis, from the genome to metacognitive representations (Figure 15.1). We believe this emerging model will provide a fruitful point of orientation for scientists from a range of disciplines to integrate their work and evaluate new experimental and therapeutic interventions as they develop this model and seek to inform social policy.

In the sections that follow, we consider the behavioral and cognitive dimensions by examining the formation and maintenance of social bonds. Then we briefly consider how bonds develop over time, how they are altered by either the loss of attachment figures or the addition of new and potentially competing attachments (intra- and inter-bond dynamics). We provide a brief review of the neural pathways involved and examine the very limited information available on the role of genetic and epigenetic mechanisms in sculpting aspects of affiliative behavior. We close with a reevaluation of our model as well as a series of conclusions and as yet unanswered questions.

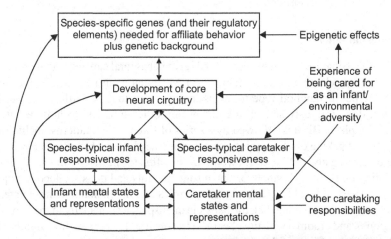

Figure 15.1 An integrative model of biobehavioral processes involved in the formation and maintenance of caretaker–child bonds and related attachment phenomena. In this framework, "bonds" are seen as tending more to the biological domains while "attachment" has a stronger psychological connotation, although some overlap was present in the formulation of most group members. "Responsiveness" includes (a) a range of perceptual, autonomic, behavioral, emotional, and cognitive responses conditioned by the absence, presence, or merely cues of the other; (b) responses conditioned by the caretaker's experience of being cared for as an infant; and (c) responses conditioned by perceived threats and adversity. Metacognitive representations and mental states correspond to internal working models and are continually updated and revised. Early experiences with caregivers can, however, powerfully shape the landscape of possible and expected interactions with others. Stranger anxiety appears when infants experience a mismatch as they compare expected caregiver stimuli and interactions with actual caregiver stimuli and interactions. These metacognitive representations and mental states can be both conscious and unconscious and can directly influence both patterns of responsiveness in the self and others as well as the core neural circuitry.

MAMMALIAN BEHAVIOR IN THE FORMATION
AND MAINTENANCE OF BONDS
(see Hrdy, Sachser, this volume)

We begin with a review of parental care and infant responsivity before turning our attention to pair bond formation and romantic love. We conclude with a discussion of the similarities and differences between parental and romantic love.

Adaptive parental behavior can be defined as any response toward a reproductively immature, genetically related, conspecific that increases the probability of the survival and eventual reproductive success of one or more of the recipients. Parental care can either be uniparental or biparental. Among mammals, uniparental care systems are the norm, with the mother being the sole provider in about 90% of the species (Eisenberg and Kleiman 1983). In some species, however, individuals who are not the biological parents provide care (Hrdy, this volume). In such species, alloparental care may be critical for the survival of the offspring.

Maternal Behavior

Maternal behavior is a highly conserved set of behavioral capacities that are crucial for reproductive success (Table 15.1). Most mammals have distinctive and stereotyped behavioral repertoires as they prepare to give birth. Mice build nests; dogs furiously scratch the dirt or any other substrate to hollow out a birthing place. Birth is followed by a series of fixed action patterns, including biting and licking off the amniotic sack, eating the placenta, biting the umbilical cord, sniffing and licking the newborn clean, often (as in sheep) olfactorily imprinting on the baby's smell, or (as in some rodents and dogs) collecting pups into the nest and huddling over them to permit suckling. In nonhuman primates, mothers eat the placenta, lick the baby clean, inspect it (especially in the genital regions), and groom it with their hands. After birth and during the first months of life, patterns of care of the newborn vary across species.

Table 15.1   Common behavioral elements of maternal care across mammalian species.

Feature
Nest-building and maintenance (place preference)
Perceptual exploration (identification of nest and/or offspring)
Retrieval (reciprocal calls)
Grooming and kissing or licking
Crouching or preferred nursing positions
Nursing and lactation and/or feeding
Prolonged physical contact/sleeping
Aggressive behavior in response to perceived threats to their offspring

Newborn altricial rodents, such as rats and mice, which are virtually immobile and incapable of body temperature maintenance, are dependent for their survival on the initiation of a specific set of maternal behaviors (Rosenblatt and Lehrman 1963). Maternal behavior in these rodents involves a complex set of activities, including nest repair, sniffing and exploration of pups, mouthing, pup retrieval, licking, grooming, and various forms of nursing (arched-back, prone, blanket; Pryce et al. 2001). In addition to caring for their own pups, recently parturient females avidly display retrieving, licking, and nursing behavior toward foster pups introduced into the cage. In contrast, adult virgin female rats do not show maternal behavior when first presented with foster pups; however, if virgin female rats cohabit with young pups, eventually they display maternal behavior after a period of 4–7 days (Rosenblatt 1967). This experimental paradigm is referred to as *sensitization* and has served as a useful tool in the assessment of maternal behavior.

Sheep, goats, and other ungulates provide other well characterized examples of maternal behavior in mammalian species that give birth to precocial young. In these species, the mother sniffs, licks, and grooms her offspring shortly after birth. The newborn is able to follow his/her mother, and the mother, in turn, selectively allows her offspring to suckle.

Among New World common marmosets, mothers may seek a tree cavity or other safe place to give birth. Once born, the baby (or babies, since twins are the common rule in marmosets) crawl up the mother, under her arm, and onto her back. Marmosets are a species with a great deal of allomaternal care (from adult males and pre-reproductives), and both sexes may compete vigorously to eat the placenta as well as to gain access to the newborn. It has been suggested that paternal consumption of the placenta in some species of marmosets may help to prime hormonally males, who within weeks of birth will be doing most of the care, apart from suckling, carrying the relatively heavy infants more than 50% of the time. In Old World cercopithecine monkeys and the Great Apes, however, exclusive maternal care of singleton young, who cling to the mother and are carried by her is the rule, and only the mother eats the placenta (Kraemer et al. 1991; Kraemer 1992). In one of the few births observed among wild gorillas, the female set the infant on the ground while she ate the placenta. Only then did she pick up and adjust her infant to her breast. Among Old World colobines (e.g., langur monkeys) mothers attempt to give birth unmolested by others, but group members are permitted to hold and carry the baby on the first day of life. In the wild, day-old langurs spend up to 50% of daylight hours being carried by females other than the mother, although at night they are retrieved by their mother and spend the night with her, presumably making up lost time suckling then.

In contrast to mammals generally and to most other primates, human mothers exhibit relatively few universal fixed behaviors apart from the labor experience itself. Universals observed across cultures include inspecting the infant, noting its condition. Like other primates, humans pay special attention to the genitals and other anatomical features. Humans are unique among those primates who give birth to singleton young (albeit not among mammals generally) in discriminating on the basis of such attributes: abandoning an infant with real or perceived defects including being the "wrong" sex; being born too close in age to an older sibling; too many or too few fingers (Hrdy 1999). Universally, the mother and/or her companions clean off the newborn, but the means by which this quite practical task is accomplished depend on available methods and customs. Licking babies clean is rare. More typically following a close visual and tactile inspection, newborns are washed with water or oil and perhaps powdered with dust, dye, charcoal, cornmeal, or even dried dung. Treatment of the placenta is highly variable (it may be discarded or ceremonially buried, but cross culturally it is the exception rather than the rule for placentas to be eaten). Many, but not all mothers hold the baby close immediately and encourage nursing. Others do so later. Colostrum may be offered to the baby or (as in many African and Haitian societies) expressed onto the ground. Usually the baby suckles first from the mother, but in some Central Africa pgymy groups a newborn may first suckle from a lactating allomother. The picture emerging for humans is of mothers for whom cognitive processes play a more important role (Keverne, this volume), although physiological changes in the mother during pregnancy and the birth process clearly prime mothers for responding maternally, and after birth, cues from the infant play a role in sustaining maternal commitment (Fleming, this volume) as do physiological processes linked to lactation.

Differences across Mammalian Species

The most striking differences across species concerns the perceptual means by which the offspring are identified. In virtually all mammalian species studied, olfactory, gustatory, tactile, auditory, and visual systems are engaged, although the relative contribution of each is species dependent. For rodents and sheep, olfactory systems are key, but they become less important for humans and other primates where visual discrimination is preeminent.

Biparental Caretaking

Although biparental care is commonplace (> 90%) among avian species, it is present in only about 10% of mammals. Note, however, that biparental care of some kind (often as rudimentary as protection) is far more common in the Order primates than in mammals generally. Typically full-fledged biparental care is seen in monogamous species with altricial young, where the male optimizes his genetic investment by caring for and defending his offspring. Ethnographic reports indicate that some level of biparental care is common in human cultures, albeit far from universal.

Nursing and feeding are those parental behaviors most associated with a new infant. Women describe breastfeeding as a uniquely close, very physical, at times sensual experience — one that brings a particular unity between the mother and her infant. Cleaning, grooming, and dressing behaviors carry a special valence inasmuch as they permit closeness between parent and infant and provide for frequent inspection of the infant's body and appearance.

Whereas behavioral fixed action patterns in humans are minimal, on a mental level birth is often viewed as a potentially dangerous, often supernaturally charged event. Mortal dangers to mother and infant are widely recognized, and may require ritual intervention. These rituals include acts of purification and supplication as well as special events surrounding the naming of the child and acknowledgement by the social group that a viable new member has safely been born and in need of their guidance and support.

At a cross-cultural level, little is known about the mental preoccupations of postpartum mothers; Leckman et al. (1999) have begun to catalog various postpartum preoccupations with care and well-being of the infant characteristic of Western (mostly middle-class) mothers. In this culture, the peripartum is associated with intense parental preoccupations (Leckman and Mayes 1999; Leckman et al. 1999; Winnicott 1956). The content of these preoccupations includes intrusive worries concerning the parents' adequacy as parents and the infant's safety and well-being. These thoughts and the harm-avoidant behavior they engender resemble those encountered in obsessive-compulsive disorder (OCD). Even before the child is born, parents preoccupy themselves with creating a safe and secure environment for the infant. Major cleaning and renovation projects are commonplace as the human form of nest-building unfolds. Uppermost among parental concerns are safety and unimpeded access. Safety issues include the cleanliness of the infant's immediate environment. After birth this same sense of heightened responsibility will compel parents to check on the baby frequently, even at times when they know the baby is fine.

In contrast to these anxious intrusive thoughts and harm-avoidant behaviors, human parents also regularly report their infant as being "perfect." For example in a recent study Leckman et al. (1999) reported that this experience peaked at three months of age, with 73% of the mothers and 88% of the fathers endorsing this experience. Exquisite and prolonged attention to physical details and similarities to one or both parents occupy considerable amounts of time. Cross-cultural studies of the first weeks following delivery also suggest that in some societies some parents perceive themselves as psychologically merging with the infant. For example, among the Siriono of northeastern Bolivia there is a lack of emphasis on personal names; in fact, parents change their name with the birth of each infant indicating their close kinship. In this way, they demonstrate a shared identity with the newborn (Scheffler and Lounsbury 1971).

Whereas human parents will typically prepare a special location (the nursery in middle-class Western societies) in anticipation of the baby's arrival, no monkey or ape mother has been observed preparing any kind of nest in preparation for birth, apart from prosimian primates (who may store babies in nests), nor is this customary among nomadic foragers. Such preparations may be more convincingly explained as outgrowths of maternal preoccupations with the infant's physical environment, safety, and well-being than actual nest-building.

Infant Responsiveness

Critical to the formation of social bonds between infant and parent is some form of social engagement (Porges, this volume). At the time of birth, mammalian young exhibit behaviors that either bring the infant into contact with the mother or serve to bring the mother into contact with her newborn. The exact behaviors exhibited differ dramatically across species and vary as well with the usual conditions at the time of birth for the species in question. As a rule, infants that are born in a mature state exhibit such behaviors as clinging (e.g., precocial primate species) or approach (e.g., guinea pigs). In species in which infants are born less well developed, characteristics of the young, including their vocalizations, typically serve to attract the mother to the infant. However, even in these species, subtle infant proximity-seeking behaviors can be apparent. Newborn rat pups, for example, attempt to direct the snout in the direction of the familiar odor of amniotic fluid (Teicher and Blass 1977). Because the mother consumes birth fluids, and then licks her own ventrum, this behavior by the pup brings it into contact with the nipple.

Behavioral mechanisms to establish contact with the mother occur in species that both do and do not establish a specific infant–mother attachment. However, in species in which attachment occurs, sooner or later the behaviors come to be directed preferentially toward the attachment object. Moreover, in species where the mother is initially identified through a particular stimulus modality, the infant begins to respond to a wider range of mother-specific stimuli.

Once in contact with the mother, the infant may also play an active role in determining the level of investment. For example, sex differences in weight gain may be due to sex differences in strength or duration of sucking. In species with multiple young, competition between siblings may affect access to resources provided by the mother (Clutton-Brock 1991).

It is also clear that infants' awareness of caretakers begins very early in life and is closely related to the maintenance of physiological homeostasis with regard to warmth, feeding, and fluid and water balance. The human infant's capacity to attend to the caregiver's face, gestures, voice, and responsiveness appears relatively early (Trevarthen, this volume) and provides the stimuli needed for human language processing to develop normally. Tzourio-Mazoyer et al. (2002) observed that 2-month-old human infants, when shown a woman's face, activate a distributed network of cortical areas including the areas that in adults are involved in facial recognition (fusiform gyrus) and language processing (left superior temporal gyrus). This suggests a close linkage between the formation of social relationships and language acquisition.

It is likely that our ancestors were cooperative breeders among whom maternal commitment was contingent on social support. Consequently, human infants have a greater need to monitor and interpret the moods and intentions of others than do other primates. Infants who could engage their mothers right from birth and respond accordingly would have an advantage over those who could not. Beyond the discomfort and separation cries characteristic of all infant apes, little humans were under greater selection pressure to appeal to both mothers and allomothers (Hrdy 1999). Perhaps not surprisingly, right from birth human infants seek out human faces and initiate contact with others. Remarkably early in development, babies imitate faces, smile, and laugh in ways that no other ape living in the wild to our present knowledge does (Meltzoff and Prinz 2002; Papousek et al. 1991; Tomasello 1999).

Early learning biases persist and are refined and reinforced through experience (Tomasello 1999), as babies become more discriminating. Visual gaze plays a key role in the attendant social engagements (Baron-Cohen 1995). Human infants seek out and fixate on eyes and preferentially respond to a direct gaze. The sociocognitive tools for monitoring others and reading their intentions by seeking out their eyes and following their gaze are more developed in humans than in other apes (Baron-Cohen 1995). Emerging evidence for chimpanzees indicates that infant apes are capable of observational learning and imitation (Tomasello and Call 1997). Some experts in primate cognition have expressed doubts whether apes are really able to imitate in the sense that they can understand the intentions of the act to be imitated; humans appear not only capable, but eager to do so, and adept at it (Caldwell and Whiten 2002).

Babbling, a stream of vocalizations with consonants and vowels, emerges in human infants after a long phase of vocalizations, about the time babies begin to accept pre-weaning foods. The onset of babbling coincides with a heightened sensitivity toward the phonemes of the mother tongue, as infants are no longer able to produce the wide variety of phonemes the different natural languages use to discriminate meanings. The onset of babbling also coincides with changes of the vocal tract, which develops more human characteristics after the third month (Ingram 1989; Kent and Miolo 1995). Far from unique, babbling is also present among the Callitrichids (marmosets and tamarins), virtually the only primates other than humans known to have full-fledged cooperative breeding. For example, in pygmy marmosets, babbling emerges between the first and third weeks, just about the time allomothers take over most of the care (Elowson et al. 1998). Hrdy (this volume) proposes that babbling in human babies, like smiling, originated for the same reason that babbling developed in Callitrichids to attract solicitude (including shared food) from caretakers. It has long been assumed that infants babble because the practice helps them learn to talk. No doubt it does, but it is likely that babbling evolved before language. Our ancestors were born clever apes who because they needed to engage caretakers babbled at them. Over the course of evolution, the best babblers were the best fed, and they eventually learned to talk, thus entering into a whole new world of possibilities.

Over the course of development, most human children become experts on other people, particularly their caretakers. Although debate continues over just how different chimps and humans are in this respect, it is clear that human infants develop the capacity to read intentions far better than infant apes (Tomasello 1999). By age two or three years, human children have developed the capacity to begin to intuit what someone else is trying to do, and why. Understanding how someone else is thinking about a task improves our ability to learn through observation and makes humans especially prone to accumulate and transmit new knowledge (Trevarthen, this volume). Hrdy (this volume) argues that it is our cooperative heritage that is responsible in part for the emergence of the human infant's abilities as a mind reader, and communicator *par excellence*.

In considering the mother–infant dyad, it is important to consider disruptions and challenges to this tie once it has been established (Table 15.2). One prominent example concerns mother–infant separation, especially in primates. Mother–infant separation can be catastrophic. Multiparous rhesus mothers are

Table 15.2 Comparison of prominent features of early parental love and infant responsiveness with romantic love (adapted from Leckman and Mayes 1999). Ratings are based on the judgments of 21 experts on bond formation and attachment (7 females and 14 males) following this Dahlem Workshop. Ratings were on a 5-point ordinal scale (0-4). Mean values rounded to the nearest integer except for mid-range values, which are presented as the two closest integers (e.g., $3.5 = +++/++++$). Male and female raters showed no differences.

Feature	Early Parental Love	Infant Responsiveness	Romantic Love
Selective recognition – exclusivity of focus	+++/++++	+++	+++/++++
Altered mental state – altered autonomic and behavioral responsivity conditioned by the absence, presence, or merely cues of the other(s)	+++/++++	+++[a]	+++
Clear onset – hedonic transformation	+++	++	+++
Intrusive thoughts and images (preoccupations):			
• Longing for reciprocity	++[*]	+++[a]	++++[*]
• Idealization of the other	+++[*]	++[a]	++++[*]
• Heightened awareness of the other	++++	+++[a]	+++
• Heightened sense of responsibility and worries about the well-being of the other	++++	++[a]	+++
• Upsetting aggressive thoughts focused on the self or the other	+[*]	+++[a]	++[b*]

[a] Initially, mental processes of the infant are ineffable and out of conscious awareness
[b] May be sexually dimorphic with males > females
[*] $p < 0.01$ Wilcoxon Signed Ranks test

always upset and agitated and "Whoo" call if their infant is taken away from them. This response is intense initially but tapers off over 2–3 days. The response of infants to separation depends largely on their age at the time of separation and the duration of the separation. All separations involve "Protest," that is, vocalizing and agitation. This can be followed by the "Despair" phase. Despair marks the "severe" response characterized by dramatic reductions in eating, drinking, and locomotor activity. This can be lethal. In general, early separations (up to three months of age) and separations beyond five months of age have less chance of producing a severe despair response and the related consequences. In rhesus monkeys the period between 3–4 months of age is the "danger zone" in which the most severe despair responses to separation can occur (Harlow et al. 1971; Kraemer et al. 1991).

Table 15.2 (*continued*)   Using a Wilcoxon Signed Ranks test (*p* < 0.01), romantic love was rated as having more longing for reciprocity, a greater tendency to idealize the other, more likely to entertain aggressive thoughts towards the other, and a greater likelihood that the relationship would end with rejection compared to early parental love. Early parental love was rated as being more focused on things being "just right" for the infant. Differences between infant responsiveness and the other two forms of love were not subjected to statistical tests, because less than half of the raters completed those ratings. Visual inspection suggests that the participating raters considered infants to harbor more aggressive thoughts toward their caretakers.

Feature	Early Parental Love	Infant Responsiveness	Romantic Love
Altered repetative behaviors:			
• Proximity seeking, physical contact, and separation distess	++++	+++	+++
• Emotionally charged caring: talking, singing, feeding, grooming	++++	+++	++
• Need for things to be safe, secure, "just right"	++++*	++	++*
• Aggressive behavior in defense of child/partner	++++	+++	++++[b]
Dichotomous resolution, either:			
• Establishment of intimate mutually satisfying reciprocal patterns of interaction, usually marked by a culturally defined ritual as well as reorganization and ongoing development of metacognitive representations, or,	+++	+++	+++
• Rejection	+*	+	+++*

[a] Initially, mental processes of the infant are ineffable and out of conscious awareness
[b] May be sexually dimorphic with males > females
* *p* < 0.01 Wilcoxon Signed Ranks test

The long-lasting effects of early separations, especially those producing a despair response, are inordinate and maladaptive responses to separations and/or social stressors occurring later in life. The most prominent social effects are tendencies to become aggressive or withdrawn, by comparison to conciliatory or prosocial behavior exhibited by monkeys not experiencing separation(s) earlier in life. Very early separations (1–3 months) generally produce mild or no persistent effects. Substantial effects are produced if the monkey is separated in the "danger zone" and/or has repeated separations early on; monkeys often do not habituate to separations, they sensitize, with the response to each separation likely to be worse than the previous one. These adverse effects of very early separations persist even if the animals are returned to their mothers.

As juveniles or young adult monkeys, previous separations in early development potentiate adverse responses to later separations, should they occur, and to social conflict. Previously separated monkeys are more likely to have "unusual" responses to separations from their social groups if these occur. When returned to their social groups, they are likely to be inordinately aggressive, or withdrawn. As yet, there are no predictors that indicate which unfortunate behavior pattern will be augmented for each individual. Indeed, with repeated separations later in life, both excessive withdrawal and aggression may be observed on different occasions. Previously separated monkeys are likely to be subordinate in social groups where other monkeys have not experienced separations early on. Females are less likely to mate successfully, and if they do mate and give birth, they tend to be physically abusive to their infants. Males are subordinate and for that reason, or because they are withdrawn or aggressive, have difficulty mating (Harlow et al. 1971; Kraemer et al. 1991).

Adult–Adult Pair Bonds and Romantic Love

The social behaviors and temporal parameters that lead to pair bond formation vary among species. In socially monogamous rodent species, a comparative short period of time may be required for the formation of a pair bond. In prairie voles (*Microtus ochrogaster*) olfactory, gustatory, and tactile exploration combined with sexual behavior, often occurring within a few hours or less, is sufficient to produce a lifelong bond characterized by selective proximity seeking and place preference, defense of mate and the nest, as well as biparental care of the young. If reinforced by association/cohabitation these bonds may be maintained for the life of the animal (Carter et al. 1995).

Another example of a pair-bonding species is found in the tree shrews (*Tupaia belangeri*), which are small diurnal mammals from Southeast Asia. In nature, treeshrews live in pairs in territories, which the males defend fiercely against intruding conspecifics. In laboratory enclosures, treeshrews are often maintained singly. Many pairs are not spontaneously compatible. In a majority of cases, if a male and a female tree shew are "paired" large enclosure fighting begins — after a few weeks or months — and can lead to the death of one partner. In about 20% of all pairings, both individuals show from the beginning intensive sociopositive behaviors, such as mutual marking and grooming, communal eating and resting, and an especially pronounced mutual mouthlicking ("kissing"), which are behavioral indicators of a strong monogamous bond. In nature these selective affiliations may be the basis of new pair bonds.

Among primates, an example of a monogamous pair bond is provided by the titi monkey. Although little is known about how these animals initially form social bonds in the wild, once formed, the bond is intense and enduring. Males and females remain together in their territory essentially indefinitely, share in infant caretaking, and spend much of their day engaged in mutual grooming or sitting quietly side-by-side with tails entwined (Mason 1974).

Of particular interest here are human pair bonds, since humans are unique in either capacity to communicate the cognitive and emotional processes associated with the formation of social bonds. Jankowiak and Fischer (1992), in a cross-cultural study, found direct evidence of romantic love in 87% of the 168 cultures studied. Prominent features include the perception of an altered mental state, the sudden and frequent intrusion into consciousness of a characteristic set of thoughts, images, and moods; state-specific behaviors; a predictable course; and a particular range of outcomes. In this period, actual and would-be lovers focus deeply on their partner to the apparent conscious exclusion of all else. This preoccupation leads to a growing ability to anticipate the other's signals, actions, and desires. If sustained and reciprocated, this process may lead to pair bonding and the formation of a new family unit.

From antiquity and from a diverse set of cultural traditions, authors have described romantic love as a malady or a form of madness. The *Song of Solomon* (Chapter 5, verse 8) records the lament, "I am sick of love," while the *Ramayana* depicts the romantic love between Rama and Sita as a reflection of a preexisting union in a heavenly realm. Tennov (1979) characterized romantic love or "limerence" as being associated with a general intensity of feelings that leaves other concerns in the background. Based on interviews with approximately 400 individuals, she reports that this altered mental state usually has a clear beginning that can be later recalled. She characterizes this state as "an essentially involuntary process" during the initial phase of which you "feel buoyant, elated, and ironically…free." This state is subjectively experienced as a distinct period during which the usual course of mental life is disrupted by alterations in perception, a broad range of intrusive thoughts, and unstable emotions ranging from elation to anxious insecurity and despair.

A core feature of romantic love, at least within the Western cultural tradition, is the emergence of time-consuming intrusive thoughts. The terms most frequently used to describe these thoughts include: preoccupations, obsessions, reveries, and brooding. In a sample of 656 college students, Shea and Adams (1984) reported that the most potent predictor of reported romantic love was the degree to which they were preoccupied (how often and how much time) with thoughts about their dating partner. Tesser and Paulhus (1976) have reported similar results. Thoughts of the other are frequently described as coming from nowhere, but it is clear that perceptual triggers play a role as well (e.g., if the person's name is mentioned or if one were to pass by the street on which the beloved lives or see a person or place associated in some way with the beloved).

Although there is abundant evidence for the presence of these intrusive thoughts in private journals, poems, fiction, theater, and popular songs, empirical thematic analysis is scant. Anecdotal accounts suggest that these reveries are exclusively focused on the beloved and predictably contain a range of sentiments, longings, and doubts. A consistent theme from antiquity concerns the importance of feelings of closeness and intimacy and the desire for reciprocity with a particular other person. Most descriptions include a longing for intimate reciprocity, the tender harmony that is anticipated if and when the beloved loves in return, and feelings of relief and ecstatic bliss if reciprocation seems likely (Beyle 1975; Tennov 1979). In one of the few descriptive empirical studies, Horton (1957) reports an analysis of the lyrics of 235 popular songs published in 1955. Among the 196 songs (83%) that were conversational songs about love, 23 contained lyrics focused on questioning or offering reassurances concerning mutual commitment. This, however, is likely to be an underestimate given the mutually exclusive categories used in the study.

Preoccupations of the lover focus on minute and "objectively trivial" aspects of the beloved. According to Beyle, "a person in love is unremittingly and uninterruptedly occupied with the image of [the] beloved...." He further suggests that this image of the beloved is distorted and has more to do with the "the wonderful inner vision...[that has been]...created" within the eye of the beholder. Beyle called this process of idealization "crystallization," a process where each aspect of the beloved comes to be admired as beautiful. In this process, "ugliness must not present an obstacle...the lover will see beauty, whatever [he/she] looks like, without giving a thought to real beauty." These idealizing thoughts and euphoric feelings are balanced by feelings of "frightful calamity," when doubts are raised that one's love will be ever returned, and these doubts can give way to fears of rejection, jealousy, hatred, vilification, revenge, murderous rage, suicidal despair "when all is not well between you and your beloved."

In addition to the mental states described above, there are a number of patterns of behaviors that are typically associated with this period. Partners and potential partners show a heightened responsiveness to one another. Feelings of attraction and the wish to be joined with the beloved often results in behavior that diminishes the physical distance between the two (Givens 1983; Perper 1985). As pointed out by Tennov (1979), one wants to be either with the beloved or where the beloved is likely to be (place preference).

Typically, the periods of self-doubt that accompany being "in love" are associated with efforts to alter one's appearance and potentially increase one's beauty and desirability to the beloved person. Grooming and dressing behaviors are heightened in the hope of attracting the beloved by appearance or dress. Perfumes, colognes, lotions, and salves gain wider use. Music and song also seem to play a special role when individuals are overtaken by limerent feelings. Beyle asserted that "perfect music has the same effect on the heart as the presence of the beloved," and Shakespeare has the Duke in *Twelfth Night* reflecting, "music be the food of love." As heightened reciprocity and pair bonding occurs, certain preferences for places, activities, and such things as shared songs may develop.

Initial success often results in a series of reciprocal behaviors: mutual gaze, "grooming talk," in which there is a distinctive change in the pitch, prosody, and content of speech, touching, and periods of synchrony as each mirrors the other in tandem movement (Givens 1983; Morris 1967; Perper 1985). Although sexual behaviors are often seen as the culmination of this process, it is also clear that sex increasingly has a place in the early phases of falling in love.

Beyle and Tennov offer complementary views on the early course of being in love. The process often begins at a particular point in time that can later be recalled. Sexual attraction per se need not be experienced, although the person is typically viewed as a possible sexual partner and the initial "admiration" may be, or seem to be, primarily based on an attraction to certain aspects of the other's appearance or behavior: how they look, walk or talk. An initial pleasurable phase is characterized by feelings of buoyancy, elation, hope, and freedom, free not only from the usual restraints of gravity, but emotionally unburdened. The individual's mental life is increasingly occupied with considering and reconsidering what is attractive about the person and replaying precious memories of being together.

At any point in the process, if reciprocation occurs, ranging from mutual gaze to sexual coupling, the anxiety and distress of being "in love" diminishes. Over time, according to Beyle, "what love loses in intensity — its fears, that is — it makes up for by the charm of complete abandon and infinite trust, becoming a gentle habit which softens the hardships of life and gives new interest to its enjoyment." As with early parental attachments, the elation, distress, and confusion of romantic love gives way to predictable habits of intimate reciprocity. Adjusting to the rhythms and expectations of the other, outcomes include "affectional bonding," in which the preoccupation subsides and is replaced by a more secure attachment and genuine love. These developments often have a significant impact on the immediate social environment including cohabitation and the eventual formation of a new family unit that are marked in most cultures with a marriage ritual (Dulaney and Fiske 1994). An element of marriage ceremonies in most cultures is an explicit statement of commitment and shared responsibility for one another. Several investigators have emphasized the role of commitment in love relationships. Kelly (1983) emphasizes that commitment concerns the stability of forces that affect an ongoing relationship whereas Sternberg (1986) focuses on the cognitive appraisal and determination to maintain one's connection with the partner.

The other common outcome is a rejection of the suitor and the attendant fantasies of reciprocity. This can occur at many points along the path — from an outright rejection at the first indication of interest to rejections that occur after some mutuality has been established. Rejection is often painfully one-sided, with one party still hoping while the other is adamant in their rejection. The emotional and behavioral trajectory for the rejected suitor or mate covers an enormous range from despair and recovery to persistent, mind-dominating obsessions that in a small minority of cases lead to stalking or other extreme behaviors such as suicide or homicide (Buteau et al. 1993; Easteal 1994; Marzuk et al. 1992).

At the level of subjective experience, the early phases of romantic love and early parental love share much in common: an altered mental state, intrusive thoughts and images associated with a heightened awareness of the other, and a complex behavioral repertoire aimed at eliciting a reciprocal response. In many instances these altered mental states lead to the same outcome: the formation of intimate interpersonal ties.

Similarities between Early Parental Love and Romantic Love

One of the landmarks of contemporary developmental psychology has been its focus on attachment between infant and parent (Ainsworth 1973; Bowlby 1969; 1973). It may be reasonable to apply the same conceptual framework in judging the nature and quality of the romantic attachments formed in adulthood, as proposed by Hazan and Shaver (1987, 1994). Both romantic love and the early phases of parental love are characterized, at least in most Western cultures, by an altered mental and emotional state (Table 15.2). Although it is difficult, some would say impossible, to compare intrapsychic states across individuals or within the same individual at different points in time, there is evidence to suggest that these altered states share much in common. For example, in both instances there is an anxious tension between the joyous reveries of being "at one" with one another and intrusive worries that something terrible will happen to place the desired outcome in jeopardy. Although studies have not yet quantified the frequency and intensity of these preoccupations, many parents anecdotally report the feeling is the same: "No one told me it was like falling in love." Other clear thematic parallels include the tendency to be preoccupied with small details of the other's appearance and the tendency to see the lover or new infant as "perfect." As one mother said after her baby was born, "I just can't believe it, here she is and she's so perfect, I can't believe she's really mine."

The similarities with regard to the behavioral repertoires of romantic love and early parental love are striking. In both instances there is a compelling urge to shape one's behavior to the perceived needs of the other. Frequently, these behavioral responses have a "just right" character, so that they exactly fit the needs of the other. The heightened sense of responsibility that usually accompanies both states leads to an increased level of vigilance and behaviors aimed at insuring the safety of infant or lover. Beyond the intimacies of the home environment, it is also worth noting that both states are marked by culturally defined rituals (Table 15.2; Leckman and Mayes 1999).

Many of the behaviors seen in courtship are borrowed from the repertoire of the early parent–child relationship or vice versa (Eibl-Eibesfelt 1971, 1989). Specific examples include parental care actions such as comforting embraces, caressing, grooming, kissing, feeding, mutual gaze, and the use of terms of endearment like "baby" in referring to a lover. Similarly, needy infant-like appeals by gesture or whimper are not uncommon elements of the lover's behavioral repertoire. In addition, neonatous features are often considered sources of feminine allure. The ethologic literature has documented these infantilisms across human cultures as well as the occurrence of comparable behaviors in other species including birds and mammals.

Vicissitudes of Bond Formation and Loss

Changes in the interpersonal landscape that occur as we make room in our lives for someone new (lover, spouse, or child) or cope with the loss of a close attachment figure demand a remarkable degree of psychological and biological flexibility as new cognitive, emotional, and homeostatic equilibria are achieved (Table 15.3). Although a full exploration of the scientific literature on this topic is beyond the scope of this review, it is notable that most empirical studies have focused on the formation or loss of one bond to the exclusion of others without examining the complex dynamics of how the formation or loss of one relationship affects the course and quality of other close relationships (Table 15.3). For example, in both romantic love and early parental love, exclusivity develops, other

Table 15.3 Bond dynamics: a listing of a variety of challenges to existing interpersonal bonds and the impact of new bond formation on existing bonds (see text for examples).

Challenge to, loss, or reestablishment of an existing bond	Formation of a new bond affecting an existing bond
• Mother–infant separation • Reunion • Death of infant (child) • Break-up of a pair bond (divorce) • Reunion of a separated couple • Death of spouse	• Addition of a new family member (first born): effect on parent–parent bond • Birth of a sibling: effect on older sibling; effect on parent–parent bond • Bond to a teacher or mentor • Bond to a closely affiliated individual (fellow combat veteran) • Remarriage after divorce • Effect on children and other relationships • Remarriage after the death of a spouse: effect on children, memory of lost spouse and other relationships

concerns diminish in importance, and mental and emotional energy becomes focused. This exclusivity is highly adaptive during courtship and early parenting; however, it may pose certain difficulties for the spouse or older siblings. For example, such a deepening sense of an exclusive relationship between mother and child may contribute to increased tension between mother and father as both alter the amount of time they spend with one another and focus more on the baby (Entwisle and Doering 1981). Indeed, the weeks following the birth of an infant are cited as a critical period for marital adjustment. In several studies, mothers have reported diminished marital satisfaction following the birth of an infant (Belsky et al. 1983). More successful transitions to parenthood occur in couples who were more prepared and closer before pregnancy; conversely, unplanned pregnancies or younger parents are at greater risk for marital difficulties after a birth (Cowan et al. 1985).

Another challenge concerns the birth of a new sibling and the psychological adjustments required to maintain close ties with each child in the family. Although the level of parental preoccupation is often less with a second child compared to the first, everyone in the family needs to adjust to the arrival of a new family member. An extreme example of this challenge comes with multiple births. In some cultures, twin births are regarded as unwelcome and unnatural and often one of the two infants is killed. Others describe how some parents of twins find it too difficult to establish clearly differentiated relationships with each infant and may attempt to merge the twins into a single unit through similar names, dress, and perceived attributes (Robin et al. 1992). In other instances, parents develop clear preferences, favoring one twin more than the other (Mann 1992; Minde et al. 1990).

KEY ELEMENTS IN THE NEURAL CIRCUITRY OF AFFILIATIVE BEHAVIORS
(see Keverne, Carter, and Fleming in this volume)

Bond formation relies on neural circuits necessary to account for (a) social motivation and subsequent engagement with a member of the same species, (b) identification of an appropriate partner, (c) formation of a bond possibly relying on neural reward systems, (d) maintenance of established bonds, even in the face of social challenges, and (e) recognition of the absence of the partner, leading in some cases to separation distress. Essential elements of social engagement (Porges, this volume) and pair bond formation (Carter, this volume; Keverne, this volume) are discussed in detail elsewhere, and summarized briefly here.

Attempts to define neural circuits involved in affiliative behavior and the eventual formation of social bonds have been limited by the number of species that have a natural predisposition to bond formation and the availability of such species for laboratory studies. In spite of these limitations, it is reasonable to assume that common neural mechanisms underlie at least some aspects of social bonding across species. Furthermore, core elements may be shared between parent–infant bonds and social bonds between adults. Social bonding also appears to be based on neural circuits that are shared with other forms of socio-sexual behavior including sexual behavior and maternal behaviors, even in species, such as rats, for which maternal behavior is nonselective (Fleming et al. 1997; this volume). Hence, to identify features that are common to all forms of social bonding, versus those that are not, it is useful initially to catalog the components of those behaviors that are necessary for social bond formation, to determine which of these components are species specific and which are common across mammalian species (Table 15.1). Commonality among these behavioral elements from mouse to human would suggest common mechanisms that can be called into play and hence common hormones, including neuropeptides and their receptors; transmitter systems and possibly genes which underpin the development and wiring of these circuits (Fleming et al. 1997). In this section we offer a tentative biobehavioral model of bonding and attachment that focuses on the interface of several neural systems involved in perception, arousal, maintenance of physiological and autonomic homeostasis, as well as reward and threat detection and response pathways. Thus far, the available empirical evidence supports a role for each of these in the development and maintenance of mammalian maternal care. How they are called into action, the contexts for these actions, the sensory components contingent on these actions probably represent the main distinctions across species.

Core Neuroanatomic Structures

Classical lesion studies, site-specific injections and methods for measuring neural activation following social experiences, conducted in rodent model systems (rats, mice, and voles) have implicated ancient brain structures in the limbic/olfactory systems including the amygdala, the medial preoptic area (MPOA) of the hypothalamus, the ventral part of the bed nucleus of the stria terminalis (BNSTv), and the lateral septum (LS) as regions pivotal for social engagement and the initial stages of bond formation (Carter and Keverne, 2002; Leckman and Herman 2002; Numan 1994; Numan and Sheehan 1997). As reviewed by Fleming (this volume) in rats repeated pup exposure leads to the activation of many of these structures (measured by the expression of the c-Fox oncogene) including the medial and cortical amygdala, MPOA, BNSTv, and the cingulate cortex. These same neural systems are activated during initial encounters between male and female prairie voles (Cushing et al. 2003). Subsequently, once the animal has gained experience (become sensitized to the pups), the MPOA and parietal cortices show heightened c-fos expression in the presence of pup-associated cues, even if animals are not actually behaving maternally. More recent work using BrdU and assessments of neurogenesis show increased cell (neuronal) proliferation in the subventricular zone when animals gain an experience and increased cell (neuronal) survival in the MPOA in experienced over inexperienced animals suggesting that the brain undergoes changes in activation and inactive neurogenesis with a maternal experience (Akbari et al. 2003).

Although information about these circuits in humans and other primate species is sparse, the available data are consistent with at least some of the same circuitry involved (Fleming et al. 1999; Lorberbaum et al. 2002). Relationships, emotional states, and pair bonding may be indirectly indexed by the measurement of blood or salivary levels of adrenal glucocorticoids (corticosterone or cortisol). Fleming and co-workers have found that first-time mothers with high levels of circulating cortisol were better able to identify their own infant's odors. In these same primiparous mothers, the level of affectionate contact with the infant (affectionate burping, stroking, poking and hugging) by the mother was associated with higher levels of salivary cortisol (Fleming et al.1997). Likewise, Lorberbaum and colleagues (2002) found increased levels of activity in the cingulate cortex as well as the midbrain, hypothalamus, dorsal and ventral striatum, and the lateral septal region. Each of these findings supports the hypothesis that our stress response systems are adaptively activated during the period of heightened maternal sensitivity surrounding the birth of a new infant.

Oxytocin and Vasopressin

Two neuropeptide hormones in particular, oxytocin and vasopressin, have been implicated in maternal behavior and social bonding. Oxytocin and vasopressin are primarily synthesized in the magnocellular secretory neurons of two hypothalamic nuclei, the paraventricular (PVN) and the supraoptic (SON) nuclei. In addition, especially in males, vasopressin can be synthesized in other brain regions including the medial amygdala/BNST. The PVN and SON project to the posterior pituitary gland where oxytocin and vasopressin are transported and released. Pituitary release of oxytocin into the bloodstream results in milk ejection during nursing and uterine contraction during labor. It has also been shown that oxytocin fibers, which arise from parvocellular neurons in the PVN, project to areas of the limbic system including the amygdala, BNST, and LS (Sofroniew and Weindl 1981). Intracerebral sources of oxytocin may be of particular importance to mammalian maternal behavior, and may be released by various social stimuli including the simple presence of an infant or other social stimulus. Vasopressin is released in the presence of various stressors, including dehydration and social stressors; under these conditions, the release of vasopressin is associated with adaptive responses which may help the individual defend itself or its family against both physical and social stressors. In addition, vasopressin may have specific effects on pair bond formation, especially in males (Carter 1998; Young, 1999).

A particularly powerful, but potentially complex instance of sociality occurs between most mothers and their infants. The endocrine changes associated with the end of gestation activate neural mechanisms regulating maternal behavior, however, it is important to note that in most laboratory rodents this relationship is not marked by individual selectivity and thus may not qualify as "social bonding" (Carter, Fleming and Keverne, this volume).

Estrogen, prolactin, opioids and oxytocin may in particular affect the limbic system, brainstem and associated neural tissue to promote maternal behavior (Bridges et al.1990; Numan et al. 1997; Pedersen and Prange 1979). Progesterone may be inhibitory to maternal behavior, as well as to the release and actions of oxytocin; the decline in this hormone that precedes parturition — in conjunction with pulses of oxytocin associated with birth — probably helps to coordinate the onset of maternal behavior with the delivery of the offspring.

Oxytocin released during lactation may serve to reinforce maternal behavior (Pedersen 1997). However, lactation is not essential for the induction or maintenance of maternal/alloparental behavior in humans and a number of other cooperatively breeding species including the highly social prairie vole. The possibility exists, and remains to be tested, that oxytocin or related neuropeptides may play a role in the willingness of nonreproductive animals to show alloparental behavior, even in the absence of birth or lactation.

There are several reports that oxytocin facilitates maternal behavior (sensitization) in estrogen-primed nulliparous female rats. Intracerebroventricular (ICV) administration of oxytocin in virgin female rats induces full maternal behavior within minutes (Pedersen and Prange 1979). Conversely, central injection of an oxytocin antagonist, or a lesion of oxytocin-producing cells in the PVN, suppresses the onset of maternal behavior in postpartum female rats (Van Leengoed et al. 1987). These manipulations have no effect on maternal behavior in animals permitted several days of postpartum mothering. This result suggests that oxytocin plays an important role in facilitating the onset of maternal interest in pups during a critical developmental window (Pedersen 1997).

In prairie voles, treatment with oxytocin quickly facilitates positive social behaviors, including maternal behavior (Bales and Carter, unpublished) and selective partner preferences (Carter, this volume). Exposure to oxytocin is capable of down regulating or buffering the adrenocorticoid response to stressors, the reactivity of the autonomic nervous system, including heart rate and blood pressure (Uvnas-Moberg 1998), and the release of adrenal hormones (Carter 1998). A possible mechanism by which stress might influence social behaviors through increased binding of oxytocin to its receptor, is facilitated in the presence of adrenal steroids, especially in the amygdala (Liberzon and Young 1997).

Data on the role of oxytocin in maternal behavior in humans is scarce and limited to peripheral measurements that correspond to oxytocin release from the posterior pituitary. Mother–infant touch and contact have been shown to stimulate oxytocin release. Newborn infants placed on the mother's chest stimulate oxytocin release by hand movement and suckling (Matthiesen et al. 2001), and mother–infant skin-to-skin contact immediately after birth elevates maternal oxytocin levels (Nissen et al.1995). Breast pumping and breastfeeding are related to a comparable increase in oxytocin levels (Zinaman et al.1992), and thus measuring exact amounts of expressed milk may serve as a proxy of oxytocin levels. Mothers of premature infants who expressed higher quantities of breast milk showed more optimal maternal behavior, in terms of higher sensitivity and more affectionate touch during interactions. The amount of breast milk also predicted the infant's cognitive and motor development and negatively correlated with maternal depression (Feldman and Eidelman 2003). Since oxytocin functions as an antidepressant/anxiolytic agent, reducing anxiety and elevating social activity in humans (Carter 1998; Heinrichs et al. 2003; Uvnas-Moberg 1998) and is increased with touch and contact, it is likely to play a role in the general complex of emotional behaviors and possibly even mental representations related to maternal caregiving.

Vasopressin

Vasopressin is a neuropeptide related to oxytocin in its genetic origins and structure. Like oxytocin, central vasopressin is involved in the regulation of several social behaviors, including social recognition and affiliation. This neuropeptide also appears to play a critical role in the regulation of social bonding in the monogamous prairie vole. Pair bonding in prairie voles normally occurs following an overnight cohabitation with mating. Central infusions of a vasopressin receptor (V1aR) antagonist prevent partner preference formation (a laboratory index of pair bond formation) while vasopressin infusions stimulate partner-preference formation in the absence of mating (Winslow et al. 1993; Cho et al. 1999). Like oxytocin, vasopressin may have the capacity to reduce anxiety in the presence of a novel social partner. Such changes in behavior could serve to facilitate both pair bonding and the response of a male toward infants (Carter 2003).

Vasopressin also has been implicated in aggression, especially in defense of a mate or territory (Carter 1998), and manipulations of vasopressin that induce partner preferences are also associated with a dramatic increase in male–male aggression. Endogenously produced vasopressin is androgen dependent and sexually dimorphic, especially in the amygdala, BNSTv, and LS. The role of vasopressin in pair bonding has been primarily explored in males (Young 1999). However, females are capable of responding to exogenous vasopressin, and it is possible that this peptide has consequences for pair bonding in both sexes (Cho et al. 1999), possibly through actions on both the tendency to show social engagement as well as enhancing the rewarding properties of a social experience.

Voles have proven especially useful for the analysis of social bonding because some species of voles, including the well-characterized prairie voles, are socially monogamous (Carter et al. 1995), while other related species, such as montane voles, typically show few indications of pair bonding or other traits of socially monogamous species (cf. Carter, this volume). The neural systems required for the production of both oxytocin and vasopressin are highly conserved and similar across most mammals (Russell et al. 2003). However, receptor distributions show distinct species-typical patterns of distribution, which may be fundamental to the capacity of any particular species (or even a particular individual) to exhibit pair bonding.

For example, receptor autoradiographic analyses indicate that the density of V1a receptors is high in the ventral in prairie voles but very low in this region in montane voles. In addition, oxytocin receptors are abundant in the nucleus accumbens of prairie voles, but not in montane voles. The nucleus accumbens and ventral pallidal systems are central components of the dopamine reward pathway in mammals. The coexistence of dopamine receptors and either oxytocin or vasopressin receptors, in the same or adjacent cells, may provide a neural substrate for reinforcing the development of selective partner preferences. Among the species that have thus far been studied, only those capable of forming selective pair bonds have shown both receptors for dopamine and either oxytocin or vasopressin in the nucleus accumbens and ventral pallidum. Whether this co-occurrence of receptors for neuropeptides and dopamine is characteristic of primates remains to be determined.

The species-specific role of peptide receptors in social behavior has led Young and his colleagues (Hammock et al. 2003) to explore the molecular mechanisms underlying the species-specific expression patterns of the V1aR. These studies revealed that a stretch of about 420 bp located 700 bp upstream of the transcription start site of the prairie vole V1aR is absent in the polygamous montane vole gene. This sequence is composed of di- and tetranucleotide repeats interspersed between nonrepetitive sequences and appears to be an expansion of a short repetitive microsatellite sequence found in the promoter of both species. The socially monogamous pine vole also has this microsatellite in its V1aR promoter; the nonmonogamous meadow vole does not.

Stress and Stress Hormones in Social Bonding

As reviewed by Carter and Fleming (both this volume), another neuropeptide implicated in stress and anxiety as well as pair bonding is corticotropin-releasing hormone (CRH), which is synthesized and released in the hypothalamus and other areas of the brain implicated in emotion and the regulation of autonomic responses. In male prairie voles, evidence suggests that treatment with moderate doses of CRH can facilitate pair bonding; pretreatment with a specific CRH antagonist can block these effects (DeVries et al. 2002). Evidence from other species indicates that the actions of CRH are synergistic with vasopressin to regulate the release of adrenocorticotropic hormone (ACTH) and adrenal steroids. It is possible that CRH and vasopressin work in conjunction to facilitate pair bonding, especially in males. Further, some species of socially monogamous mammals have exceptionally high levels of adrenal steroids, and it is possible that these steroids have behavioral consequences related to the development and expression of the traits of monogamy (DeVries et al. 1996; Carter 1998; Carter and

Keverne 2002). Thus far these findings are mostly correlative. It remains to be seen whether other systems, such as the endogenous opioid system, are also boosted concurrently to induce a causative effect.

Perceptual Systems

Social bonds are by definition selective and thus require individual recognition through one or more sensory modalities. Even if bonding is to a litter of pups or to a nest (in the case of birds or some mammalian species), this form of attachment also requires recognition. Since recognition involves learning and memory, there will always be a time course involved in the full development of the system. Likewise, following consolidation of the bond, sensory recognition cues themselves may be sufficient to evoke the behaviors or emotional states characteristic of social bonding.

Olfactory signals are frequently involved in mammalian social bond formation. To accommodate its role in social bonding, the olfactory system has to undergo radical reorganization in its relationship with the "emotional" brain. Animals must overcome aversive (neophobic) responses to strangers (mate or pups) and may even be willing to ingest a normally aversive object, such as placenta (a behavioral change that is especially striking in herbivores). Specific olfactory recognition requires the release of catecholamines and neuropeptides (oxytocin, vasopressin, and opioids), some of which are synchronously active in the olfactory bulbs and its relay to the amygdala. These transmitters are released in response to tactile stimuli (mating, parturition, grooming, licking) and in some cases arousing, fearful stimuli. How and where these transmitters have their action depends on receptors and their distribution in the brain, including accessory and olfactory bulb, medial amygdala, BNST, MPOA, arcuate nucleus, ventral striatum, and brainstem nuclei. These peptides are often released as neurohumors into cerebrospinal fluid and reach receptors that have no direct terminals. Many of these receptors that are sensitive to neuropeptides have been up-regulated by hormonal priming appropriate to the biological condition (mating, parturition, fear, and anxiety). As described above, there is commonality in brain areas involved in maternal care, mating behavior, as well as aggressive and social behavior at the limbic level; it is possible that the differences between these bonds at the neural level may simply involve the addressing mechanism (sensory stimuli and hormonal priming). Olfactory recognition permits proximity through familiarity, which enables other behaviors to occur that sustain the bond. In this context, integral to bonding is a "reward," which involves the ventral striatum (including the ventral pallidum and nucleus accumnbens) and the mesolimbic dopamine projection that detects reward-predicting stimuli and discrepancies from such predictions, thus enabling "updating."

In reflecting on the shift from predominantly olfactory cues in rodent and ungulates to visual cues on Old World monkeys, apes, and humans, Liman and Innan (2003) offer an intriguing hypothesis that the vomeronasal organ was functional in the common ancestor of New World monkeys, Old World monkeys, and apes but then became vestigial in the common ancestor of Old World monkeys and apes. It is postulated that this shift in function occurred at the same time that color vision was emerging as a new sensory modality which then largely replaced signaling by pheromones.

Visual, auditory, and somatosensory infant-related inputs likely involve projections from primary sensory areas to the orbitofrontal cortex (OFC). Recent work in animals has highlighted the functional importance of the OFC in affective and motivational behavior. Primates appear to be particularly good at attending to and integrating all sensory cues from all modalities in recognizing and bonding to their newborn. This integrative process likely requires neocortical processing in the OFC and other cortical limbic areas including the cingulate cortex as well as auditory and visual association areas in order for rapid recognition and bonding to occur. For example, it is well documented that the fusiform gyrus responds preferentially to faces (Haxby et al. 1999; Kanwisher et al. 1997). Given the obsessive attention to anatomical details of the hands, face, and genitalia (that show most variance across primates) during the grooming of offspring and bonded conspecifics, it is likely that these cortical regions play an important role in the maintenance of selective social bonds. Some of these same regions are also involved in the detection and appraisal of threats as well as the recognition of bonded conspecifics (see below). Auditory and visual association areas are also likely to be integral in processing relevant sensory information.

In rats, brain areas have also been identified that inhibit maternal behavior (Sheehan et al. 2000). For example, the vomeronasal and primary olfactory systems have been identified as brain regions that mediate avoidance behavior in virgin female rats exposed to the odor cues of pups (Fleming et al. 1980). This suggests that sensory cues may be key indicators of the hedonic transformation (a shift from a set of stimuli being aversive to rewarding) that occurs when a selective social bond is formed.

Reward

Ascending dopaminergic and noradrenergic systems associated with reward pathways appear to play a crucial role in facilitating maternal behavior (Koob and Le Moal 1997). Rat dams given microinfusions of the neurotoxin 6-hydroxydopamine (6-OHDA) in the ventral tegmental area (VTA) to destroy catecholaminergic neurons during lactation showed a persistent deficit in pup retrieval but were not impaired with respect to nursing, nest-building, or maternal aggression (Hansen et al.1991). As described above, there also appears to be an important interaction between dopaminergic neurons and oxytocin pathways. Specifically, pup retrieval and assuming a nursing posture over pups were blocked in parturient dams by infusions of an oxytocin antagonist into either the VTA or MPOA (Pedersen et al. 1994).

What makes affiliative motor patterns of behavior and the sensory cues that represent the object of the bond special (i.e., a primary motivated behavior) is the reward system of the brain to which others are linked. The birth process not only initiates learning and maternal care but also the brain's reward system. Regardless of what is being recognized, activation of this ventral striatal reward system may be another system common to maternal care and bonding in all species. The object of recognition and bonding is usually not fixed and static; it continually grows and changes with respect to phenotype and sensory cues emitted. To adapt to these phenotypic changes and sustain maternal care, it is important that attention be given to the sensory inputs provided by the offspring. Hence this system serves as an error detector crucial to sensory motor integration permitting affiliative behavior to be sustained to an evolving set of stimuli.

Arousal and Threat Detection

Unless our forbearers were acutely attuned to potential external threats posed by other humans, predators, the external manifestations of microbial disease, or periods of privation due to drought, natural disasters, or internecine conflict, our species would not have survived. As described by Porges in his Polyvagal Theory (this volume), social engagement behaviors associated with nursing, reproduction and the formation of strong pair bonds require immobilization; immobilization in turn requires a "neuroception" of safety. The social engagement system has a control component in the cortex (i.e., upper motor neurons) that regulates brainstem nuclei (i.e., lower motor neurons) to control eyelid opening (e.g., looking), facial muscles (e.g., emotional expression), middle ear muscles (e.g., extracting human voice from background noise), muscles of mastication (e.g., ingestion), laryngeal and pharyngeal muscles (e.g., vocalization and language), and head-turning muscles (e.g., social gesture and orientation). Collectively, these muscles function as filters that limit social stimuli (e.g., observing facial features and listening to human voice) and determinants of engagement with the social environment. Neural control of these muscles is a crucial element in social experiences.

Other Cortical Regions

Key neocortical and striatal regions involved in social bond formation include the OFC, caudate nucleus, and anterior cingulate cortex (ACC), all of which are thought to work together to inhibit or terminate inappropriate responses and to select and monitor preferred behavioral sequences. The OFC, in particular, appears to have a specific role in decision making based on emotional cues (Anderson et al.1999; Bechara et al.1994; Rolls 2000). As such, the OFC appears to be directly involved in both threat detection and appraisal. It is reciprocally connected with the amygdala, hippocampus, LC, and VTA, as well as brainstem autonomic nuclei. As emphasized by Porges, these connections can also facilitate the initiation and regulation of the endocrine response to stress that is mediated by the hypothalamic–pituitary–adrenal (HPA) axis.

In summary, the initiation and maintenance of bonding involves a specific set of neural circuits. With pregnancy, repeated exposure to infants, and the formation of pair bonds, structural and molecular changes occur, most of which are not yet completely understood, in specific limbic, hypothalamic, and midbrain regions that reflect, in part, an adaptation to the various homeostatic demands associated with maternal care. Remarkably, many of the same cell groups implicated in the control of maternal behavior have been implicated in the control of ingestive (eating and drinking) behavior, thermoregulatory (energy homeostasis), social (defensive and sexual) behaviors, as well as general exploratory or foraging behaviors (with locomotor and orienting components) that are required to obtain any particular goal object. Many of these same structures are also intimately involved in stress response. Swanson (2000) conceptualized this set of limbic, hypothalamic, and midbrain nuclei as a "behavioral control column" that is voluntarily regulated by cerebral projections. Consistent with this formulation, it is readily apparent that motherhood presents a major homeostatic challenge within *each* of these behavioral domains.

GENETIC DETERMINANTS OF MATERNAL BEHAVIOR

Gene knockout technology has provided new insights into the molecular basis of maternal behavior that are congruent with the existing neurobiological literature. At least ten of the 30,000 or so genes in the mammalian genome have been identified that are necessary for the expression of one or more aspects of maternal behavior. These genes encode for three transcription factors, including nerve growth factor; three enzymes, including dopamine beta hydroxylase and neuronal nitric oxide synthase; three receptors, including the prolactin and the estrogen α receptor; the dopamine transporter; and one neuropeptide, oxytocin (Leckman and Herman 2002; Numan and Insel 2003). By way of illustration, we briefly review two of these genes, dopamine beta hydroxylase (*Dbh*) and parentally expressed gene 3 (*Peg3*).

Dopamine Beta Hydroxylase

Noradrenergic neurons in the brain project from brainstem nuclei and innervate virtually all areas of the brain and spinal cord. Along with dopamine and serotonergic pathways, these noradrenergic projections are part of our vertebrate salience and reward systems. The enzyme Dbh synthesizes the adrenergic receptor ligands norepinephrine (NE) and epinephrine. Thomas et al. (1995) disrupted the *Dbh* gene in mice. In a subsequent study, Thomas and Palmiter (1997) demonstrated impaired maternal behavior across virtually all domains evaluated. Pups were observed scattered within the bedding around the nest.

Often pups were not cleaned, and their placentas remained attached. Remarkably, milk was not detected in the stomachs of most pups born to *Dbh* –/– females, even though these females can nurse and their lactation is not impaired. The impairment in maternal behavior in the *Dbh* –/– animals could reflect a developmental deficit caused by NE deficiency or a physiological deficit. To distinguish between these possibilities, DOPS (L–threo–3, 4–dihydroxyphenyl-serine, a synthetic precursor of NE) was used to restore NE transiently to the mutant females. When mutant females were injected with DOPS on the morning after birth, maternal behavior was not restored, and all pups subsequently died; however, when mutant females were injected with DOPS on the evening prior to birth, more than half of the litters survived. Even more pups survived when DOPS was injected both in the evening before and on the morning after birth. These findings suggest that NE may play a key role in initiating a realignment of the dam's sense of what is salient and important in the environment. Interestingly, in 85% of the mutant females, the rescue of maternal behavior by DOPS extended to the mother's subsequent pregnancies even in the absence of DOPS injections. These data are consistent with our model that central reward pathways are intimately involved in aspects of parental care.

Paternally Expressed Gene 3

Peg3 is an imprinted gene. Imprinted autosomal genes display differential expression in a haploid condition according to parental origin. Some of the genes we inherit from our parents are only expressed when they pass through the matriline, others when they are inherited through the patriline. Among vertebrates, imprinting is unique to mammals. Many of these genes are expressed in the placenta and influence fetal development; others are expressed in the brain and influence brain development and behavior.

Peg3 is a paternally expressed gene that is expressed both in the placenta and the brain that has been shown to influence brain development and maternal behavior. *Peg3* contains two zinc finger motifs and two proline or acidic amino acid-rich repeat domains, which suggest its involvement in DNA binding and protein–protein interactions (Kuroiwa et al.1996).

Li et al. (1999) disrupted *Peg3* by inserting a βgeo selection cassette into its 5' coding exon. Pups born to *Peg3* –/– mutant mothers failed to survive. Whereas only 8% of litters born to mutant mothers grew to weaning age, 83% of litters born to wild-type females survived. The offspring of mutant females and wild-type males (+/– X +/+) also failed to thrive, suggesting that the genotype of the mother, not the father, was relevant for their survival. Because these pups inherited the active paternal *Peg3* allele and the silent maternal allele, they should develop as normal adults. The fact that so few pups survived suggested that there was a defect in maternal behavior. Mutant primiparous mothers were subjected to a behavioral assay of nurturing behaviors. These animals were found to be deficient in nest-building, pup retrieval, and nursing. During the first three weeks, surviving offspring of *Peg3* mutant females gained less weight compared with the offspring of wild-type mothers. These offspring were also smaller at birth and had problems suckling and were found to have a late onset of thermogenic regulation; thus their entry into puberty was delayed.

Normally in rodent brain, high levels of *Peg3* expression are present in a number of hypothalamic nuclei (MPOA and PVN) as well as the MA, BNST, hippocampus, and olfactory bulb that have been implicated in maternal behavior. Histologic examination revealed that the mutant mothers had fewer oxytocin-positive neurons in the PVN. These findings suggest that *Peg3* is required for oxytocin-related nurturing behavior but do not exclude the possibility of more general defects in the mice, such as deficits in cognitive abilities, olfaction, and hypothalamic function.

The *Peg3* story may offer an additional insight. Because there is a matching of phenotypes through very different pathways (placenta and brain), this may be an example of mother–infant coevolutionary adaptation. Since it is extremely unlikely that a father could sire both a mother and her daughter, these paternally expressed *Peg3* alleles may represent transgenerational patrilineal cooperation; that is, male pups which extract maximum resources from their mothers will also provide the means for their offspring to do likewise.

In sum, gene-targeting studies have demonstrated that at least ten specific genes, including *Dbh* and *Peg3*, are necessary for the development of maternal behavior. We conclude that the basic microcircuitry responsible for mediating maternal behavior is at least, in part, genetically determined. Indeed, the limbic–hypothalamic–midbrain circuit implicated by the gene knockout studies is the same circuit identified by the classical lesion studies. Strikingly, some of the genetically mediated deficits in maternal behavior can be restored through early environmental manipulations.

EPIGENETIC INFLUENCES ON AFFILIATIVE BEHAVIOR

A growing body of work indicates that the neural "programs/circuits" contributing to subsequent maternal behavior are influenced by the intrauterine environment (Francis et al. 2003) as well as the care received in the days following birth Further, the pups' level of hypothalamic–pituitary–adrenal responsiveness to stress (Denenberg et al.1969; Francis et al. 1999; 2002; Heim and Nemeroff 2001; Levine 1975; Newport et al. 2002) seems to be established at these early stages. This complex programming also appears to influence aspects of learning and memory. Many of the brain regions implicated in these experimental interventions are the same as those identified in the knockout gene and earlier lesioning studies of maternal behavior (Leckman and Herman 2002; Numan and Insel 2003). Evidence from investigations of social primates also highlights the importance of early mothering in determining how the daughters will ultimately mother (Harlow 1963; Suomi and Ripp 1983). It is also clear that the effects of early maternal deprivation in primates may be difficult to reverse, as many maternally deprived monkeys, as adults, are able to function normally under usual conditions but are unable to cope with psychosocial stressors (Suomi et al.1976; Kraemer et al.1991). Alternatively, in rodent models environmental enrichment in the peripubertal period appears to compensate for the effects of early maternal separation (Francis et al. 2002).

One particularly compelling set of studies concerns the differential outcomes associated with the naturally occurring variations that rodent mothers display in maternal licking/grooming and arched-back nursing (Francis et al. 1999). Since the licking/grooming behavior occurs most frequently before or during arched-back nursing, the frequencies of these two behaviors are closely correlated among mothers. In a subsequent cross-fostering study, investigators determined that the amount of licking and grooming that a female pup receives in infancy is associated with how much licking and grooming she provides to her offspring as a new mother. Francis et al. (1999) reported that the low-licking and grooming dams could be transformed into high-licking and grooming dams by handling. Most impressively they also found that this change was passed on to the next generation; that is, female offspring of the low-licking, grooming dams became high-licking, grooming mothers if they were either cross-fostered by high-licking, grooming dams or if they were handled. The converse was also true, namely that the female offspring of the high-licking and grooming dams became low-licking and grooming mothers if they were cross-fostered by low-licking and grooming dams.

These naturally occurring variations in licking, grooming, and arched-back nursing have also been associated with the development of individual differences in behavioral responses to novelty in adult offspring. Adult offspring of the low-licking, grooming, and arched-back nursing mothers show increased startle responses, decreased open-field exploration, and longer latencies to eat food provided in a novel environment.

In the neurobiological arena, Francis and coworkers have demonstrated that the influence of maternal care on the development of stress reactivity was mediated by changes in gene expression in regions of the brain that regulate stress responses. For example, adult offspring of high-licking, grooming, and arched-back nursing dams showed increased hippocampal glucocorticoid receptor mRNA expression as well as increased expression of NMDA receptor subunit and brain-derived neurotrophic factor mRNA, and increased cholinergic innervation of the hippocampus. In the amygdala there are increased central benzodiazepine receptor levels in the central and basolateral nuclei. There is decreased CRH mRNA in the PVN. These adult pups also show a number of changes in receptor density in the locus coeruleus including increased α_2 adrenoreceptors, reduced GABA A receptors, and decreased CRH receptors (Caldji et al. 1998; 2000). In another study, oxytocin receptor binding levels were examined in brain sections from high- and low-licking, grooming, and arched-back nursing animals sacrificed either as nonlactating virgins or during lactation (Francis et al. 2000). Examination of the MPOA and the intermediate and ventral regions of the lateral septum disclosed that oxytocin receptor levels were significantly higher in lactating females compared with nonlactating females. Lactation-induced increases in oxytocin receptor binding were greater in high compared with low-licking, grooming, and arched-back nursing females in the BNST and ventral region of the septum. Francis and colleagues suggest, therefore, that variations in maternal behavior in the rat may be reflected in, and influenced by, differences in oxytocin receptor levels in the brain.

In the prairie vole model, there is also strong evidence that epigenetic influences can have long-lasting, possibly permanent effects on subsequent social behaviors (Carter 2003, and this volume). Even routine colony procedures, such as cage cleaning, can influence later behavior. Male prairie voles that are reared with minimal intervention during the pre-weaning period appear to be fearul in later life, which translates into deficiencies in social behaviors including reductions in alloparental behavior. Conversely, prairie voles that received additional handling, i.e., were picked up (handled, Day 1–7) once daily during the first week of life, were highly social when compared to animals handled on Day 1; after the first week of life, all animals were routinely cleaned on a weekly basis. At the age of weaning (Day 21) oxytocin levels in the PVN in animals handled daily for the first week were significantly higher animals than in animals that were handled only on Day 1 (Carter et al. 2003).

In sum, despite genetic constraints, the nature of early caregiving experiences can have enduring consequences on individual differences in subsequent maternal behavior, anxiety regulation, and patterns of stress response. Data from animal studies indicate that the interval surrounding the birth of the rat pup or the rhesus infant is a critical period in the life of the animal that likely has enduring neurobiological and behavioral consequences (Figure 15.1).

EARLY LIFE EXPERIENCE, RISK AND RESILIENCY IN HUMANS
(see Trevarthen, O'Connor, Hennighausen and Lyons-Ruth, this volume)

Building on the early work of Bowlby and colleagues (1969; 1973), efforts to characterize the reciprocal interaction in the early caregiver–infant dyad and to assess its impact have provided a powerful theoretical and empirical framework in the fields of social and emotional development (Leckman et al. 2004; Cassidy and Shaver 1999). Over the past thirty years, clear evidence has emerged that significant disturbances in the early parent–child relationship (reflected in such behavior as child abuse, neglect, or insecure attachments) contribute to an increased risk for developing both internalizing and externalizing disorders (Sroufe et al.1999). Although early adversity and insecure attachment may not be a proximal cause of later psychopathology, it appears to confer risk. Conversely, longitudinal studies of high-risk infants suggest that the formation of a special relationship with a caring adult in the perinatal period confers a degree of resiliency against the development of psychopathology later in life (Werner and Smith 2001). It is likely that in addition to affecting the key elements in the neural circuitry of affiliative behaviors, these early interactions have a profound effect on the individual's view of the world and the multiplicity of the social relationships it contains (Figure 15.1).

A growing body of evidence also indicates that human caregivers' levels of responsivity to their children can be traced in part to the caregivers' own childrearing histories and attachment-related experiences (Miller et al. 1997). Caregivers' attachment-related experiences are hypothesized to be encoded as "internal working models" of self and others that establish styles of emotional communication that either buffer the individual in times of stress or contribute to maladaptive patterns of affect regulation and behavior (Belsky, this volume; Bretherton and Munholland 1999). For example, Adult Attachment Interviews about mother's recollections of attachment-related memories (Main and Hesse 1990) were searched for indications of traumatic experiences, such as separations (e.g., hospitalization, evacuation from war-endangered cities into children camps) or loss of family members (fathers, grandparents, etc). Then their children were observed in Ainsworth's Strange Situation procedure to classify their strategies of reestablishing contact with the mother after two brief separations, each of which was no longer than three minutes. Indications of disturbance/disorganization attachment strategies were observed more frequently among the infants whose mothers had indicated the presence of such traumatic experiences in their past (Grossmann 1999).

It is important to recognize that some behaviors typically viewed as psychopathological may indeed be adaptive under certain situations. For example, an aggressive insecurely attached infant (perhaps later to become conduct disordered or remorseless) may receive more support in a neglectful environment and survive while a meek sibling would not under the same circumstances (Belsky, this volume). Indeed, such scenarios are commonplace in other primate species.

Of special interest in this context is recent theoretical and empirical work on the role of secure attachment relationship in shaping the experience and expectancies of the infant (Fonagy et al. 2002). By entering into a synchronous affective communication with the infant, the caregiver provides an external support for the infant's developing bioregulatory abilities and thereby conveys resilience to stress-coping capacities throughout life. The experience of caregiver and a child's micro-level matching of affective states and level of arousal during face-to-face interactions, which begin around the second month of life, provides the basis for children's social development, empathy, and moral internalization (Feldman et al. 1999). Maternal gaze matching, facial expressions, vocalizations, and regulation of arousal states during face-to-face play provide critical environmental inputs during the sensitive period of maturation of the visual cortex. Furthermore, by synchronizing with infant arousal state, mothers entrain the infant's biological rhythms (Lester et al.1985; Feldman, unpublished paper, Society for Research in Child Development 2003), providing a "resonance" (Trevarthen 1993, this volume) of internal and external experience, self and other, brain and behavior. Work on the detailed nature of these developmental sensitive periods of risks or resiliency enhancement for affect regulation may inform intervention programs after trauma (Heim and Nemeroff 2001; Pine and Cohen 2002), or with high-risk families (see below).

EARLY INTERVENTIONS ENHANCE PARENTAL SENSITIVITY AND CHILD ATTACHMENT SECURITY

Attachment security is a resiliency factor across the life span. In a recent meta-analysis of 88 intervention studies Bakermans-Kranenburg and colleagues (2003) found that interventions were effective in enhancing parental sensitivity and child attachment security. Interventions focused on parenting skills, social supports, or maternal well-being were significantly more successful. So were interventions that included both mother and father. Thus, the body of research on early interventions underscores the importance of devising clear-cut, short-term, behavioral interventions for a variety of at-risk populations. One caveat of this important study is that the time since the termination of treatment was not systematically evaluated. It is thus impossible to determine whether the improvement observed immediately after treatment was short-lived or had a long-term impact on risk and resiliency to later psychopathology.

Thus far there have been at least three selective intervention studies with *random assignment*, prenatal initiation, and at least one-year duration that focused on child behavioral adjustment (Leckman et al. 2004). The first set of studies was based on an intervention model that included home visits, parent meetings, and medical care (Brooks-Gunn et al. 1993; McCarton et al.1997). This intervention showed early effects at two and three years of age that attenuated by five years of age. A second intervention that also included home visits by nurses, parent meetings, and medical care showed less of an effect early on at four years of age but became significant at five and six years of age (Gutelius et al. 1972, 1977). A third set of studies, which relied on home visits by nurses, focused on low-income, unmarried mothers (that began prenatally and continued for 30 months) has shown a remarkable number of positive outcomes as late as 15 years of age including a reduced number of subsequent pregnancies, reduced use of welfare, lower rates of child abuse and neglect, and fewer arrests for criminal behavior among the offspring (Olds et al. 1997, 1998, 1999, 2002). These studies provide some of the strongest evidence to date that early intervention can make a difference in the lives of high-risk children. Although the mechanism by which these effects are achieved is unknown, Olds et al. argue that one key element is the length of time between the first and second pregnancies by the mothers participating in the home visitation program. On average, the time to the second pregnancy was more than 60 months in the experimental group that participated in the home visitation program versus less than 40 months in the comparison group. This suggests that there was the potential for a greater maternal investment in the children who were in the nurse home visitation program compared to the children born to the control-group mothers.

A recent study based in Denver by the same group of investigators documented that new mothers visited by nurses had fewer subsequent pregnancies (29% vs. 41%) and births (12% vs. 19%); they delayed subsequent pregnancies for longer intervals; and during the second year after the birth of their first child, they worked more than women in the control group (6.83 vs. 5.65 months). Nurse-visited mother–child pairs interacted with one another more responsively than those in the comparison group. At six months of age, nurse-visited infants were also less likely to exhibit emotional vulnerability in response to fearful stimuli (16% vs. 25). Remarkably at 21 months, nurse-visited children born to women with low psychological resources were less likely to exhibit language delays (7% vs. 18%); at 24 months, they exhibited superior mental development to their control-group counterparts.

In sum, data from selective early intervention programs indicate that the interval surrounding the birth of the infant is a critical period in the life of the human infant and that this likely has enduring behavioral consequences. The most compelling data suggest that these early intervention programs reduce a variety of maladaptive outcomes such as early involvement in the juvenile justice system. Less clear is the impact of these early interventions on the later rates of depression and anxiety disorders as these children reach maturity. Nor is it clear what effect these early intervention programs have on an individual's stress responsivity, susceptibility to drug abuse, or on their capacity as parental caregivers. It is also worth noting that none of these selective early intervention programs has monitored maternal preoccupations as a possible proximal predictor of individual differences in outcome (Table 15.2).

CRITIQUE OF PROPOSED MODEL

At the beginning of this chapter we offered a tentative biobehavioral model of bonding and attachment that focuses on the interface of several highly conserved neural systems involved in perception, arousal, maintenance of physiological and autonomic homeostasis, as well as reward and threat detection and response pathways. Based on the available animal and human data and while details are lacking, it appears that a compelling case can be made concerning the inherent validity of this model. In our estimation the full utility of this integrative model will only be appreciated when we are able to identify which of these biobehavioral components are active in any one range of adaptive and maladaptive outcomes. We encourage investigators to continue to explore how these systems interact with each other at each level of analysis, from the genome to metacognitive representations (Figure 15.1). Finally, the available data supports our view that this emerging model will provide a fruitful point of orientation for scientists from a range of disciplines to integrate their work and evaluate new experimental and therapeutic interventions as they develop this model and seek to inform social policy. Some specific unanswered questions include:

- What is the physiological basis of individual discrimination vis-à-vis bond formation?
- Why are some characteristics preferred over others; does the physiological status of the individual (child or adult) influence their social preferences?
- What are the molecular events that occur when there is a shift in an individual's hedonic homeostasis (as they bond to a new individual)? More specifically, how does the neurobiology of ventral striatal reward and its strong connections with prefrontal neocortex and amygdala embrace "reward" in the context of bonding?
- In humans, is the period from puberty to late adolescence the most sensitive period for forming social bonds with same-age individuals of the same and opposite sex? What physiological changes might underlie the initiation and termination of such a sensitive period?
- Why do we fall in love with a particular person and not another? What is the adaptive value of specific bonds?

Although the physiological basis and the adaptive value of a bond between a mother and her offspring is evident, it is less clear, how other bonds are adaptive (e.g., between adults of the same sex):

- How can we best study the multiplicity and dynamic interrelationships between bonds using all of the tools available to the biobehavioral scientist (Table 15.3)? Will *in vivo* neuroimaging studies have sufficient resolution to examine precisely the dynamics of bond formation, maintenance, and dissolution in humans? What are the best stimuli and ligands? There is a clear need to study the distribution of oxytocin and vasopressin receptors in humans at different points in time in the formation and maturation of parental and romantic bonds. How different are the patterns of activation for parental bonds versus romantic bonds? What is the best way to deepen our understanding of the metacognitive representations?
- Which strategies can be mobilized to respond to potential conflicts between bonds?
- Will a deeper understanding of the biology of attachment and bonding advance our understanding of religion and altruism? Will we be able to develop interventions that will reduce conflicts between larger social groups by promoting altruism and the recognition that such conflicts are self perpetuating in part through the metacognitive representations and narratives of groups in conflict?

- Will a deeper understanding of the biology of attachment and bonding advance our understanding of mentorship and teaching?
- Will a deeper understanding of the biology of attachment and bonding advance our understanding and treatment of human psychopathology? For example, it appears likely that in humans and other animals, direct applications of oxytocin can reduce both behavioral and physiological measures of stress and anxiety (Heinrichs et al. 2003).

AN URGENT PUBLIC HEALTH CONCERN

Most research by attachment theorists interested in assessing caretaking regimens have compared care at home by mother with care out of home by others, although some of this research has also looked at small home care settings. It is now time to look much more carefully at how infants respond to different kinds of allomothers in both home, but especially in out-of-home care settings. What are the attributes (including minimum attributes) of allomothers that provide infants a secure base? Ongoing work by K.E. and K. Grossmann, L. Ahnert, and W. Tietze (pers. comm.) are currently addressing such questions, yet a broader range of researchers, using various methods, is needed to pursue these topics.

A TROUBLING TREND

The current fact that approximately 15% of all children (based on U.S. statistics) fall at into the disorganized attachment category, not counting other avoidantly attached categories, is sobering (Hennighausen and Lyons-Ruth, this volume). Knowing that attachment strategies are, in many instances, passed on transgenerationally, it seems likely — even without factoring in further social chaos in the world — that the number of children in this category is going to increase. Placed in an evolutionary perspective, this ought to prompt serious self-reflection as disorganized attachment strategies are associated with a lack of empathy.

Most anthropologists define *Homo sapiens* as a bipedal hominid with language and an enormous potential for learning and culture. They speak of our human (and humane) capacity to empathize, to put ourselves cognitively and emotionally in someone else's place, even to identify emotionally with someone we have never seen (Hrdy 2002). Presumably, empathy was useful to our ancestors: it enhanced our ability to read the moods and intentions of others, increased our cooperative abilities, and played an important role in sharing, joint ventures, and reproduction. From the work of Zahn-Waxler et al. (1992), we know that this empathetic capacity is partially heritable, but it also depends on the expression of particular rearing environments (Emde et al. 1992).

So here is the problem: Heritable traits not expressed in phenotypes are invisible to selection. No matter how useful this trait has been to humans, it is not possible for selection to favor empathy if it is not expressed. In the past, children whose mothers abandoned them, or even retrenched somewhat on investment (producing disorganized or avoidantly attached kids), were unlikely to survive, although some probably did. Today, however, large predators have been eliminated and other methods for substituting aspects of maternal behavior (i.e., baby bottles and infant formulas) are in place; thus, children manage to survive a greater rate. Added to this is the probability that benefits of empathy are frequency dependent in any given population; that is, altruism is most likely to pay if one lives in a society with other altruists, not in one with a disproportionate number of "takers." This raises the question about whether our descendants' — who presumably will still be bipedal and very clever — will be "human" in the same way that we apply the term today. If we really are changing the terms of human existence in this way, perhaps we should be more aware of it. That said, it is important to recall the pogroms, ethnic cleansing, the Holocaust, fire bombing of large cities, the use of nuclear weapons against population centers, etc., as these acts are part of our cultural heritage. Part of the blame for these events rests with individuals and policy makers within governments, as they seek to acquire or hold onto power through the use of propaganda and other incentives, in an effort to manipulate human nature. It appears to be part of this nature that humans are, in turn, susceptible to the influences of such individuals; their manipulation of social bonds unites members into one group — often at the expense of other members or groups. The worry is that with less empathy and compassion, such catastrophes will become even more commonplace.

PHYSICAL HEALTH AND IMMUNE FUNCTION: AN UNDERSTUDIED AREA

Preliminary data support the view that positive bonding experiences will have a beneficial impact on physical as well as mental health. The literature on social support in humans clearly indicates that physiological changes induced by psychosocial processes (e.g., lack of social bonds or loss of a bonded person) contribute to a wide spectrum of somatic, psychosomatic, and psychiatric disorders. Positive social relationships are second, only to genetics, in predicting health and longevity in humans (Uchino et al. 1996; Seeman et al. 2002). The physiological base for these effects is, however, not really clear. Most attempts to explain these findings implicate social bonds as a source of security, with a consequent reduction in the physiological stress responses, anxiety, or arousal in challenging situations. A decreased activation of the HPA and sympathetic–adrenomedullary systems in the presence of bonded individuals during acute challenges has been demonstrated in several studies with humans and subhuman mammals compared to situations without another individual or in presence of an unbonded one. It must be pointed out that most studies have focused only on glucocorticoid secretion and/or indicators of sympathetic–adrenomedullary activity (e.g., changes in heart rate and blood pressure). Response of an organism to a challenge, however, may well include all systems, from those responsible for body growth rate and fertility to disease resistance due to immunomodulation. This stress-buffering effect of social bonds alone cannot explain the dramatic effects of intact social bonds on the health of mammals, since after the end of an acute challenge bodily functions quickly return to the former state. It is possible that social bonds exert a tonic influence on the physiological state of an organism that allows buffer the adversities of life.

Three examples are briefly discussed. In the first, consider the mating behavior of the monogamous tree shrews discussed above. What was not mentioned in earlier was that, in parallel to their mating behavior, the physiological state of both animals changes dramatically. The heart rate of both individuals decreases by up to 20%, the serum levels of glucocorticoids and the adrenocortical responsiveness to acute challenges is reduced by about 50%, the gonadal activity is increased in both individuals, and notable changes occur in all parameters of the immune system, suggesting improved resistance to disease resistance. Specifically, one finds an increase of the number of granulocytes, monocytes, lymphocytes, and their subpopulations in the blood; the phagocytotic activity of the macro- and microphages and the proliferation capacity of the T- and B-cells after mitogen-stimulation is increased by more than 100%; the production of interferon-γ and interleukin-1 is heightened; and furthermore the production of immunglobulins and the activity of the complement system are improved. Although under controlled laboratory conditions the impact of these immunological changes for the health of the animals cannot be demonstrated, under natural conditions the better immunological state might serve to protect the animals from disease or control the parasites which are thought to be the most important cause of death in all mammals under natural conditions.

Second, whereas it has been known for sometime that separation from the mother or prenatal stress can induce immunological changes in primate young (Coe 1993; Coe et al. 2002), recent evidence suggests that the mother's influence on immune function may, in turn, affect the adaptive behavior of the infant. In guinea pigs, behavior seen during the second, "despair," phase of separation appears to represent "stress-induced sickness behaviors" mediated by cytokines (Hennessy et al. 2001). In other words, nonspecific inflammatory responses typically seen during the early period of infection may also be induced by maternal separation and, through interaction of proinflammatory cytokines with neural structures, lead to reduced activity and postural changes. In unpublished work, Schiml-Webb, Hennessy, Deak, and Greenlee found that ICV administration of α melanocyte-stimulating hormone, which has widespread antiinflammatory effects, reversed the passive responses observed during prolonged separation. The mother's presence, therefore, may exert tonic influences on adaptive behavior through an indirect route involving the immune system.

The last example comes from a long-term study of European rabbits (*Oryctolagus cuniculus*) living under natural conditions in a 22,000 m^2 enclosure in Bayreuth, Germany. Rabbits live in small groups of 1–3 males and there are about twice as many females in each territory, which the males defend against intruders. The groups are kept stable by dominance hierarchies and social bonds between the males and females. Each female produces about 20 offspring per year, but about 95% of the young die in the year following their birth, before they gain reproductive maturity. Juvenile mortality during the winter period is especially important and may be regulated by social bonds. All males and about 50% of the female juveniles leave their home group in autumn and attempt to gain acceptance in other groups. At first all juveniles are attacked and driven out of the territories by the adults, but after a few days some succeed in their attempts to integrate into an existing group of adults. The immigrant juveniles form bonds (mostly with an adult female), aggressive behaviors decline, and sociopositive behavior is primarily observed towards the juveniles. Only individuals who become socially integrated in a group survive the winter. Nonintegrated juveniles die in the early winter as a result of parasitic diseases (mainly intestinal coccidiosis). The underlying physiological mechanism necessary for survival is a socially induced immunomodulation. Animals that are integrated into the social network of a group improve their immune status and are thus able to keep the ever-present parasites at a low, non-life-threatening level. In nonintegrated juveniles, the immunological resistance is greatly reduced such that after 4–6 weeks, high parasitic load is reached and death eventually results.

The mechanisms underlying these effects are not well understood. Various neuroendocrine systems known to be networked with the immune system are thought to play an immunomodulatory role. These neuroendocrine–immune interactions are bidirectional. For example, stimulated immunocytes, including B and T lymphocytes, splenocytes, and monocytes produce factors that closely resemble peptide hormones including ACTH, whereas neuropeptides such as CRH act as an inflammatory cytokine (Karalis et al. 1991; Moll 1997; Smith and Blalock 1988). Immunocytes are also known to respond with fidelity to hypothalamic-releasing factors. For example, CRH is known to stimulate the production of ACTH and endorphin in lymphocytes, which is suppressable by dexamethasone (Smith et al. 1986). A full understanding of the role of oxytocin in this bidirectional set of processes may be particularly important given its early and persistent presence in the thymus and its likely involvement in T-cell development (Geenen et al. 1999), as well as its pervasive actions throughout the nervous system, on the pituitary gland and on peripheral tissue that allows an integrated reduction of reactivity to stressors, including physical challenge and perceived threats (Carter 1998).

CONCLUSIONS

Behavioral, genetic, and neurobiological studies in model mammalian systems have the potential to inform biomedical research, clinical practice, and particularly early intervention programs for high-risk expectant parents. "Good enough" genes combined with "good enough" parental care are needed to insure positive outcomes in childhood and beyond. Among these positive outcomes is a resiliency to subsequent adversities in life, the capacity to be a good enough parent for the next generation, and possibly improved physical health. Consequently, it is possible that effective early intervention programs may have positive consequences for generations. Measures of "primary parental preoccupations" may be useful in future early intervention programs as an index of change within a key domain of functioning.

Close collaborations between clinicians and the designers of model intervention programs have been long standing. These collaborations are now beginning to include neuroimagers, developmental and behavioral neuroscientists, geneticists, and immunologists. Our capacity to study genes, the development of the brain, and the determinants of immunological health has never been stronger. Future studies should permit the examination of how successful early intervention programs influence brain development, problem-solving abilities, stress responses, as well as altering vulnerability to later mental and physical illnesses.

REFERENCES

Ainsworth, M.D.S. 1973. The development of infant–mother attachment. In: Review of Child Development Research, ed. B. Caldwell and H. Ricciuti, vol. 3, pp. 1–94. Chicago: Univ. of Chicago Press.

Akbari, E.M., D. Chatterjee, F. Levy, and A.S. Fleming. 2003. The effects of artificial rearing ("pup-in-a-cup") and maternal experience on neurogenesis in the "maternal circuit." Program No. 728.17. Washington, D.C.: Soc. for Neuroscience.

Anderson, S.W., A. Bechara, H. Damasio et al. 1999. Impairment of social and moral behaviour related to early damage in human prefrontal cortex. *Nature Neurosci.* **2**:1032–1037.

Bakermans-Kranenburg, M.J., M.H. van IJzendoorn, and F. Juffer. 2003. Less is more: Meta-analyses of sensitivity and attachment interventions in early childhood. *Psychol. Bull.* **129**:195–215.

Baron-Cohen, S. 1995/2001. Mind-Blindness: An Essay on Autism and Theory of Mind. Cambridge, MA: MIT Press.

Bechara, A., A.R. Damasio, H. Damasio et al. 1994. Insensitivity to future consequences following damage to human prefrontal cortex. *Cognition* **50**:7–15.

Belsky, J., G.B. Spanier, and M. Rovine. 1983. Stability and change in marriage across the transition to parenthood. *J. Marr. Fam.* **45**:567–577.

Beyle, M.H. 1822/1975. Love. London: Penguin.

Bowlby, J. 1969. Attachment. Attachment and Loss, vol. 1. London: Hogarth.

Bowlby, J. 1973. Separation: Anxiety and Anger. Attachment and Loss, vol. 2. New York: Basic.

Bretherton, I., and K. Munholland. 1999. Internal working models in attachment relationships: A construct revisited. In: Handbook of Attachment: Theory, Research, and Clinical Applications, ed. J. Cassidy and P. Shaver, pp. 89–111. New York: Guilford.

Bridges, R.S., M. Numan, P.M. Ronsheim et al. 1990. Central prolactin infusions stimulate maternal behavior in steroid-treated, nulliparous female rats. *PNAS* **87**: 8003–8007.

Brooks-Gunn, J., P.K. Klebanov, F. Liaw et al. 1993. Enhancing the development of low-birthweight, premature infants: Changes in cognition and behavior over the first three years. *Child Dev.* **64**:736–753.

Buteau, J., A.D. Lesage, and M.C. Kiely. 1993. Homocide followed by suicide: A Quebec case series, 1988–1990. *Can. J. Psychiatry* **38**:552–556.

Caldji, C., D. Francis, S. Sharma et al. 2000. The effects of early rearing environment on the development of GABAA and central benzodiazepine receptor levels and novelty-induced fearfulness in the rat. *Neuropsychopharm.* **22**:219–229.

Caldji, C., B. Tannenbaum, S. Sharma et al. 1998. Maternal care during infancy regulates the development of neural systems mediating the expression of fearfulness in the rat. *PNAS* **95**:5335–5340.

Caldwell, C.A., and A. Whiten. 2002. Evolutionary perspectives on imitation: Is a comparative psychology of social learning possible? *Anim. Cogn.* **5**:193–208.

Carter, C.S. 1998. Neuroendocrine perspectives on social attachment and love. *Psychoneuroendocrin.* **23**:779–818.

Carter, C.S. 2003. Developmental consequences of oxytocin. *Physiol. Behav.* **79**:383–397.

Carter, C.S., A.C. DeVries, and L.L. Getz. 1995. Physiological substrates of mammalian monogamy: The prairie vole model. *Neurosci. Biobehav. Rev.* **19**:303–314.

Carter, C.S., and E.B. Keverne. 2002. The neurobiology of social affiliation and pair bonding. In: Hormones, Brain, and Behavior, ed. D.W. Pfaff, vol. 1, pp. 299–337. San Diego: Academic.

Carter, C.S., Y. Yamamoto, K.M. Kramer et al. 2003. Long-lasting effects of early handling on hypothalamic oxytocin-immunoreactivity and responses to separation. *Soc. Neurosci. Absts.* 191.14.

Cassidy, J., and P.R. Shaver, eds. 1999. Handbook of Attachment: Theory, Research, and Clinical Applications, pp. 89–111. New York: Guilford.

Cho, M.M., A.C. DeVries, J.R. Williams et al. 1999. The effects of oxytocin and vasopressin on partner preferences in male and female prairie voles (*Microtus ochrogaster*). *Behav. Neurosci.* **113**:1071–1080.

Clutton-Brock, T.H. 1991. Evolution of Parental Care. Princeton: Princeton Univ. Press.

Coe, C.L. 1993. Psychosocial factors and immunity in nonhuman primates: A review. *Psychosom. Med.* **55**:298–308.

Coe, C.L., M. Kramer, C. Kirschbaum, P. Netter, and E. Fuchs. 2002. Prenatal stress diminishes the cytokine response of leukocytes to endotoxin stimulation in juvenile rhesus monkeys. *J. Clin. Endocrinol. Metab.* **87**:675–681.

Cowan, C.P., P.A. Cowan, G. Heming et al. 1985. Transitions to parenthood: His, hers, and theirs. *J. Fam. Iss.* **6**:451–481.

Cushing, B.S., N. Mogekwu, W.W. Le, G.E. Hoffman, and C.S. Carter. 2003. Cohabitation induced Fos immunoreactivity in the monogamous prairie vole. *Brain Res.* **965**:203–211.

Denenberg, V.H., K.M. Rosenberg, R. Paschke et al. 1969. Mice reared with rat aunts: Effects on plasma corticosterone and open-field activity. *Nature* **221**:73–74.

DeVries, A.C., M.B. DeVries, S.E. Taymans et al. 1996. Stress has sexually dimorphic effects on pair bonding in prairie voles. *PNAS* **93**:11,980–11,984.

DeVries, A.C., T. Guptaa, S. Cardillo et al. 2002. Corticotropin-releasing factor induces social preferences in male prairie voles. *Psychoneuroendocrin.* **27**:705–714.

Dulaney, S., and A.P. Fiske. 1994. Cultural rituals and obsessive-compulsive disorder: Is there a common psychological mechanism? *Ethos* **22**:243–283.

Easteal, P. 1994. Homocide-suicides between adult sexual intimates: An Australian study. *Suicide Life Threat Behav.* **24**:140–151.

Eibl-Eibesfelt, I. 1971. Love and Hate: The Natural History of Behavior Patterns. New York: Holt, Rinehart and Winston.

Eibl-Eibesfelt, I. 1989. Human Ethology. New York: Aldine de Gruyter.

Eisenberg, J.F., and D.G. Kleiman 1983. Advances in the Study of Mammalian Behavior. Shippensburg, PA: Am. Soc. Mammalogists.

Elowson, A.M., C. Snowdon, and C. Lazaro-Perea. 1998. "Babbling" and social context in infant monkeys: Parallels to human infants. *Trends Cogn. Sci.* **2**:31–37.

Emde, R.N., R. Plomin, J.A. Robinson et al. 1992. Temperament, emotion, and cognition at fourteen months: MacArthur Longitudinal Twin Study. *Child Dev.* **63**:1437–1455.

Entwisle, D.R., and S.G. Doering. 1981. The First Birth: A Family Turning Point. Baltimore: Johns Hopkins Univ. Press.

Feldman, R., and A.I. Eidelman. 2003. Direct and indirect effects of breast milk on the neurobehavioral and cognitive development of premature infants. *Dev. Psychobiol.* **43**:109–119.

Feldman, R., A. Weller, J.F. Leckman et al. 1999. The nature of the mother's tie to her infant: The formation of parent–infant bonding in healthy and at-risk dyads. *J. Child Psychol. Psychiat.* **40**:929–939.

Fleming, A.S., D.H. O'Day, and G.W. Kraemer. 1999. Neurobiology of mother–infant interactions: Experience and central nervous system plasticity across development and generations. *Neurosci. Biobehav. Rev.* **23**:673–685.

Fleming, A.S., M. Steiner, and C. Corter. 1997. Cortisol, hedonics, and maternal responsiveness in human mothers. *Horm. Behav.* **32**:85–98.

Fleming, A.S., F. Vaccarino, and C. Luebke. 1980. Amygdaloid inhibition of maternal behavior in the nulliparous female rat. *Physiol. Behav.* **25**:731–743.

Fonagy, P., G. Gergely, E.L. Jurist et al. 2002. Affect regulation, mentalization, and the development of the self. New York: Other Press.

Francis, D.D., F.C. Champagne, and M.J. Meaney. 2000. Variations in maternal behavior are associated with differences in oxytocin receptor levels in the rat. *J. Neuroendocrin.* **12**:1145–1148.

Francis, D., J. Diorio, D. Liu et al. 1999. Non-genomic transmission across generations of maternal behavior and stress responses in the rat. *Science* **286**:1155–1158.

Francis, D.D., J. Diorio, P.M. Plotsky et al. 2002. Environmental enrichment reverses the effects of maternal separation on stress reactivity. *J Neurosci.* **22**:7840–7843.

Francis, D.D., K. Szegda, G. Campbell et al. 2003. Epigenetic sources of behavioral differences in mice. *Nature Neurosci.* **6**:445–446.

Geenen, V., O. Kecha, F. Brilot, C. Charlet-Renard, and H. Martens. 1999. The thymic repertoire of neuroendocrine-related self antigens: Biological role in T-cell selection and pharmacological implications. *Neuroimmunomod.* **6**:115–125.

Givens, D.B. 1983. Love Signals: How to Attract a Mate. New York: Crown.

Grossmann, K.E. 1999. The impact of collective education on the development of children and youth: Traumatic experiences and the development of inner working models of attachment relationships. In: The Transformation of Collective Education in the Kibbutz: The End of Utopia?, ed. W. Fölling and M. Fölling-Albers, pp. 179–191. Frankfurt: Peter Lang.

Gutelius, M.F., A.D. Kirsch, S. MacDonald et al. 1972. Promising results from a cognitive stimulation program in infancy: A preliminary report. *Clin. Pediatr.* **11**:585–593.

Gutelius, M.F., A.D. Kirsch, S. MacDonald et al. 1977. Controlled study of child health supervision: Behavioral results. *Pediatrics* **60**:294–304.

Hammock, E.A.D., M.M. Lim, H.P. Nair, and L.J. Young. 2003. Genetic control of variability in brain vasopressin receptor V1a expression and behavior in prairie voles. Prog. No. 200.15. Washington, D.C.: Soc. for Neuroscience.

Hansen, S., C. Harthon, E. Wallin et al. 1991. Mesotelencephalic dopamine system and reproductive behavior in female rat: Effects of ventral tegmental 6-hydroxy-dopamine lesions on maternal and sexual responsiveness. *Behav. Neurosci.* **105**:588–598.

Harlow, H.F. 1963. The maternal affectional system of rhesus monkeys. In: Maternal Behavior in Mammals, ed. H.L. Rheingold, pp. 254–281. New York: Wiley.

Harlow, H.F., M.K. Harlow, S.J. Suomi et al. 1971. From thought to therapy: Lessons from a primate laboratory. *Am. Scientist* **59**:538–549.

Haxby, J.V., L.G. Ungerleider, V.P. Clark et al. 1999. The effect of face inversion on activity in human neural systems for face and object perception. *Neuron* **22**:189–199.

Hazan, C., and P. Shaver. 1987. Romantic love conceptualized as attachment process. *J. Pers. Soc. Psychol.* **52**:511–524.

Hazan, C., and P. Shaver. 1994. Attachment as an organizational framework for research, on close relationships. *Psychol. Inq.* **5**:1–22.

Heim, C., and C.B. Nemeroff. 2001. The role of childhood trauma in the neurobiology of mood and anxiety disorders: Preclinical/clinical studies. *Biol. Psych.* **49**:1023–1039.

Heinrichs, M.T., T. Baumgartner, C. Kirschbaum, and U. Ehlert. 2003. Social support and oxytocin interact to suppress cortisol and subjective responses to psychosocial stress. *Biol. Psych.* **54**:1389–1398.

Hennessy, M.B., T. Deak, and P.A. Schiml-Webb. 2001. Stress-induced sickness behaviors: An alternative hypothesis for responses during maternal separation. *Dev. Psychobiol.* **39**:76–83.

Horton, D. 1957. The dialog of courtship in popular songs. *Am. J. Sociol.* **62**:569–578.

Hrdy, S.B. 1999. Mother Nature: A History of Mothers, Infants and Natural Selection. New York: Pantheon.

Hrdy, S.B. 2002. On why it takes a village: Cooperative breeders, infant needs and the future, Part II of: The Past, the present and the future of the human family. In: Tanner Lectures on Human Values, vol. 23, pp. 57–110. Salt Lake City, UT: Utah Press.

Ingram, D. 1989. First Language Acquisition: Method, Description, and Explanation. Cambridge: Cambridge Univ. Press.

Jankowiak, W.R., and E.F. Fischer. 1992. A cross-cultural perspective on romantic love. *Ethnology* **31**:149–155.

Kanwisher, N., J. McDermott, and M.M. Chu. 1997. The fusiform face area: A module in human extrastriate cortex specialized for face perception. *J. Neurosci.* **17**:4302–4311.

Karalis, K., H. Sano, J. Redwine et al. 1991. Autocrine or paracrine inflammatory actions of corticotropin-releasing hormone in vivo. *Science* **254**:421–423.

Kelly, H.H. 1983. Love and commitment. In: Close Relationships, ed. H.H. Kelly, pp. 265–314. New York: Freeman.

Kent, R.D., and G. Miolo. 1995. Phonetic abilities in the first year of life. In: Handbook of Child Language, ed. P. Fletcher and B. MacWhinney, p. 303–334. Oxford: Blackwell.

Koob, G.F., and M. Le Moal. 1997. Drug abuse: Hedonic homeostatic dysregulation. *Science* **278**:52–58.

Kraemer, G.W. 1992. A psychobiological theory of attachment. *Behav. Brain Sci.* **15**:493–511.

Kraemer, G.W., M.H. Ebert, D.E. Schmidt, and W.T. McKinney. 1991. Strangers in a strange land: A psychobiological study of infant monkeys before and after separation from real or inanimate mothers. *Child Dev.* **62**:548–566.

Kuroiwa, Y., T. Kaneko-Ishino, F. Kagitani et al. 1996. *Peg3* imprinted gene on proximal chromosome 7 encodes for a zinc finger protein. *Nature Genet.* **12**:186–190.

Leckman, J.F., R. Feldman, J.E. Swain et al. 2004. Primary parental preoccupation: Neurohormonal circuits, genes, and the crucial role of the environment. *J. Neur. Trans.* **111**:753–771.

Leckman, J.F., and A. Herman. 2002. Maternal behavior and developmental psychopathology. *Biol. Psych.* **51**:27–43.

Leckman, J.F., and L.C. Mayes. 1999. Preoccupations and behaviors associated with romantic and parental love: Perspectives on the origin of obsessive-compulsive disorder. *Child Adoles. Psych. Clins. N. Am.* **8**:635–665.

Leckman, J.F., L.C. Mayes, R. Feldman et al. 1999. Early parental preoccupations and behaviors and their possible relationship to the symptoms of obsessive-compulsive disorder. *Acta Psychiatrica Scand.* **396(100)**:1–26.

Lester, B.M., J. Hoffman, and T.B. Brazelton. 1985. The rhythmic structure of mother–infant interaction in term and preterm infants. *Child Dev.* **56**:15–27.

Levine, S. 1975. Psychosocial factors in growth and development. In: Society, Stress and Disease, ed. L. Levi, pp. 43–50. London: Oxford Univ. Press.

Li, L.L., E.B. Keverne, S.A. Aparicio et al. 1999. Regulation of maternal behavior and offspring growth by paternally expressed *Peg3*. *Science* **284**:330–333.

Liberzon, I., and E.A. Young. 1997. Effects of stress and glucocorticoids on CNS oxytocin receptor binding. *Psychoneuroendocrin.* **22**:411–422.

Liman, E.R., and H. Innan. 2003. Relaxed selective pressure on an essential component of pheromone transduction in primate evolution. *PNAS* **100**:3328–3332.

Lorberbaum, J.P., J.D. Newman, A.R. Horwitz et al. 2002. A potential role for thalamocingulate circuitry in human maternal behavior. *Biol. Psych.* **51**:431–445.

Main, M., and E. Hesse. 1990. Parents' unresolved traumatic experiences are related to infant disorganized attachment status: Is frightened and/or frightening parental behavior the linking mechanism? In: Attachment in the Preschool Years: Theory, Research and Intervention, ed. M. Greenberg, D. Cicchetti, and E.M. Cummings, pp. 161–184. Chicago: Univ. of Chicago Press.

Mann, J. 1992. Nurturance or negligence: Maternal psychology and behavior preference among pre-term twins. In: The Adapted Mind, ed. J. Barkow et al., pp. 367–390. New York: Oxford Univ. Press.

Mason, W.A. 1974. Differential grouping patterns in two species of South American monkey. In: Ethology and Psychiatry, ed. N.F. White, pp. 153–169. Toronto: Univ. of Toronto Press.

Marzuk, P.M., K. Tardiff, and C.S. Hirsch. 1992. The epidemiology of murder-suicide. *JAMA* **267**:3179–3183.

Matthiesen, A.S., A.B. Ransjo-Arvidson, and E. Nissen. 2001. Postpartum maternal oxytocin release by newborns: Effects of infant hand massage and sucking. *Birth* **28**:13–19.

McCarton, C.M., J. Brooks-Gunn, I.F. Wallace et al. 1997. Results at age 8 years of early intervention for low-birth-weight premature infants: The Infant Health and Development Program. *JAMA* **277**:126–132.

Meltzoff, A.N., and W. Prinz. 2002. The Imitative Mind: Developmental, Evolution and Brain Bases. Cambridge: Cambridge Univ. Press.

Miller, L., R. Kramer, V. Warner et al. 1997. Intergenerational transmission of parental bonding among women. *J. Am. Acad. Child Adoles. Psych.* **36**:1134–1139.

Minde, K., C. Corter, S. Goldberg et al. 1990. Maternal preference between premature twins up to age four. *J. Am. Acad. Child Adoles. Psych.* **29**:367–374.

Moll, U.M. 1997. Functional histology of the neuroendocrine thymus. *Microsc. Res. Tech.* **38**:300–310.

Morris, D. 1967. Intimate Behavior. New York: Bantam.

Newport, D.J., Z.N. Stowe, and C.B. Nemeroff. 2002. Parental depression: Animal models of an adverse life event. *Am. J. Psych.* **159**:1265–1283.

Nissen, E., G. Lilja, A.J. Widstrom et al. 1995. Elevation of oxytocin levels early post partum in woman. *Acta Obstet. Gynecol. Scand.* **74**:530–533.

Numan, M. 1994. Maternal behavior. In: The Physiology of Reproduction, ed. E. Knobil and J.F. Neill, pp. 221–301. New York: Raven.

Numan, M., and T.R. Insel. 2003. The Neurobiology of Maternal Care. New York: Springer.

Numan, M., J.S. Rosenblatt, and B.R. Kiminsaruk. 1997. Medial preoptic area and onset of maternal behavior in the rat. *J. Comp. Physiol. Psychol.* **91**:146–164.

Numan, M., and T.P. Sheehan. 1997. Neuroanatomical circuitry for mammalian maternal behavior. *Ann. NY Acad. Sci.* **807**:101–125.

Olds, D.L., J. Eckenrode, C.R..Henderson, Jr., et al. 1997. Long-term effects of home visitation on maternal life course and child abuse and neglect: Fifteen-year follow-up of a randomized trial. *JAMA* **278**:637–643.

Olds, D., C.R. Henderson, Jr., R. Cole et al. 1998. Long-term effects of nurse home visitation on children's criminal and antisocial behavior: 15-year follow-up of a randomized controlled trial. *JAMA* **280**:1238–1244.

Olds, D.L., C.R. Henderson, Jr., H.J. Kitzman et al. 1999. Prenatal and infancy home visitation by nurses: Recent findings. *Future Child* 9:44–65; 190–191.

Olds, D.L., J. Robinson, R. O'Brien et al. 2002. Home visiting by paraprofessionals and by nurses: A randomized, controlled trial. *Pediatrics* **110**:486–496.

Papousek, H., U. Jurgens, and M. Papousek, eds. 1991. Nonverbal Vocal Communication: Comparative and Developmental Approaches. Cambridge: Cambridge Univ. Press.

Pedersen, C.A. 1997. Oxytocin control of maternal behavior: Regulation by sex steroids and offspring stimuli. *Ann. NY Acad. Sci.* **807**:126–145.

Pedersen, C.A., J.D. Caldwell, C. Walker et al. 1994. Oxytocin activates the postpartum onset of rat maternal behavior in the ventral tegmental and medial preoptic areas. *Behav. Neurosci.* **108**:1163–1171.

Pedersen, C.A., and A.J. Prange. 1979. Induction of maternal behavior in virgin rats after intracerebroventricular administration of oxytocin. *PNAS* **76**:6661–6665.

Perper, T. 1985. Sex Signals: The Biology of Love. Philadelphia: ISI Press.

Pine, D.S., and J.A. Cohen. 2002. Trauma in children and adolescents: Risks and treatment of psychiatric sequelae. *Biol. Psych.* **51**:519–531.

Pryce, C.R., D. Bettschen, and J. Feldon. 2001. Comparison of the effects of early handling and early deprivation on maternal care in the rat. *Dev. Psychobiol.* **38**:239–251.

Robin, M., H. Kheroua, and I. Casati. 1992. Effects of early mother–twin relationships from birth to age 3, on twin bonding. *Acta Genet. Med. Gemellol.* **41**:143–148.

Rolls, E.T. 2000. The orbitofrontal cortex and reward. *Cereb. Cortex* **10**:284–294.

Rosenblatt, J.S. 1967. Nonhormonal basis of maternal behavior in the rat. *Science* **158**:1512–1514.

Rosenblatt, J.S., and D.S. Lehrman. 1963. Maternal behavior in the laboratory rat. In: Maternal Behavior in Mammals, ed. H.L. Rheingold, pp. 8–57. New York: Wiley.

Russell, J.A., G. Leng, and A.J. Douglas. 2003. The magnocellular oxytocin system, the fount of maternity: Adaptations in pregnancy. *Front. Neuroendocrin.* **24**:27–61.

Scheffler, H.W., and F.G. Lounsbury. 1971. A Study in Structural Semantics: The Sirionó Kinship System. Englewood Cliffs, NJ: Prentice-Hall.

Seeman, T.E., B.H. Singer, C.D. Ryff, G. Dienberg Love, and L. Levy-Storms. 2002. Social relationships, gender, and allostatic load across two age cohorts. *Psychosom. Med.* **64**:395–406.

Shea, J.A., and G.R. Adams. 1984. Correlates of romantic attachment: A path analysis study. *J. Youth Adoles.* **13**:27–44.

Sheehan, T.P., J. Cirrito, M.J. Numan et al. 2000. Using c-fos immunocyto-chemistry to identify forebrain regions that may inhibit maternal behavior in rats. *Behav. Neurosci.* **114**:337–352.

Smith, E.M., and J.E. Blalock. 1988. A molecular basis for interactions between the immune and neuroendocrine systems. *Intl. J. Neurosci.* **38**:455–464.

Smith, E.M., A.C. Morrill, W.J. Meyer, and J.E. Blalock. 1986. Corticotropin releasing factor induction of leukocyte-derived immunoreactive ACTH and endorphins. *Nature* **321**:881–882.

Sofroniew, M.V., and A. Weindl. 1981. Central nervous system distribution of vasopressin, oxytocin, and neurophysin. In: Endogenous Peptides and Learning and Memory Processes, ed. J.L. Martinez et al., pp. 327–369. New York: Academic.

Sroufe, L.A., E.A. Carlson, A.K. Levy et al. 1999. Implications of attachment theory for developmental psychopathology. *Dev. Psychopathol.* **11**:1–13.

Sternberg, R.J. 1986. A triangular theory of love. *Psychol. Rev.* **93**:119–135.

Suomi, S.J., R. Delizio, and H.F. Harlow. 1976. Social rehabilitation of separation-induced depressive disorders in monkeys. *Am. J. Psych.* **133**:1279–1285.

Suomi, S.J., and C. Ripp. 1983. A history of motherless mothering at the University of Wisconsin Primate Laboratory. In: Child Abuse: The Non-human Data, ed. M. Reite and N. Caine, pp. 49–78. New York: A.R. Liss.

Swanson, L.W. 2000. Cerebral hemisphere regulation of motivated behavior. *Brain Res.* **886**:113–164.

Teicher, M.H., and E.M. Blass. 1977. First suckling response of the newborn albino rat: The roles of olfaction and amniotic fluid. *Science* **198**:635–636.

Tennov, D. 1979. Love and Limerence: The Experience of Being in Love. New York: Stein and Day.

Tesser, A., and D.L. Paulhus. 1976. Toward a causal model of love. *J. Pers. Soc. Psychol.* **34**:1095–1105.

Thomas, S.A., A.M. Matsumoto, and R.D. Palmiter. 1995. Noradrenaline is essential for mouse fetal development. *Nature* **374**:643–646.

Thomas, S.A., and R.D. Palmiter. 1997. Impaired maternal behavior in mice lacking norepinephrine and epinephrine. *Cell* **91**:583–592.

Tomasello, M. 1999. The Cultural Origins of Human Cognition, chap. 6: Discourse and representational redescription. Cambridge, MA: Harvard Univ. Press.

Tomasello, M., and J. Call. 1997. Primate Cognition. Oxford: Oxford Univ. Press.

Trevarthen, C. 1993. The self born in intersubjectivity: The psychology of an infant communicating. In: The Perceived Self: Ecological and Interpersonal Sources of Self-knowledge, ed. U. Neisser, pp. 121–173. New York: Cambridge Univ. Press.

Tzourio-Mazoyer, N., S. De Schonen, F. Crivello et al. 2002. Neural correlates of woman face processing by 2-month old infants. *NeuroImage* **15**:454–461.

Uchino, B.N., J. Holt-Lunstad, D. Uno, R. Betancourt, and T.S. Garvey. 1996. Social support and age-related differences in cardiovascular function: An examination of potential mediators. *Ann. Behav. Med.* **21**:135–142.

Uvnas-Moberg, K. 1998. Oxytocin may mediate the benefits of positive social interaction and emotions. *Psychoneuroendocrin.* **23**:819–835.

Van Leengoed, E., E. Kerker, and H.H. Swanson. 1987. Inhibition of postpartum maternal behavior in the rat by injecting an oxytocin antagonist into the cerebral ventricles. *J. Endocrinol.* **112**:275–282.

Werner, E.E., and R.S. Smith. 2001. Journeys from Childhood to Midlife: Risk, Resilience, and Recovery. Ithaca, NY: Cornell Univ. Press.

Winnicott, D.W. 1956/1975. Primary maternal preoccupation. In: Collected Papers: Through Paediatrics to Psycho-Analysis, pp. 300–305. New York: Basic.

Winslow, J.T., N. Hastings, C.S. Carter, C.R. Harbaugh, and T.R. Insel. 1993. A role for central vasopressin in pair bonding in monogamous prairie voles. *Nature* **365**:545–548.

Young, L.J. 1999. Frank A. Beach Award: Oxytocin and vasopressin receptors and species-typical social behaviors. *Horm. Behav.* **36**:212–221.

Zahn-Waxler, C., J.L. Robinson, and R.N. Emde. 1992. The development of empathy in twins. *Dev. Psychol.* **28**:1038–1037.

Zinaman, M.J., V. Hughes, J.T. Queenan et al. 1992. Acute prolactin and oxytocin responses and milk yield to infant suckling and artificial methods of expression in lactating women. *Pediatrics* **89**:437–440.

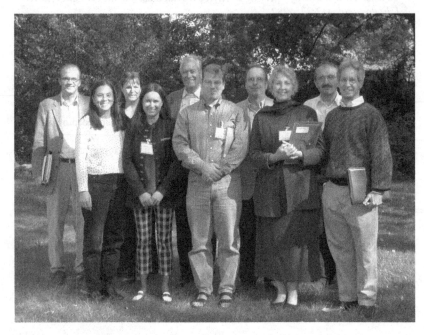

Back, left to right: Markus Heinrichs, Heidi Keller, Klaus Grossmann, Eckart Voland,
   Gottfried Spangler
Front, left to right: Sheila Wang, Katharina Braun, Tom O'Connor, Megan Gunnar,
   Ross Thompson

16

Group Report: Early Social Attachment and Its Consequences

The Dynamics of a Developing Relationship

R. A. THOMPSON, Rapporteur

K. BRAUN, K. E. GROSSMANN, M. R. GUNNAR, M. HEINRICHS,
H. KELLER, T. G. O'CONNOR, G. SPANGLER,
E. VOLAND, and S. WANG

ABSTRACT

The origins and consequences of early social attachments are long-standing interests of developmental scientists that have been enlivened through the integrative contributions of psychobiological research. Among the issues to emerge in this integrative work are:

- A better understanding of the behavioral and biological prerequisites for forming first attachments in infancy, and how these are reorganized when first attachments must develop later than is species-typical, or under atypical conditions.
- A better understanding of how attachment develops in different cultural settings within the context of the biologically adaptive requirements of inclusive fitness.
- A clearer conceptualization of the interaction between behavioral experience and psychobiological development with respect to how early caregiving shapes infant regulatory capacities, and how these influences become progressively updated through new caregiving experiences.
- Greater theoretical clarification of how attachment continues to develop beyond infancy, and the representations associated with this developmental process, in concert with the development of new measures and methods for assessing attachment at later ages.
- More systematic inquiry into the internal and external processes mediating continuity and change in attachment relationships over time, and the identification of the expectable consequences of early attachment relationships for both behavioral and psychobiological organization.
- The integration of biological and behavioral insights into the most compelling question of all: How does early experience influence later behavior?

INTRODUCTION

The origins and consequences of infant–mother attachment have consumed the interest of philosophers for centuries and of developmental scientists through-out psychology's short history. This is because the developmental dynamics of this primary relationship provide a forum for examining questions of enduring interest: How formative are early experiences for psychological development? What are the influences underlying continuity and change in early personality growth? How does the first relationship shape later relational experience? In addressing these questions, the formulations of developmental theory can be integrated with the findings of biobehavioral studies that examine attachment development from the perspective of the psychobiological systems in the infant and mother. Results of this integrative work form the basis for new insights and inquiry addressed in this chapter.

UNDERSTANDING EARLY ATTACHMENT

Forming relationships with primary caregivers is one of the most important developmental tasks of the early months in many species. These relationships are bidirectional; that is, characteristics of both infant and caregiver are important in forming and maintaining the relationship, and the relationship affects the development of both partners. A central facet of the relationship between an infant and primary caregiver is their "attachment." However, the diversity in how specific attachment relationships are formed for members of different species, and for humans of different cultures, requires a careful examination of what is meant by this term. Are there specific, unique defining features of attachment relationships (distinct from other kinds of social affiliations) that are shared across species and cultures? If we can identify common elements, then we can begin to explore their common (or shared) neurobiology, and this information can provide insights into the ontogeny of these behavioral patterns and their association with other adaptive systems. What makes an individual an attachment figure for another individual? What are the behavioral or physiological indices that reliably indicate that an attachment relationship exists for an infant or young animal? What are the functions served by attachment figures? In many species, and especially in humans, attachment figures serve many roles (e.g., protector, playmate, teacher), but these roles are also assumed by other individuals to whom a child may not be attached. Is it possible to identify the specific, unique functions that attachment figures alone provide the child and caregiver?

In addressing these questions, it is important to distinguish different facets of the term *attachment*. First, there is an *attachment system*, which may be conceived as a behavioral or motivational system (in attachment theory) or a module (in modularity theory) with specific information-processing functions serving attachment functioning. An attachment system evaluates and integrates information, for example, concerning (a) the partner in the relationship, such as a baby or caregiver, (b) one's internal state relevant to relational activity (e.g., competing or complementary motives and needs), and (c) environmental conditions (e.g., social support, material and emotional resources). Second, there are *attachment behaviors*, which are the behavioral results of the functioning of the attachment system: how attachment figures act in relation to each other. Third, there is an *attachment relationship*, which is the interpersonal history and functioning of attachment behavior. Individual differences in the quality or security of attachment relationships have been of particular interest to students of human attachments in childhood. Because the term *attachment* is commonly used to refer to each of these facets, however, it is easy for developmental scientists to be needlessly confused about the use of the term.

Attachment and bonding are related concepts (Ainsworth 1985). *Bonding* typically refers to the establishment of an emotional connection of the mother to the infant, often shortly after birth, that is closely tied to the hormonal processes associated with birth. As we discuss below, the release of oxytocin and other hormones at parturition biologically primes many physical and behavioral aspects of caregiving in adults of many animal species, including humans. The process of bonding, especially of the mother to the baby, shortly after birth sets the stage for the development of attachment, which develops later in infancy as a mutual relationship shared by caregiver and offspring. Bonding is not essential to attachment (as studies of adoptive parents show) but typically leads to attachment in most mother–infant dyads.

Developmental scientists from different disciplines typically approach the phenomenon of attachment from various orientations. Scientists studying the neurobiological substrates of attachment or attachment relationships in nonhuman populations are interested in attachment as a normative phenomenon and seek to clarify its origins and outcomes. Researchers studying humans more often focus on individual differences in attachment relationships and their consequences. In each case, conceptualizations of attachment permit analyses of how these relationships contribute to support, security, and the regulation of one or both partners. Ethological studies of pair bonding emphasize analyses of whether two animals have established a pair bond and the processes (behavioral and neurobiological) that contribute to the formation of the bond. Both behavioral and neurobiological approaches are required to understand the disturbances in relationship formation of individuals whose early environments and experiences deviate sufficiently from the expectable environment that they cannot form a normal attachment relationship at the species-typical time.

Attachment in Mothers

The formation of a specific, unique relationship between an infant and an adult begins before birth, and its bidirectional character is evident early. In mammals, for example, there is a biological priming of the physical and behavioral aspects of becoming a mother. Progesterone levels are high during pregnancy and decrease toward the end of pregnancy; estrogen levels increase to promote the synthesis of oxytocin receptors (Keverne, this volume). Oxytocin[1] is critical for stimulating uterine contractions during labor and for the ejection of milk. During birth, there is a massive release of oxytocin, a hormone which has also been shown to facilitate maternal behavior (Pedersen and Prange 1979) and formation of selective social bonds in some mammals (Carter 1998).

A major factor in establishing maternal behavior in mammals appears to be the shift in motivational processes toward selective reinforcement of maternal behavior (e.g., nursing, infant grooming, infant retrieval, physical contact, and protection of the infant), which are relevant to the infant's early physiological regulation, well-being, and survival. Research on the endogenous opioid, dopamine, and oxytocin systems in relation to maternal behavior and the formation of social bonds indicates that these three systems are likely to be involved in the predisposition to bond, which is related to a dramatic change in the reinforcing properties of mother–infant interaction for the mother (e.g., Aragona et al. 2003). Blocking opioid receptors with naloxone in postpartum rhesus monkeys reduces maternal initiation of caregiving and protective behavior toward the infant, including grooming and infant retrieval (Martel et al. 1993). Blocking opioids in sheep also blocks oxytocin release (Keverne, this volume). Blocking oxytocin receptors has been shown to decrease maternal behavior in mammals, including decreasing the percentage of time a mother rat grooms her infant compared to the time she grooms herself (Pedersen and Boccia 2002). Dopamine–oxytocin interactions have been implicated in the formation of social bonds in some mammals, and it has been proposed (Insel 2003) that the rewarding effects of dopamine could be related to the strong positive emotional feelings associated with the formation of social bonds.

In primates, compared to smaller-brained animals, there may be less exclusive reliance on these hormonal systems and more reliance on experiential and cognitive influences to initiate a shift to preferential reinforcement of caregiver–infant interactions; this may also allow nonbiological mothers and other individuals to provide high-quality caregiving. However, pregnancy and birthing still supply significant biological priming in all primates to facilitate the mother–infant bonding process. But understanding better the nature of the interaction between neurohormonal systems and the influences of particular

---

[1] Oxytocin is synthesized in magnocellular neurons of the paraventricular and supraoptic nuclei of the hypothalamus (Swaab et al. 1975; Vandesande and Dierickx 1975). It is processed from precursor forms, together with carrier proteins, along the axonal projection to the posterior pituitary, from which the peptide is secreted into the systemic circulation (Brownstein et al. 1980). Oxytocin is widely distributed throughout the central nervous system from smaller parvocellular neurons and influences many neurobehavioral functions (de Wied et al. 1993; McCarthy and Altemus 1997).

experiences and related cognitions and attributions is an important task of research concerning the development of maternal behavior in humans. This is particularly so since experiential influences (e.g., the absence of social support) and cognitive factors (e.g., the self-attributions associated with maternal depression) may function contrarily to the biological primes that would ordinarily help to activate maternal behavior, resulting in more troubled early mother–child interactions and disruptions in the bonding process.

Attachment in Offspring

The development of an attachment relationship is an extended developmental process for offspring, and research in this area has focused more on behavioral than hormonal processes (for reviews, see Cassidy and Shaver 1999; Colin 1996; Lamb et al. 1985; Thompson 2006). The extended process of attachment owes not only to the child's physical and socio-emotional immaturity. If one of the distinctive features of attachment entails an individualized relationship from which the baby can predict and form expectations for the partner's behavior, cognitive advances are necessary before the child can generalize broader social expectations from specific event representations of a particular partner. Several achievements must occur: Cognitively, the infant must be capable of recognizing the adult's voice, face, and/or other features, integrate these features into a perceptual whole, and identify the attachment figure consistently across different contexts. Affectively, the infant must begin to associate the caregiver's presence with distress relief, heightened pleasure or joy, and/or other qualities that contribute to a preference for the attachment figure's stimulus characteristics. In this respect, the child must also develop an awareness of the contingencies that exist between the child's behavior and social responses from the adult. A history of shared experiences is required to enable infants to develop these cognitive capacities and affective expectancies, of course, but there is evidence that this begins to develop quite early. Between three and six months of age, for example, infants reveal a generalized expectancy that others will respond to their initiatives in the "still face" paradigm (in which infants respond positively to their mothers' interactive behavior but become withdrawn, more sober, and behaviorally provocative when their mothers are instructive to be impassive to them). During the second half of the first year, a distressed infant will sooth to the sound of the mother's distinctive footsteps as she approaches to provide comfort (Cohn et al. 1991; Gekoski et al. 1983; Lamb and Malkin 1986). In general, infants respond with positive emotion to their perception of social contingency from early in the first year (Watson 1972, 1979).

All of these prerequisites for developing attachment relationships are evident in the young infant's responses to attachment figures, but some of these responses are also displayed with familiar figures to whom the baby is not attached. There are other elements to attachment formation that are likely to be more specific to the attachment figure. One is the adult's privileged influence over the infant's developing neurobiological regulatory systems, which arises through repeated shared interactions: feeding, soothing, play, and other experiences involving arousal and its regulation. Owing to the frequency with which the caregiver manages the baby's positive and negative arousal, the adult's responsiveness becomes a salient and important influence on the child's biobehavioral regulation and experience of well-being (Gunnar, this volume; Gunnar 2000; Gunnar and Donzella 2002). Together with the cognitive expectancies in the baby created by these recurrent (daily) experiences, this contributes to the qualities that may make attachment relationships distinct from others to the baby: they are individualized relationships from which the infant develops expectancies for the partner's behavior that help to define the affective quality of their relationship, afford security, and contribute to the child's self-regulation.

Other potentially important developmental influences also contribute to the initial creation of attachment relationships. Joint attention is probably central to the interactive experiences leading to attachment, especially as it relates to the child's growing capacity for intersubjectivity and developing understanding of the mother as a person (e.g., Harris 1996; Tomasello 1999). The role of self-produced locomotion, which has been shown to be an important influence on affective development and parent–child relations late in the first year, may also be relevant to the development of attachment as well as to the growth of security or insecurity within this relationship (Campos et al. 1992). In short, although attachment researchers have devoted considerable attention to the origins of individual differences in attachment, much more work is needed to elucidate how and why attachment develops initially and the ontogenetic processes in brain and behavior that cause infants to become attached to their caregivers.

What are the behavioral indicators of attachment in the young? It appears that behaviors such as recognizing the mother (her face, voice, and/or smell) and joint attention — and the experiences of intersubjectivity with which they are associated — may contribute to the development of an attachment relationship but are not, in themselves, definitive because they are also displayed with non-attachment figures. On the other hand, a large literature on attachment in infancy has developed during the past thirty years that enlists the 12-month-old baby's responses to separation and reunion with the mother (within the Strange Situation procedure) as an index of attachment (for reviews, see Cassidy and Shaver 1999; Lamb et al. 1985). The problem here is the variability in cultural child-rearing conditions that make short separations differentially stressful for one-year-olds (indeed, to mothers of some cultures, the extent of normative separation between mother and baby required in most Western societies might be regarded as abusive) (Thompson 2006). Other indices of attachment that are likely to be differential to the attachment figure include monitoring the physical location of the adult, developing strategies for reestablishing proximity and contact with that figure when needed (with "psychological access" substituting for physical contact with increasing age), the reallocation of attention and effort from other interests to reestablishing contact or access when it is precluded, and preferentially seeking contact or access to the attachment figure under conditions of threat or stress. These reflect how the attachment figure functions as a "secure base" as well as a haven of safety for the child under stress. In addition, the child's "affective sharing" (i.e., making social contact for purposes of conveying pleasure in a discovery or achievement) may also be an important marker of the existence of an attachment relationship in infants and young children (Ainsworth et al. 1978).

It is clear that the behavioral markers of an attachment relationship will be developmentally flexible and somewhat different in the years from birth to adolescence based on the changing cognitive, social, and emotional capabilities of the child, but they are likely to share in common reliance on attachment figures as supportive havens for exploration, a secure base during stress, and assistance in developing self-regulation. Indeed, although attachment theorists vary in their underlying conceptions of the psychological qualities definitive of attachment relationships (e.g., the emphasis on secure base behavior of theorists like Waters and Cummings [2000] compared with the focus on the adult as a haven of safety by others; see Thompson and Raikes [2003]), children are likely to rely on attachment figures for all of these reasons. Candidate indices for the development of an attachment relationship in older children are important both for normative reasons (children often form new attachments to individuals like stepparents) and for clinical reasons (such as indexing attachment in children whose aberrant early experiences have precluded the creation of reliable adult relationships). Such behaviors might include: (a) monitoring the well-being of the attachment figure (e.g., concern over that person's health, injury or harm), (b) motivation to maintain the self as a valued figure to the adult (e.g., sharing accomplishments with that person and the salience of the adult's expressions of pride or disinterest in those accomplishments), and (c) competition for the attention of the attachment figure in preference to others of interest to the adult (such as other offspring or adult partners). Although we might colloquially call the latter "jealousy," the activation of attention-seeking behaviors in these circumstances probably reflects the development of a differentiated, exclusive emotional attachment to a specific, valued person.

Clearly, considerable theoretical and empirical work is needed to understand better the indicators that an attachment relationship has developed between a caregiver and a child. It is apparent, however, that there is no rich literature on the developing biological foundations of human attachment in the infant, comparable to the extensive understanding of the hormonal determinants of bonding in the mother. It would be especially desirable, therefore, to have greater knowledge of specific brain systems whose maturation is relevant to the unfolding of attachment relationships early in life, and which humans may share with other primate species and, indeed, with other mammalian species. This constitutes a pressing research need for the future.

Development of a Bidirectional Relationship

Cross-culture research of humans instructs us that infants develop attachment relationships with multiple caregivers and that, in many cultures, caregivers other than the mother care for the young and elicit responses consistent with an attachment to them. The behavioral propensities that cause a caregiver to become an attachment figure vary across species and, within humans, cross-culturally because of the variety of ecological and cultural constraints and incentives that define caregiving. Among these influences are the availability of cooperative conspecifics who can function as alloparents (Hrdy, this volume), subsistence strategies and workload (Blurton Jones 1993; Hurtado et al. 1992; Panter-Brick 1995), and the condition and needs of the infant. All of these shape the environmental context in which care occurs. What remains unclear in many studies is the degree to which the childcare strategies found in different cultures represent adaptive choices or environmental constraints. To clarify this, detailed knowledge of the costs and benefits of various childcare options are necessary to determine more precisely parents' trade-off problems. This knowledge is necessary to recognize the outcomes of parenting favored by natural selection: maximization of production of offspring, of their survivorship, or of their social and material endowment (Blurton Jones 1993).

In the human attachment literature, particular attention has been devoted to variations in maternal responsiveness and sensitivity as a major proximate (or psychological) determinant of the formation of attachment relationships and, especially, of variations in the child's sense of security within those attachments (Ainsworth et al. 1978; De Wolff and van IJzendoorn 1997). Most recently, a cognitive construct called maternal "mind-mindedness" has been studied as a complement of maternal sensitivity (Meins et al. 2001). Although maternal sensitivity must itself be expressed in culturally specific ways, its importance reflects the safe haven/secure base/supporting self-regulation features of attachment relationships highlighted above.

Beyond this, it is apparent that the attachment system is robust or, in evolutionary terms, highly canalized. Even in aberrant and abusive conditions of care (e.g., those of Romanian orphanage children or others subjected to neglectful institutional care), the majority of children manage to create attachments to new caregivers after their rescue (indexed by criteria like those discussed above), often long after the normative developmental period for creating first attachments has passed, although many children still have lingering sequelae (O'Connor, this volume). This reflects a system that is both resilient and, in the context of cultural variability in normative conditions of child care, flexible.

EARLY ATTACHMENT AND INCLUSIVE FITNESS

Behavioral and neurobiological studies of attachment in mother and infant are theoretically framed by the assumption that attachment evolved as an adaptation to promote the inclusive fitness of each partner. It is thus important to inquire about how attachment processes relate to the reproductive success and inclusive fitness of mother and baby.

In the case of the infant, the answer seems clear. It is beneficial to remain close to, and to elicit the proximity of, mature conspecifics who are likely to provide protection, nurturance, developmental guidance, and other survival-related forms of assistance when nearby. It follows, therefore, that infants are likely to be biologically organized to strive to obtain maximal resources from the caregiver, assuming that the caregiver is both willing and capable of providing these resources for her offspring.

Fitness considerations for the mother in forming attachments to offspring are more complicated. Promoting the survival, health, and well-being of each child contributes to the mother's lifetime reproductive success. However, maternal energy and other resources to invest in reproduction are finite and must be divided between the demands of multiple offspring and the mother's own physical requirements, including her own future reproductive potential. Consequently, the determinants of maternal investment in any particular offspring are complex, based in part on characteristics of the child (health, intactness), the presence of other offspring, environmental resources (e.g., social support), and the mother herself.

Norms for infant care vary across cultures, but within populations, mothers may also vary in their commitment to offspring depending on their circumstances. In adversity, mothers may retrench their investment or even terminate it altogether by abandoning or even eliminating offspring through infanticide. Across traditional societies, rates of infanticide vary from a low of around 1 per 100 births in the nomadic hunting and gathering !Kung to rates as extreme as 40% or higher in groups like the Eipo of highland New Guinea, where there is a strong preference for sons that leads mothers to expose daughters (Schiefenhoevel 1989). The conditions and determinants of infanticide in these and other cultures merits further study, especially in relation to the theoretically predicted determinants of maternal investment outlined above. The occurrence of infanticide in the past (reviewed in Hrdy 1999) suggests that whenever other forms of birth control were not available, mothers who lacked what they needed to rear offspring resorted to infanticide. This suggests that infanticide as a means of birth spacing was likely to have been an option among our human ancestors in the Pleistocene environment of evolutionary adaptedness (EEA). Newborns were and are at high risk of not being accepted by their mothers. The contingent nature of maternal solicitude in our species has meant that infants are biologically selected to look appealing to mothers from birth onward and to act in ways that demonstrate their health and vitality, including robust crying, limb movements, facial engagement, and visual gazing. Mothers are highly sensitive to these cues in the baby during the immediate postpartum period. Because of the time lag until the onset of lactation and full engagement of bonding, neonates may be especially vulnerable during the 72 hours or so immediately after birth, which is the period when most abandonment or infanticide committed by mothers occurs. Once breastfeeding has been established and the mother has begun to recognize her baby as an individual, the decision to terminate investment becomes much more difficult.

One lesson deriving from this discussion of maternal fitness considerations is that the mother's adaptive interests do not always coincide with those of the baby. In certain circumstances (perhaps commonly, if not always, associated with infanticide in traditional societies), it may be in the mother's lifetime reproductive success to withdraw care from an infant in order to invest in other (perhaps more healthy) offspring or in other ways that improve her chances of producing more offspring in the future. This, of course, is not in the adaptive interests of the baby. Divergence of fitness considerations means that maternal solicitude cannot always be expected and that maternal sensitivity is a highly contingent phenomenon when viewed within the context of biological adaptation. This is not only true during the postpartum period but in other developmental periods as well. Trivers (1974, 1985) states that weaning conflicts later in infancy reflect a divergence of the fitness interests of mother and baby. During weaning conflicts, the child's interests in maximizing and maintaining the mother's investment in feeding conflicts with the mother's interests in withdrawing resources for the sake, for example, of preparing for future offspring (Blurton Jones and Da Costa 1987). There are likely other developmental periods when the interests of mothers and offspring diverge to create conflict between them and, in another sense, constitute biologically adaptive forms of maternal insensitivity. The conclusion that maternal disinvestment, withdrawal, and/or insensitivity is, at times, biologically adaptive conflicts with the underlying assumption of many developmental theories, including attachment theory, that parental investment is biologically prepared and that departures from maternal sensitivity are adaptively anomalous. It remains for developmental theorists within psychology to explore more fully the implications of the fitness considerations of mother and baby, especially early in life, for understanding the conditions in which maternal solicitude can and should be expected, and when it should not, and the consequences of this for the mother–child relationship. It is especially important to understand and distinguish processes that may be biologically adaptive for the mother and baby from those that are psychologically adaptive for either partner.

Humans are reproductive strategists, and there are many other considerations that shape maternal investment decisions (for a review, see Voland 1998). These include the infant's health, gender, the type of birth (single vs. twin), maternal age and previous reproductive history, and social support from others in the human community. Thus inter- and intra-individual variability in investment decisions can be expected and is fully consistent with an evolutionary perspective on attachment and bonding. Among these considerations, the importance of social support merits further examination, especially because of its associations with maternal retrenchment, infanticide (Hrdy 1994), and postnatal maternal depression (Hagen 1999). If it is true that human communities in the EEA involved cooperative caregiving (Hrdy, this volume), then judgments of the extent of social support available are probably another important source of information relevant to inter- and intra-individual variation in maternal investment and attachment.

Indeed, social support may be significant not only because of its relevance to inclusive fitness considerations but, more proximally, as it interacts with the neurohormonal priming of maternal behavior after birth. There is, of course, substantial evidence indicating that psychosocial risk factors (e.g., lack of social support) contribute to a wide spectrum of somatic, psychosomatic, and psychiatric disorders with major public health significance, such as depression (Bruce 2002; Kraemer et al. 2001; Rozanski et al. 1999). In animals, oxytocin has been shown to exert behavioral and physiological stress-attenuating effects and, as noted earlier, to promote positive social interaction and attachment (Carter 1998; Legros 2001; McCarthy and Altemus 1997; Pedersen 1997; Pedersen and Boccia 2002). The specific effects of oxytocin as a biological mechanism for the reduction of stress and anxiety as well as the promotion of positive social interactions are yet to be determined in humans. In one study, however, oxytocin appeared to enhance the efficacy of social support in coping with stress (Heinrichs et al. 2003). Here, 37 healthy men were subjected to a stress test: participants were randomly assigned to receive either intranasal oxytocin[2] or a placebo shortly before the test, and they received either social support from their best friend or no support during the preparation period. The findings revealed that the combination of oxytocin and social support was associated with the lowest subsequent cortisol concentrations as well as enhanced calmness and decreased anxiety during the stress test (social support was also directly associated with lower cortisol, and oxytocin was directly associated with reduced anxiety). In this sense, oxytocin seemed to enhance the buffering effects of social support on stress responsiveness. These results are in accord with data from animal research, which suggests an important role of oxytocin as an underlying biological mechanism for stress protective effects of positive social interactions.

There are thus significant biological, social, and cognitive contributions to the development of attachment consistent with species fitness requirements, and

---

[2] Some studies on the central effects of oxytocin and vasopressin in healthy humans and clinical patients have been conducted with exogenous stimulation using intranasal administration (Born et al. 1998; Bruins et al. 1992; Heinrichs 2000; Pitman et al. 1993). Neuropeptides have recently been shown to enter the cerebrospinal fluid directly following nasal administration (Born et al. 2002).

these multidetermined influences introduce considerable flexibility to the attachment system, especially in the context of substantial cultural variability in childcare practices. In this sense, cultural variability usually reflects adaptive phenotypic plasticity. This is important, especially in light of the differences between Eastern and Western prototypical conceptions of self (Greenfield et al. 2003; Markus and Kitiyama 1991) and the parenting strategies and child-rearing goals with which they are associated. Although attachment theory may primarily reflect Western approaches to parenting and child development (particularly emphasizing practices that contribute to the development of independent agency and self-respect in offspring), considerable variability in parenting practices and child-rearing goals can be accommodated within attachment formulations and broader biological models of the parent–child relationship. This is because a general species-typical repertoire of parenting practices can be activated in different compositions or styles in response to ecocultural demands (Keller 2000, 2002). As one illustration, a network of institutional and personal sources of social support and a broad variety of reproductive options (including birth control) may be one reason why rates of infanticide are much lower in Western industrialized nations compared to those observed in more traditional hunter–gatherer and horticulturalist societies. Although not all cultural systems are necessarily consistent with the adaptive requirements of infant care and well-being, it is clear that evaluating these cultural practices requires understanding the broader ecological and material circumstances affecting parenting practices within these niches.

BIOLOGY–BEHAVIOR MECHANISMS MEDIATING EARLY ATTACHMENT

Attachment is a biologically based behavioral system (Bowlby 1969, 1973). Within a systems view, such a behavioral system integrates biological substrates with behavioral control processes that exist within the child and the environment. Attachment theorists believe that the attachment system is one of several behavioral systems deeply rooted in our biological heritage. An exploratory system, for example, functions interactively with the attachment system such that exploratory interest decreases when children become concerned with reestablishing contact with an attachment figure (see Grossmann and Grossmann, this volume). A fear/wariness system is believed to have evolved to guide a child's reactions to circumstances of potential danger or threat. Importantly, morphologically similar behaviors may be motivated by different behavioral systems: a baby's cry may be a signal to a caregiver to reestablish proximity (attachment) or a distress response to an unexpected event (fear/wariness), and in many circumstances both systems may be activated simultaneously. The value of a behavioral systems perspective is that it permits developmental scientists to understand the complementary and conflicting motivational processes that exist from an early age, each of which has adaptive value.

The complexity of behavioral systems is based, in part, on the complex relations between biological functioning and behavioral responding within and across each system. For example, Spangler and Schieche (1998) recently showed that cortisol levels increased with distress in insecurely attached infants, but cortisol had no relation to crying for securely attached infants when each group was observed in standard stress procedures. Understanding these interrelations requires considering the behavioral systems that might be involved in each case (with fear/wariness perhaps evoked along with attachment for insecure infants), and the influence of attachment relationships on children's developing emotional self-regulatory skills. Concerning the latter, the attachment figure appears to contribute to modulating the functioning of the child's stress response in secure relationships, but this does not occur in insecure attachment relationships (Hertsgaard et al. 1995; Spangler and Grossmann 1993). This influence is especially prominent in infants who are behaviorally inhibited, for whom the internal resources for coping with stress may be more limited (Nachmias et al. 1996; Spangler and Schieche 1998).

Relations between biological functioning and behavioral development are thus complex and interesting. There is now abundant evidence from the animal literature of how early caregiving experiences tone the dynamics of stress response. The work of Michael Meaney, Seymour Levine, Paul Plotsky, and others shows, for example, that early maternal deprivation (and the reduction of maternal licking and grooming) during the pre-weaning period for rat pups has a number of significant consequences on the rat's subsequent physiological and behavioral functioning (Bredy et al. 2003; Francis et al. 2002; Rosenfield et al. 1992; Sanchez et al. 2001). These include heightened neophobia and fearfulness, increased corticotropin-releasing hormone (CRH) in the amygdala and locus coeruleus, a reduced number of glucocorticoid receptors, and increased and more prolonged corticoid and adrenocorticotropic hormone (ACTH) responses to psychosocial or progressive stressors. The continued sensitivity of these behavioral and physiological systems to further experience is revealed in subsequent research that shows considerable recovery in these functions when the rats were subsequently placed in cages affording complex social and physical stimulation (similar to a "complex environment"). When compared with pre-weaning- deprived rats who continued in deprived circumstances, those in the pre-weaning-deprived condition who subsequently lived in complex environments showed diminished neophobia and fearfulness, diminished corticoid and ACTH responses to stressors, and other indications of enhanced coping. Their outcome functioning was, indeed, more comparable to those of rat pups who had experienced early handling without maternal deprivation. Nonetheless, they still exhibited reduced numbers of corticoid receptors in regions of the brain involved in feedback regulation of the system.

Recent studies of rhesus monkeys and human infants reared in aberrant, species-atypical conditions tell a similar story: early experiences of deprivation and neglect are associated with disturbances in the diurnal rhythm in cortisol[3] levels (Boyce et al. 1995; Carlson et al. 1995). The effect is most easily identified at the peak of the cycle, when deprived human infants frequently show a blunting of the peak and, for some, there may be relatively unvarying levels of cortisol throughout the day (Gunnar and Vazquez 2001). These atypical diurnal rhythms do not constitute, however, a fixed characteristic of the child: changing the caregiving context alters these patterns. In one study (P. Fisher, pers. comm.), children entering foster care were monitored for the first six months of their placements. Those children living in homes where their foster parents had been given special support and training to manage the needs of traumatized children tended to establish a robust diurnal cortisol rhythm over time, whereas those children in unsupported foster care placements did not improve and sometimes showed a worsening of the diurnal pattern.

One of the contemporary challenges of denoting biology–behavior connections in psychology that is relevant to the study of attachment concerns how we conceptually organize our understanding of physiological and behavioral systems. As research on the functional organization of the brain reveals, there is no direct connection between the complex psychological functions we seek to understand (e.g., categories of thoughts, feelings, and motives) and the functional development of specific brain regions. Indeed, there is no reason to expect that this would be so, given that the ways which scientists have classified psychological experience during the past century derive more from influences from

---

[3]   The cortisol system is often interpreted as a simple physiological measure of stress, a view that leads to considerable confusion about the meaning of cortisol findings. Instead, it might be more accurately viewed as reflecting a dynamic balance between opposing arousal and anti-arousal mechanisms. Under conditions of threat and loss of control, elevated cortisol is related to loss of safety and the arousal of fear and anxiety, whereas low cortisol appears to be a compensatory defensive response to heightened arousal associated with emotional withdrawal, including emotional numbing, avoidance, and other disengagement strategies (Wolff et al. 1964; Mason et al. 2001). The latter may also be associated with diminished interpersonal sensitivity and compassion (Henry 1993). Under conditions of safety (from which social engagement and attachment behavior emerge), elevated cortisol is related to arousal and active engagement, but not fear, and has been associated with increased social competence (Hart et al. 1995) and sensitivity (Fleming et al. 1997). Lower cortisol under safe conditions is related to low arousal states and passive engagement (Handlon et al. 1962). This framework, which considers the perception of safety and level of engagement as important factors in determining the "meaning" of cortisol findings, may help us interpret apparently contradictory findings, such as high cortisol being related to fear and anxiety, on one hand, and increased competence and sensitivity, on the other, as well as low cortisol being associated with maladaptive behavior and also with increased relaxation and well-being in different circumstances. It also provides an orientation for understanding the response of individuals who have experienced early trauma or deprivation, which may create a bias toward heightened perception of threat and make it more difficult for them to engage in a mode of safety and relaxation associated with social engagement and attachment behavior (Henry and Wang 1998).

Western philosophy than from cognitive neuroscience.[4] Contrary to the tendency of popular psychology to denote specific brain regions as the centers for complex psychological motives, neuroscientists are increasingly emphasizing the complex interconnections between multiple brain areas related to ordinary as well as sophisticated psychological processes. This poses a challenge, however, to efforts to identify interconnections between biological and behavioral functioning in psychological development, and suggests that it may become necessary to reconsider conventional ways of conceptualizing psychological processes to accord better with the developmental organization of the brain. With respect to attachment, for example, it may be necessary to "unpack" conceptually the complex cognitive, affective, and motivational elements of attachment functioning (see above) before developmental associations with the functional emergence of specific brain processes can be revealed. Similarly, it may be necessary to reconsider early behavioral organization in terms of broad motivational systems (e.g., attachment, exploration, fear/wariness) when the neurobiological substrates are likely to be organized much differently. Such an effort is worthwhile, however, for the potential it affords to understand better the ontogeny of this important social phenomenon in a concertedly integrated biobehavioral manner.

DEVELOPMENT OF ATTACHMENT EARLY IN LIFE

Attachment theorists have identified several stages in the development of attachment relationships during the first year of life that accord with the earlier discussion of the cognitive and affective origins of attachment in offspring (Ainsworth et al. 1978; Bowlby 1969; Lamb et al. 1985). During the initial months of life, a young infant typically responds in an undifferentiated social manner, with clear social discriminations later emerging at about 3–4 months of age as the child responds uniquely to familiar social partners. According to attachment theorists, another important transition occurs early in the second half of the first year, when infants begin to focus preferentially on specific partners, and this is reflected in the emergence of separation protest and, to a lesser extent, stranger wariness. As infants acquire locomotor skills, they begin to search for the caregiver when absent and follow the caregiver when present, which further reflect the baby's active engagement with a specific partner who is becoming an attachment figure for the child. This developmental sequence culminates by the end of the first year, when theorists believe a differentiated attachment relationship has fully developed.

---

[4] The same problem applies to the nosology of psychiatric diagnosis and efforts to denote connections between diagnostic categories and neurobiological processes. Indeed, the normative comorbidity among psychiatric diagnoses and the complexity of symptomatology together suggest that the diagnostic categories of clinical practice require considerable reexamination, hopefully informed by the emerging insights of the neurosciences.

Although there is evidence that infants identify familiar figures earlier than Bowlby and Ainsworth had hypothesized, and research on joint attention highlights the greater sophistication of young infants in inferring mental states in adults, this general developmental framework has held up well to the tests of time and empirical inquiry (Thompson 2006). Most research concerned with attachment in infancy has focused not on its normative development but rather on individual differences in the security of attachment, distinguishing infants who are securely attached from those who are insecurely attached. This research has been guided by a general theoretical expectation that secure attachment promotes more confident exploration in infants as mothers function as a secure base for the child and as a haven of safety when the baby is threatened or alarmed (Ainsworth et al. 1978).

Bowlby's (1969, 1973) developmental theory of attachment also posited another stage in the development of attachment relationships after the first birthday. In toddlerhood, he proposed, children become capable of engaging in a "goal-corrected partnership" with the attachment figure based on their growing comprehension of the caregiver as a psychological figure with needs, interests, and feelings of her own. At the same time, other aspects of mental representation become increasingly important in their relationship as attachment security changes from an exclusively behavioral system to a representational system in which security becomes mediated by the child's expectations and representations of the caregiver's behavior. These representations, or "internal working models" (IWMs), arise out of the simpler behavioral expectations that underlie attachment security in infancy, and become more elaborated and complex with increasing age and the growing sophistication of the child's representational skills (Bretherton and Munholland 1999). Indeed, according to one formulation (Grossmann and Grossmann, this volume), different forms of IWMs emerge developmentally as new representational capacities emerge and as children become capable of sharing and comparing their representations of experience with others through language (Thompson 2000, 2006). By adulthood, attachment is a fully representational system that has become associated with self-understanding, relational intimacy, and caregiving of offspring.

These developmental formulations are important and provocative, but they raise new problems for the study of early attachment and its consequences. One basic challenge is that there is little theoretical guidance concerning the development of attachment relationships beyond the phase of the "goal-corrected partnership." General developmental formulations exist, however, that have been broadly accepted by attachment researchers (Thompson and Raikes 2003). Attachment security increasingly becomes an attribute of the person rather than of a specific relationship with increasing age (e.g., as children's representations of relationships become generalized across different partners). The IWMs underlying security of attachment also become more complex and multidimensional but internally coherent over time, consistent with advances in intellectual growth. Attachment theorists also tend to agree that parent–child relationships change over time with the child's psychological maturity and that the requirements of parental responsiveness evolve even as the adult's sensitivity has a continuing influence on the maintenance of a secure attachment. In adolescence, for example, the parent–child relationship must accommodate the concurrent psychological needs for relatedness and autonomy in young people and the dynamic balance between these needs shapes the security of attachment (Allen and Land 1999).

Beyond these general ideas, theory development is critically important to clarify, for example, how other changes in the relationship shared by a child with a caregiver occur as a consequence of the child's psychological growth, how IWMs evolve with the development of cognitive skills, and the bases for consistency and change in attachment representations over time. Understanding the development of IWMs in relation to concurrent growth in cognition is especially important. For example, from the perspective of current ideas about domain-specific conceptual skills (e.g., Hirschfeld and Gelman 1998), the IWM might be conceptualized as a "theory of attachment" (G. Spangler and A. Delius, pers. comm.) that includes representations, assumptions, and expectations concerning attachment, behavioral strategies, and attachment figures. Such a "theory" is based on early experiences with the attachment figure but would be expected to change and become more complex with later experiences and advances in conceptual growth, as do other intuitive "theories" of mind, biological kinds, and other conceptual domains in early childhood. Another approach describes the development of IWMs within a neo-Vygotskian framework in which implicit features of the conversations shared by parents with young children shape emergent representations of relationships, self, and psychological understanding, consistent with the literatures on event representation, autobiographical memory, and theory of mind (Thompson 2000, 2006; Thompson et al. 2003).

Further development of attachment formulations is also needed to elucidate the defining features of attachment relationships that exist in middle childhood, adolescence, and adulthood, and how they are associated with attachment relationships formed in infancy and early childhood (Raikes and Thompson 2004). Absent theoretical guidance, attachment researchers who have been interested in exploring these issues have had to work inductively, bootstrapping theoretical explanations onto empirical findings, and have had to develop methods and procedures that presuppose theoretical clarity that does not yet exist.

Theoretical development should be a guide to the development of measures and methods in the study of attachment, rather than the reverse. Thus another challenge raised by the developmental study of attachment is the need for theoretically based, valid, and reliable assessments of attachment after infancy (Thompson and Raikes 2003). There has been a proliferation of attachment assessments in recent years for research into attachment in middle childhood, adolescence, and adulthood. With the exception of the concerted validational work on the Adult Attachment Interview (AAI), researchers have not tended to focus on their validation. There have been no efforts comparable to the careful validation of the Strange Situation for measures of attachment security in childhood or adolescence. This is unfortunate, because it means that there have been critical assumptions incorporated into the creation of attachment assessments that merit more careful examination.

For example, several widely used assessments of attachment after infancy rely on the quality of children's narrative discourse in response to incomplete story stems or doll-play prompts (Solomon and George 1999). Children's responses are often evaluated in terms of their coherence, in a manner similar to how narrative coherence is a central feature in assessing adult security from AAI responses. In adult studies using the AAI, lack of coherence is assumed to reflect the influence of defensive processes in adults' recollections of early childhood care (Hesse 1999). Where children are concerned, there are important questions concerning whether children's semiprojective story responses and the quality of their narrative stories can be comparably interpreted. Can "coherence" be similarly interpreted as reflecting unconscious defenses in a child's account compared to an adult's? Are children of age 5, 8, or 13 comparably capable of reflecting on the quality of their relationships with their attachment figures or of projecting onto story stems the affective features of their relationships with their caregivers? These are especially important questions in light of concerns, related to the AAI, that Grice's maxims of communicative coherence are a limited and culturally focused approach to discourse analysis. In the same way that individuals from dissimilar cultures have different narrative styles for which "coherence" must be interpreted distinctly, so too do children of different ages have various narrative skills to make "coherence" mean something particular for them. In the developmentally downward extension of the methodology of the AAI to research with children and adolescents, there may be important developmental differences in a variety of capabilities that require greater consideration in the interpretation of children's narrative discourse.

Another issue concerns how individual differences in attachment security should be characterized. It is remarkable that the adult attachment categories yielded by the AAI are so closely comparable to the fourfold classification categories of the Strange Situation, as though no further developmental changes in the organization of attachment from infancy to adulthood were expected. With few exceptions, researchers have devised attachment assessments for children of different ages that yield security delineations that are also quite similar to the Strange Situation classifications (Thompson and Raikes 2003). In the developmentally upward extension of the classifications of the Strange Situation to research with children and adults, important theoretical assumptions about the consistency of the organization of attachment security and insecurity are made that seem, in some respects, contrary to the wealth of psychological changes that occur from infancy to adulthood.

This is particularly surprising because in other ways, attachment in adults and infants is much differently conceptualized. In infancy, attachment security is relationship-specific, behaviorally oriented, and focused on current relational experience in which secure base behavior is a central index. For adults, attachment security is thought to be an attribute of the person rather than of specific relationships, representationally oriented, with assessments focusing on past relational experience (primarily in childhood) in which discourse coherence is a central index. There is a developmental account that is inherent in these differences in conceptualization and assessment that attachment theorists have yet to articulate and develop fully. Such an account would clarify how IWMs grow from infancy to adulthood, and how attachment transitions from a behavioral system early in life to a fully representational system in adolescence and adulthood. It would also articulate the dynamics of stability and change in the organization of the attachment system over life, and clarify expectations for whether early attachment security is expected to lead to security throughout life, or whether change is possible or likely.

How the development of attachment is theoretically conceptualized also has implications for expectations of stability or change in attachment relationships over the life course. In general, attachment theory has had strong claims, based on its object relations theory progenitors, that because attachment initially emerges during a formative early period of psychological development in infancy, its effects are likely to be long-lasting. Thus if the first and primary mother–infant relationship is secure, it is likely to remain so and will, furthermore, bias the infant to expect security and to elicit warmth and sensitivity from other relational partners, partly because of the influence of security on the child's developing IWMs (e.g., Sroufe and Fleeson 1986). In a sense, early developing attachment security becomes self-perpetuating because of how it shapes the internal representations that the child brings to new relationships and new opportunities for relational intimacy. The same is true, of course, of early attachments that are insecure.

Below, we discuss research evidence concerning this theoretical view. Theoretical expectations still need to be elaborated, however, to guide research as to the development of attachment. In a sense, attachment scientists have a valuable opportunity to extend systematically Bowlby's provocative formulations to the development of attachment in childhood, adolescence, and adulthood to give clarity and coherence to empirical efforts, and to do so in light of emerging findings in developmental neuroscience.

CONSEQUENCES OF EARLY ATTACHMENT FOR CHILD AND MOTHER

Studying continuity and change in psychological functioning presents developmental scientists with the formidable challenge of documenting heterotypic continuity. When studying the consistency of psychological functioning in rapidly changing organisms over time, or the consequences of early functioning for later behavior, researchers must find ways to index psychological processes that are believed to remain continuous over time but are manifested in different, developmentally appropriate ways. In this sense, their search for continuity is "heterotypic": its manifestations will be different at various ages.

Consequences for the Child

This challenge is especially apparent when considering the consequences of attachment for the child. There are two senses in which one might be concerned with the consequences of attachment relationships for a child's development (Thompson 2001). First, one might ask: What are the consequences for the child *having become attached* to a caregiver? From an adaptive standpoint, the answer is likely to focus on the child's survival to maturity and reproductive success; from the perspective of psychological growth, an attachment relationship provides a child with a socio-emotional connection to another individual that influences self-understanding, social competence, and self-regulation. These are issues that merit further exploration. Second, attachment research has been concerned with a different question: What are the consequences for the child of *individual differences* in the security of attachment? Do securely attached children show different forms of self-understanding, emotional understanding, friendship and peer relationships compared with insecurely attached children? The challenges of heterotypic continuity are encountered in seeking to understand whether a secure attachment early in life leads to security in later years and to other sequelae (e.g., social competence, self confidence, emotional understanding) that might be expected from secure versus insecure attachment.

As considered earlier, one expected outcome of a secure parent–child attachment is that the parent–child relationship will remain secure in years to come. This concerns the stability of individual differences in attachment over the life course. Belsky (this volume) reviewed research evidence and concluded that attachment security exhibits modest but significant stability from infancy to adulthood, and that there are theoretical reasons to expect that attachments will be stable over time for some individuals, but not for others. In light of the remarkable variability in research findings on this issue, with some studies indicating that a high proportion of children are consistent in remaining secure or insecure for many years and others showing that infants and young children change dramatically in the security of attachment over a matter of months (Thompson 2000, 2006), the proper question is perhaps not to inquire about the average consistency of individual differences in the security of attachment over time. Rather, the better question might be: *Under what conditions is attachment security likely to remain stable, and under what conditions is it likely to change?*

Research evidence (Thompson 2006) on this issue suggests two provisional conclusions. First, children with secure attachments and (perhaps) those with the disorganized classification are more likely to remain consistent in their attachment status over time than are children with the two insecure classifications (avoidant and resistant). This is likely to be true for different reasons (e.g., secure relationships are stable because they are mutually rewarding; disorganized relationships are stable because their atypicality becomes self-perpetuating in the responses children and their caregivers elicit and provoke). Second, children and parents in more stable living circumstances are likely to enjoy more stable relationships, while those who experience disruptive family events are more likely to change because of the impact of those events on their relationship.

Research support for the importance of stability in living circumstances is suggestive but not conclusive (Thompson 2000, 2006). It remains for researchers to identify clearly the kinds of events that are likely to provoke change in attachment security over time. In their taxonomy of attachment-altering experiences, for example, most researchers would include manifestly traumatic events (e.g., death or loss of a parent). Many would also include stressors such as parental separation or divorce (see Grossmann and Grossmann, this volume), which is an important consideration in light of the high proportion of children in countries like the U.S. who have experienced parental separation or divorce by middle childhood. There is evidence that the birth of a sibling can provoke alterations in the security of attachment between firstborns and the mother, and some suggestions that events like parental employment changes or family difficulty may also be influential (Teti et al. 1996; Thompson et al. 1982; Vaughn et al. 1979). Surprisingly, little systematic research has been devoted to elucidate the origins of change (and consistency) in attachment relationships over time (cf. Belsky et al. 1991). This is a topic meriting further inquiry because of its relevance to understanding the dynamic influences on parent–child relationships over time. For example, although family experiences are likely to be most influential, outside events might also affect the security of parent–child attachments if they impose stress on either partner that the other cannot accommodate. Conversely, extrafamilial sources of social support might buffer difficulties in the parent–child relationships and can thus provide avenues to the development of greater security. There are also many provocative new hypotheses warranting exploration. For example, to what extent do normative developmental transitions in a child's life create opportunities for the renegotiation of parent–child relationships, leading to enhanced security for some and diminished security for others because of the challenges these transitions present to the adult? To what extent are culturally normative practices that alter children's relational experiences (e.g., changes in childcare providers or the transition to school) influential in changing parent–child attachment because of the challenges and new relational experiences afforded the child? To what extent is the impact of changing circumstances and stressors contingent on the maturity of the brain at the time they occur (e.g., the vulnerability of developing psychobiological systems relevant to attachment or stress)? In a sense, systematic study of the factors contributing to change and continuity in attachment relationships across the life course provides another window into the factors influencing attachment security.

Until relevant research is conducted, attachment researchers are left with the conclusion that attachments change for some children and remain consistent for others (Thompson 2000). Even so, this has important implications for understanding the consequences of early parent–child relationships. For example, developmental formulations that assume long-term influences from early attachment relationships must accommodate the fact that attachment relationships themselves often change over time, and thus the consequences of early attachment may also be malleable (see the evolutionary formulation of Belsky et al. 1991). Moreover, such a conclusion underscores the dynamic nature of parent–child relations, which is consistent with the cascade of developmental changes occurring in the child and the changing parent and family ecology that constitutes the child's home.

Attachment theory also predicts that early secure parent–child relationships will yield other beneficial consequences later in life and that an early insecure attachment inaugurates children on developmental pathways that are likely to be less successful in other ways. In a large, expanding empirical literature, attachment researchers have explored the relations between attachment security and a wide variety of expected outcomes, studied either in consequent or contemporaneous relations to the security of attachment. Predicted outcomes have included teacher–child relationships; cognitive and language development; frustration tolerance; self-recognition; behavioral problems; relations with peers, friends, and siblings; interactions with unfamiliar adults; exploration and play; competence in preschool and kindergarten; curiosity; psychopathology; ego resiliency; and math achievement. Although researchers in this field disagree over the scope of the theoretically predicted sequelae of attachment security, this is because attachment theory is not especially clear about the range of consequences that could reasonably be anticipated from early security. Consequently, researchers have been guided alternatively by broader or narrower views of the range of outcomes under the umbrella of a general expectation that a secure attachment should be related to more optimal later functioning than an insecure attachment. Greater theoretical clarity is thus needed to inform hypotheses and the design and interpretation of findings. How can the claims of attachment theory be properly evaluated if researchers are unclear about its central hypotheses concerning the consequences of early attachment?

A large empirical literature examining the contemporaneous and predictive correlates of attachment security in infancy and early childhood yields, however, several conclusions (Thompson 1999, 2006). First, a secure attachment seems to be associated with greater competence and success in close relationships. Most notably, a secure attachment in infancy foreshadows a more harmonious parent–child relationship in the immediate years to come, which heightens the child's receptiveness to the parent's socialization incentives and fosters mutual cooperation and responsiveness (Waters et al. 1991). Securely attached young children are also more successful in other close relationships, such as with friends, teachers, and counselors, although it is unclear whether this is due to social skills, social expectations (such as IWMs of relationships), maternal support, or other reasons. Attachment security is not strongly associated with children's interactions with unfamiliar partners. Second, there is also evidence that securely attached young children have different ways of thinking about the social world, reflected in a more acute emotional understanding, more positive friendship conceptions, and advances in conscience development, although this evidence is limited. Third, there is little systematic evidence that attachment security is associated with personality characteristics, such as ego resiliency, or with behavioral problems and other potential precursors of clinical difficulties (although research indicates that the disorganized classification may be a risk factor for later clinical problems).

The strongest evidence for the broader influences of a secure or insecure attachment arises from contemporaneous assessments of attachment and other behaviors which do not permit unequivocal causal conclusions. In predictive studies, short-term associations between attachment and outcomes are stronger than longer-term predictive associations but, at best, the strength of the relation between attachment security and its psychological correlates is modest (although some studies show a small, enduring effect for some children; see e.g., Sroufe et al. 1990). There are many reasons for this (Thompson 1999). The sequelae with which attachment security is associated are themselves multidetermined and are likely to be affected by a variety of influences besides the parent–child relationship. Moreover, children typically experience multiple attachment relationships that may have complementary or conflicting influences on aspects of the child's later psychological growth. Parent–child relationships also change over time, such that later relational experience at home may confirm the influences of early attachment security or may alter earlier developmental influences. Taken together, therefore, the security of attachment is an important but modest influence on children's subsequent relational experience; its broader effects have yet to be systematically established.

The central hypothesized mediator between early attachment security and its expected outcomes is the IWM of attachment in the mind of the child. In most current research, scientists seek to evaluate hypothesized consequences in relation to the nature of the IWMs that are presumed to result from secure or insecure attachments. As earlier noted, there is considerable uncertainty about what an IWM really is, how it changes with development, and how it relates to other cognitive constructs that have also been studied by psychologists (e.g., schemas, attributions, autobiographical representations). Part of the confusion is attributable, again, to lack of clarity within attachment theory. In some regards, the IWM is conceptualized in a manner resembling the dynamic unconscious, initially formed based on relational experiences through the perceptual-affective schemas of infancy, and remaining influential throughout life but largely inaccessible to subsequent linguistic-representational influences. In other respects, the IWM is conceptualized in a manner consistent with other conscious, representational models; it functions like a script or relational schema, incorporating motivational attributions, elements of event representation, and autobiographical memory. These alternative conceptualizations are not entirely inconsistent, of course, but the differences between them have significant implications for how IWMs might be thought to develop, how they would influence behavior, or how they might be measured (Spangler and Zimmermann 1999). Without greater clarity on these and other central theoretical issues, researchers have been enticed by the powerful heuristic value of the IWM construct to create hypotheses based on their own conceptualization of the IWM (Thompson and Raikes 2003). It is unlikely that a clear and coherent research literature on the consequences of early attachment will be possible without greater theoretical clarity on this and other central issues.

There are other conceptual challenges to studying the consequences of early attachment for the child. First, although researchers have commonly examined the direct effects of attachment on other aspects of psychological development, it is also likely that attachment has indirect and interactive consequences. For instance, attachment security may enhance the efficacy of other forms of social support for the child. Although insecure attachment is not generally a direct risk factor for later psychopathology (with the possible exception of the D classification), it is likely to be influential within a constellation of additional risks to early mental health. Second, because cultural systems vary so significantly in parental belief systems, child-rearing goals and parenting practices, the interaction of parental sensitivity, attachment security, and developmental sequelae is likely to vary somewhat in different societies. Several decades ago, attachment researchers engaged in cross-cultural research on the Strange Situation situation and found that they were required to understand indigenous child-rearing practices to interpret infant attachment classifications properly (van IJzendoorn and Sagi 1999); similar processes of cultural understanding (within the context of the biologically adaptive needs of the human species) will likely be necessary to design and interpret properly studies of the consequences of early attachment in non-Western cultures. Third, if the stability of attachment security is contingent on influences such as the consistency in living conditions for parent and child, the same factors may be important in understanding the conditions when later outcomes of early attachment may be evident, and the conditions in which later sequelae will be hard to find. Thus, children living in markedly changing circumstances may show fewer long-term correlates of early attachment security than children living in more stable conditions, when the initial tendencies fostered by a secure or insecure attachment are more likely to be maintained.

This brings us back to the central question: How important are early experiences for psychological development? There have been at least four broad models of the influence of early experiences on long-term development (O'Connor 2003; Thompson 2001):

1. The "programming" model argues that early experiences exert a lasting effect because of the early malleability of biological (or personality or conceptual) systems that become subsequently less plastic. Supportive evidence for such a model often derives from studies of animals or human infants exposed to antenatal or early postnatal stressors (e.g., Barker 1998; O'Connor, Heron et al. 2003).

2. The "developmental sensitivity" model argues that the effects of particular events or experiences depends on the developmental period in which they occur. Contrary to the programming model, early experiences are not necessarily formative, and influences occuring at later ages (such as parturition) can have a comparably profound developmental influence.

3. The "cumulative experience" model argues that both early and later influences are important, and early experiences have an enduring effect when they are maintained or supported by subsequent experiences. Conversely, early adversity does not necessarily impair healthy development if it is corrected and replaced by supportive care, which is consistent with the literature on psychological resiliency (Clarke and Clarke 2000).

4. The "cognitive/affective processing" model argues that effects of early experiences on long-term development depends on how these events are interpreted and/or internalized by the individual. Like the cumulative experience model, the relations between early influences and later development is not deterministic but probabilistic.

It is difficult, of course, to design empirical tests that would set one model against another because of the difficulties of distinguishing the effects of early experience from later experience. The best opportunities to compare these alternative formulations arise from studies of the long-term effects of early deprivation, in which depriving conditions are followed by adequate, supportive care. One such study is the English and Romanian Adoptees (ERA) study (O'Connor et al. 2000; O'Connor, Marvin et al. 2003; Rutter et al. 2001, 2004), which examined long-term effects of early institutional deprivation for a sample of Romanian orphanage children who were subsequently adopted into well-functioning homes in the U.K.

The ERA study has yielded several conclusions concerning the effects of early deprivation. First, a number of disadvantageous outcomes were reliably associated with institutional deprivation, including cognitive delay, attachment problems, and difficulties with inattention and hyperactivity. These problems developed in a dose-response manner: prolonged early institutional experience was associated with severe outcomes. Other common behavioral problems (e.g., conduct disturbances) were not found, at least in the earlier follow-up assessments. Second, there was evidence of substantial recovery in some developmental domains, most notably increases in weight and height. Third, and most interestingly, where later outcomes of institutionalization were identified, the strength of the effect was as marked at age 11 years as at earlier assessments at four and six years of age; that is, the relative impact of institutional deprivation did not dissipate with time, even though children improved after adoption and were continuing to live in supportive, developmentally appropriate care settings. Finally, there were marked individual differences in outcome that were not easily explained either by characteristics of the adoptive placements or by other factors. Simply, some children showed severe impairment while other children showed relatively few disturbances in developmental functioning.

Findings such as these are not easily accommodated within any of the developmental models outlined above. The persistence of disturbance in the context of recovery but in the absence of continuing adversity, the wide range of individual differences in outcomes, and the dose-response association of early adversity with later outcomes are not fully consistent with any of the current formulations of the effects of early experiences. This suggests that newer, more complex models — or combinations of models — may be necessary to comprehend more adequately the effects of early experiences on children's development. Such a conclusion is also consistent with the larger literature on the outcomes of attachment security in early childhood, which reveals sequelae in some developmental domains but not others, multidetermined developmental outcomes, and influences from early experiences that wane but, for some, leave a lingering legacy.

Such a conclusion is also consistent with research into the psychobiological foundations of early attachment, which provides a view of plasticity as well as consistency in the biobehavioral systems related to attachment. Limbic system structures related to social reward, for example, are early-maturing but are also modified by experience throughout most of life, with some limbic structures maturing into the third decade of life. In a manner consistent with psychobiological studies reviewed earlier, it is clear that early experiences of marked abuse, neglect, and other chronic stressors can meaningfully alter the functioning of this reward system. In work with rodents, for example, repeated parental separation experiences transiently elevated dopaminergic receptors and serotonergic receptors in the prefrontal cortex, hippocampus, and amygdala (Ziabreva, Schnabel et al. 2003; Ziabreva, Poeggel et al. 2003). Long-term alterations of the limbic system deriving from chronic social isolation include reduced dopaminergic innervation in the anterior cingulate and orbitofrontal cortex (Braun et al. 2000; Poeggel, Nowicki et al. 2003), which are each related to social reward. Serotonin, which during early brain development also has a neurotrophic function to stimulate synaptic development, is also altered in these cortical regions as well as the amygdala (Braun et al. 2000; Poeggel, Helmeke et al. 2003). Thus early experiences can significantly alter limbic-mediated social reward systems, albeit interventions that are species-atypical. Experiential "training" or "imprinting" of the limbic system's development in early years, however, involves continuous "updating" in light of current experience (e.g., during vocal communication between the mother and offspring; see Poeggel and Braun 1996; Braun and Poeggel 2001; Braun et al. 2003), and this is mediated by dopaminergic reward mechanisms. Human and rodent studies (Bredy et al. 2003; Francis et al. 2002) document this story by showing how subsequent caregiving can alter effects of earlier influences of care on psychobiological systems related to stress and coping. In a sense, early experiences (especially with a primary caregiver) help create a "grammar of emotion" that may be enduring, even though the language of emotion continues to unfold in the years to come.

Attachment is more than the limbic system, of course, and the multiple brain regions and behavioral regulators related to attachment confer additional flexibility to this developing system. There are limits to this flexibility, as continuing research into the developmental outcomes of Romanian orphanage children adopted into well-functioning British families thoughtfully documents. In the end, the conclusion that early experiences are important but not determinative, that later experiences are also influential, and that individual differences in outcomes are a significant consideration, probably constitutes a useful general working hypothesis to guide further inquiry.[5]

Consequences for the Mother

In contrast to the rich literature on the consequences of early attachment for the child's psychological development, theory and research concerning consequences for the mother are more sparse. It is apparent that as a counterpart to her enormous investment in infant care (energic costs, vulnerability, and inability to invest resources alternatively), mothers derive rewards from caregiving. Aside from the well-known role of breast milk for infant health, breastfeeding seems to

---

[5] At this Dahlem Workshop, we had the opportunity to ponder issues of early attachment and its long-term consequences with the artistic catalysts provided by a delightful evening of viewing Prokofiev's ballet, "Romeo and Juliet" at the *Deutsche Oper*. It raised many questions concerning the developmental dynamics of the young, central figures in this drama. How much, for example, was Juliet's sudden infatuation with a boy from the other side of town named Romeo anticipated by her uncertain attachment to her mother (about whom very little is said in Shakespeare's play or the ballet)? To what extent was her current troubled relationship with her father, characterized by his coercive overcontrol, prognostic of a potentially troubled marriage to Romeo (assuming, of course, that both had managed to live long enough to share a married life together)? What does it mean that the nurse who cares for Juliet in Shakespeare's play became transformed into a priest in Prokofiev's staging, and what does this reflect about Prokofiev (or, for that matter, Shakespeare)? How were the somewhat disturbing peer relational dynamics of the adolescent subculture related to the interfamilial conflict of the Montagues and Capulets, and the possibility of insecure attachments within each family? We leave these questions for the reader to ponder.

have protective effects for the mother and directly promotes attachment behavior. During lactation, the sucking stimulus of the newborn increases both oxytocin and prolactin release and decreases basal plasma levels of ACTH and cortisol, suggesting an inhibitory influence of both peptides on stress-responsive neurohormonal systems (Amico et al. 1994; Russell et al. 2001). As earlier indicated, data from several species implicate oxytocin in social attachment and related prosocial behaviors (Carter 1998; Insel and Young 2001; Pedersen 1997). Together, the inhibitory effect of intracerebral oxytocin on stress-induced activity of the hypothalamic–pituitary–adrenocortical (HPA) axis responsiveness points to its key role in social behavior and stress management.

Consistent with these animal findings, pituitary–adrenal reactivity to psychosocial stress is attenuated after endogenous stimulation of oxytocin following breastfeeding in postpartum lactating mothers (Heinrichs et al. 2001). Moreover, lactating women had reduced plasma ACTH, cortisol, and glucose responses to physical stress in comparison with postpartum nonlactating women (Altemus et al. 1995). In addition to physiological measurements, psychometric measures were also assessed in some studies. Both breastfeeding and holding the infant for a 15-minute period, for example, led to decreased state anxiety in lactating women (Heinrichs et al. 2001).

There may also be broader consequences of the lactating mother's short-term hyporesponsiveness to stress that facilitate attachment to the infant, including (a) lower cortisol levels that could conserve energy required for lactation, (b) suppression of the secretion of stress-responsive hormones that could inhibit lactation, (c) lower glucocorticoid levels to facilitate enhanced immune functioning for the mother, (d) enhanced sensitivity and responsiveness to the infant owing to fewer competing responses (Heinrichs et al. 2002). Beyond these psychobiological concomitants, breastfeeding in many cultures is regarded by mothers as a primary avenue to bonding with the baby and, for some, as a way of creating cultural identity.

Breastfeeding constitutes one exemplary illustration of the bidirectional influences that promote mutual attachment by mother and baby. Although maternal and offspring interests are not always concordant in an ultimate sense, especially in families with siblings close in age, it is striking how often the behavioral systems guiding attachment processes yield shared benefits for the mother and baby who are finding each other in a developing relationship.

CONCLUSION

At present, the integration of behavioral and psychobiological perspectives to early attachment and its consequences is more promise than realization. Our discussion has highlighted discoveries that are emerging in this integrative work and, more important, avenues for essential further exploration. Among the latter identified in this discussion are:

- Understanding better the behavioral and biological prerequisites for forming first attachments in infancy, and how these are reorganized when first attachments must develop later than is species-typical, or in circumstances that are atypical. More concerted research attention to attachment *development* will integrate attachment and bonding processes with other normative psychobiological growth processes and yield greater insights into the causes of attachment dysfunction.
- Understanding better how attachment develops in different cultural settings within the context of the biologically adaptive requirements of inclusive fitness. Attachment is both biologically imperative and context sensitive.
- Conceptualizing more clearly the interaction of behavioral experience and psychobiological development with respect to how early caregiving shapes infant regulatory capacities, and how these influences become progressively updated through new caregiving experiences. Current research shows that prevailing models of the effects of early experience on long-term development are inadequate to the complexity of psychobiological growth.
- Greater theoretical clarification of how attachment continues to develop beyond infancy, and the representations associated with this developmental process, in concert with the development of new measures and methods for assessing attachment at later ages. In this manner, the development of attachment can be better understood in the context of concurrent advances in cognition, relationships, social skills, personality, and the growth of self-understanding.
- More systematic inquiry into the internal and external processes mediating continuity and change in attachment relationships over time, and what are the expectable consequences of early attachment relationships for both behavioral and psychobiological organization, and the role of IWMs in the regulation of attachment functioning.
- Integration of biological and behavioral insights into the most compelling question of all: How does early experience influence later behavior?

REFERENCES

Ainsworth, M.D.S. 1985. Attachment across the life span. *Bull. NY Acad. Med.* **61**: 792–812.

Ainsworth, M.D.S., M.C. Blehar, E. Waters, and S. Wall. 1978. Patterns of Attachment. Hillsdale, NJ: Erlbaum.

Allen, J.P., and D. Land. 1999. Attachment in adolescence. In: Handbook of Attachment: Theory, Research, and Clinical Applications, ed. J. Cassidy and P.R. Shaver, pp. 319–335. New York: Guilford.

Altemus, M., P.A. Deuster, E. Galliven, C.S. Carter, and P.W. Gold. 1995. Suppression of hypothalamic–pituitary–adrenal axis responses to stress in lactating women. *J. Clin. Endocrinol. Metab.* **80**:2954–2959.

Amico, J.A., J.M. Johnston, and A.H. Vagnucci. 1994. Suckling-induced attenuation of plasma cortisol concentrations in postpartum lactating women. *Endocr. Res.* **20**: 79–87.

Aragona, B.J., Y. Liu, J.T. Curtis, F.K. Stephan, and Z. Wang. 2003. A critical role for nucleus accumbens dopamine in partner preference formation in prairie voles. *J. Neurosci.* **23**:3483–3490.

Barker, D.J. 1998. *In utero* programming of chronic disease. *Clin. Sci.* **95**:115–128.

Belsky, J., S.B. Campbell, J.F. Cohn, and G. Moore. 1996. Instability of infant–parent attachment security. *Dev. Psychol.* **32**:921–924.

Belsky, J.L., L. Steinberg, and P. Draper. 1991. Childhood experience, interpersonal development and reproductive strategy: An evolutionary theory of socialization. *Child Dev.* **62**:647–670.

Blurton Jones, N.G. 1993. The lives of hunter–gatherer children: Effects of parental behavior and parental reproductive strategy. In: Juvenile Primates: Life History, Development, and Behavior, ed. M.E. Pereira and L.A. Fairbanks, pp. 309–326. New York: Oxford Univ. Press.

Blurton Jones, N.G., and E. Da Costa. 1987. A suggested adaptive value of toddler night waking: Delaying the birth of the next sibling. *Ethol. Sociobiol.* **8**:135–142.

Born, J., T. Lange, W. Kern et al. 2002. Sniffing neuropeptides: A transnasal approach to the human brain. *Nature Neurosci.* **5**:514–516.

Born, J., R. Pietrowsky, and H.L. Fehm. 1998. Neuropsychological effects of vasopressin in healthy humans. *Prog. Brain Res.* **119**:619–643.

Bowlby, J. 1969. Attachment. Attachment and Loss, vol. 1. New York: Basic.

Bowlby, J. 1973. Separation: Anxiety and Anger. Attachment and Loss, vol. 2. New York: Basic.

Boyce, W.T., M. Champoux, S.J. Suomi, and M.R. Gunnar. 1995. Salivary cortisol in nursery-reared rhesus monkeys: Reactivity to peer interactions and altered circadian activity. *Dev. Psychobiol.* **28**:257–267.

Braun, K., P. Kremz, W. Wetzel, T. Wagner, and G. Poeggel. 2003. Influence of parental deprivation on the behavioral development in Octodon degus: Modulation by maternal vocalizations. *Dev. Psychobiol.* **42**:237–245.

Braun, K., E. Lange, M. Metzger, and G. Poeggel. 2000. Maternal separation followed by early social isolation affects the development of monoaminergic fiber systems in the medial prefrontal cortex of *Octodon degus. Neurosci.* **95**:309–318.

Braun, K., and G. Poeggel. 2001. Recognition of mother's voice evokes metabolic activation in the medial prefrontal cortex and thalamus of *Octodon degus* pups. *Neurosci.* **103**:861–864.

Bredy, T.W., R.A. Humpartzoomian, D.P. Cain, and M.J. Meaney. 2003. Partial reversal of the effect of maternal care on cognitive function through environmental enrichment. *Neurosci.* **118**:571–576.

Bretherton, I., and K.A. Munholland. 1999. Internal working models in attachment relationships: A construct revisited. In: Handbook of Attachment: Theory, Research, and Clinical Applications, ed. J. Cassidy and P. Shaver, pp. 89–111. New York: Guilford.

Brownstein, M.J., J.T. Russell, and H. Gainer. 1980. Synthesis, transport, and release of posterior pituitary hormones. *Science* **207**:373–378.

Bruce, M.L. 2002. Psychosocial risk factors for depressive disorders in late life. *Biol. Psych.* **52**:175–184.

Bruins, J., R. Hijman, and J.M. Van Ree. 1992. Effect of a single dose of des-glycinamide-[Arg8]vasopressin or oxytocin on cognitive processes in young healthy subjects. *Peptides* **13**:461–468.

Campos, J.J., R. Kermoian, and M.R. Zumbahlen. 1992. Socioemotional transformations in the family system following infant crawling onset. In: Emotion and Its Regulation in Early Development, ed. N. Eisenberg and R. Fabes, pp. 25–40. San Francisco: Jossey-Bass.

Carlson, M., C. Dragomir, F. Earls et al. 1995. Effects of social deprivation on cortisol regulation in institutionalized Romanian infants. *Soc. Neurosci. Abst.* **21**:524.

Carter, C.S. 1998. Neuroendocrine perspectives on social attachment and love. *Psychoneuroendocrin.* **23**:779–818.

Cassidy, J., and P.R. Shaver, eds. 1999. Handbook of Attachment: Theory, Research, and Clinical Applications. New York: Guilford.

Clarke, A.M., and A.D.B. Clarke. 2000. Early Experience and the Life Path. London: Kingsley.

Cohn, J.F., S.B. Campbell, and S. Ross. 1991. Infant response in the still-face paradigm at 6 months predicts avoidant and secure attachment at 12 months. *Dev. Psychopathol.* **3**:367–376.

Colin, V.L. 1996. Human Attachment. New York: McGraw-Hill.

de Wied, D., M. Diamant, and M. Fodor. 1993. Central nervous system effects of neurohypophyseal hormones and related peptides. *Front. Neuroendocrin.* **14**:251–302.

de Wolff, M.S., and M.H. van IJzendoorn. 1997. Sensitivity and attachment: A meta-analysis on parental antecedents of infant attachment. *Child Dev.* **68**:571–591.

Fleming, A., M. Steiner, and C. Corter. 1997. Cortisol, hedonics, and maternal responsiveness in human mothers. *Horm. Behav.* **32**:85–98.

Francis, D.D., J. Diorio, P.M. Plotsky, and M.J. Meaney. 2002. Environmental enrichment reverses the effects of maternal separation on stress reactivity. *J. Neurosci.* **22**: 7840–7843.

Gekoski, M.J., C.K. Rovee-Collier, and V. Carulli-Rabinowitz. 1983. A longitudinal analysis of inhibition of infant distress: The origins of social expectations? *Infant Behav. Dev.* **6**:339–351.

Greenfield, P.M., H. Keller, A. Fuligni, and A. Maynard. 2003. Cultural pathways through universal development. *Ann. Rev. Psychol.* **54**:461–490.

Gunnar, M.R. 2000. Early adversity and the development of stress reactivity and regulation. In: The Effects of Adversity on Neurobehavioral Development, ed. C.A. Nelson, pp. 163–200. Minnesota Symposia on Child Psychology 31. Mahwah, NJ: Erlbaum.

Gunnar, M.R., and B. Donzella. 2002. Social regulation of the LHPA axis in early human development. *Psychoneuroendocrin.* **27**:199–220.

Gunnar, M., and D.M. Vazquez. 2001. Low cortisol and a flattening of the expected daytime rhythm: Potential indices of risk in human development. *Dev. Psychopathol.* **13**:516–538.

Hagen, E.H. 1999. The functions of postpartum depression. *Evol. Hum. Behav.* **20**:325–359.

Handlon, J.H., R.W. Wadeson, J.R. Fishman et al. 1962. Psychological factors lowering plasma 17-hydroxycorticosteroid concentration. *Psychosom. Med.* **24**:535–542.

Harris, P.L. 1996. Between Strange Situation and false beliefs: Working models and theories of mind. In: Early Mother–child Interaction and Attachment: Old and New Approaches, ed. W. Koops, J. Hoeksma, and D. van den Boom, pp. 187–199. Amsterdam: Elsevier.

Hart, J., M. Gunnar, and D. Cicchetti. 1995. Salivary cortisol in maltreated children: Evidence of relations between neuroendocrine activity and social competence. *Dev. Psychopathol.* **7**:11–26.

Heinrichs, M. 2000. Oxytocin and Behavior: Psychobiological Effects of Oxytocin on Human Cognitive Performance and Stress Reactivity. Gottingen: Cuvillier.

Heinrichs, M., T. Baumgartner, C. Kirschbaum, and U. Ehlert. 2003. Social support and oxytocin interact to suppress cortisol and subjective responses to psychosocial stress. *Biol. Psych.* **54**:1389–1398.

Heinrichs, M., G. Meinlschmidt, I. Neumann et al. 2001. Effects of suckling on hypothalamic–pituitary–adrenal axis responses to psychosocial stress in postpartum lactating women. *J. Clin. Endocrinol. Metab.* **86**:4798–4804.

Heinrichs, M., I. Neumann, and U. Ehlert. 2002. Lactation and stress: Protective effects of breast-feeding in humans. *Stress* **5**:195–203.

Henry, J.P. 1993. Psychological and physiological responses to stress: The right hemisphere and the hypothalamo–pituitary axis, an inquiry into problems of human bonding. *Integ. Physiol. Behav. Sci.* **28**:368–386.

Henry, J.P., and S. Wang. 1998. Effects of early stress on adult affiliative behavior. *Psychoneuroendocrin.* **23**:863–875.

Hertsgaard, L., M. Gunnar, M.F. Erickson, and M. Nachmias. 1995. Adrenocortical responses to the strange situation in infants with disorganized/disoriented attachment relationships. *Child Dev.* **66**:1100–1106.

Hesse, E. 1999. The Adult Attachment Interview: Historical and current perspectives. In: Handbook of Attachment: Theory, Research, and Clinical Applications, ed. J. Cassidy and P.R. Shaver, pp. 395–433. New York: Guilford.

Hirschfeld, L.A., and S.A. Gelman. 1998. Toward a topography of mind: An introduction to domain specificity. In: Mapping the Mind: Domain Specificity in Cognition and Culture, ed. L.A. Hirschfeld and S.A. Gelman, pp. 3–35. Cambridge: Cambridge Univ. Press.

Hrdy, S.B. 1994. Fitness tradeoffs in the history and evolution of delegated mothering with special reference to wet-nursing, abandonment and infanticide. In: Infanticide and Parental Care, ed. S. Parmigiani and F.S. Vom Saal, pp. 3–41. Chur: Harwood.

Hrdy, S.B. 1999. Mother Nature: Maternal Instincts and How They Shape the Human Species. New York: Ballantine.

Hurtado, A.M., K. Hill, H. Kaplan, and I. Hurtado. 1992. Trade-offs between female food acquisition and child care among Hiwi and Ache foragers. *Hum. Nat.* **3**:185–216.

Insel, T. 2003. Is social attachment an addictive process? *Physiol. Behav.* **79**:351–357.

Insel, T.R., and L.J. Young. 2001. The neurobiology of attachment. *Nat. Rev. Neurosci.* **2**:129–136.

Keller, H. 2000. Human parent–child relationships from an evolutionary perspective. *Am. Behav. Sci.* **43**:957–969.

Keller, H. 2002. The role of development for understanding the biological basis of cultural learning. In: Between Culture and Biology, ed. H. Keller, Y. Poortinga, and A. Schoelmerich, pp. 215–240. Cambridge: Cambridge Univ. Press.

Kraemer, H.C., E. Stice, A. Kazdin, D. Offord, and D. Kupfer. 2001. How do risk factors work together? Mediators, moderators, and independent, overlapping, and proxy risk factors. *Am. J. Psych.* **158**:848–856.

Lamb, M.E., and C.M. Malkin. 1986. The development of social expectations in distress-relief sequences: A longitudinal study. *Intl. J. Behav. Dev.* **9**:235–249.

Lamb, M.E., R.A. Thompson, W.P. Gardner, and E. Charnov. 1985. Infant–mother Attachment. Hillsdale, NJ: Erlbaum.

Legros, J.J. 2001. Inhibitory effect of oxytocin on corticotrope function in humans: Are vasopressin & oxytocin ying-yang neurohormones? *Psychoneuroend.* **26**:649–655.

Markus, H.R., and S. Kitiyama. 1991. Culture and the self: Implications for cognition, emotion and motivation. *Psychol. Rev.* **98**:224–253.

Martel, F.L., C.M. Nevison, M.D.A. Simpson, and E.B. Keverne. 1993. Opioid receptor blockade reduces maternal affect and social grooming in rhesus monkeys. *Psychoneuroend.* **18**:307–321.

Mason, J.W., S. Wang, R. Yehuda et al. 2001. Psychogenic lowering of urinary cortisol levels linked to increased emotional numbing and a shame-depressive syndrome in combat-related posttraumatic stress disorder. *Psychosom. Med.* **63**:387–401.

McCarthy, M.M., and M. Altemus. 1997. Central nervous system actions of oxytocin and modulation of behavior in humans. *Molec. Med. Today* **3**:269–275.

Meins, E., C. Fernyhough, E. Fradley, and M. Tuckey. 2001. Rethinking maternal sensitivity: Mothers' comments on infants' mental processes predict security of attachment at 12 months. *J. Child Psychol. Psychiat.* **42**:637–648.

Nachmias, M., M. Gunnar, S. Mangelsdorf et al. 1996. Behavioral inhibition and stress reactivity: The moderating role of attachment security. *Child Dev.* **67**:508–522.

O'Connor, T.G. 2003. Early experiences and psychological development: Conceptual questions, empirical illustrations, and implications for intervention. *Dev. Psychopathol.* **15**:671–690.

O'Connor, T.G., J. Heron, J. Golding, V. Glover, and the ALSPAC study team. 2003. Maternal antenatal anxiety and behavioural/emotional problems in children: A test of a programming hypothesis. *J. Child Psychol. Psychiat.* **44**:1025–1036.

O'Connor, T.G., R.S. Marvin, M. Rutter, J. Olrick, P.A. Britner, and the English and Romanian Adoptees Study Team. 2003. Child–parent attachment following early institutional deprivation. *Dev. Psychopathol.* **15**:19–38.

O'Connor, T.G., M. Rutter, and the English and Romanian Adoptees Study Team. 2000. Attachment disorder behavior following early severe deprivation: Extension and longitudinal follow-up. *J. Am. Acad. Child Adoles. Psych.* **39**:703–712.

Panter-Brick, C. 1995. Child-care strategies in Nepal: Responses to ecology, demography, and society. In: Human Populations: Diversity and Adaptation, ed. A.J. Boyce and V. Reynolds, pp. 174–188. Oxford: Oxford Univ. Press.

Pedersen, C.A. 1997. Oxytocin control of maternal behavior: Regulation by sex steroids and offspring stimuli. *Ann. NY Acad. Sci.* **807**:126–145.

Pedersen, C.A., and M.L. Boccia. 2002. Oxytocin links mothering received, mothering bestowed and adult stress responses. *Stress* **5**:259–267.

Pedersen, C.A., and A.J. Prange. 1979. Induction of maternal behavior in virgin rats after intracerebroventricular administration of oxytocin. *PNAS* **76**:6661–6665.

Pitman, R.K., S.P. Orr, and N.B. Lasko. 1993. Effects of intranasal vasopressin and oxytocin on physiologic responding during personal combat imagery in Vietnam veterans with posttraumatic stress disorder. *Psychiatry Res.* **48**:107–117.

Poeggel, G., and K. Braun. 1996. Early auditory filial learning in degus (*Octodon degus*): Behavioral and autoradiographic studies. *Brain Res.* **743**:162–170.

Poeggel, G., C. Helmeke, T. Schwabe et al. 2003. Juvenile emotional experience alters synaptic composition in the rodent prefrontal cortex, hippocampus and lateral amygdala. *PNAS* **100**:16,137–16,142.

Poeggel, G., G. Nowicki, and K. Braun. 2003. Early social deprivation alters monoaminergic afferents in the orbital prefrontal cortex of *Octodon degus. Neurosci.* **116**:617–620.

Raikes, H.A., and R.A. Thompson. 2004. Attachment in middle childhood: Issues of theory and method. In: Attachment in Middle Childhood, ed. K.A. Kerns and R.A. Richardson, pp. 255–282. New York: Guilford.

Rosenfield, P.D., S. Suchecki, and S. Levine. 1992. Multifactorial regulation of the hypothalamic–pituitary–adrenal axis during development. *Neurosci. Biobehav. Rev.* **16**: 553–568.

Rozanski, A., J.A. Blumenthal, and J. Kaplan. 1999. Impact of psychological factors on the pathogenesis of cardiovascular disease and implications for therapy. *Circulation* **99**:2192–2217.

Russell, J.A., A.J. Douglas, and C.D. Ingram. 2001. Brain preparations for maternity: Adaptive changes in behavioral and neuroendocrine systems during pregnancy and lactation: An overview. *Prog. Brain Res.* **133**:1–38.

Rutter, M., J. Kreppner, T.G. O'Connor, and the English and Romanian Adoptees Study Team. 2001. Specificity and heterogeneity in children's responses to profound deprivation. *Brit. J. Psychiatry* **179**:97–103.

Rutter, M., T.G. O'Connor, and the English and Romanian Adoptees Study Team. 2004. Are there biological programming effects for psychological development? Findings from a study of Romanian adoptees. *Dev. Psychol.* **40**:81–94.

Sanchez, M.M., C.O. Ladd, and P. Plotsky. 2001. Early adverse experience as a developmental risk factor for later psychopathlogy: Evidence from rodent and primate models. *Dev. Psychopathol.* **13**:419–449.

Schiefenhoevel, W. 1989. Reproduction and sex-ratio manipulation through preferential female infanticide among the Eipo, in the highlands of west New Guinea. In: The Sociobiology of Sexual and Reproductive Strategies, ed. A.E. Rasa, C. Vogel, and E. Voland, pp. 170–193. London: Chapman and Hall.

Solomon, J., and C. George. 1999. The measurement of attachment security in infancy and childhood. In: Handbook of Attachment: Theory, Research, and Clinical Applications, ed. J. Cassidy and P.R. Shaver, pp. 287–316. New York: Guilford.

Spangler, G., and K.E. Grossmann. 1993. Biobehavioral organization in securely and insecurely attached infants. *Child Dev.* **64**:1439–1450.

Spangler, G., and M. Schieche. 1998. Emotional and adrenocortical responses of infants to the Strange Situation: The differential function of emotional expression. *Intl. J. Behav. Dev.* **22**:681–706.

Spangler, G., and P. Zimmermann. 1999. Attachment representation and emotion regulation in adolescents: A psychobiological perspective on internal working models. *Attach. Hum. Dev.* **1**:270–290.

Sroufe, L.A., B. Egeland, and T. Kreutzer. 1990. The fate of early experience following developmental change: Longitudinal approaches to individual adaptation in childhood. *Child Dev.* **61**:1363–1373.

Sroufe, L.A., and J. Fleeson. 1986. Attachment and the construction of relationships. In: Relationships and Development, ed. W. Hartup and Z. Rubin, pp. 51–71. Hillsdale, NJ: Erlbaum.

Swaab, D.F., C.W. Pool, and F. Nijveldt. 1975. Immunifluorescence of vasopressin and oxytocin in rat hypothalamo–neurohypophyseal system. *J. Neur. Trans.* **36**:195–215.

Teti, D.M., J.W. Sakin, E. Kucera, K.M. Corns, and R. Das Eiden. 1996. And baby makes four: Predictors of attachment security among preschool-age firstborns during the transition to siblinghood. *Child Dev.* **67**:579–596.

Thompson, R.A. 2006. The development of the person: Social understanding, relationships, self, conscience. In: Handbook of Child Psychology, ed. W. Damon and R.M. Lerner, Vol. 3: Social, Emotional, and Personality Development (N. Eisenberg, vol. ed.). New York: Wiley, in press.

Thompson, R.A. 1999. Early attachment and later development. In: Handbook of Attachment: Theory, Research, and Clinical Applications, ed. J. Cassidy and P.R. Shaver, pp. 265–286. New York: Guilford.

Thompson, R.A. 2000. The legacy of early attachments. *Child Dev.* **71**:145–152.

Thompson, R.A. 2001. Sensitive periods in attachment? In: Critical Thinking about Critical Periods, ed. D.B. Bailey, J.T. Bruer, F.J. Symons, and J.W. Lichtman, pp. 83–106. Baltimore: Brookes.

Thompson, R.A., D.J. Laible, and L.L Ontai. 2003. Early understanding of emotion, morality, and the self: Developing a working model. In: Advances in Child Development and Behavior, ed. R.V. Kail, vol. 31, pp.137–171. San Diego: Academic.

Thompson, R.A., M.E. Lamb, and D. Estes. 1982. Stability of infant–mother attachment and its relationship to changing life circumstances in an unselected middle-class sample. *Child Dev.* **53**:144–148.

Thompson, R.A., and H.A. Raikes. 2003. Toward the next quarter-century: Conceptual & methodological challenges for attachment theory. *Dev. Psychopathol.* **15**:691–718.

Tomasello, M. 1999. The Cultural Origins of Human Cognition. Cambridge, MA: Harvard Univ. Press.

Trivers, R.L. 1974. Parent–offspring conflict. *Am. Zoologist* **14**:249–264.

Trivers, R. 1985. Social Evolution. Menlo Park, CA: Benjamin Cummings.

Vandesande, F., and K. Dierickx. 1975. Identification of the vasopressin producing and of the oxytocin producing neurons in the hypothalamic magnocellular neurosecretory system of the rat. *Cell Tiss. Res.* **164**:153–162.

van IJzendoorn, M.H., and A. Sagi. 1999. Cross-cultural patterns of attachment: Universal and contextual dimensions. In: Handbook of Attachment: Theory, Research, and Clinical Applications, ed. J. Cassidy and P. Shaver, pp. 713-734. New York: Guilford.

Vaughn, B.E., B. Egeland, L.A. Sroufe, and E. Waters. 1979. Individual differences in infant–mother attachment at twelve and eighteen months: Stability and change in families under stress. *Child Dev.* **50**:971–975.

Voland, E. 1998. Evolutionary ecology of human reproduction. *Ann. Rev. Anthropology* **27**:347–374.

Waters, E., and E.M. Cummings. 2000. A secure base from which to explore close relationships. *Child Dev.* **71**:164–172.

Waters, E., K. Kondo–Ikemura, G. Posada, and J.E. Richters. 1991. Learning to love: Mechanisms and milestones. In: Self Processes and Development, ed. M.R. Gunnar and L. Sroufe, pp. 217–255. Minnesota Symp. Child Psych. 23. Hillsdale: Erlbaum.

Watson, J.S. 1972. Smiling, cooing, and "the game." *Merrill-Palmer Qtly.* **18**:323–339.

Watson, J.S. 1979. Perception of contingency as a determinant of social responsiveness. In: Origins of the Infant's Social Responsiveness, ed. E.B. Thoman, pp. 33–64. Hillsdale, NJ: Erlbaum.

Wolff, C.T., S.B. Friedman, M.A. Hofer, and J.W. Mason. 1964. Relationship between psychological defenses and mean urinary 17-OHCS excretion rates: A predictive study of parents of fatally ill children. *Psychosom. Med.* **26**:576–591.

Ziabreva, I., G. Poeggel, R. Schnabel, and K. Braun. 2003. Separation–induced receptor changes in the hippocampus and amygdala of Octodon degus: Influence of maternal vocalizations. *J. Neurosci.* **23**:5329–5336.

Ziabreva, I., R. Schnabel, G. Poeggel, and K. Braun. 2003. Mother's voice "buffers" separation–induced receptor changes in the prefrontal cortex of Octodon degus. *Neurosci.* **119**:433–441.

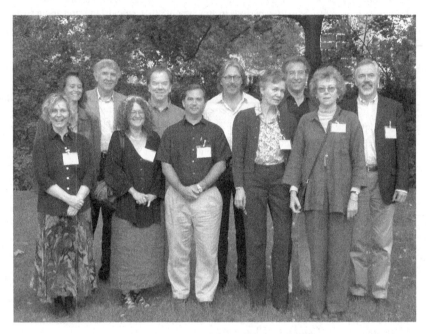

Back, left to right: Simone Sommer, Wolfgang Tietze, Cort Pedersen, Norbert Sachser,
    Jay Belsky, Gustl Anzenberger
Front, left to right: Lilo Ahnert, Alison Fleming, Larry Young, Karin Grossmann,
    Patricia Draper

17

Group Report: Beyond Infant Attachment

The Origins of Bonding in Later Life

C. A. PEDERSEN, Rapporteur

L. AHNERT, G. ANZENBERGER, J. BELSKY, P. DRAPER,
A. S. FLEMING, K. GROSSMANN, N. SACHSER,
S. SOMMER, D. P. TIETZE, and L. J. YOUNG

ABSTRACT

Older children, adolescents, and adults form close social bonds that are more diverse and mutual than the infant's attachment to his/her mother. This chapter examines our current understanding, drawing on animal and human studies, of factors that give rise to and shape social bonds later in life as well as the functional significance of those bonds. Etiological factors will be considered at multiple levels. We begin with the neurobiological mechanisms of two prominent adult social bonds: parental bonding to infants and monogamous pair bonding between sexual partners. The focus then turns to the effects of experience at different ontogenetic periods on adult social bonding and other social behaviors, an area in which dramatic advances have occurred in recent years. The considerable influence of social structure and culture on social bonds, especially between parents and children and between marital partners, is illustrated by comparing characteristics of these relationships between Western and non-Western societies. Evolutionary mechanisms that have selected for social bonding are discussed. It is argued that a modern evolutionary perspective raises issues that differ from the traditional mental health perspective on attachment and bonding and, thereby, contributes significantly to the understanding of human development. Current childcare and school policies and practices in Western Europe and the United States are compared with what is known about optimal conditions to meet children's social bonding needs. Finally, it is speculated that bonding may be an important factor contributing to the physical and mental health benefits of social support as well as commitments that are not strictly social, such as religious belief.

INTRODUCTION

Although we summarize current knowledge and theory about the etiology and regulation of social bonding after infancy and early childhood, our primary objective was to identify gaps in knowledge and promising perspectives that are either emerging or have been underemphasized. Our hope is to stimulate creative thinking and productive new lines of research. Before we begin, however, consideration must be given to the characteristics and scope of human bonds later in life as well as how social bonding is measured in animal research.

Characteristics and Scope of Bonding Later in Life

Attachment is the term used by John Bowlby (1969) and Mary Ainsworth (1979) to refer to their hypothesized motivational system in infants/children that compels them to seek and maintain close contact with their primary caretaker, who in most cases is their mother. Based on research and theoretical considerations, a number of components and characteristics have been incorporated into the attachment concept by the Bowlby/Ainsworth schools (Cassidy and Shaver 1999; Grossmann and Grossmann, this volume). In the securely attached infant/child, these include distress upon separation from the caretaker, confidence in the reliability of help from the caretaker in stressful situations, feelings of safety/tranquility in the presence of the caretaker, external organization by the caretaker of internal processes, attentional guidance by the caretaker (e.g., alerting to dangers, meaning of stimuli/events, right and wrong), developmental effects that enhance relatedness to others, intrapsychic processes and coping ability later in life, and jealousy when attachment is perceived to be threatened, sometimes resulting in efforts to defend against or attack that threat. Infancy and early childhood are viewed as a sensitive period during which attachment to the caretaker occurs more readily and vulnerability is greatest to long-term consequences of the quality of caretaking received.

The evolution of dependency and the attachment motivational system in infants and toddlers has required the complementary evolution in parents of the caregiving motivational system. The latter assures provision of basic needs to infants, food, warmth, shelter, as well as vigorous defense against potential threats. The infant–caretaker bond is a highly asymmetric relationship between a weaker, more vulnerable, less knowledgeable, experienced individual (the infant/child) and a stronger, more experienced/knowledgeable individual (the primary caretaker). In this relationship, the infant/child demands and receives, but does not give, whereas the caretaker gives without receiving.

In animals and humans, other emotionally close relationships develop during later childhood, adolescence, and adulthood that are generally more mutual. These include dyadic (individual to individual) bonds, such as love between parents and their older/adult children, sibling bonds, friendships in childhood and adulthood, bonds between sexual partners, and love between other biological relatives. It has been hypothesized that the motivation drawing bonded individuals to significant others is similar to the attachment motivational system exhibited by infants/young children toward their caretakers (see Carter, this volume). Romantic love relationships have been studied fruitfully from an attachment perspective; both secure and insecure patterns have been identified (Feeney 1999; Hazan and Zeifman 1999). These bonds, however, also include some degree of mutual caregiving. Thus, the dyadic bonds that emerge after early childhood may be based on a combination of infant-like attachment and parental-like caregiving motivation.

Bonding, however, is not restricted to dyadic relationships. Individuals are often strongly emotionally committed to their social group/troupe. In humans, this sort of bond can be extended to very large groups, such as tribes and nations. Individuals form strong bonds to many entities besides other humans, including animals, inanimate objects (e.g., homes, property), and goal-directed activities (work, play). Our species has the unprecedented ability to generate an almost unlimited number of mental constructs. Some of these become important elements of culture (spiritual concepts like God, ideals like freedom/truth/honor/ beauty, traditions, institutions) and are objects of considerable emotional investment for many people. Thus the mental world provides outlets for emotional bonding that are unique to *Homo sapiens*. Human intelligence also enhances the quality of dyadic bonds. Awareness of the inner selves of others (theory of mind) and spoken language vastly increases the degree to which individuals can understand each other and express mutual affection. Human and animal bonds to their larger social group as well as human bonds to culture may be extensions of early primary social bonds because they are usually forged during childhood/adolescence within the context of relationships with parents and other close family and social group members.

Social and nonsocial bonds formed later in life have many of the same characteristics as infant attachment and parental bonding and provide similar benefits (Figure 17.1). Loss of close family members, friends, or the social group produce emotional distress similar to that of the infant separated from its mother. In humans, losing valued entities (e.g., property, wealth) or purposeful

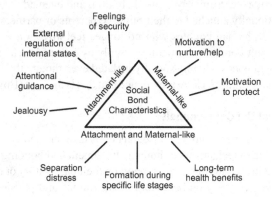

Figure 17.1 Human social bonds formed later in life feature a mixture of infant attachment-like and maternal-like characteristics.

enterprise (e.g., employment) and even disillusionment with beliefs or alien-ation from associated religious or ideological groups can be as emotionally up-setting as the death of a close friend. Bonds to individuals, social groups, and (among humans) culturally based beliefs, traditions, values, and institutions also provide a sense of security, solace in stressful situations, guidance in deci-sion making, physiological regulation, as well as long-term mental and physical health benefits (Henry and Stephens 1977; Sagi-Schwartz et al. 2003; Uvnas-Moberg 1997). Jealousy and retaliation can also be sparked by the per-ception of threats to these bonds. After early childhood, some bonds may be more likely to occur during specific phases of life (e.g., peer bonding during la-tency, commitment to social/cultural values during adolescence, pair bonding after puberty). Later life bonds to other individuals or the social group are also characterized by parental-like desires to be helpful and protective. Humans ex-perience similar nurturing impulses toward their culture's belief systems, tradi-tions, values, and associated institutions. Of course people also avidly protect and take care of their homes, lands, possessions, and other valued entities.

Do formation and maintenance of infant attachments and social bonds later in life require hedonic reward? Evidence from animal and human research sug-gests that these close relationships may form and persist despite aversive conse-quences or lack of positive reward. Learning and becoming attached to their mother's odor is crucial to the survival of young rat pups because they depend upon olfactory cues to locate their mother and her nipples. Recent findings sug-gest that preference for maternal odors can develop even if the mother is abusive to her pups. Prior to ten days of age, pairing odors with painful electroshock ac-tually increases rat pups' preference for locations scented with those odors (Sullivan et al. 2000). By ten days of age, pups have developed the ability to learn to avoid odors paired with aversive stimuli, possibly because of maturation of the amygdala which is necessary for fear conditioning. However, preferences for odors previously paired with shock persist after pups have become able to learn odor avoidance. Similarly, abused children and even adults often remain strongly emotionally attached to their punitive parents or partners. Frequently, bonds persist in human couples who no longer feel affection for each other. Could some adult bonds be maintained simply by fear of loneliness and other negative consequences of being socially isolated even though they are not plea-surable or even soothing? There is evidence that this is the case (Bowlby 1988).

Defining Social Bonds in Animals

Investigation of the neurobiology of social bonds in other species is essential for understanding the mechanisms of human attachment and bonding. To measure social bonding in animals that cannot report on their past history or internal emo-tional state, we must rely on behavioral observations and physiological mea-surements. Wickler (1976) proposed some parsimonious behavioral traits for a

Table 17.1 Ethological criteria for defining a social bond (adapted from Wickler 1976).

---

* Maintenance of close proximity with the bonding partner
* Synchronization of behaviors between partners
* Exclusive or more frequent positive social behavior directed toward partner
* Proximity, synchronization, and exclusivity are maintained over time

---

bond that could be applied to any species (Table 17.1). Neuroscientists studying social behavior in mammals have incorporated and elaborated upon these "bare bones" criteria (Carter and Keverne 2002). Bonded individuals usually maintain close proximity to each other, synchronize their behaviors, and interact in ways that differ from the social behavior they direct toward others (Wickler 1976). In addition, socially bonded individuals experience positive affective states, at least from time to time. Loss of, or separation from, a bonding partner will elicit behavioral signs of stress (e.g., distress vocalizations) and physiological stress responses (increased glucocorticoid and catecholamine release, alterations in heart/respiration rate, gastrointestinal motility). Correspondingly, reunion with the bonding partner will bring about the opposite effect. The presence of a bonding partner in a challenging situation may attenuate or suppress behavioral and physiological stress responses (Sachser et al. 1998; Hennessy 1999; Carter and Keverne 2002). In addition, preference tests, in which an experimental animal is allowed a choice between individuals, can be used to detect social bonds (Anzenberger 1988; Carter and Keverne 2002). Avid protection and caregiving behaviors, such as grooming and food sharing, are also selectively provided to the bonding partner. These aspects of animal social bonds bear striking similarities to the characteristics of human attachments and bonds discussed above.

CAUSES OF LATER LIFE BONDING

Here we examine factors that motivate and shape social bonding later in life (after early childhood) at multiple levels. More is known about the neurobiology of maternal behavior and monogamous pair bonds than any other close social relationships, including infant attachment to the caretaker. Aspects of this large body of experimental evidence that may be relevant to other social bonds are summarized below. Much has been learned in recent years about the influence of experiences at different stages of life on social behavior and the underlying neurobiological mechanisms. Comparisons of non-Western and Western societies demonstrate that social structure strongly influences the types of relationships in which close emotional bonds are formed. At the evolutionary level, bonding appears to have provided selection advantages in several ways.

Proximate Mechanisms of Parental Bonding

We briefly summarize current knowledge of the neurobiological basis of parental (primarily maternal) behavior under headings that correspond to major themes that have emerged in this field of research. Characteristics of maternal behavior are compared among rats, sheep, primates, and humans (Table 17.2). Recent reviews provide more comprehensive coverage of the experimental literature in this area (Gonzalez-Mariscal and Poindron 2002; Kendrick 2000; Numan and Insel 2003). Primary references are thus cited sparingly below.

Bonding Selectivity

As in most subprimate mammalian species, nulliparous rats and sheep avoid, threaten, or even attack newborns. During or just prior to parturition, females of these species undergo a marked transformation in their responses to young from avoidant and/or hostile to nurturing and protective behavior. Rats and sheep, however, differ in the selectivity of their maternal behavior. Rat mothers exhibit no preference for their own offspring. They care for other rat mothers' pups with as much gusto as their own. It can be argued that rat mothers "bond" to young pups in general but not their own litters, and certainly not to individual offspring. Parturient sheep, in contrast, rapidly form selective bonds to their own lambs during the first several hours postpartum and remain hostile toward other lambs. In primate species, nulliparous females are attracted to infants in general and readily exhibit pro-nurturant behavior if given the opportunity. Although

Table 17.2 Comparison of maternal behavior characteristics among species (for details see text). — = lacking; + = lowest; ++ = mid range; +++ = highest; ? = unknown.

	Rat	Sheep	Primates	Humans
Selectivity of bond to offspring	—	+++	+++	+++
Nurturing by nullipara	—	—	+++	+++
Importance of early experience/ learning	+	?	++	+++
Activational role of ↑ estrogen, ↓ progesterone	+++	+++	+	+
Role of oxytocin	++	+++	?	?
Role of prolactin	++ (maternal)	?	+ (paternal)	+ (paternal)
Role of dopamine	+++	++	?	?
Role of opioids	+	++	++	?
Role of glucocorticoids	++	?	?	+
Role of vaginocervical stimulation	+	+++	?	—
Decreased anxiety during lactation	++	?	?	++
Increased protective aggression	+++	+++	+++	+++

their postpartum maternal behavior is quantitatively greater and selective for their own infant, a complete turn around from avoidant/hostile to nurturing/protective does not occur in most subprimate species. This is much closer to the human parental behavior pattern than the rat or sheep model.

Onset of Maternal Behavior: The Roles of Hormones, Neuropeptides, and Neurotransmitters

In rats and sheep, the sex hormone changes during pregnancy (especially high estrogen and declining progesterone levels) that initiate parturition and stimulate mammary tissue to produce milk also trigger the postpartum onset of maternal behavior. Estrogen and progesterone exert these effects by increasing the release and/or receptor concentrations of other hormones, neuropeptides, and neurotransmitters in specific brain areas. Prolactin, oxytocin, and dopamine all play important roles within the brain in mediating the effects of sex steroids on maternal behavior activation. Distention of the cervix and vagina during delivery of the offspring is critical for activating maternal behavior in the sheep but not in the rat. Oxytocin neurons in the hypothalamic paraventricular nucleus have long axons that project to numerous other areas within the brain (Gimpl and Fahrenholz 2001). Vaginocervical stimulation in sheep with high estrogen levels activates ascending neural pathways, which increases the firing rate of paraventricular nucleus oxytocin neurons thereby causing simultaneous release of oxytocin in multiple brain areas (Figure 17.2). Oxytocin exerts specific effects in each brain area, resulting in coordinated activation of pro-nurturant behaviors, while suppressing hostile and other incongruent behaviors (Kendrick 2000). This involves interactions with local norepinephrine release. In some brain areas, oxytocin activates nurturing behaviors such as nuzzling the lamb, low-pitched bleating, and allowing the lamb to suckle. In other brain areas, oxytocin inhibits aggressive actions toward the lamb (butting, high-pitched bleats) or suppresses behaviors that would distract attention away from the lamb (e.g., sexual behavior). Oxytocin interactions with other neurotransmitters in some of these brain areas have been linked to the initiation of maternal behavior.

In rats, the medial preoptic area is the core of the motivational neural circuitry for maternal behavior (Numan and Insel 2003) (Figure 17.2). Projections from this area to brainstem nuclei are critical for both the motivation to mother and the execution of specific maternal behaviors. Inputs to the medial preoptic area from limbic brain areas convey processed sensory information, which regulates maternal behavior. Estrogen and prolactin effects in this area are necessary for the postpartum onset of maternal behavior. The medial preoptic area is also critical for maintaining maternal behavior after the hormonally dependent initiation of mothering during the early postpartum period. The onset of rat maternal behavior is facilitated by oxytocin in some of the same brain areas implicated in sheep, including the medial preoptic area, ventral tegmental area, and olfactory bulbs (Pedersen et al. 1994; Yu et al. 1996). Vasopressin activity in the medial

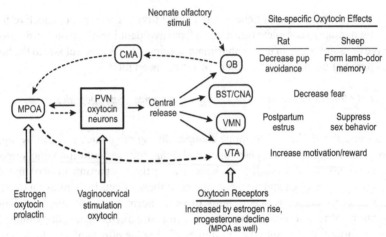

Figure 17.2 A model of oxytocin activation of maternal behavior drawing on findings in rats and sheep (adapted from Figure 6.5 in Numan and Insel 2003). Oxytocin neurons in the paraventricular nucleus (PVN) are stimulated by vaginocervical stimulation and ovarian steroid-induced oxytocin release within the PVN resulting in oxytocin release in projection sites within the brain (solid lines and arrows), including the medial preoptic area (MPOA), olfactory bulbs (OB), bed nucleus of the stria terminalis (BST), central nucleus of the amygdala (CNA), ventromedial nucleus (VMN), and ventral tegmental area (VTA). Oxytocin receptor expression is up-regulated in these sites by the rising estrogen and declining progesterone concentrations that trigger parturition. Oxytocin exerts site- and species-specific effects that result in coordinated mobilization of various aspects of species typical maternal behavior. Several other key features of maternal behavior neural circuitry and neuroendocrinology are also included: processing of neonate olfactory stimuli in the corticomedial amygdala (CMA) before projection to the MPOA (dashed line and arrow), prolactin-activating effects in the MPOA, MPOA projections to the VTA that probably stimulate ascending dopaminergic reward pathways. The vertical arrow indicating estrogen, oxytocin, and prolactin effects in the MPOA mainly summarizes findings in the rat. The vertical arrow indicating vaginocervical stimulation and oxytocin effects on PVN oxytocin neurons summarizes findings in sheep.

preoptic area also appears to play a significant activating role (Pedersen et al. 1994). Oxytocin neurons in the paraventricular nucleus, which give rise to projections to these areas, very likely initiate rat maternal behavior by orchestrating coordinated oxytocin release in multiple brain areas, as in the sheep. Lesions of the paraventricular nucleus during late pregnancy severely disrupt the postpartum onset of maternal behavior (Insel and Harbaugh 1989). The mesolimbic dopamine projection from the ventral tegmental area to the nucleus accumbens, which has been implicated in reward and addiction, is vital for the postpartum onset of rat maternal behavior (Gaffori and LeMoal 1979; Hansen et al. 1991a, b). Evidence that oxytocin in the ventral tegmental area contributes to maternal behavior activation suggests that oxytocin stimulation of mesolimbic dopamine projections may be important in making mothering rewarding. Although there is evidence for interactions between oxytocin and prolactin (Popeski et al. 2003;

Zhu and Onaka 2003), their relationship in the initiation of maternal behavior remains unexplored.

Maintenance of Maternal Behavior

Once maternal behavior is initiated in rats and sheep, maintenance of maternal responses to offspring rapidly becomes independent of sex steroids and much less dependent on the neuropeptide and neurotransmitters that are critical for the onset. For example, central administration of an oxytocin receptor blocker or paraventricular nucleus lesioning, which interferes with the postpartum onset of all components of rat maternal behavior, does not eliminate any pup-directed components of established maternal behavior. Recent, more quantitative studies of the effects of central administration of a receptor antagonist in dams which had been nursing for several days indicate that oxytocin continues to stimulate a significant proportion of pup-licking and kyphotic nursing (during which the mother maintains an upright, arched-back posture over pups) but not other components of established maternal behavior (Champagne et al. 2001; Pedersen and Boccia 2002, 2003). These particular maternal behaviors influence the development of stress responses, pup-licking, and arched-back nursing frequencies and central oxytocin receptor expression in adult female offspring (Caldji et al. 1998; Francis, Caldji et al. 1999; Francis, Diorio et al. 1999; Francis et al. 2000; Champagne et al. 2001).

An enhancing role of corticosterone during the maintenance phase of rat maternal behavior has also been demonstrated. In the postpartum, lactating rat dam, removal of corticosterone by adrenalectomy results in a reduction in pup-licking and crouching, whereas administration of corticosterone reverses these effects in a dose-dependent manner (Rees et al., in prep). Given the interactions between oxytocin and the adrenal axis (Neumann 2001; Windle et al. 1997), it will be of great interest to determine if their effects on these components of established maternal behavior are interrelated.

Offspring Stimulus Regulation of Maternal Behavior

As discussed above for sheep and below for rats (see next section), olfactory stimuli from newborns can be either aversive or attractive to mothers. Somatosensory stimuli from pups are critical for eliciting appropriate maternal responses in rats (Stern and Lonstein 2001). Selective interference with somatosensory but not other components of pup stimuli (olfactory, auditory, visual), by isolating her litter in a basket within the dam's cage maintains high levels of maternal motivation but alters the underlying neurochemistry (Pedersen et al. 1995). After three or more days in this condition (proximal separation), all components of maternal behavior are again controlled by oxytocin; that is, their resurgence when dams are again given unimpeded access to pups is blocked by central administration of an oxytocin receptor antagonist.

Changes in Stress Reactivity Associated with Maternal Behavior

Stress activation of the hypothalamic–pituitary–adrenal (HPA) axis is markedly suppressed during lactation in rodents and humans (Altemus et al. 1995; Carter et al. 2001). In rats, anxious and fearful responses to novel and other stressful stimuli also decline during late pregnancy and lactation. It has been speculated that this emotional change has evolved so that parturient females, especially those giving birth for the first time, will not run away from or attack unfamiliar newborns (Fleming and Li 2002). In other species, it remains unclear whether a general decline in anxiety/fear accompanies the lactational decline in HPA axis activation. Evidence suggests that central oxytocin contributes to these emotional and behavioral changes during lactation (Consiglio and Lucion 1996; Lubin et al. 2003).

Changes in Maternal-like Responsivity to Newborns across the Life Span

The rapidity and quality of maternal-like responsivity to newborns shifts considerably over the life course of rats. During the pre-weaning period, juvenile females and males readily lick, retrieve, group, and crouch over newborns. As puberty approaches, at the end of the adolescent period, juveniles become avoidant of pups — an aversion that is largely olfactory-based and mediated in the corticomedial amygdala. The postpartum onset of maternal behavior involves inhibition of the female's aversive perception of pup odors. After acquiring postpartum mothering experience, however, females subsequently exhibit more rapid reactivation of maternal behavior, even following long periods of separation from pups. These observations imply that the neural program for maternal behavior is present early in development but is actively inhibited during juvenile and adult life when rats cannot nurse pups. After postpartum activation of the program and alteration of pup odor perception, inhibition of maternal behavior remains much diminished. The neurobiology of post-weaning and postpartum experience-induced changes in maternal responsivity is poorly understood (cf. Fleming, this volume).

From an evolutionary perspective, it is of interest that newborn caregiving behavior is relatively uninhibited in the pre-weaning juvenile period, just when the rat mother would have her next litter if she is impregnated the evening after giving birth, which is the usual pattern in the wild. Perhaps the maternal-like behavior of juvenile rats has a beneficial effect on the survival and reproductive success of their half-siblings, thereby increasing the juvenile's inclusive fitness.

The Neurobiology of Nonhuman and Human Primate Maternal Behavior

A limited number of studies suggest that estrogen may enhance maternal behavior in monkeys and apes (Maestripieri and Zehr 1998; Pryce et al. 1993). Pharmacological blockade of opioid receptors with naloxone diminishes interactions of monkey mothers with their infants. One small study found central administration of oxytocin increased infant-directed nurturing behavior in nulliparous female rhesus monkeys (Holman and Goy 1995). In many primate species, mothers and their offspring, especially daughters, maintain close, supportive relationships throughout life. Are these life-long bonds an extension of mother–infant bonds and are they maintained by similar neurobiological mechanisms?

In humans the role for hormones in the onset of maternal responsiveness is necessarily based on correlational studies. However, it is reasonable to predict that the initial feelings of attachment (associated with onset) and the extent of sensitive interactions (ongoing behavior once maternal) will be linked to endocrine changes similar to those implicated in other mammals. Clearly, however, causal statements about the role of these hormones in the regulation of human maternal behavior cannot be made. There is now evidence that the quality of mothers' feelings at birth (how nurturant mothers feel, based on responses on Likert-like scales) is related to the ratio of estrogen to progesterone during the pregnancy, such that those with higher postpartum nurturance exhibit higher estrogen/progesterone ratios in late compared to early pregnancy, with the low nurturant group showing the opposite pattern (Fleming et al. 1997).

In terms of glucocorticoid–maternal behavior relations, findings in women parallel those from animal studies. On postpartum day 2, mothers with higher concentrations of circulating cortisol exhibit more affectionate behavior towards their infants; they are also more attracted to infant body odors and more sympathetic to the infant cries (Corter and Fleming 2002; Stallings et al. 2001; Fleming, this volume). Recent work by Spangler (in prep.) supports these findings and shows, in addition, that the cortisol concentrations in mothers and infants are correlated. By 4 months postpartum, however, concentrations are negatively correlated with positive maternal responses to infants. Connecting cortisol concentrations with maternal motivation in humans is fraught with complications. During pregnancy, baseline concentrations rise well above the normal nonpregnant range. Concentrations decline postpartum but do not level out within the normal range until approximately 6–9 weeks after delivery (Pedersen et al. 1993). Stress activation of the HPA axis is suppressed by lactation (Altemus et al. 1995). Cortisol concentrations are positively correlated with good mood on postpartum day 2 but later are higher in women with postpartum depression and in nondepressed women with histories of prior major depressions (Fleming, this volume; Pedersen et al. 1993). In addition, teenage mothers have higher cortisol concentrations than older mothers, possibly because they are experiencing more stress (Krpan et al. 2005). Thus, correlations and perhaps causal relationships of cortisol concentrations with behavior and emotion can be "positive" or "negative" but certainly not linear.

With advances in imaging techniques, it is increasingly feasible to examine which areas of the human brain are activated when parental emotions are evoked. Indeed, a recent fMRI study found that listening to infant cries increased activity in the medial thalamus, medial prefrontal, and right orbitofrontal cortices, hypothalamus, anterior cingulate cortex, dorsal, and ventral striatum and midbrain of nursing women (Lorberbaum et al. 2002).

Paternal Behavior

In monogamous species, fathers contribute a significant proportion of the parental care. In some bird species, prolactin appears to facilitate paternal behavior (Buntin 1996). Prolactin levels in several monogamous New World monkey species have been reported to correlate positively with paternal care, although it is unclear whether hormone concentrations are a cause or a consequence of paternal care (Schradin and Anzenberger 1999; Schradin et al. 2003). In human fathers, nurturing responses to infant cries have been linked to higher prolactin and lower testosterone levels (Fleming et al. 2002; Storey et al. 2000). Men living with pregnant partners occasionally develop the couvade syndrome, in which their prolactin levels rise and they gain weight in a pattern similar to that occurring during pregnancy (Munroe et al. 1981; Trethowan 1972). The neuropeptide, vasopressin, which stimulates male pair bonding in the monogamous prairie vole (see below), also stimulates paternal behavior (Wang et al. 1994). Vasopressin is very similar in structure to oxytocin.

Proximate Mechanisms of the Adult Pair Bond

Neurobiology of Monogamous Pair Bonding

Studies examining the mechanisms underlying the formation of pair bonds in monogamous species have provided significant insight into the neurobiology of social bond formation (Insel and Young 2001). Approximately 3–5% of mammalian species are socially monogamous; that is, a preferential bond forms between pairs of breeding females and males. The neurobiology of the adult pair bond has been most extensively studied in the monogamous prairie vole (Carter and Getz 1993; Carter 1998; Insel and Young 2001). In this species, mating facilitates the formation of the pair bond, although a pair bond can be established without mating in some circumstances. Interestingly, both oxytocin and vasopressin play critical roles in the formation of the bond. Although there is some overlap, it appears that oxytocin plays the predominant role in the bonding of the female to the male, whereas vasopressin is more critical for the bonding of the male to the female. Central infusion of oxytocin into the female or vasopressin into the male facilitates pair bond formation even when the period of cohabitation with the partner is too short for bonding to occur normally (Winslow et al. 1993; Cho et al. 1999). This effect occurs in the absence of copulation. In contrast, central infusion of an oxytocin receptor antagonist in females and vasopressin receptor antagonist in males prior to mating or extended cohabitation prevents the establishment of the pair bond. Aggression against other males that approach the bonded male's partner is also activated by central vasopressin (Winslow et al. 1993). Prairie voles copulate repeatedly during the first several hours of cohabitation, resulting in extensive vaginocervical stimulation, as seen during parturition, which may be the stimulus for oxytocin release within the female's brain. Thus, in the case of prairie vole pair bonding, it appears that central oxytocin and vasopressin systems may act in a manner similar to the facilitation of the onset of maternal bonding.

By what neurobiological mechanisms do these crucial neuropeptides facilitate pair bonding? The first clues were the significantly higher densities of oxytocin receptors in the nucleus accumbens and V1a vasopressin receptors in the ventral pallidum of monogamous compared to nonmonogamous vole species (Insel and Shapiro 1992; Young et al. 2001) (Figure 17.3b). The nucleus accumbens and ventral pallidum are interconnected nuclei of the mesolimbic dopamine reward pathway, which is thought to be involved in addiction (Kalivas 2000; Lim et al. 2004). Site-specific pharmacological studies demonstrate that these structures are, in fact, critical for the formation of the pair bond. Infusion of oxytocin antagonist into the nucleus accumbens of female prairie voles and infusion of vasopressin antagonist into the ventral pallidum of males completely prevents pair bond formation (Young et al. 2001; Lim and Young 2004). Dopamine neurotransmission in these brain regions is also essential for pair bond formation, suggesting an interaction between these neuropeptides and dopamine systems in the development of social bonds (Gingrich et al. 2000; Aragona et al. 2003). When these findings are combined with observations that oxytocin and vasopressin are involved in the processing of social cues involved in individual recognition (e.g., in knockout mice models [Bielsky et al. 2004] and maternal bonding in the parturient ewe, as discussed above) and dopamine release in the ventral striatum mediates rewarding aspects of copulation (Becker et al. 2001; Hull et al. 2002), a potential model of pair bonding begins to emerge. Perhaps the convergence of oxytocin or vasopressin receptor activation and dopaminergic stimulation in the nucleus accumbens or ventral pallidum result in the animal forming an association between the rewarding aspects of mating and the specific social cues of the partner, resulting in a selective partner bond (Figure 17.3a). It should be noted that mating is not absolutely necessary for pair bond formation; it is possible that nonsexual social stimulation may also activate these pathways, albeit to a lesser extent than that of mating.

Based on the extensive research into the neurobiology of maternal behavior, a number of unresolved questions regarding pair bonding emerge that should be addressed as this field develops. First, *are there more sophisticated measures of pair bond formation than time spent in contact or in close contact with the partner or stranger?* Although these variables are easily quantified, are there not other partner-directed behavioral dimensions to pair bonding, such as mutual grooming or ultrasonic vocalizations? If so, they may be foci for fruitful future investigations (see, e.g., Sachser et al. 1998). Second, *are oxytocin, vasopressin,*

398   C. A. Pedersen et al.

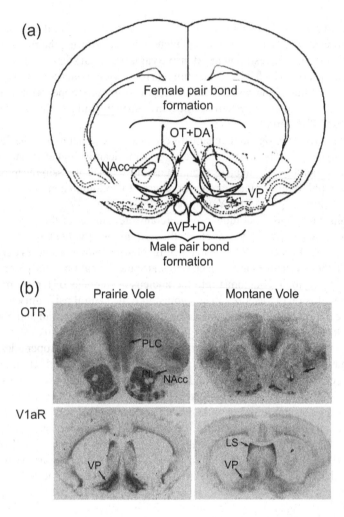

Figure 17.3   (a) Portrayal of combined oxytocin (OT) and dopamine (DA) effects in the prairie vole nucleus accumbens (NAcc) that are hypothesized to stimulate female pair bonding and combined arginine vasopressin (AVP) and DA effects in the ventral pallidum (VP) hypothesized to stimulate male pair bonding. (b) Autoradiograms illustrating differences between the monogamous prairie vole and the promiscuous montane vole in OT receptor (OTR) concentrations in the NAcc and in AVP receptor (V1aR) concentrations in the VP. PLC = prelimbic cortex, LS = lateral septum. After Young et al. (2001, Figures 1 and 4).

and dopamine involved in maintaining as well as initiating pair bonds? Do these factors as well as glucocorticoids regulate the amount of pair bonding-related behavior after partner preference formation is established? If onset and maintenance mechanisms differ, will proximal separation that selectively prevents physical contact (but not other stimuli from the partner) reinstate the onset mechanism? Third, *what are the key stimuli involved in pair bond formation?* Current theory about the neurobiology of pair bond formation stresses the importance of mating. Copulation is thought to trigger neuroendocrine systems which produce a persistent preference for the mating partner. In addition to their unique odors and possibly vaginocervical stimulation during mating, are there other sensory cues from partners that are important in the onset and/or maintenance of selective pair bonds (e.g., somatosensory or thermal stimulation of specific cutaneous areas, vocalizations)? Are proximity, side-by-side contact, and other behavior components of pair bonding elicited by stimuli other than odor? Is it possible that the key stimuli required for pair bond formation vary among species, since in some species strong and persistent bonds develop well before the first copulation occurs? Finally, *what is the relationship between pair bond formation and stress responses?* Stress responses can be ameliorated by the presence of members of the same species (Henry and Stephens 1977; von Holst 1998; Sachser et al. 1998). This phenomenon is called social support. Frequently such social support cannot be provided by any conspecific, but rather the ability to give social support is restricted to bonding partners (see Sachser, this volume). It remains undetermined whether anxiety and fear levels in general are diminished by pair bond formation. Increased aggressiveness, which is often inversely related to anxiety, of the male partner toward other males implies that this might be the case. Diminished emotional stress (e.g., greater feelings of safety) may be a mechanism that promotes and maintains pair bonding; it may operate independently of the reward pathways involved in bond formation. Interestingly, in humans there is evidence for gender-related differences in the effects of social relationships on stress responses (Kirschbaum et al. 1995).

New Frontiers in Bonding Research

The neurobiology of human pair bonding.   Oxytocin, vasopressin, and dopamine pathways in the brain may also be involved in human pair bonding. Both oxytocin and vasopressin levels rise during genital stimulation and orgasm in humans (Carmichael et al. 1994; Murphy et al. 1987). Central release of these neuropeptides may also increase in humans during sexual activity. Unlike females of many species, which mate only during periods of fertility, women show sexual interest in all phases of the ovarian cycle. Perhaps more frequent oxytocin release caused by more regular sexual intercourse strengthens the human pair bond, especially in women. In females of all other mammalian species, breasts become prominent only during lactation. Women's breasts remain protuberant during all postpubertal reproductive states and breast stimulation is a unique feature of human lovemaking. Breast stimulation in this intimate situation may also release oxytocin within the human female's brain and thereby facilitate emotional bonding to her sex partner. Other forms of intimate touch, such as massage, have also been reported to increase oxytocin levels in women

(Uvnas-Moberg 1997). A recent fMRI study found greater activity in the mesolimbic reward pathways when subjects viewed photographs of partners with whom they reported being deeply in love (Bartels and Zeki 2000). The authors noted that the brain activation patterns were similar to those seen in subjects after an infusion of cocaine or opiates.

The relationship between love and sex in human pair bonds. Particular features of human female sexuality (e.g., sexual receptivity across the menstrual cycle, face-to-face copulations, kissing, mutual and often quite elaborate and innovative genital stimulation, and the psychophysiological pleasure experienced during female orgasm) appear to enhance and maintain pair bonds. It is unlikely, however, that these capacities originally evolved for this reason, since they are not unique to humans and are exhibited by primate species that do not form pair bonds (Hrdy and Whitten 1987). Although females of most nonprimate mammalian species confine sexual behavior to the period around ovulation, females of many primate species are receptive during much of the menstrual cycle (e.g., bonobos) or in specific situations outside the fertile period (wild *Macaca fascicularis* or wild langur monkeys) or exhibit elaborate mutual genital stimulation and engage in face-to-face copulations (orangutans and capuchin monkeys). Still, none of these species form exclusive pair bonds. Phylogenetic analyses through evolutionary time suggest that situation-dependent receptivity and nonadvertised (or "concealed") ovulation tends to emerge first, prior to speciation into primates with exclusive long-term pair bonds and monogamy (Sillen-Tullberg and Moller 1993). Similarly, linguistic communication and theory of mind (the ability to think about what the partner is thinking about) clearly play important roles in the formation and maintenance of relationships and intimacy, as do social/mental constructs and ideals such as "love" and "commitment." However, even though these capacities really can be said to be uniquely human, it is not yet known whether they evolved to cement human pair bonds or were secondarily incorporated into facilitating and maintaining them. Most likely, they served as "preadaptations" for the formation and maintenance of intimate and prolonged personal relationships, in general, rather than evolving specifically to promote pair bonding. Nevertheless, other aspects of human sexuality are unique and harder to explain outside of the contexts of sexual advertisement, mate selection, and pair bonding. These include a longer and broader (relative to other apes) penis and prominent female breasts that develop at puberty, before giving birth or lactating, and serve as erotic stimuli as well as erogenous zones. It is tempting to speculate (as we have above) that oxytocin release during copulation and orgasm throughout the menstrual cycle as well as during precopulatory breast stimulation and other types of foreplay may contribute to the formation and maintenance of human pair bonds.

Neurobiology of other types of bonds. It seems clear that somewhat similar mechanisms, or at least neurochemical mediators, may be involved in both mother–infant and adult pair bond formation. To what extent, however, do these play roles in other types of bond formation? For example, some species form strong bonds among females within families or among other members of the group (see Sachser, this volume). Do these mechanisms play any role in more subtle relationships, such as friendships? To date, these issues have not been addressed but may be tractable in some animal models. One study suggests that oxytocin deficiencies could be a factor in psychopathologic disorders involving social deficits. Modahl et al. (1998) and Green et al. (2001) reported that autistic patients have lower plasma levels of oxytocin but higher levels of extended (by 1 or 2 amino acids) and presumably less biologically active oxytocin, suggesting that oxytocin synthesis or processing may be abnormal in this disorder.

Contextual flexibility in bonding. Within many species, social structure varies considerably with environmental circumstances (Lott 1984). Such flexibility may have evolved in small rodent species to facilitate adjustment to a wide range of habitats, population densities, and seasonal conditions (Eisenberg 1966). In domestic guinea pigs, social structure and, in particular, social bonds between males and females differ between low and high population conditions (Sachser, this volume). When the population is low, a strictly dominance-structured system exists. When animal numbers are high, long-lasting bonds are predominant. Meadow voles provide another example of situational flexibility in social structure. In this species, males are promiscuous and nonpaternal during the summer but form selective pair bonds, cohabitate with their partners, and care for offspring under the harsher conditions of winter (Madison et al. 1984; Parker et al. 2001). The duration of daylight may be a factor that regulates these changes in sexual and parental behavior (Parker et al. 2001; Parker and Lee 2001). Parker and Lee (2001) have demonstrated that, as in male prairie voles, vasopressin activity in the brain promotes male meadow vole pair bonding under short photoperiod conditions.

These observations raise several questions which may guide future investigations: What are the specific stimuli associated with population change or season that alter social organization in species (e.g., photoperiod in meadow voles and population density-dependent increase in the number of agonistic encounters in guinea pigs), and by what mechanisms do those stimuli regulate the activity of the motivational systems generating male–female bonds and parental behavior? Do neurobiological mechanisms similar to those underlying persistent pair bonds in monogamous prairie voles also promote selective but polygynous male–female bonds that form under high population conditions in guinea pigs and short photoperiod-related monogamous bonds in meadow voles? The role of vasopressin in male meadow voles suggests that this may be the case, but what about oxytocin (especially in females) and dopamine?

Finally, if adult social bonding emerged in our ancestors as a behavioral strategy to help the individual adapt to his/her environment and if we still bear the ancient motivational system underlying the formation of adult social bonds, then changes in the social and physical environment may cause changes in adult social bonding patterns in humans as well (Sachser, this volume). It would be interesting to elucidate which modern-day environmental condition may favor adult social bonding and which might promote an alternative way to live.

  Major histocompatibility complex and mate selection. The vertebrate major histocompatibility complex (MHC) is a cluster of approximately 200 genes primarily involved in immune response regulation (MHC is also referred to as H-2 in mice and HLA [human leucocyte antigen] in humans). The genes of the MHC are one of the most polymorphic known in vertebrates, with individuals carrying different combinations of theses genes (Klein 1986). There is now substantial evidence in mice, rats, and humans that individuals prefer sexual partners who have different MHC genes to their own (for recent reviews, see Bernatchez and Landry 2003; Penn and Potts 1999). Preference for mates with nonmatching MHC genes may have been selected for because of the immune benefits of MHC heterozygosity in offspring (Apanius et al. 1997; Penn 2002). Also, females mating with a male with the same MHC haplotype suffer increased fetal loss in humans (Schacter et al. 1984; Ober et al. 1997) and nonhuman primates (Knapp et al. 1996). How individuals choose a mate with a particular MHC haplotype is unclear, although it is likely that genes controlling olfactory function located within the region are responsible. The MHC plays a role in individual odor, both through production of soluble proteins or proteins, which bind volatile molecules, and the influence on bacterial gut flora. Coupled with the high variability of the MHC, this provides a basis for individual and kin recognition (reviewed in Brown and Eklund 1994). In humans, polymorphic olfactory receptor genes are located in the MHC (Fan et al. 1995), and both males and females prefer the odor of MHC-dissimilar individuals (Wedekind et al. 1995; Wedekind and Füri 1997). MHC preference in mice has a learned component (Beauchamp and Yamazaki 1997). By rearing individuals in foster families with a MHC haplotype different to their own, MHC preferences can be eliminated (e.g., Eklund 1997; Arcaro and Eklund 1999) or even reversed (Beauchamp et al. 1988; Penn and Potts 1998). These observations suggest that the memory of sibling and mother odors from early life may, in adulthood, inhibit sexual behavior from being directed toward members of the opposite sex that exude similar odors. In summary, current knowledge suggests that MHC plays an important role in the mate choice of vertebrates. Hence, it may be crucial for the formation and maintenance of the adult pair bond as well.

Ontogenetic Experiences and Bonding

Attachment of infant to mother and the bonding of mother to infant or between individuals later in life result from a variety of endocrine, neural, and experiential mechanisms. Here we discuss the role of experience in the formation of attachments and social bonds. Experiences acquired across the life span do not act on naive substrates. Instead they occur within the context of a prior genetic and experiential history, which imposes constraints on how susceptible individuals will be to the effects of experiences. In the mother–infant relationship, influences of experience are greatest during periods of rapid brain development and endocrine change. During these periods of heightened sensitivities to the environment, an animal learns important features of its social and ecologic environment that contribute to its later social bonding and provide the substrate for subsequent learning.

Life periods of most importance for the development of infant–mother attachment and later life bonds include the prenatal period, the early postnatal period, weaning, puberty, and the postpartum period itself, and these have been demonstrated in animals (mammals) and humans alike (Table 17.3). Despite the clear importance for development of the prenatal period (see, e.g., Hofer and Sullivan 2001; Kaiser, Heemann et al. 2003; Kaiser, Kruijver et al. 2003), we restrict our discussion to the very extensive ontogenetic influences through life after birth and provide a few examples from animals and humans to illustrate how learning during specific periods contributes to the mother–infant relationship.

Postnatal Period

Specific and general effects of the environment on infant–maternal attachment/bonding and social–sexual behavior have been studied more extensively. In rats, for instance, exposure to a mother's odors during the first few days of life enhances an infant's attraction to the nest and to mother's odors, which keep the young in close proximity to the mother during the nursing period. An infant readily develops preference for odors associated with its mother's presence. Interestingly, oxytocin in the pup brain has been reported to facilitate these associations (Nelson and Panksepp 1996). There is also now evidence that these olfactory experiences have effects on later life, when the male offspring grow up to be attracted to female odors that resemble the maternal odors (presumably non-MHC associated odors; see above) and females grow up to be more attracted to pups scented with mother-like odors (Fleming and Li 2002; Fleming, this volume). These hedonic changes come about through effects of these odors on the development of the olfactory bulbs, producing long-term changes to the properties of cells that specifically encode the particular odors (Wilson and Sullivan 1994). In humans, as well, there is evidence that infants with brief experience with their mother develop an attraction to the breast-pads of lactating over nonlactating women, which narrows down over time to a selective attraction to their own mothers' odors (Schaal and Porter 1991; MacFarlane 1975). This shift in attraction illustrates how specific attachments can develop from a more general attraction to preference for an individual.

Nonspecific postnatal influences on subsequent development are also pervasive. It is now well established that pups which receive more licking stimulation from their mothers during the early postnatal period show both short-term and long-term changes in the development and functioning of their HPA axes, emotionality, attentional systems, learning ability, and maternal behavior (Francis,

Table 17.3 Short- and long-term effects on social bonds of specific perceptions and general experiences during various stages of life.
r = rat, s = sheep, p = primate, h = human.

Life Stages	Experiences	Short-term Effects	Long-term Effects
Specific Perceptions			
Postnatal	Mother stimuli—amniotic fluid, taste and smell, vocalizations, appearance (r, s, p, h)	Orientation to milk line (r), recognition and development of preference for mother (s, p, h)	Preference for conspecifics/environment with mother-associated odors (r)
	Sibling stimuli (r, h)	—	Suppression of sexual attraction to related conspecifics (r, h)
Postpartum	Offspring stimuli—taste, odor, vocalizations, appearance (r, s, p, h)	Location, recognition of, preference for neonates in general (r) or mother's own neonates (s, p, h)	Persistent heightened maternal responsivity to neonates in general (r) or mother's own offspring (s, p, h)
General Experiences			
Postnatal	Lower maternal licking, arched-back nursing (r), maternal deprivation (r, p), abuse, neglect (p, h)	Depression-like behavior (p, h), distorted development of internal working model (h)	Increased acute stress responses (r, p), decreased maternal and social behavior (r, p, h), increased aggression, antisocial behavior (p, h)
Juvenile	Play (r), care-taking of neonates (r, marmosets)	Decreased aggression (marmosets)	Increase parental and other social behavior (r, marmosets)
Puberty	Agonistic encounters with mature males (guinea pigs)	—	Ability to interact with unfamiliar conspecifics in a nonaggressive and nonstressful way; respect for other males' females and social rank
Postpartum	Hormone changes, nursing stimulation, other physical contact with offspring, mothering experience (r, s, p, h)	—	Persistent heightened maternal responsivity to neonates in general (r) or mother's own offspring (s, p, h)

Caldji et al. 1999; Liu et al. 1997, 2000). The importance of the postnatal environment for normal development can be illustrated most clearly by the effects on development of depriving animals of those experiences, through isolation rearing or limited maternal deprivation (Fleming, this volume).

In humans, the importance of early postnatal stimulation for infant health and development seems to be obvious. Mothers in most cultures nurse, cradle, and provide kinesthetic and somatosensory stimulation to the infant as part of their daily caregiving (Corter and Fleming 2002; Gottschalk-Batschkus and Schuler 1996). Lullabyes are sung in many cultures, and cross-cultural similarities exist in the rhythm, cadence, and frequency properties, suggesting a more or less universal form of vocal stimulation (Trehub and Trainor 1998). What the specific or singular effects of these early forms of stimulation may be is unknown.

Since the work on institutionalized infants (Spitz 1945) and, more recently, infants and children from Romanian orphanages (O'Connor, this volume), we have been able to see the devastating impact of little or no early relational stimulation on emotional, attentional, social, and cognitive development. In addition, work by Rutter, O'Connor, and Gunnar shows that these institutionalized children experience alterations in the regulation of the HPA axis and that some of these effects persist even after infants are adopted into high socio-economic status, stimulating homes (O'Connor, this volume). By acting on the brain and neuroendocrine axes at a time of enhanced plasticity, postnatal social experiences or the lack thereof can either enhance or impoverish the ability to engage in subsequent social interactions (see below).

Weaning and Post-weaning Period

It is generally accepted that experience obtained by playing with conspecifics shapes an animal's adult social behavior. Rats that are deprived of juvenile play experience show poorer attention, hyperactivity, increased fear, alterations in performance on a variety of learning tasks (Dalley et al. 2002), and disordered social behavior, including decreased licking of their own pups (Rees and Fleming 2001; Fleming, this volume). Numerous reports from a variety of primate species suggest that infant handling by juvenile females enhances their later rearing success (Hrdy 1999; Snowdon 1996). Compared to firstborn or only children, children with older siblings appear to acquire a theory of mind that may facilitate sensitive social interactions at an earlier age (Perner et al. 1994). A number of researchers have found positive correlations between infant–parent attachments and peer interactions (e.g., Lyons-Ruth et al. 1993; Park and Waters 1989). Securely attached infants are able to respond more sensitively towards peers' communication efforts than are insecurely attached infants (Fagot 1997).

Puberty

During puberty, social relationships change dramatically. Conspecifics of the same sex frequently become rivals, and animals of the opposite sex become attractive as mating and bonding partners. Thus, in some species it is not surprising to find that the time around puberty is crucial for the acquisition of significant coping patterns needed later in life. Male guinea pigs, for example, raised in large mixed-sex colonies experience agonistic encounters with older dominant males around puberty, whereby they acquire the social skills needed to adapt to conspecifics in a nonaggressive and nonstressful way (Sachser et al. 1994). Similarly, it might be speculated that the ability to form and maintain adult social bonds also depends on social experiences at about this time. Some data, indeed, point in this direction: The "respect" that males show for the social bonds of other males under high-density living conditions (Sachser, this volume) does not seem to develop without certain social experiences around puberty. For Syrian hamsters, a two-stage model for maturation of male social behaviors has been proposed: a perinatal critical period for sexual differentiation of neural circuits, followed by the pubertal period during which gonadal steroids are agents of further organizational change that enhances behavioral responsiveness to hormones in adulthood (Romeo et al. 2002).

Social experience influences in the postpubertal period are much more complicated in humans. The impact of peer contact on social development depends on the sort of peers with which an adolescent associates, which in turn depends on their relation with their parents or teachers (Collins et al. 1997). If adolescents aggregate with antisocial peers, they become less socially competent and at greater risk for delinquency, teenage pregnancy, and dropping out of school (Cairns and Cairns 1994). The absence of a father or an adult male in the home has been associated with increased oppositional and antisocial tendencies in adolescent boys, although undesirable outcomes do not necessarily ensue if compensatory social influences and structures are in place (Cooley 1998; Lim and Howard 1998). It may be that boys reared with regular contact with investing adult males are more likely to learn nonconflictual ways to negotiate a male hierarchy. Some studies of boys reared in the absence of a father have found they harbor disparaging attitudes toward women and girls and pursue a "fast" reproductive strategy rather than one that courts slowly and leads to investment in children. Draper and Harpending (1982) have speculated about the evolutionary basis of this male social pattern.

Postpartum Period

The postpartum period is a very plastic period, during which time experiences have long-term effects on responsiveness to subsequent young (see all Group Reports, Belsky as well as Fleming, this volume). During this period, mothers become familiar with their offspring and in some species develop a selective, exclusive attraction to them. Through experience with young, mother rats come to recognize their own litters' odors and male offspring from female offspring, although individual recognition does not occur. Nonetheless, experiences obtained by the mother of infant odors and through somatosensory stimulation, derived while nursing young, produce changes in the sensory (parietal cortex), emotional (amygdala), and maternal (hypothalamic) systems within the brain. Although this does not constitute a traditional "learning system," as a result of experience, these limbic and hypothalamic sites show elevations in the expression of certain proto-oncogenes (c-fos, FosB), astroglial proteins, and in neurogenesis (see Fleming as well as Leckman et al., both this volume). Thus, the brain is quite plastic in adulthood and shows evidence of real structural change with experience.

During the early postpartum period, sheep mothers (ewes) come to recognize their own lambs' odors and will thereafter selectively accept their own lambs and reject alien lambs. In contrast to the rat, where individual recognition does not develop, this odor learning is clearly mediated by very specific changes in the olfactory bulbs of these animals and shares many behavioral and neurochemical properties with the effects in the olfactory bulbs of young rat pups when they learn about their mothers' odors. Similar to this early learning, these effects can be quite long-term and influence how the mother responds to subsequent litters (Gonzalez-Mariscal and Poindron 2002).

Human mothers, like ewes, develop an attraction to their infants' odors and come to recognize their own babies, using olfactory, touch, auditory cues and our species' highly developed visual ability (Corter and Fleming 2002). This identification is probably not critical during the early postpartum period when mother and altricial young remain in close contact with one another. Nevertheless, the ability to discriminate exists very early on and varies as a function of how much experience mothers have had with their offspring. For example, in the olfactory domain, Porter et al. (1983) and Schaal et al. (1980) demonstrated that within a couple of days of birth, mothers can discriminate their own infants' soiled T-shirts from the T-shirts of same-age infants and they come to prefer their own. The odors are also assessed to be more attractive by mothers than by non-mothers, indicating that mothers' emotional states are being affected by these odors (Fleming et al. 1993).

Conclusions

Taken together, these examples of specific perceptual learning and diffuse experience effects at different stages of life illustrate that the organism is not fixed in its behavior at any point; it is flexible and, with new information and experiences, it can alter the direction of behavioral development. Since conditions at the time of birth are not necessarily the same as those that prevail during adulthood, adaptation may be involved. Thus, learning can set the stage for the later time, but does not determine it in a rigid linear fashion. Each stage of plasticity sets the stage for the next. However, animals are not infinitely flexible, and phases exist during which certain experiences and kinds of learning occur most easily; that is, there are constraints on what is learned, when it is learned, when it is expressed, and how long it is retained.

In addition, there are large individual differences in susceptibility to the effects of experience. Constraints on susceptibility are imposed both by prior experiences during development and by genetics. For instance, interactions with very young pups during the juvenile period will have positive effects on later maternal behavior in rats that had undisturbed contact with their mothers, but negative effects in rats that had been maternally deprived (Gonzalez-Mariscal and Poindron 2002; Rees and Fleming 2001). Thus, the same stimulus complex experienced during the juvenile period has effects on later behavior that vary considerably with pre-weaning experience. The genotype of the animal can also alter how experiences are expressed. This has been demonstrated in both monkeys and humans, where possessing one form of a genetic polymorphism (short form of the serotonin transporter gene) results in negative prenatal stress effects on juvenile behavior and physiology, whereas the same prenatal stress is much less deleterious in animals with the long form of this gene (G. Kraemer, pers. comm.). Also, men with a specific polymorphism of the monoamine oxidase A gene, which causes reduced monoamine oxidase activity, are more likely to exhibit excessive aggressiveness, but only if they were abused as children (Caspi et al. 2002).

We are clearly at an early stage in understanding gene–environment interactions in the development of attachment and bonding processes in nonhuman and human mammals. These studies have been made possible through the development of new genetic assessment technologies, and we expect to see major advances in the near future. Imaging techniques such as fMRI and PET may permit investigation in children as to which brain areas and neurochemical systems are altered by extreme conditions of inadequate/abusive parenting and how therapies, interventions, and placement in enriched environments may alter brain structure and function during early and later life stages.

Cultural and Societal Influences on Bonding

Mother–infant bonding and romantic love have been idealized in Western societies. These biases have certainly contributed to the central attachment theory premise that the infant's relationship with his/her mother (or primary caretaker) is the major influence on the quality of close relationships later in life and the assumption that monogamous, emotionally close male–female relationships are the most important bonds during adult life. Social organization systems in many non-Western societies, however, de-emphasize and even discourage emotional attachments between reproductive partners. These social institutions appear to have arisen for economic, security, and religious reasons. They include customs regarding the segregation of the sexes, norms about relations between spouses, and rules governing the form of marriage and residence practices.

In some societies, particularly horticultural societies of lowland tropical South America and highland New Guinea, the sexes are largely segregated in their familial work and leisure roles (e.g., Chagnon 1988; Gelber 1986; Herdt 1993; Kelly 1993). Men and women, even when they both do agricultural work, for example, do their work in same-sexed groups and at different phases of the agricultural cycle. Although involved as marital partners and living in the same village, men and women often do not eat together in the same place and will often not sleep together. Instead, women and children have their cooking and eating places in one part of the village, while men and older boys spend their time in other designated places. The genders are not only separated but are ranked hierarchically. Men have higher prestige and are credited with ritual knowledge: roles that women are specifically denied. Often there are strong values of taboo and contamination associated with mature females such that women must be restricted from certain areas and activities belonging to males, lest some violation of the supernatural order may occur.

In other societies, the spatial and symbolic segregation of the sexes is less marked, yet the structure of the family is organized in such a way that the wife is strongly subordinated to the structure of the husband's family. In cases where families are organized patrilineally, patrilocally, and patriarchally, a wife's ability to make a successful adjustment to her marriage depends not primarily on her relationship with her husband but on her ability to do productive work in the company of other women of the household and to accept the dominance of her husband's mother as well as other senior women of the household. Her relationship with her husband is likely to be formal, particularly in the early years of her marriage, and the nature of her emotional attachment to her husband is less important for the "success" of the marriage. Their relationship is, of course, sexual and reproductive but does not necessarily involve mutual sensitivity, consideration, or cooperation. These characteristics usually apply to but are not restricted to polygynous marital systems.

Extramarital love affairs, however, do occur within social structures like those described above, in which emotional distance between spouses is the norm. This is particularly true in societies in which older men take much younger wives. For example, among the pastoral, gerontocratic Masaai and other East African peoples like the Nuer and Turkana, women are married according to the wishes of their fathers to older men. At marriage, men are 30 years or older, while their brides are typically around menarche. Premenarcheal girls and even married women sometimes enter into intense "affairs" with young men who are not yet of marriageable age, though in terms of physical maturation they are fully adult. These relationships have all the earmarks of romantic love and are described as such in the ethnographies (e.g., Dickerson-Putman and Brown 1998; Hodgson 2000).

In many areas of sub-Saharan Africa it is common for children of various ages to be fostered out of their natal households into households of relatives or nonrelatives for a variety of reasons. There is a substantial descriptive literature on this topic that covers many aspects of fostering including its function in terms of kinship, education, and occupational training (Bledsoe 1995; Draper 1989; Isiugo-Abanihe 1985). Other studies focus on the health and well-being of fostered children compared with non-fostered children of the household (Bledsoe 1995; Castle 1995; Draper 1989; Isiugo-Abanihe 1985; Sudre et al. 1990). For example, a child will sometimes be sent away as a foster child at age two or three, in part to promote weaning, to free the mother to attend to a new infant, to provide a childless couple with a child, or to provide a grandmother with a companion. At older ages, such a child may be retrieved by its parents, kept "at home" for a few months, and then sent out again to a different household where, as an older child, she/he can do useful work. In other cases, a child will be fostered out to friends or family living in more urban areas where there are better opportunities for schooling or for being apprenticed for professional training. It is important to note that fosterees are often sent away to different villages and are effectively separated socially and physically from their parents and siblings. In the Trobriand Islands, Papua New Guinea, older siblings from the age of six years on are frequently observed to carry their infant siblings. When a mother gives birth to her first child, she will ask a niece of appropriate age to stay with her to help her with the baby. Draper and Harpending (1987) describe various social systems in which children are reared primarily by peers rather than parents. Thus, in a number of non-Western societies, it is the norm and not the exception for children to undergo a change in primary caretaker, often several times, before they reach adulthood. The parents who help to arrange these transfers of their children believe that what they are doing is in the best interest of the child, as well as of the household into which the child is transferred. Westerners who read about the custom of fostering, as practiced in sub-Saharan Africa, should understand that, unlike adopted children in the West, fosterees do not lose contact with their natal family and do not surrender rights of inheritance and group membership because of their various "postings" to other households. These practices raise important research questions: Despite being separated from their biological mothers and reared by a succession of other, sometimes immature, caretakers, do secure attachment styles and stable internal working models develop in infants and young children in these societies? What are the consequences for the quality of their relationships later in life? Answers to these questions may require some adjustments in current attachment theory.

Social stratification is another sociocultural factor that can produce powerful effects on social attachment style, especially parental treatment of offspring. Parents that are of higher/wealthier social classes (humans) or higher rank in the dominance hierarchy (animals) may be more indulgent and less punitive of their offspring because this does not adversely affect their survival (Altmann 1987). However, parents of a lower class or rank may be compelled to be much stricter and more restrictive to optimize their offspring's survival in their more constrained social environment, where there is less access to resources and greater risk of being harmed by higher class/rank individuals.

Human Social Bonding and Evolutionary Theory

General Considerations

Infant attachment and later life social bonding are the products of evolutionary forces. The central concept of evolutionary theory is that genes coding for traits that increase the relative reproductive success of individuals or their offspring will become more prevalent through successive generations, leading over time to phenotypic changes within species and the emergence of new species. The success of individuals in transmitting their genes to successive generations is referred to as *reproductive fitness*. Several mechanisms of selection for traits and their associated genes have been hypothesized. *Natural selection*, first described by Darwin in 1859, is the increase in prevalence over successive generations of traits that enhance survival of individuals or their offspring until they reproduce. *Sexual selection* is a form of natural selection that occurs when individuals differ in their ability to compete with others for mates or to attract members of the opposite sex (Darwin 1871; Alcock 1998; Miller 2000). *Kin selection* increases the prevalence of traits that enhance the reproductive success of close relatives who have many of the same genes as the individual (Hamilton 1964). *Reciprocal altruism* refers to traits that promote mutual assistance among unrelated individuals thereby amplifying their reproductive fitness (Trivers 1971). Natural selection, sexual selection, kin selection, and reciprocal altruism are ultimate mechanisms that drive evolutionary change. They are distinguished from proximate mechanisms that are the specific genetic, physiological, and behavioral alterations brought about by ultimate mechanisms that result in greater reproductive success of individuals, kin, and/or allies.

Brain systems underlying attachment and bonding have evolved because they provide selective advantages by all of the evolutionary mechanisms described above. Attachment to their mother motivates young to maintain protective proximity to their mothers and/or to emit signals that elicit maternal attention, thereby increasing their natural selection advantage. Maternal and paternal bonding, which motivate parents to feed and protect their offspring, provide enormous kin selection advantages. Avid parental protection and sustenance also permit longer periods of immaturity during which offspring can learn skills that increase their survival rate when they have to fend for themselves. Affectional bonding between family members increases mutual aid and protection, thereby increasing kin selection advantages. The capacity to form social bonds with unrelated conspecifics enhances the probability of gaining selective advantage by reciprocal altruism and may also increase mating opportunities. Monogamous pair bonding is an excellent example of unrelated individuals mutually enhancing each others' reproductive fitness.

Relationships between Early Attachment and Later Life Bonding

It would be a mistake to presume that all theorized linkages between early attachment security in humans and later social and emotional development are

Table 17.4 Phases of intergenerational transmission of secure and insecure attachment styles. Evidence, summarized by Belsky (this volume), indicates that parents' internal working model determines the quality of their parenting, which in turn affects their children's attachment style (secure vs. insecure) and social behavior during infancy, subsequent development, and adulthood, including the quality of their parenting. Compared below are the classical "mental health" and evolutionary views of the different trajectories that perpetuate secure and insecure attachment styles across generations.

Parents' Internal Working Model	Dismissing	Autonomous	Preoccupied
Parents' Quality of Infant/Child Care	Insensitive Rejecting Intrusive	Sensitive Consistent	Insensitive Inconsistent
	↓	↓	↓
Infant/Child's Attachment Style	Avoidant ↓	Secure ↓	Resistant ↓
Children's Later Social Behavior	Aggressive Behavioral problems	Social competence Better emotional regulation Good friendships	Dependent Helpless Isolated
	↓	↓	↓
Adult Offspring's Attachment Style	Dismissing	Autonomous	Preoccupied
Adult Offspring's Social and Parental Behavior	Avoids social closeness Insensitive parenting	Intimacy Skilled, sensitive parenting	Inconsistent Dependent social relationship Insensitive parenting

Classical View: Secure attachment is optimal, facilitates mental health. Insecure attachment patterns are fallback strategies when secure attachments are not available.

Evolutionary View: All three attachment patterns are primary strategies depending on contextual and ecological circumstances.

well established or particularly strong. Although many studies report findings from which one can construct a developmental story line (Table 17.4; Belsky, this volume), the data could be construed differently by open-minded scholars.

There is considerable evidence that infants and children learn from and about their mothers and social environment in the home and, in that process, develop many kinds of relationships with their caregivers; these are discussed throughout this volume and thus will only be briefly mentioned here to provide organizational closure. Although longitudinal studies spanning more than one generation have not yet been done, prospective studies show significant correlations between the quality of attachment of mothers as infants and the attachment status of their infants (Levy 1999) and between quality of caregiving of both parents and their child's security in social relations and secure autonomy as adults, as determined by the "Adult Attachment Interview," hence closing the circle of relations between mother and infant (Grossmann and Grossmann, this volume). In addition, many other closer relationships (with siblings, alloparents, peers), the larger social environment, and the ecology in which the infant lives no doubt exert significant influences on infant social and emotional development (Belsky, this volume).

If the effect sizes that record linkages between early attachment and later development are appraised, few contemporary students of social development would presume that this linkage will inevitably be thick and strong, as it will always be contingent upon experiences and events that intervene between the assessment of early attachment and later measurements of child functioning.

Despite expectations that early secure attachment will forecast better mental health and some correlational evidence consistent with this prediction (e.g., better stress regulation, closer friendships, increased tolerance of frustration), there is actually very little data linking attachment security/insecurity to formal assessments of mental health or mental disorders. Perhaps the strongest support for such linkage comes from Carlson (1998), who shows that a particular form of insecure attachment in the 12–18 month period (namely, disorganized attachment) forecasts dissociative mental states at age 19 years (see below).

Where the traditional mental health perspective and the evolutionary perspective on attachment security differ is in terms of whether — at least once upon a time in the environment of evolutionary adaptatedness (EEA), and even perhaps today — one would expect attachment security processes to be related to reproductive fitness. This is an assumption underlying the modern evolutionary perspective articulated by Belsky (1999) but most certainly not of the traditional developmental perspective. This is not to say that attachment processes, especially those established early in life, would necessarily be expected to predict fitness outcomes in the modern environment, which deviates so greatly from the presumed EEA. This is also not to say that such could not be the case. Ultimately, it is an empirical case.

A modern evolutionary perspective also raises other issues with respect to the traditional mental health perspective on attachment security/insecurity: Why has nature seemingly designed development so as to link early experiences in the infant–parent relationship with later developmental outcomes, as theorized by attachment researchers, such as emotion regulation/dysregulation, stress regulation, friendship bonds, the capacity for intimacy, and even patterns of parenting when rearing the next generation? After all, nature could have shaped development so that these putative outcomes of early relationships were not at all related to early relationships or even related in just the opposite manner theorized by students of attachment theory.

If one combines data on the thousands of "strange situations" conducted around the world to date, or at least many of the cases, it appears that about two thirds to three quarters of children studied emerge with secure attachment classifications (van IJzendoorn and Sagi 1999). Why is this the case? Could it be that attachment security and insecurity could be frequency dependent; that is, the rate of insecurity could be a function of the rate of security (and vice versa)?

Certainly inconsistent with the possibility of frequency-dependent selection is Michael Lamb's informal observation during this group's deliberations that at least within the few hunter–gatherer groups he and his associates have observed, a full 100% of infant–mother relationships look secure. One has to wonder, however, whether what looks secure to the "naked eye," so to speak, would emerge as secure in the "strange situation" were it possible to carry out such assessment in this population. Perhaps noteworthy in this context is that informal observations made by Grossmann et al. (2005) of toddlers on the Trobriand Islands, who are in almost constant bodily contact with their mother or kin during their first year of life, could have tempted these investigators to suppose 100% secure attachments; however, formal assessments of 20 toddlers in the "strange situation" revealed that 20% were insecurely attached to their mothers.

Consistent with much general developmental thinking, traditional attachment theory presumes that all children are equally susceptible to rearing experience. Thus, maternal sensitivity should foster security and maternal insensitivity should foster insecurity. However, although experimental data confirm this causal process and a meta-analysis of correlational studies also provides evidence in favor of the causal role of sensitivity, the absolute effect size is modest with respect to the relation between sensitivity and security (De Wolff and van IJzendoorn 1997). Could this be because some children are more affected by sensitivity or insensitivity of maternal care relative to others, at least with respect to the development of attachment security, as Belsky (this volume) argues from an evolutionary perspective using the notion of bet hedging on an uncertain future?

Emerging evidence indicates that infants who are high in negative emotionality may be particularly susceptible to rearing influence and perhaps the security-promoting effects of sensitive maternal care (Belsky 2004). Indeed, such evidence raises the prospect that the children studied by Kagan who show high fear (and low activity), who he refers to as inhibited children, may be especially susceptible to the effects of rearing in general and sensitive care in particular. What is certainly clear is that Kagan has been mistaken in arguing that security–insecurity evaluations reflect main effects of temperament (for compelling evidence, see van den Boom 1994).

CHILDCARE AND SCHOOL: CONTRASTS BETWEEN CHILDREN'S SOCIAL NEEDS AND PUBLIC POLICY

Is it possible for society to set up ideal care environments where children can easily form and maintain social bonds? Research has demonstrated that sensitive and stable early care environments enhance the mental and psychological development of children. An increasingly large percentage of preschool children receive out-of-home childcare. Public schools educate the vast majority of children. Rarely has the best available knowledge about optimal social environments for children shaped the organization of these institutions.

Classical attachment theory clearly defines the "ideal" childcare environment: caretakers are the biological parents, their numbers are limited, they are readily available, and their care is continuous (Bowlby 1969). As a result of profound changes in social structure over the past several decades, today's care environments for children have diverged from this ideal in many ways (Table 17.5). The traditional family embedded in an extended family network and a close-knit community is no longer the predominant model. Nuclear families more commonly live and work far from parents and other relatives. Divorce and out-of-wedlock births have increased single-parent families. Children of divorced couples are often shuttled between contrasting family environments. The rise in the percentage of mothers of young children who are employed and the diminished availability of relatives has markedly increased the demand for childcare providers who are not kin. Caretakers in those environments are not always available and there is considerable discontinuity in care.

Despite deviations from the theoretically ideal childcare environment, a large body of research has produced a number of positive and reassuring findings. Children clearly maintain attachments to their mothers, although the mothers are not able to provide continuous care (NICHD Early Child Care Network 1997). Children readily form attachments to care providers who enhance security, especially when the children are very young. Child–care-provider relationships, however, are not determined by the security of child–parent attachment and reflect that child–parent and child–care-provider attachments develop in care environments with different demands (Ahnert and Lamb 2000). Peer interactions can increase social skills among children who are shy and reluctant to communicate (Fox et al. 2001).

Table 17.5 Deviations from ideal childcare environment with the rise of nonfamilial childcare and nontraditional families.

Traditional Family Childcare Environment	Aspects of Nonfamilial Childcare Environments	Nontraditional Families
Caretakers are most likely the biological parents	Caretakers are not biological parents	Single parents
Small number of caretakers	Multiple caretakers	"Patchwork" families resulting from divorce
Caretakers are readily available	Caretaker availability varies	Reliance on alloparenting
Continuity of caretakers	Frequent changes in caretaker	Foster care and adoption

Concurrent to these potential positive effects on children's social life, research also indicates that childcare environments also pose a number of risks. Poor childcare amplifies the effects of poor parenting on children's social development, but does not hardly affect good mother–child relationships. Large contrasts between the home and childcare environments can be quite stressful. This may account for the finding that cortisol levels remain high over the first two weeks after entering childcare, decrease by the fifth month, but are still higher than pre-entry baseline levels (Ahnert et al. 2004). Early peer interactions can be conflictual with more dominant children bullying others. High-quality supervision is necessary to prevent these potentially psychologically damaging situations from arising (Lamb 1998).

Childcare and education are planned environments in almost all modern societies. Although attachment and social bonding are crucial for optimal development, both societal norms and the way these environments are organized rarely address the needs of children adequately.

Although transition models are available to help small children form secondary attachments when they enter childcare environments outside the home, such models are rarely practiced. Childcare workers and teachers often receive little or no training in psychosocial development and the application of this knowledge in their work environments. Elementary school teachers can become bonding figures for young children, yet the importance this role can play, especially for children who receive inadequate nurturing in their home environments, is often not appreciated. If teachers become attachment figures, permanent separation from them may be perceived by the child as rejection or abandonment and precipitate aggressive behavior. More research is needed to understand the full impact of childcare and primary school environments on children to maximize benefits and avoid negative consequences in these settings.

SPECULATIONS ON THE SIGNIFICANCE
OF BONDS IN LATER LIFE

An exciting challenge for future research will be to determine the relevance of biologically based bonds to health and social stability, on one hand, and disease and social conflict, on the other. A large number of studies have found that social support mitigates a wide variety of disease processes (e.g., Berkman et al. 2000; Cohen 1988; House et al. 1988; Krantz and McCeney 2002). Are bonding systems in the brain engaged by social support, and do they produce physiological effects that enhance health? Uvnas-Moberg (1998), for instance, has hypothesized that oxytocin mediates some of the health benefits of positive social interactions. In the social support research literature, there is considerable variability among studies in the frequency, duration, and quality of interpersonal contact that has been considered to be social support. Measurements of the quality and strength of interpersonal relationships in future studies may clarify the role of bonding in the health benefits of social support (Berkman et al. 2000).

Religious belief and practice have been linked to improved health (Hill and Pargament 2003; Powell et al. 2003; Seeman et al. 2003). Earlier in this chapter we speculated that bonding systems may contribute to the emotional commitment inherent in religious and other beliefs. Might activation of bonding systems associated with religious belief have health-enhancing physiological effects? Pet ownership also has health benefits that may involve mobilization of bonding systems (Beck and Meyers 1996; Brasic 1998). Odendaal and Meintjes (2003) reported that oxytocin, β-endorphin, and dopamine concentrations rose in dogs and their owners during affectionate interactions. Experiments testing behavior in bargaining games have consistently found a bias in subjects toward initial generosity and trust that runs counter to the assumptions of classic economic/game theory that individuals always act to maximize personal gain and minimize risk (McCabe et al. 2003). Levels of interpersonal trust have been linked to levels of economic development in surveys of a wide variety of nations (Zak and Knack 2001). Is the capacity to be generous and trust others related to bonding systems? Interestingly, plasma oxytocin concentrations were significantly higher in trust game subjects who received generous offers and then reciprocated in kind (Zak et al. 2003).

Further research into the basis of later life bonding, especially the underlying neurobiology, may provide greater understanding of the consequences of disrupting important relationships and the pathophysiology of disorders in which sociality is adversely affected. The loss of loved ones or other emotional investments (e.g., job, wealth, reputation) can trigger depression and anxiety. Diminished interest in social interactions and confidence in the positive regard of others are prominent symptoms of depressive and anxiety disorders. Conversely, excessive and inappropriate feelings of closeness to others often occur during manic episodes. Diminished interpersonal relatedness is among the most common negative symptoms of schizophrenia. Abnormal development of bonding systems related to neglect, abuse, or other pathological early life experiences may give rise to personality disorders in which the capacity to form stable, caring, and trusting relationships is severely impaired (antisocial, borderline, narcissistic, histrionic) or there is excessive dependency on others. Genetically based defects in bonding systems may cause the severe social deficits found in autism and other developmental disorders. All too often acceptance within some social groups and adherence to some beliefs require demonizing those outside the group or nonbelievers. In this paradoxical way, bonding systems may have contributed to the sectarian bigotry, persecution, and violence that have plagued humankind throughout history.

REFERENCES

Ahnert, L., M.R. Gunnar, M.E. Lamb, and M. Barthel. 2004. Transition to child care: Association of infant–mother attachment, infant negative emotion and cortisol elevations. *Child Dev.* **75**:629–650.

Ahnert, L., and M.E. Lamb. 2000. Infant–careprovider attachments in contrasting German child care settings. II. Individual-oriented care after German reunification. *Infant Behav. Dev.* **23**:211–222.

Ainsworth, M. 1979. Attachment as related to mother–infant interaction. *Adv. Stud. Behav.* **9**:1–49.

Alcock, J. 1998. Animal Behavior. 6th ed. Sunderland, MA: Sinauer.

Altemus, M., P. Deuster, G. Galliven, C. Carter, and P. Gold. 1995. Suppresssion of hypothalamic-pituitary-adrenal responses to stress in lactating women. *J. Clin. Endocrinol. Metab.* **80**:2954–2959.

Altmann, J. 1987. Life span aspects of reproduction and parental care in anthropoid primates. In: Parenting across the Life Span, ed. J. Lancaster, J. Altman, A.S. Rossi, and L.R. Sherrod, pp. 15–29. Hawthorne, NY: Aldine de Gruyter.

Anzenberger, G. 1988. The pairbond in the titi monkey (*Callicebus moloch*): Intrinsic versus extrinsic contributions of the pairmates. *Folia Primatol.* **50**:188–203.

Apanius, V., D. Penn, P. Slev, L.R. Ruff, and W.K. Potts. 1997. The nature of selection on the major histocompatibility complex. *Crit. Rev. Immunol.* **17**:179–224.

Aragona, B.J., Y. Lui, J.T. Curtis, F.K. Stephan, and Z. Wang. 2003. A critical role for nucleus accumbens dopamine in partner-preference formation in male prairie voles. *J. Neurosci.* **23**:3483–3490.

Arcaro, K.F., and A. Eklund. 1999. A review of MHC-based mate preferences and fostering experiments in two congenic strains of mice. *Genetica* **104**:241–244.

Bartels, A., and S. Zeki. 2000. The neural basis for romantic love. *NeuroReport* **11**: 3829–3834.

Beauchamp, G.K., and K. Yamazaki. 1997. HLA and mate selection in humans: Commentary. *Am. J. Hum. Genet.* **61**:484–496.

Beuchamp, G.K., K. Yamazaki, J. Bard, and E.A. Boyse. 1988. Pre-weaning experience in the control of mating preferences by genes in the major histocompatibility complex of the mouse. *Behav. Genet.* **18**:537–547.

Beck, A.M., and N.M. Meyers. 1996. Health enhancement and companion animal ownership. *Ann. Rev. Publ. Hlth.* **17**:247–257.

Becker, J., C. Rudick, and W. Jenkins. 2001. The role of dopamine in the nucleus accumbens and striatum during sexual behavior in the female rat. *J. Neurosci.* **21**: 3236–3241.

Belsky, J. 1999. Modern evolutionary theory and patterns of attachment. In: Handbook of Attachment: Theory, Research and Clinical Applications, ed. J. Cassidy and P.R. Shaver, pp. 151–173. New York: Guilford.

Belsky, J. 2004. Differential susceptibility to rearing influence: An evolutionary hypothesis and some evidence. In: Origins of the Social Mind: Evolutionary Psychology and Child Development, ed. B. Ellis and D. Bjorklund. New York: Guilford.

Berkman, L.F., T. Glass, I. Brissette, and T.E. Seeman. 2000. From social integration to health: Durkheim in the new millennium. *Soc. Sci. Med.* **51**:843–857.

Bernatchez, L., and C. Landry. 2003. MHC studies in nonmodel vertebrates: What have we learned about natural selection in 15 years? *J. Evol. Biol.* **16**:363–377.

Bielsky, I.F., S.B. Hu, K.L. Szegda, H. Westphal, and L.J. Young. 2004. Profound impairment in social recognition and reduction in anxiety-like behavior in vasopressin V1a receptor knockout mice. *Neuropsychopharm.* **29**:489–493.

Bledsoe, C.H. 1995. Marginal members: Children of previous unions in Mende households in Sierra Leone. In: Situating Fertility: Anthropology and Demographic Inquiry, ed. S. Greenhalgh, pp. 130–153. Cambridge: Cambridge Univ. Press.

Bowlby, J. 1969. Attachment. Attachment and Loss, vol. 1. London: Hogarth.

Bowlby, J. 1988. A Secure Base: Clinical Applications of Attachment Theory. London: Travistock/Routledge.

Brasic, J.R. 1998. Pets and health. *Psychol. Rep.* **83**:1011–1024.

Brown, J.L., and A. Eklund. 1994. Kin recognition and the major histocompatibility complex: An integrative review. *Am. Naturalist* **143**:435–461.

Buntin, J. 1996. Neural and hormonal control of parental behavior in birds. *Adv. Stud. Behav.* **25**:161–213.

Cairns, R., and B.D. Cairns. 1994. Life-lines and Risks: Pathways of Youth in Our Time. Cambridge: Cambridge Univ. Press.

Caldji, C., B. Tannenbaum, S. Sharma et al. 1998. Maternal care during infancy regulates the development of neural systems mediating the expression of fearfulness in the rat. *PNAS* **95**:5335–5340.

Carlson, E.A. 1998. A prospective longitudinal study of attachment disorganization/disorientation. *Child Dev.* **69**:1107–1128.

Carmichael, M., V. Warburton, J. Dixen, and J. Davidson. 1994. Relationships among cardiovascular, muscular, and oxytocin responses during human sexual activity. *Arch. Sex. Behav.* **23**:59–79.

Carter, C. 1998. Neuroendocrine perspectives on social attachment and love. *Psychoneuroendocrin.* **23**:779–818.

Carter, C., M. Altemus, and G. Chrousos. 2001. Neuroendocrine and emotional changes in the post-partum period. In: Progress in Brain Research: The Maternal Brain, ed. J. Russell, A. Douglas, R. Windle, and C. Ingram, pp. 241–249. Amsterdam: Elsevier.

Carter, C., and L.L. Getz. 1993. Monogamy and the prairie vole. *Sci. Am.* **268**:100–106.

Carter, C., and E.B. Keverne. 2002. The neurobiology of social affiliation and pair bonding. In: Hormones, Brain and Behavior, ed. D. Pfaff et al., vol. 1, pp. 299–337. San Diego: Academic.

Caspi, A., J. McClay, T. Moffitt et al. 2002. Role of genotype in the cycle of violence in maltreated children. *Science* **297**:851–854.

Cassidy, J., and P.R. Shaver, eds. 1999. Handbook of Attachment: Theory, Research, and Clinical Applications. New York: Guilford.

Castle, S.E. 1995. Child fostering and children's nutritional outcomes in rural Mali: The role of female status in directing child transfers. *Soc. Sci. Med.* **40**:679–693.

Chagnon, N. 1988. Life histories, blood revenge, and warfare in a tribal population. *Science* **239**:985–992.

Champagne, F., J. Diorio, S. Sharma, and M. Meaney. 2001. Naturally occurring variations in maternal behavior in the rat are associated with differences in estrogen-inducible central oxytocin receptors. *PNAS* **98**:12,736–12,741.

Cho, M.M., A.C. De Vries, J.R. Williams, and C.S. Carter. 1999. The effects of oxytocin and vasopressin on partner preferences in male and female prairie voles (*Microtus ochrogaster*). *Behav. Neurosci.* **11**:1071–1079.

Cohen, S. 1988. Psychosocial models of the role of social support in the etiology of physical disease. *Health Psychol.* **7**:269–297.

Collins, W.A., T. Gleason, and A. Sesma. 1997. Internalization, autonomy and relationships: Development during adolescence. In: Parenting and Children's Internalization of Values: A Handbook of Contemporary Theory, ed. J.E. Grusec and L. Kuczynski, pp. 78–94. New York: Wiley.

Consiglio, A., and A. Lucion. 1996. Lesion of hypthalamic paraventricular nucleus and maternal aggressive behavior in female rats. *Physiol. Behav.* **59**:591–596.

Cooley, R.L. 1998. Children's socialization experiences and functioning in single-mother households: The importance of fathers and other men. *Child Dev.* **69**: 219–230.

Corter, C., and A.S. Fleming. 2002. Psychobiology of maternal behavior in human beings. In: Handbook of Parenting: Biology and Ecology of Parenting, ed. M.H. Borstein, pp. 141–182. Mahwah, NJ: Erlbaum.

Dalley, J.W., D.E. Theobald, E.A. Pereira, P.M. Li, and T.W. Robbins. 2002. Specific abnormalities in serotonin release in the prefrontal cortex of isolation-reared rats measured during behavioral performance of a task assessing visuospatial attention and impulsivity. *Psychopharm.* **164**:329–340.

Darwin, C. 1859. On the Origin of Species by Means of Natural Selection, or the Preservation of Favoured Races in the Struggle for Life. London: Atheneum.

Darwin, C. 1871. The Descent of Man, and Selection in Relation to Sex. London: Princeton Univ. Press.

De Wolff, M., and M.H. van IJzendoorn. 1997. Sensitivity and attachment: A meta-analysis on parental antecedents of infant attachment. *Child Dev.* **68**:571–591.

Dickerson-Putman, J., and J.K. Brown. 1998. Women among Women: Anthropological Perspectives on Female Age Hierarchies. Urbana: Univ. of Illinois Press.

Draper, P. 1989. African marriage systems: Perspectives from evolutionary ecology. *Ethol. Sociobiol.* **10**:145–170.

Draper, P., and H. Harpending. 1982. Father absence and reproductive strategy: An evolutionary perspective. *J. Anthropol. Res.* **38**:255–273.

Draper, P., and H. Harpending. 1987. Parent investment and the child's environment. In: Parenting across the Life Span: Biosocial Dimensions, ed. J.S. Lancaster, A.S. Rossi, J. Altmann, and L.R. Sherrod, pp. 207–238. Chicago: Aldine.

Eisenberg, J. 1966. The social organization of mammals. *Handb. Zool.* **10**:1–92.

Eklund, A. 1997. The major histocompatibility complex and mating preferences in wild house mice. *Behav. Ecol.* **8**:630–634.

Fagot, B.I. 1997. Attachment, parenting, and peer interactions of toddler children. *Dev. Psychol.* **33**:489–499.

Fan, W., Y.C. Liu, S. Parimoo, and S.M. Weismann. 1995. Olfactory receptorlike genes are located in the human major histocompatibility complex. *Genomics* **27**:119–123.

Feeney, J.A. 1999. Adult romantic attachment and couple relationships. In: Handbook of Attachment: Theory, Research, and Clinical Applications, ed. J. Cassidy and P.R. Shaver, pp. 355–377. New York: Guilford.

Fleming, A.S., C. Corter, P. Franks et al. 1993. Postpartum factors related to mother's attraction to newborn infant odors. *Dev. Psychobiol.* **26**:115–132.

Fleming, A.S., C. Corter, J. Stallings, and M. Steiner. 2002. Testosterone and prolactin are associated with emotional responses to infant cries in new fathers. *Horm. Behav.* **42**:399–413.

Fleming, A.S., and M. Li. 2002. Psychobiology of maternal behavior and its early determinants in nonhuman mammals. In: Handbook of Parenting, ed. M.H. Borstein, vol. 2, pp. 263–284. Mahwah, NJ: Erlbaum.

Fleming, A.S., D. Ruble, H. Krieger, and P.Y. Wong. 1997. Hormonal and experiential correlates of maternal responsiveness during pregnancy and the puerperium in human mothers. *Horm. Behav.* **31**:145–158.

Fox, N.A., H.A. Henderson, K.H. Rubin, S.D. Calkins, and L.A. Schmidt. 2001. Continuity and discontinuity of behavioral inhibition and exuberance: Psychophysiological and behavioral influences across the first 4 years of life. *Child Dev.* **72**:1–21.

Francis, D., C. Caldji, F. Champagne, P. Plotsky, and M. Meaney. 1999. The role of corticotropin-releasing factor-norepinephrine systems in mediating the effects of early experience on the development of behavioral and endocrine responses to stress. *Biol. Psychiatry* **46**:1153–1166.

Francis, D., F. Champagne, and M. Meaney. 2000. Variations in maternal behaviour are associated with differences in oxytocin receptor levels in the rat. *J. Neuroendocrin.* **12**:1145–1148.

Francis, D., J. Diorio, D. Liu, and M. Meaney. 1999. Nongenomic transmission across generations of maternal behavior and stress responses in the rat. *Science* **286**:1155–1158.

Gaffori, O., and M. Le Moal. 1979. Disruption of maternal behavior and appearance of cannibalism after ventral mesencephalic tegmentum lesions. *Physiol Behav.* **23**:317–323.

Gelber, M.G. 1986. Gender and society in the New Guinea Highlands: An anthropological perspective on antagonism toward women. Boulder, CO: Westview Press.

Gimpl, G., and F. Fahrenholz. 2001. The oxytocin receptor system: Structure, function and regulation. *Physiol Rev* **81**:629–683.

Gingrich, B., Y. Liu, C. Cascio, Z. Wang, and T.R. Insel. 2000. Dopamine D2 receptor in the nucleus accumbens are important for social attachment in female prairie voles (*Microtus ochrogaster*). *Behav. Neurosci.* **114**:173–183.

Gonzalez-Mariscal, G., and P. Poindron. 2002. Parental care in mammals: Immediate internal and sensory factors of control. In: Hormones, Brain and Behavior, ed. D.W. Pfaff, A.P. Arnold, A.M. Etgen, S.E. Fahrbach, and R.T. Rubin, pp. 215–298. New York: Academic.

Gottschalk-Batschkus, C.E., and J. Schuler, eds. 1996. Ethnomedizinische Perspektiven zur frühen Kindheit. Berlin: Verlag für Wissenschaft und Bildung.

Green, L., D. Fein, C. Modahl et al. 2001. Oxytocin and autistic disorder: Alterations in peptide forms. *Biol. Psychiatry* **50**:609–613.

Grossmann, K.E., K. Grossmann, and A. Keppler. 2005. Universal and culturally specific aspects of human behavior. In: Culture and Human Development: The Importance of Cross-cultural Research to the Social Sciences, ed. W. Friedlmeier, P. Chakkarath, and B. Schwarz. Amsterdam: Swetz and Zeitlinger.

Hamilton, W.D. 1964. The genetical evolution of social behavior. *J. Theor. Biol.* **7**:1–52.

Hansen, S., C. Harthon, E. Wallin, L. Loftberg, and K. Svensson. 1991a. The effects of 6-OHDA-induced dopamine depletions in the ventral or dorsal striatum on maternal and sexual behavior in the female rat. *Pharmacol. Biochem. Behav.* **39**:71–77.

Hansen, S., C. Harthon, E. Wallin, L. Loftberg, and K. Svensson. 1991b. Mesotelencephalic dopamine system and reproductive behavior in the female rat: Effects of ventral tegmental 6-hydroxydopamine lesions on maternal and sexual responsiveness. *Behav. Neurosci.* **105**:588–598.

Hazan, C., and D. Zeifman. 1999. Pair bonds as attachments: Evaluating the evidence. In: Handbook of Attachment: Theory, Research, and Clinical Applications, ed. J. Cassidy and P.R. Shaver, pp. 336–354. New York: Guilford.

Hennessy, M.B. 1999. Social influences on endocrine activity in guinea pigs, with comparisons to findings in nonhuman primates. *Neurosci. Biobehav. Rev.* **23**:687–698.

Henry, J.P., and P.M. Stephens. 1977. Stress, Health, and the Social Environment: A Sociobiologic Approach to Medicine. New York: Springer.

Herdt, G.S. 1993. Sexual repression, social control, and gender hierarchy in Sambia culture. In: Sex and Gender Hierarchies, ed. B. Miller, pp. 193–211. Cambridge: Cambridge Univ. Press.

Hill, P.C., and K.I. Pargament. 2003. Advances in the conceptualization and measurement of religion and spirituality: Implications for physical and mental health research. *Am. Psychol.* **58**:64–74.

Hodgson, D.L. 2000. Pastoralism, patriarchy and history among Maasai in Tanganyika. In: Rethinking Pastoralism in Africa: Gender, Culture and the Myth of the Patriarchal Pastoralist, ed. D.L. Hodgson, pp. 97–120. Oxford: James Currey.

Hofer, M.A., and R. Sullivan. 2001. Toward a neurobiology of attachment. In: Handbook of Developmental Cognitive Neuroscience, ed. C.A. Nelson and M. Luciana, pp. 599–616. Cambridge, MA: MIT Press.

Holman, S., and R. Goy. 1995. Experiential and hormonal correlates of care-giving in rhesus macaques. In: Motherhood in Human and Nonhuman Primates, ed. C. Pryce, R. Martin, and D. Skuse, pp. 87–92. Basel: Karger.

House, J.S., K.R. Landis, and D. Umberson. 1988. Social relationships and health. *Science* **241**:540–545.

Hrdy, S.B. 1999. Mother Nature: A History of Mothers, Infants, and Natural Selection. New York: Pantheon.

Hrdy, S.B., and P. Whitten. 1987. Patterning of sexual behavior. In: Primate Societies, ed. B. Smuts, D. Cheney, R. Seyfarth, R. Wrangham, and T. Struhasker, pp. 370–384. Chicago: Univ. of Chicago Press.

Hull, E., R. Meisel, and B. Sachs. 2002. Male sexual behavior. In: Hormones, Brain, and Behavior, ed. D. Pfaff, A. Arnold, A. Etgen, S. Fahrbach, and R. Rubin, pp. 1–138. San Diego: Elsevier.

Insel, T., and C. Harbaugh. 1989. Lesions of the hypothalamic paraventricular nucleus disrupt the initiation of maternal behavior. *Physiol. Behav.* **45**:1033–1041.

Insel, T.R., and L.E. Shapiro. 1992. Oxytocin receptor distribution reflects social organization in monogamous and polygamous voles. *PNAS* **89**:5981–5985.

Insel, T.R., and L.J. Young. 2001. The neurobiology of attachment. *Nat. Rev. Neurosci.* **2**:129–135.

Isiugo-Abanihe, U.C. 1985. Child fosterage in West Africa. *Pop. Dev. Rev.* **11**:53–73.

Kaiser, S., K. Heemann, R.H. Straub, and N. Sachser. 2003. The social environment affects behaviour and androgens, but not cortisol in pregnant female guinea pigs. *Psychoneuroendocrin.* **28**:67–83.

Kaiser, S., F.P.M. Kruijver, D.F. Swaab, and N. Sachser. 2003. Early social stress in female guinea pigs induces a masculinization of adult behaviour and corresponding changes in brain and neuroendocrine function. *Behav. Brain Res.* **144**:199–210.

Kalivas, P.W. 2000. A role for glutamate transmission in addiction to psychostimulants. *Addiction Biol.* **5**:325–329.

Kelly, R.C. 1993. Constructing Inequality: The Fabrication of a Hierarchy of Virtue among the Etoro. Ann Arbor: Univ. of Michigan Press.

Kendrick, K. 2000. Oxytocin, motherhood, and bonding. *Exp. Physiol.* **85**:111S–124S.

Kirschbaum, C., T. Klauer, S.H. Filipp, and D.H. Hellhammer. 1995. Sex-specific effects of social support on cortisol and subjective response to acute psychological stress. *Psychosom. Med.* **57**:23–31.

Klein, J. 1986. Natural History of the Major Histocompatibility Complex. New York: Wiley.

Knapp, L.A., J.C. Ha, and G.P. Sackett. 1996. Parental MHC antigen sharing and pregnancy wastage in captive pigtail macaques. *J. Reprod. Immunol.* **32**:73–88.

Krantz, D.S., and M.K. McCeney. 2002. Effects of psychological and social factors on organic disease: A critical assessment of research on coronary heart disease. *Ann. Rev. Psychol.* **53**:341–369.

Krpan, K., R. Coombs, D. Zinga, M. Steiner, and A.S. Fleming. 2005. Experiential and hormonal correlates of maternal behaviour in teen and adult mothers. *Horm. Behav.*, in press.

Lamb, M.E. 1998. Nonparental child care: Context, quality, correlates and consequences. In: Handbook of Child Psychology, ed. W. Damon, I.E. Sigel, and K.A. Renninger, vol. 4, pp. 73–133. New York: Wiley.

Levy, A. 1999. Continuities and Discontinuities in Parent-child Relationships across Two Generations: A Prospective Longitudinal Study. Ph.D. diss., Univ. of Minnesota.

Lim, S., and R. Howard. 1998. Antecedents of sexual and non-sexual aggression in young Singaporean men. *Pers. Ind. Diffs.* **25**:1163–1182.

Lim, M.M., A.Z. Murphy, and L.J. Young. 2004. Ventral striatopallidal oxytocin and vasopressin V1a receptors in the monogamous prairie vole (*Microtus ochrogaster*). *J. Comp. Neurol.* **468**:555–570.

Lim, M.M., and L.J. Young. 2004. Vasopressin-dependent neural circuits underlying pair bond formation in the monogamous prairie vole. *Neurosci.* **125**:35–45.

Liu, D., J. Diorio, J.C. Day, D.D. Francis, and M.J. Meaney. 2000. Maternal care, hippocampal synaptogensis and cognitive development in rats. *Nature Neurosci.* **3**:799–806.

Liu, D., J. Diorio, B. Tannenbaum et al. 1997. Maternal care, hippocampal glucocorticoid receptors, and hypothalamic-pituitary-adrenal responses to stress. *Science* **277**: 1659–1662.

Lorberbaum, J., J. Newman, A. Horwitz et al. 2002. A potential role for thalamocingulate circuitry in human maternal behavior. *Biol. Psychiatry* **51**:431–445.

Lott, D. 1984. Intraspecific variation in the social-systems of wild vertebrates. *Behaviour* **88**:266–325.

Lubin, D., J. Elliott, M. Black, and J. Johns. 2003. An oxytocin antagonist infused into the central nucleus of the amygdala increases maternal aggressive behavior. *Behav. Neurosci.* **117**:195–201.

Lyons-Ruth, K., L. Alpern, and B. Repacholi. 1993. Disorganized infant attachment classification and maternal psychosocial problems as predictors of hostile-aggressive behavior in the preschool classroom. *Child Dev.* **64**:572–585.

MacFarlane, A. 1975. The Psychology of Childbirth. Cambridge: Harvard Univ. Press.

Madison, D., R. Fitzgerald, and W. McShea. 1984. Dynamics of social nesting in overwintering meadow voles (*Microtus pennsylvanicus*): Possible consequences for population cycling. *Behav. Ecol. Sociobiol.* **15**:9–17.

Maestripieri, D., and J. Zehr. 1998. Maternal responsiveness increases during pregnancy and after estrogen treatment in macaques. *Horm. Behav.* **34**:223–230.

McCabe, K.A., M.L. Rigdon, and V.L. Smith. 2003. Positive reciprocity and intention in trust games. *J. Econ. Behav. Org.* **52**:267–275.

Miller, G. 2000. The Mating Mind: How Sexual Choice Shaped the Evolution of Human Nature. New York: Random House.

Modahl, C., L.A. Green, D. Fein et al. 1998. Plasma oxytocin levels in autistic children. *Biol. Psychiatry* **43**:270–277.

424   *C. A. Pedersen et al.*

Munroe, R.L., R.H. Munroe, and J.W.M. Whiting. 1981. Male sex-role resolutions. In: Handbook of Cross-cultural Human Development, ed. R.L. Munroe, R.H. Munroe, and J.W.M. Whiting, pp. 611–632. New York: Garland.

Murphy, M., J. Seckl, S. Burton, S.A. Checkley, and S.L. Lightman. 1987. Changes in oxytocin and vasopression secretion during sexual activity in men. *J. Clin. Endocrinol. Metab.* **65**:738–741.

Nelson, E., and J. Panksepp. 1996. Oxytocin and infant-mother bonding in rats. *Behav. Neurosci.* **110**:583–592.

Neumann, I. 2001. Alterations in behavioral and neuroendocrine stress coping strategies in pregnant, parturient and lactating rats. In: The Maternal Brain: Neurobiological and Neuroendocrine Adaptation and Disorders in Pregnancy and Post Partum, ed. J. Russell, A. Douglas, R. Windle, and C. Ingram, pp. 143–152. Amsterdam: Elsevier.

NICHD Early Childcare Network. 1997. The effects of infant child care on infant-mother attachment security: Results of the NICHD study of early child care. *Child Dev.* **68**:860–879.

Numan, M., and T. Insel. 2003. The Neurobiology of Parental Behavior. New York: Springer.

Ober, C., L.R. Weitkamp, N. Cox et al. 1997. HLA and mate choice in humans. *Am. J. Hum. Genet.* **61**:497–504.

Odendaal, J.S.J., and R.A. Meintjes. 2003. Neurophysiological correlates of affiliative behaviour between humans and dogs. *Vet. J.* **165**:296–301.

Park, K.A., and E. Waters. 1989. Security of attachment and preschool friendships. *Child Dev.* **60**:1076–1081.

Parker, K., and T. Lee. 2001. Central vasopressin administration regulates the onset of facultative paternal behavior in *Microtus pennsylvanicus* (meadow voles). *Horm. Behav.* **39**:285–294.

Parker, K., K. Phillips, and T. Lee. 2001. Development of selective partner preferences in captive male and female meadow voles, *Microtus pennsylvanicus*. *Anim. Behav.* **61**:1217–1226.

Pedersen, C., and M. Boccia. 2002. Oxytocin links mothering received, mothering bestowed and adult stress responses. *Stress* **5**:259–267.

Pedersen, C., and M. Boccia. 2003. Oxytocin antagonism alters rat dams' oral grooming and upright posturing over pups. *Physiol. Behav.* **80**:233–241.

Pedersen, C., J. Caldwell, C. Walker, G. Ayers, and G. Mason. 1994. Oxytocin activates the postpartum onset of rat maternal behavior in the ventral tegmental area and medial preoptic areas. *Behav. Neurosci.* **108**:1163–1171.

Pedersen, C., J. Johns, I. Musiol et al. 1995. Interfering with somatosensory stimulation from pups sensitizes experienced, postpartum rat mothers to oxytocin antagonist inhibition of maternal behavior. *Behav. Neurosci.* **109**:980–990.

Pedersen, C., R. Stern, J. Pate et al. 1993. Thyroid and adrenal measures during late pregnancy and the puerperium in women who have been major depressed or who become dysphoric postpartum. *J. Affect. Disord.* **29**:201–211.

Penn, D.J. 2002. The scent of genetic compatibility: Sexual selection and the major histocompatibility complex. *Ethology* **108**:1–21.

Penn, D.J., and W.K. Potts. 1998. MHC-disassortative mating preferences reversed by cross-fostering. *Proc. Roy. Soc. Lond. B* **265**:1299–1306.

Penn, D.J., and W.K. Potts. 1999. The evolution of mating preferences and major histocompatibility complex genes. *Am. Naturalist* **153**:145–164.

Perner, J., T. Ruffman, and S.B. Leekam. 1994. Theory of mind is contagious: You catch it from your sibs. *Child Dev.* **65**:1228–1238.

Popeski, N., S. Amir, J. Diorio, and B. Woodside. 2003. Prolactin and oxytocin interaction in the paraventricular and supraoptic nuclei: Effects on oxytocin mRNA and nitric oxide synthase. *J. Neuroendocrin.* **15**:687–696.

Porter, R.H., J.M. Cernoch, and F.J. McLaughlin. 1983. Maternal recognition of neonates through olfactory cues. *Physiol. Behav.* **30**:151–154.

Powell, L.H., L. Shahabi, and C.E. Thoresen. 2003. Religion and spirituality: Linkages to physical health. *Am. Psychol.* **58**:36–52.

Pryce, C., M. Dobeli, and R. Martin. 1993. Effects of sex steroids on maternal motivation in the common marmoset (*Callithrix jacchus*): Development and application of an operant system with maternal reinforcement. *J. Comp. Psychol.* **107**:99–115.

Rees, S., and A. Fleming. 2001. How early maternal separation and juvenile experience with pups affect maternal behavior and emotionality in adult postpartum rats. *Anim. Learn. Behav.* **29**:221–233.

Romeo, R.D., H.N. Richardson, and C.L. Sisk. 2002. Puberty and the maturation of the male brain and sexual behavior: Recasting a behavioral potential. *Neurosci. Biobehav. Rev.* **26**:381–391.

Sachser, N., D. Hierzel, and M. Dürschlag. 1998. Social relationships and the management of stress. *Psychoneuroendocrin.* **23**:891–904.

Sachser, N., C. Lick, and K. Stanzel. 1994. The environment, hormones and aggressive behaviour: A five-year study in guinea pigs. *Psychoneuroendocrin.* **23**:891–904.

Sagi-Schwartz, A., M.H. van IJzendoorn, K.E. Grossmann et al. 2003. Attachment and traumatic stress in female Holocaust child survivors and their daughters. *Am. J. Psych.* **160**:1086–1092.

Schaal, B., H. Montagner, E. Hertling et al. 1980. Les stimulations olfactives dans les relations entre l'enfants et la mère. *Reprod. Nutr. Dev.* **20**:843–858.

Schaal, B., and R.H. Porter. 1991. Microsmatic humans revisited: The generation and perception of chemical signals. *Adv. Stud. Behav.* **20**:135–199.

Schradin, C., and G. Anzenberger. 1999. Prolactin, the hormone of paternity. *News Physiol. Sci.* **14**:223–231.

Schradin, C., D.M. Reeder, S.P. Mendoza, and G. Anzenberger. 2003. Prolactin and paternal care: Comparison of three monogamous New World monkey species (*Callicebus cupreus, Callithrix jacchus*, and *Callimico goeldii*). *J. Comp. Psychol.* **117**:166–175.

Seeman, T.E., L.F. Dubin, and M. Seeman. 2003. Religiosity/spirituality and health: A critical review of the evidence for biological pathways. *Am. Psychol.* **58**:53–63.

Sillen-Tullberg, B., and A.P. Moller. 1993. The relationship between concealed ovulation and mating systems in Anthropoid primates: A phylogenetic analysis. *Am. Naturalist* **141**:1–25.

Snowdon, C. 1996. Infant care in cooperatively breeding species. *Adv. Stud. Behav.* **25**:643–689.

Spitz, R. 1945. Hospitalism: An inquiry into the genesis of psychiatric conditions in early childhood. In: The Psychoanalytic Study of the Child, ed. R. Eissler, vol. 1, pp. 53–74. New York: Intl. Univ. Press.

Stallings, J., A.S. Fleming, C. Corter, C. Worthman, and M. Steiner. 2001. The effects of infant cries and odors on sympathy, cortisol, and autonomic responses in new mothers and nonpostpartum women. *Parenting Sci. Prac.* **1**:71–100.

Stern, J., and J. Lonstein. 2001. Neural mediation of nursing and related maternal behaviors. *Prog. Brain Res.* **133**:263–278.

Storey, A.E., C.J. Walsh, R.L. Quinton, and K.E. Wynne-Edwards. 2000. Hormonal correlates of paternal responsiveness in new and expectant fathers. *Evol. Hum. Behav.* **21**:79–95.

Sudre, P., M. Serdula, N. Binkin, N. Staehling, and M. Kramer. 1990 Child fostering, health and nutritional status: The experience of Swaziland. *Ecol. Food Nutr.* **24**: 181–188.

Sullivan, R.M., M. Landers, B. Yeaman, and D.A. Wilson. 2000. Good memories of bad events in infancy. *Nature* **407**:38–39.

Trehub, S., and L. Trainor. 1998. Singing to infants: Lullabies and play songs. *Adv. Infancy Res.* **12**:43–77.

Trethowan, W.H. 1972. The couvade syndrome. In: Modern Perspectives in Psycho-Obstetrics, ed. J.G. Howells, pp. 84–85. New York: Brunner/Mazel.

Trivers, R. 1971. The evolution of reciprocal altruism. *Qtly. Rev. Biol.* **46**:35–57.

Uvnas-Moberg, K. 1997. Physiological and endocrine effects of social contact. *Ann. NY Acad. Sci.* **807**:146–163.

Uvnas-Moberg, K. 1998. Oxytocin may mediate the benefits of positive social interaction and contact. *Psychoneuroendocrin.* **23**:819–835.

van den Boom, D.C. 1994. The influence of temperament and mothering on attachment and exploration: An experimental manipulation of sensitive responsiveness among lower-class mothers with irritable infants. *Child Dev.* **65**:1449–1469.

Van IJzendoorn, M.H., and A. Sagi. 1999. Cross-cultural patterns of attachment. In: Handbook of Attachment: Theory and Research, ed. J. Cassidy and P.R. Shaver, pp. 713–734. New York: Guilford.

von Holst, D. 1998. The concept of stress and its relevance for animal behavior. *Adv. Stud. Behav.* **27**:1–131.

Wang, Z., C.F. Ferris, and G.J. De Vries. 1994. Role of septal vasopressin innervation in paternal behavior in prairie vole (*Microtus ochrogaster*). *PNAS* **91**:400–404.

Wedekind, C., and S. Füri. 1997. Body odour preferences in men and women: Do they aim for specific MHC combinations or simply heterozygosity? *Proc. Roy. Soc. Lond. B* **264**:1471–1479.

Wedekind, C., T. Seebeck, F. Bettens, and A. Paepke. 1995. MHC-dependent mate preferences in humans. *Proc. Roy. Soc. Lond. B* **260**:245–249.

Wickler, W. 1976. The ethological analysis of attachment. *Z. Tierpsychologie* **42**:12–28.

Wilson, D.A., and R.M. Sullivan. 1994. Review: Neurobiology of associative learning in the neonate: Early olfactory learning. *Behav. Neur. Biol.* **61**:1–18.

Windle, R.J., N. Shanks, S. Lightman, and C. Ingram. 1997. Central oxytocin administration reduces stress-induced corticosterone release and anxiety behavior in rats. *Endocrinology* **138**:2829–2834.

Winslow, J., N. Hastings, C.S. Carter, C.R. Harbaugh, and T.R. Insel. 1993. A role for central vasopressin in pair bonding in monogamous prairie voles. *Nature* **365**:545–548.

Young, L.J., M.M. Lim, B. Gingrich, and T.R. Insel. 2001. Cellular mechanisms of social attachment. *Horm. Behav.* **40**:133–148.

Yu, G., H. Kaba, F. Okutani, S. Takahashi, and T. Higuchi. 1996. The olfactory bulb: A critical site of action for oxytocin on the induction of maternal behaviour. *Neurosci.* **72**:1083–1088.

Zak, P.J., and S. Knack. 2001. Trust and growth. *Econ. J.* **111**:295–321.

Zak, P.J., R.O. Kurzban, and W.L. Matzner. 2003. The neurobiology of trust. Center for Neuroeconomics Studies Working Paper. Claremont, CA: Claremont Graduate Univ.

Zhu, L., and T. Onaka. 2003. Facilitative role of prolactin-releasing peptide neurons in oxytocin cell activation after conditioned-fear stimuli. *Neurosci.* **118**:1045–1053.

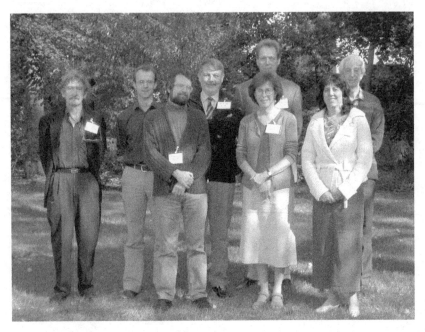

Back, left to right: Gary Kraemer, Gunther Meinlschmidt, Giovanni Liotti,
       Axel Schölmerich, Colwyn Trevarthen
Front, left to right: Michael Lamb, Karlen Lyons-Ruth, Miriam Steele

18

Group Report: Adaptive and Maladaptive Outcomes

G. W. KRAEMER, Rapporteur

M. E. LAMB, G. A. LIOTTI, K. LYONS-RUTH, G. MEINLSCHMIDT,

A. SCHÖLMERICH, M. STEELE, and C. TREVARTHEN

INTRODUCTION

In the preface to his book, *A Secure Base,* John Bowlby (1988) lamented that his theory of attachment had not had much effect on the approaches to treatment of children with behavioral disorders related to early mother–infant separation, or to depression and anxiety disorders related to disrupted attachment. He felt that clinicians had not made sufficient effort to put theory into practice. This concern continues today and was a key issue in our deliberations. Although Bowlby's views were not the only ones considered by our group, they served as a foundation for our discussions, and much of the terminology used herein can be traced back to his publications.

We began our discussions by considering evidence supporting the idea that disrupted attachment is a cause of later behavioral disorders, depression, and anxiety disorders: Is disrupted attachment a primary and substantial factor in the development of psychopathology in childhood, adolescence, and adulthood, or is it but one among many factors that may come into play? If certain kinds of psychopathology are expressed by adolescents and adults, can we reason backwards that attachment disruptions must have existed?

In our review of contemporary attachment theories and their relation to adaptive and maladaptive outcomes, we considered conscious as well as neurobiological processes not included in the Bowlby paradigm. One can view the child as having "motives," rather than "motivation," and as a seeker of information as well as an explorer. This view adds a new dimension and richness to the ways in which the functions of attachment behavior might be characterized. An infant's motives usually lead to interactions with the caregiver and integration into the larger social environment. Seeking and attending to action and sensation, whether in relation to the caregiver or others, transfers information about the social and cultural environment that has emotional and moral meaning. One implication is that compromised infants (i.e., those who do not share the intrinsic characteristics of most infants) will have difficulty integrating into an attachment relationship and the larger society (Trevarthen, this volume).

We also discussed whether Bowlby's construct of an "internal" attachment mechanism could be framed in terms of understanding the behavioral and neurobiological mechanisms that were not known at the time. Bowlby's contributions have promoted considerable progress in understanding social behavior and brain function per se, but there have been areas in which control systems theory accounts for neither the behavioral nor neurobiological data. Thus, a new theory needs to be set in place.

A second major discussion topic concerned the relationship of early and ongoing attachment to the usual progression of continuity and change in behavioral, cognitive/emotional, and social development. Is the quality of childhood attachment related to attachment styles as well as social affiliation and competence in adulthood? A premise is that salutary attachments and affiliation among adults contribute substantially to individual well-being and quality of life. Conversely, the inability to establish and maintain such relationships appears to be associated with emotional, mood, and possibly even personality disorders and, hence, reduced quality of life and a diminished sense of well-being. The idea is that *secure* attachment may be associated with later exhibition of nurturing care, companionship, and achievement; *insecure* attachment with self-protection, less flexibility, fear and anxiety; and, *disorganized* attachment with uncertainty, and contradictory and disordered social behavior.

A third topic involved the probable biological substrates (i.e., neurobiological mechanisms) that support attachment behavior and are themselves formed or altered as a result of attachment and then malformed or adversely affected by distortions or disruptions of caregiving. Neurobiological mechanisms are viewed as underpinning behavioral and cognitive/emotional systems. Disrupted attachment may interfere with the formation or function of brain mechanisms necessary for social competence. These include cognitive functions associated with motivation, planning, and problem solving, as well as mechanisms that maintain emotional stability. This would leave the individual more vulnerable to environmental problems or adversity that may not affect others experiencing more secure early attachment relationships, and hence less likely to follow a predictable developmental trajectory. We considered two major views: Bowlby's construct of "internal working models" (IWMs) of the environment and caregiver, and Hofer's construct of "internal regulators." We also discussed whether attachment plays into persisting changes in the regulation of the autonomic nervous system and/or the hypothalamic–pituitary–adrenal (HPA) axis, thereby affecting an individual's stress responsiveness and/or ability to cope cognitively and emotionally with stressors. In addition, we considered whether disrupted attachment in childhood has substantial effects on later parenting/ caregiving, and thus could propagate across generations. Many of the presumed effects of early attachment disruption would leave the adult less able to cope with the demands of caregiving and less able to establish attachments to off-spring. Such effects, if substantial, could lead to disrupted attachment in the next generation, because the parent is unable to provide what the child needs as part of an adequate attachment relationship. Hence, disrupted maternal care in one generation may produce unfortunate effects on maternal care in the next. Physi-cally nondeprived offspring in the second generation may be exposed to a strangely behaving caregiver and encounters with the environment that they would not have had otherwise. This could be a mechanism underlying intergenerational transmission of maladaptive behavior.

Our fourth topic addressed issues surrounding the probable roots of maladaptive behavior and the concept of "self-repair":

1. Quantitative and qualitative differences exist in early attachment and can profitably be viewed as usual variation, perhaps producing individuals with quite different patterns of attachment and affiliative behavior. Some individuals may do better in some environments than others.

2. All individuals may exhibit some maladaptive behavior during periods of development, under various circumstances, or in response to life situa-tions. The majority are able to self-repair to a point where they continue as functional, if not content, beings. Some individuals, however, persis-tently express behavior that would be considered to be maladaptive in any context and environment, i.e., behavior clearly harmful to the self or others, with no redeeming value to the self or society in a conceivable context. Expression of maladaptive behavior is often attributed to states of internal conflict, lack of a sense of well-being, and persistent negative affect. Self-repair involves resolution or reversal of these internal states.

3. Individuals who cannot self-repair are set off on a trajectory of persistent and perhaps increasing maladaptive behavior, eventually requiring men-tal health or criminal justice intervention by the family or the society. We also considered why certain individuals cannot self-repair.

Our final topic concerned approaches to intervention and treatment of maladaptive outcomes that may be related to disrupted attachment. We consid-ered issues surrounding the assessment of behavior and a perspective on cogni-tive/emotional characteristics of the adult, as these might be characterized in psychiatric terminology. Prevention of attachment disruption at the societal and cultural level is a key issue. Given the focus of our group, we addressed issues that relate primarily to problems in-the-making. Early intervention is considered in relation to characteristics of the caregiver or family environment which might be modified. Both intervention and treatment considerations include interrupt-ing the progression of negative emotionality and attribution and finding ways to modify or alter both internal and environmental regulatory processes, whether cognitive/emotional, neurobiological, or physiological.

This chapter is not meant to provide a comprehensive review of the literature but rather to engage a contemporary consideration of what attachment is.

Throughout our deliberations, we were mindful of an issue that transcends the topics considered at this workshop: Biologists as well as behavioral and clinical scientists do not speak the same language, especially with regard to basic concepts concerning attachment. "Attachment" and "bonding" seem to have slippery and catch-as-catch-can definitions which vary across disciplines and between individuals within them (or even within individuals at different times and in different contexts). This poses a major barrier to future progress in any endeavor that seeks to integrate behavior, biology, and genetics, and perhaps especially so on the general topic of attachment and social affiliation. The key to a new synthesis may be a general psychobiological mind-and-body theory, and a common working language to accompany it. We feel that a beginning was achieved at this Dahlem Workshop.

THREE VIEWS OF ATTACHMENT: ADAPTATION, MALADAPTATION, AND PSYCHOPATHOLOGY

Human culture provides the opportunity for emergent social processes within human families or small social groups to surface, and may lead to the expression of increasingly diverse forms of social behavior across generations. Some behavior does not appear to be adaptive in any obvious way (e.g., genetic risk for schizophrenia). Manifestation of a behavioral disorder does not necessarily contribute to the fitness of the individual or social group in the larger cultural and environmental context. Indeed, it may remain "silent" for one generation only to resurface in the next, under circumstances propitious for its expression.

In the Darwinian or evolutionary sense, genetic variability is the ultimate adaptive mechanism. Genetic combination and recombination, and occasionally mutation, produce variation among living beings. Encounters with the vagaries of environmental reality (selection) determine which individuals survive and reproduce. A "genetic rolling of the dice" brings diverse genotypes and then phenotypes into existence. Human cultural systems provide buffers that allow multiple patterns of human ecological adaptation to be expressed by and within cultures. Diversity blossoms in the absence of any true external challenge, which would dictate that one social or cultural system is more "fit" than another. For humans, the challenges to survival appear to be ourselves and the ecology of the Earth: war or conflict, economic competition, natural disaster, famine, and disease are major selection factors. Phenotypes left "unselected," under the shelter of culture, can however effect both positive and negative results.

"Adaptive" and hence "maladaptive" consequences can also be defined in a social behavioral and psychobiological sense. Adaptation to a social environment implies that an individual exhibits behaviors compatible with the expectations of other individuals; through social participation and support, these behaviors promote individual well-being and acceptance in the group. Similar rules translate to how a smaller social group fits into a larger one. Maladaptation implies that the individual or group is not well accepted in the larger surround. The consequences of maladaptation for the individual or group often fall short of death but certainly may include ostracism; a socially "maladapted" individual, however, is not necessarily less fit in biological terms.

Within the broad range of human behaviors, there are those that can be expressed and supported as adaptive in a local context but not necessarily as such in an extended or "surrounding" context. For instance, individual behavioral adaptation to the family and social group of origin per se seems to have a positive value. Behavior compatible with a small social group may be evaluated (e.g., by peers, teachers, or coworkers from the larger society) as maladaptive if this small social group, for example, is a gang of habitual miscreants and liars.

Adaptive behavior in urban societies and environments may follow different rules than in rural areas and vice versa. Cultural settings thus have a defining role. Take, for example, an almost reflexive and seemingly adaptive social behavior — smiling — in Western European cultures and contrast it to what is deemed meaningful in many Asian cultures. In addition, unfortunate treatment for an individual may be adaptive for the group as a whole (e.g., declining to respond to the infant's attachment expressive behaviors may increase demands on the infant but free the caregiver to undertake other tasks necessary for survival). In this way, "disturbed" maternal behavior can be viewed as having a strategic function to signal the need for more support from other members of the community (see Hrdy and Belsky, both this volume). Tantrums and other obtrusive or intrusive behaviors on the part of offspring might also be viewed as an adaptive response to a caregiving style, such that the behavior is rewarded by attention from the caregiver. In a larger social context, however, the behavior could be evaluated as maladaptive because of the social consequences to the child, with the concomitant blaming of the caregiver for failure to control the child. Criminal behavior or social phobia might be "adaptive" for the individual in a circumscribed social context, but not in a larger setting. Indeed, viewed from this perspective, behavioral patterns cannot be labeled as adaptive or maladaptive on the basis of their morphology.

Behavioral "adaptation," therefore, defined in a nonevolutionary social environmental sense, is the process by which the individual integrates profitably into a surround. The expanse of that surround and the demands placed on the individual are variable. Invariant requirements include the ability to maintain internal regulation of physiological homeostasis, behaving appropriately in relation to a social and environmental context, and a compatibility with the present or future demands of the social and inanimate environment. Adaptation to the surround allows the capacities of the individual to be expressed in relation to the resources and constraints of the environment. Adaptation in this social sense may lead to increased fitness in the evolutionary sense by producing progeny or increasing the survival of relatives' progeny. The distinction between "adaptation" in the social functional sense and in terms of evolutionary fitness is important. We use "adaptation" to refer to the immediate and future social environmental context.

"Maladaptation" means that an individual is not able to express itself fully, that the expression is not valued, or that the expression is harmful to the individual or to the social and/or environmental surround. Typical examples include when an individual is killed, persecuted, isolated, or ostracized. Further distinctions relate to the quality and quantity of maladaptive behavior. Some behavior is counterproductive for the individual and others in proximity (e.g., insulting a new acquaintance, neglecting or physically or psychologically abusing offspring). Other behaviors can become maladaptive when they are emitted at an extraordinary duration or frequency: if handshaking or bowing is a form of salutary greeting, then it is important to stop after an appropriate interval.

Maladaptive Behavior versus Psychopathology

What distinguishes maladaptive behavior from the usual mistakes or social faux pas that we all commit? Why do some maladaptive behaviors seem so intractable, persistent, and impervious to change, even in the face of adverse consequences or intervention? One explanation is that such behavior constitutes "psychopathology": a disorder that is expressed, in part, by abnormal behavior. Typically, this has unfortunate consequences for the individual and often for others. The Diagnostic and Statistical Manual, edition IV (DSM-IV) of the American Psychiatric Association lists criteria for abnormal internal states: mental states, perceptions, or feelings (emotions) that are reported by the individual. Recent advances in neuroscience technologies, including fMRI, may soon be able to associate brain states with DSM classifications of psychopathology. Although this will advance biological psychiatry, it will not resolve the dualism between "internal conscious mechanisms," referred to in psychology, and structural neurochemical mechanisms, considered in neuroscience.

It is important to note that DSM diagnostic criteria rely solely on verbal reports of mental states, which are treated as behaviors. Diagnosis does not depend on any theory concerning the relationship between "mental states" and behavior. The focus of the assessment is on the individual's mental illness, i.e., clinical disorders (psychopathology, Axis I), co-present personality disorders or mental retardation, medical illness, social and environmental problems, and functional status (Axes II–V, respectively). Psychopathology is viewed as being a characteristic of the individual and is usually expressed in a "context." Social context, however, is not an intrinsic part of the definition.

The constructs of adaptation and maladaptation include the idea of a "surround" (context or environmental setting), whereas "psychopathology" focuses on deviance of the individual's behavior from those of others in the same surround. Some forms of psychopathology are related to somewhat distinctive early relational patterns but are not caused by them (e.g., schizophrenia). Some forms of disturbed or atypical attachment relationships would not fit into standard classifications of psychopathology (e.g., forms of controlling behavior).

Earlier theories regarding constructs (e.g., the "ice-cold mother" as a substantial causal factor for schizophrenia) have not withstood the application of controlled research methods. Current research findings agree, though, that there are substantial environmental risk factors for the development of some forms of psychopathology, as defined in DSM-IV, and that poor attachment relationships count as a risk factor.

A more rigorous approach is needed to describe and qualitatively or quantitatively distinguish early attachment relationships. In our discussions, we used the Bowlby/Ainsworth theory of attachment and qualitative functional categorization of attachment styles as a starting point.

Bowlby/Ainsworth and Offspring

Since the late 1960s, the preeminent theory of attachment has been that propounded by John Bowlby in collaboration with Mary Ainsworth (Kraemer 1992a). The Bowlby/Ainsworth ethological control systems theory (ECST) of attachment asserts that secure infant–caregiver attachment is necessary for optimal psychosocial development of the infant. Viewed from the other direction, psychopathological behavior exhibited by juveniles, adolescents, and adults may be causally related to a disruption of early attachment (Bowlby 1988). Deemed controversial when it was first formally proposed (Bowlby 1951), it is currently viewed as common sense by many health care professionals and academicians. Perhaps, as with many things, the truth lies somewhere in the middle.

ECST is based on the premise that an inherited imprinting-like behavioral system exists, enabling an infant to attach to an object that is also a secure base and a caregiver (Bowlby 1969, p. 45). The person (or animal) serving as a *secure base* must exhibit at least three characteristics: he/she is reliable; he/she shields the infant from environmental threats; and, he/she is able to sooth distress states and provide the infant with resources (e.g., nutrition). *Attachment behavior* involves (at least) visual tracking, maintaining proximity, and seeking contact with the secure base. This behavior is regulated by "goal-corrected" homeostatic mechanisms in the infant and by IWMs of the external world (i.e., of the caregiver and environment). Having a secure base maximizes chances of survival, permits the infant to develop veridical IWMs of the external world, explore the environment, and develop optimally (Bowlby 1988).

Disruption in attachment to a caregiver means that a child does not have a secure base and is prone to incorporate conflicting IWMs of attachment figures and the environment. A child lacks soothing and may not explore, acquire knowledge, or develop as it would otherwise. Bowlby cited disrupted attachment as a cause of previously unrecognized childhood depression and anxiety disorders, later vulnerability to adverse responses to usual stressors, and inadequate caregiving when the child becomes a parent. Thus, disrupted attachment produces a form of developmental psychopathology which can propagate across generations (Bowlby 1988).

Attachment Classifications and Risk for Maladaptive Outcomes

How can one assess the quality and nature of the child's IWMs? If a typical infant/juvenile encounters fear-producing stimuli while exploring, then it retreats to the caregiver. A core premise of ECST is that this behavior occurs because of the IWM of the caregiver as being a "secure base."

The "Strange Situation," devised by Ainsworth, assesses the quality of attachment and nature of the child's IWM of the caregiver by providing mild stress to the infant. It consists of a series of episodes in which the infant can also explore or interact with an unfamiliar adult in the presence or absence of the mother. Observations are made on the effect of maternal absence on infant exploration and the quality of comfort seeking of the child when the caregiver returns (Ainsworth et al. 1978). Ainsworth described three patterns of the infant's response to reunion episodes (Ainsworth et al. 1978; Sroufe 1986):

A. Avoidant/Insecurely attached: this group appeared to reject the mother.
B. Securely attached: this group sought contact or greeted the mother.
C. Ambivalent/Insecurely attached: this group alternated between being angry and emitting attachment behavior toward the mother.

Later, a "Disorganized" (D) category was established for children whose behaviors did not fit into the A, B, or C categories — behaviors that appeared to be contradictory, undirected, dysphoric, or helpless (Main and Solomon 1990).

The reunion response of the infant appears to be related to the caregiving style of the mother. *Securely attached* children generally had mothers who were "more sensitive, accepting, cooperative, and psychologically accessible to their babies." *Insecurely attached* children generally had mothers who were inconsistent, unresponsive, or rejecting (Ainsworth et al. 1978, pp. 144–146). Later studies suggest that secure versus insecure attachment is related to adaptive and maladaptive behavior, which surfaces as the children mature.

From this theoretical standpoint, the clear expectation is that the ability of a child to explore the environment freely, manage fear and anxiety, and develop cognitively must be affected by the secure or insecure base characteristics of the caregiver. Many research reports characterize insecurely attached children as having low self-reliance, low enthusiasm for academic tasks, difficulty with integration into school social structures, and low resilience in the face of real or imagined stressors (Lewis 1990; Hennighausen and Lyons-Ruth, this volume). Research results, however, have not always conformed rigorously to theoretical expectation. Whereas Matas et al. (1978) reported better problem-solving skills of securely attached children, Main (1983) found no differences between secure and insecure children in the duration of symbolic play. Maslin-Cole and Spieker (1990) observed that both A- and B-classified children engaged in symbolic play longer than C-children. McElwain et al. (2003) reported similar degrees of exploratory behavior during solitary play among A- and B-classified children. Especially A-classified children appear to be more oriented toward the nonsocial world (Schölmerich and Lengning 2005) and can be even more persistent in an exploratory task (Frodi et al. 1985). Thus, within the range of typical development, uncertainty remains as to how firmly early attachment experiences play out in expression of cognitive abilities and social development.

Attachment Variability and Consequences

Does classifying children as A, B, C, or D aid our understanding of their later exhibition of typical adaptive behavior, maladaptive behavior, or psychopathology? A current view is that category D is most clearly associated with later persistent maladaptive or even pathological behavior, and one wonders whether it may have a substantial genetic loading.

About 15% of children tested on the Strange Situation in the U.S.A. are classified as disorganized. If category D does prove to have a strong genetic foundation, such that it is almost certainly expressed, then selection appears to be at work. On the other hand, if category D has a weak genetic loading and only occurs under specific environmental and social developmental circumstances, then the capacity to express it is there, but only under the right social circumstances. Indeed, it appears that children are adversely affected with disorganized attachment when it occurs simultaneously with very high-risk ecological circumstances (Belsky, this volume). What kind of environments exists for disorganized adolescents and young adults? Does disorganization repeat across successive siblings or generations?

From this theoretical viewpoint and in this classification system, there is no implication that something is "malfunctioning" in the child's nervous system. More specifically, the presumption is that all characteristics of A, B, C, and D performance can be and are exhibited by a fully functional nervous system; that is, a nervous system not compromised in any way other than that it has not incorporated adequate IWMs of the external world or appropriate "set-goals," which would motivate future exploration and updating of IWMs. There is also no evidence to indicate that persisting variations in attachment styles impact function or development of neurobiological systems in the child's brain. The clinical implication is obvious: a child/juvenile/adult needs to incorporate more effective IWMs and set-goals, and the role of the therapist is to encourage just that.

Psychobiology

ECST does not encompass many problems and neurobiological/physiological phenomena that are of current concern to clinicians. Research on the presumed neurobiological substrates of attachment behavior in animals has produced results that are at least not accounted for by ECST. This has led to formulation of "psychobiological attachment theory" (PAT) (Hofer 1987; Kraemer 1992a, b).

If one assumes that the only, or most significant, long-term effects of attachment are on cognitive working models of the social environment, then any behavioral effects that might be attributed to altered body physiology are outside of the theory. Indeed, undeniable constitutional, temperamental, and/or biological variation, which may be observed and cited as a factor in behavior, may be assigned to the wrong causal domain (i.e., attributable to genetic causes), even though the cause of such variation is actually social or environmental in origin.

If one attributes enduring maladaptation to only two domains of causality — altered cognition (working models) and/or temperament (another construct) — then the idea of a third or "interface" domain with equal stature may be overlooked (Kraemer 1992a, b). ECST is silent on what the persisting physiological effects of attachment might be. Yet, environmentally produced alteration of primary physiological responsiveness to stressors counts as an interface domain between cognitive regulation of behavior and more basic regulation of response proclivities which may be genetic in origin. Alteration of basic physiologic responses in offspring could be one way that maternal responsiveness persistently affects their behavior.

Hofer's Internal Regulators

Separation distress (vocalization, locomotion: protest) and reduction of that distress by contact comfort are observable in the rat pup and similar to behaviors perceived to be indicative of attachment in many species (Hofer 1987). A critical question concerns what the pup recognizes as maintaining a state of behavioral homeostasis and quiescence while it is in the nest.

Specific stimuli presented by the rat mother and nest (body contour, warmth, furry texture, nest odor, and breathing) reduce separation distress. However, the attachment schemata of the rat pup do not distinguish between the sustaining mother and the sensory environment surrounding the nest and littermates. Hofer suggests that the rat pup employs a strategy of adding cues in different sense modalities and thus comes to regard littermates as more or less complete surrogates for the mother (Hofer 1987). The mother, on the other hand, appears to provide a multimodal set of sensory stimuli (thermal, olfactory, somatosensory, visual), which selectively regulate an equally broad and multimodal physiological and behavioral homeostatic system in the infant. This littermates cannot do.

If the pup is separated from the mother for a prolonged period, a set of changes slowly develops that is comparable to the despair response observed in other species. Such changes include decreased body temperature, altered heart rate, sleep disturbance, and changes in brain catecholamine neurotransmitter mechanisms (Hofer 1987; Stone et al. 1976). These effects surface even when the protest response is blocked by the presence of an effective surrogate (e.g., littermates). Hence, only protest is directly related to the separation event. Despair appears to be a composite dysregulation that occurs if all the *regulatory* characteristics of the mother are removed (Hofer 1987).

Attachment, Perception, Physiology, and Behavior

A neonate reflexively seeks an attachment object with particular stimulus characteristics and has a repertoire of behavior that it will emit towards that object (Bowlby 1969, pp. 166–171, 180–194). The first "stimulus characteristics" that an infant can detect are visual, auditory, somatosensory, olfactory, and gustatory temporal and spatial patterning of interactions. This synchronous and harmonious difference becomes the example upon which the first working model of "what should be" is constructed. Thereafter, the only developmental requirement is the ability to recognize the "self," detect disparity between what should be and what exists, and act to reduce that disparity. One can change subsequent action in relation to what exists and what should be, as long as one maintains a representation of what has happened (i.e., a memory). These biological requirements for central nervous system function are not unusual; they also apply to the immune system (Edelman 1989).

The neonate must also come to regulate its own behavior and physiology. We now know that just as cognitive working models develop in relation to the caregiver, so do homeostatic mechanisms, which become increasingly more like those of the caregiver by virtue of shared genetic endowment and the exposure of the infant's neurobiological systems to the caregiver (Hofer 1987). This is revealed by studying the behavior and physiology of individuals that cannot have such an underlying structure because they did not have a mother.

Psychobiological studies thus indicate that the monkey mother is usually a potent regulator of the infant's behavior through exhibition of stimuli that the infant is set to respond to in a particular way. It would be a mistake to think of this as a "reflex," in the way we typically view spinal chord mechanisms. Instead, the idea is that the infant's behavior usually becomes entrained to the mother's, and vice versa, in a transactional relationship occurring over time. If all goes well, the infant internalizes a dynamic multimodal temporal and spatial sensory "image" of the regulatory systems of the caregiver. Thus, the most fundamental regulatory mechanisms of the infant, while genetically mandated, are nevertheless formed in relation to an external object. The continuing ecological role of that external object must also be considered.

In mammals, regulatory interactions between caregiver and infant persist into life stages where offspring are capable of fending for themselves. Hofer suggested that the long rearing period with the mother may preadapt offspring to the particular environment in which they happen to live. In species with more complex cortical function (e.g., juvenile monkey or human, and even in more mature rats) regulators may become increasingly "internalized." This might involve a shift from sensorimotor to higher-order associative and symbolic functions as well as from a dependence on interaction with the mother to a more flexible dependence on a variety of different social interactions (Hofer 1987).

A link between the views of Hofer and Bowlby is that selection pressure leading to the differences in brain function between primates and other species may have been primarily social, rather than ecological (Cheney et al. 1986; Vygotsky 1987). In the rhesus monkey society, for instance, protocol is often strict; most of the aggression within a social group is directed at infant or fledgling juvenile kin (Bernstein and Ehardt 1986). Sapolsky (1990) has likened the social order of baboons to a Machiavellian landscape of intrigue, subterfuge, deceit, and betrayal. In many species, contests for social dominance and access to mates involve the formation and disruption of complex and often tenuous alliances, the value of which plays out in protracted maneuverings that may culminate in combat. Defeat often carries with it the penalty of death or ostracism. Hapless bystanders can become the focus of redirected aggression and may themselves be killed or ostracized. Thus, the infant must adapt to the social environment in order to survive and procreate. The neurobiological mechanisms that enable the individual to cope cognitively and emotionally with a social environment usually form in relation to a caregiver.

When addressing maladaptation from a psychobiological point of view, it is important to highlight two aspects of Bowlby's foundational assumptions that have been revised in PAT in relation to contemporary findings in developmental neurobiology. First, an infant's physiological and behavioral regulatory systems can be understood as being analogous to cybernetic control systems; if so, their functional structure (neuroanatomy and neurochemistry) is determined by an inherited (genetic) plan (Bowlby 1969, pp. 38–50). Second, the infant is "preset" in conjunction with fear mechanisms to seek a secure base (Ainsworth et al. 1978; Bowlby 1969, pp. 215–216; Bowlby 1988, pp. 81–82). It has now been clearly established that the neonates' physiology and neurobiology are much more plastic and self-modifying than could be appreciated even a decade ago, and that the sensory systems of the infant do not select for "secure base" characteristics of the caregiver, only its stimulus characteristics. Furthermore, the aversive versus attractive nature of stimulus characteristics is not immutable, neither is it determined by the physical nature of the stimuli themselves.

It is possible for mammalian infants to attach to objects (caregivers) that are not secure bases — objects likely to increase pain and risk to the infant rather than shielding it. This has been clearly demonstrated by Hofer (1987) and Harlow et al. (1971): mammalian neonates will attach to inanimate objects bearing some of the sensory characteristics of a mother (e.g., surface texture, warmth), but are in no way, shape, or form a secure base. Indeed, rhesus monkey infants exhibit exaggerated and persistent attempts to gain and maintain contact with mothers that are aggressive and abusive. When frightened, infants will seek these objects although they offer no protection to the infant and may indeed present a greater objective danger than that from which the infant is retreating.

Hence, stimuli that initially produce pain and/or fear may be intrinsically linked to the expression of attachment behavior, as noted in ECST. "Painful" or "aversive" are not intrinsic characteristics of different kinds of stimuli, however, as one might suppose from observing the behavior of typically developing individuals. It is possible for the nervous system to organize, or reorganize, such that stimuli which are aversive for typically developing individuals may serve as rewards or reinforcers of behavior in atypically developing individuals. Seeking a secure base and protection is not an immutable goal of attachment behavior for some. In such cases, and in the absence of usual interactions with a caregiver, the nervous system develops, but the organization that would have existed if a caregiver were present does not form. Instead, an alternate organization or lack thereof occurs (Kraemer 1992a, b)

Character and Quality of the Mother–Infant Relationship

Reasoning from animal models, we hypothesize that the human caregiving relationship usually involves mechanisms for damping the infant fear response. It promotes long-term changes in mechanisms regulating the infant's fear responses to events in the surrounding environment, thereby promoting social engagement and communication.

Overall, the attachment system needs to be re-contextualized within a broader evolutionary, biological base than the fear–social awareness system alone. This is because the regulation of fearful affect involves more than just comforting and soothing around distress. More fundamentally, it involves preventing states of distress. Thus, physiological systems other than those involved in defense and fear behavior must play a role. One clear nominee for such a mechanism, with research support, is the establishment of a positively valenced sharing of communicative signals with close others early in development. Since this function may relate to biological systems mediating reward rather than fear, it cannot easily be conceptually separated from the central functions of an attachment relationship (Hennighausen and Lyons-Ruth, this volume).

The mother acts as a selective filter for information coming from the environment to the actively information-seeking neonate. Beyond the neonatal period, mammalian infants enter an exploratory phase of development and spend increasing amounts of time away from the mother. In Bowlby's terminology, they develop an IWM of the surrounding environment. As surprises arrive, infants experience fear, which is viewed as being intrinsically aversive. According to Bowlby, the built-in behavioral response is to return to the mother as a base of security. Usually, regaining contact or proximity to the mother reduces fear. Human attachment theory has focused on elaborating the caregiver's role in regulating the fear/wariness system in child development. Because of the foundational and preemptory role of fear, this function must exert a variety of further effects on the freedom to explore the social and nonsocial environment.

Due to the foundational nature of the attachment system, and as alluded to above, we need to consider what happens when the infant attaches to a neglectful, abusive, or perhaps dismissing parent. When there is little comfort offered to the infant and child, other biologically based relational and nonrelational systems may be recruited for fear-reducing functions (e.g., aggression, with-drawal, sexual behavior, substance use). A supposition is that this appears as dis-organized attachment when observed in the Strange Situation.

At this level of analysis, and also from an evolutionary perspective, it is evi-dent that our body plans, nervous systems, behavioral repertoires, and mental states are constrained. Darwin's principle of natural selection posits (a) the exis-tence of variation among individuals, (b) differential reproductive success for those individuals who exhibit traits that are useful in "the struggle for life," and (c) differential inheritance of those factors that gave rise to the favorable traits. Thus, our species has more or less species-typical potentialities, including such behaviors (and associated mental states) as purposive reaching and holding, lo-comotion, grooming, feeding, communication (gestures, species-specific vo-calizations, and language), and alarm systems activated by perceived threats (e.g., separation from an attachment object, courtship and pair bonding, and re-productive and parental behaviors).

These patterns of behavior, often associated with attachment, are persistent in human populations. Indeed they are evidently adaptive when attachment to a secure base is achieved. On the other hand, if early attachment goes awry, then these same built-in species-specific behaviors and mental states, which are es-sential for survival and reproductive success, may be disorganized in their ex-pression and finally associated with maladaptive or psychopathological states. Thus, the very characteristics that are fundamental to the development of attach-ment, bonding, social function, and well-being are also also the substrates of vulnerability to maladaptive states if attachment fails, or the infant attaches to an abusive or neglectful caregiver (Leckman and Mayes 1998).

Human Motives: The Psychobiology of Meaning

A more expansive view of attachment has been forwarded by Trevarthen (this volume). In distinction to the ECST and psychobiology viewpoints, this ap-proach focuses on the aspects of brain function and mind that most would con-sider distinctly human (i.e., not likely to be found in animals with the possible exception of the higher primates). This view also addresses issues surrounding attachment — language, consciousness, emotion, and motives (not motivations) — that are not part of either ECST or psychobiological theory. Hence, in draw-ing lines between the topics of "attachment" and "adaptation and maladap-tation," this view is difficult to fit in with the others. Just as there was no neurophysiology in ECST, there is no appeal to consciousness, self-awareness, and emotion (with the exception of fear) in psychobiology. Clearly a step for-ward needs to be taken.

Meaning-making requires both fellow feeling and cooperation. *Joint atten-tion* alone does not explain how it arises (Tomasello 1988; Trevarthen and Hubley 1978). People exchange memories, plans of events, and sympathetic emotional states, not just executive and cognitive engagements with objects and "facts" in a shared world (Damasio 1999; Donald 2001). Knowing one another's ideas requires *mutual attention* to internal interests and value states (self-other awareness) (Reddy 2001, 2003), and this governs moral relationships in consciously acknowledged friendships (Trevarthen 2001a). Intersubjectivity guides the development of meaning (Bruner 1990). Processes of "intent participation" and "self esteem" in "narratives of collaborative awareness" are an inextricable part of the culture of education, whatever its form (Rogoff 2003).

Human minds are born to share action and experience by sympathetic mimicry, taking initiative in reciprocal engagement. Stern (1999, 2000) describes the matching of expression between a mother and her infant as "attunement" by "vitality contours," terms which convey the essential "communicative musicality" of this signaling through modulations of the intensity of movement (Malloch 1999). Some infant expressions are adapted to elicit parental care for internal physiological homeostasis. Others (smiling, gaze approach/avoidance, vocalizations, certain hand gestures) transmit "relational" affects (Stern 2000), regulate intersubjective contact, and create narratives of relationship. A two-month-old's behaviors demonstrate "primary intersubjectivity" (Trevarthen 1979).

Perturbation tests, the "still- or blank-face test" (Murray and Trevarthen 1985; Tronick et al. 1978) and the "video interaction replay experiment" (Murray and Trevarthen 1985; Nadel et al. 1999) demonstrate how failure of intimate and responsive caregiver support is potentially harmful (Tronick et al. 1978). The first three months is a period of high susceptibility for lasting effects of maternal postnatal depression, especially in boys (Murray et al. 1993; Trevarthen and Aitken 2001), and this may limit a child's grasp of meaning (Murray et al. 1999). However, shared pride and shame in demonstrations of knowledge and skill depend on others' appreciation and are important at all ages.

A child comes to use words in relationships. Words gain "meaning" through their expression in collaborative action, in sharing interests, goals, purposes, and feelings. A rapid "explosion" of vocabulary begins about 20–30 months after birth, when the child has a new eagerness to share items and narratives of experience (Tomasello 1988). There are large individual differences in word knowledge, as there are in temperament, at this "difficult" transitional age (Locke 1993). A "theory of mind" may be articulated in a four-year-old's talk about other persons' mental states (Astington and Jenkins 1999), but there are individual, subcultural, and cultural differences in talk about mind states and emotions (Taylor and Carlson 1997).

Human peer play is imaginative, creating invented worlds and narratives of adventure that range far beyond present circumstances (Harris 1998). Child games and pedagogy show an "executive suite" of "domain general skill clusters" (including metacognition, "self reminding," "autocuing," or self-triggering of memory, "whole body imitation," "symbolic invention," "complex skill hierarchies") that are absent or poorly developed in apes (Donald 2001).

Cultural learning sets human beings apart. All historically contrived communities of meaning and belief, including languages, depend on motives and passions of companionship different from those involved in primary regulation of a
child's attachments (Trevarthen, this volume). Thus, a mother's play with her infant is a "cradle of thought" (Hobson 2002) as well as a nurturant external regulator of need or stress. Importantly, her role as playmate and companion in
meaning can be taken over by any other sympathetic person, even a child, whom
the baby has learned to trust. A six-month-old can negotiate interests, intentions,
and feelings with two same age peers, with no adult help (Selby and Bradley
2003). Infants are ready for "allo-companionship" in a community. These facts
of human motivation, self–other awareness, and the emotions for meaning in relationships have crucial implications for understanding socio-emotional adaptations of children, and the appropriate clinical or educational response to
pathologies or maladaptations in a child's behavior (Trevarthen 2001a). They
explain why therapies that foster the development of trusting communication in
any form may bring beneficial change.

The Neurobiology of Cultural Learning

Psychological evidence from infancy implies that the neural arrays for
self-maintenance and self-coordination and those for perceiving objects have
evolved with a third system, which regulates self–other intercoordination and
"alteroception" (Trevarthen 2001a, b). More than in any other species, human
brain and behavior development make no sense if the individual is considered in
isolation, or if the impress of stimulation on "plastic" neural circuitry is taken as
the principle process driving development. We intuitively get into other people's minds by actively sensing the motives in their brains that make them move
the way they do (Trevarthen 2001a, b). The brain activity adapted for language
is present in protoconversation with an infant, long before the lexicon and a
frame of rules and conventions for cognition and reasoning have been learned
(Trevarthen and Aitken 2003; Tzourio-Mazoyer et al. 2002).

Developments in the mesolimbic cortices of the temporal and frontal lobes
and orbito–frontal–hypothalamic connections in infants and toddlers transform
autonomic self-regulation, emotions in communication, and the "affective core"
that evaluates attachment, action, and experience (Freeman 1999; Schore 1994).
Later, maturing limbic and neocortical circuits emerge in reciprocal involvement with the multimodal regulatory systems of the brainstem Intrinsic Motive
Formation (IMF) (Trevarthen and Aitken 1994).

Human visceral sensory and motor functions are unique both in their neural
foundations in brainstem nuclei with anatomical relations to the cerebral cortex
and in their peripheral sensory and motor organs (Porges 1997). Bioaminergic
neurons of the reticular formation innervate the growing brain from embryo
stages (Holstege et al. 1996). These regulate cortical morphogenesis, then the

global state of brain functions, initiating purposeful movement and focusing awareness, and are themselves regulated by caregiver–infant interaction (Trevarthen and Aitken 1994). They offer the means for recovery from dysregulation of the self (Schore 2003 a, b). In infancy, the right brain and frontal lobes play a major role in communication of emotions and regulation of the relationship to a parent (Schore 1994). Consolidating a "working model" of mutual regulation of emotions with others, in both protective "attachment" and adventurous "companionship," motivates the child's growing brain to collaborate a response to the environment (Trevarthen and Aitken 2003).

The power of a child's brain to find regulation from sensitive communication with other persons gives a lifetime opportunity for assisting those in whom feelings and thoughts have become dysregulated by inherited or acquired damage to their motives for attachment and companionship.

Proposals regarding Meaning-making and the Fear System

Because of the elaborate meaning-making capacities of the human infant in communication with others, the infant's fear system is likely to involve:

- A hierarchy of attachment figures based on which figure best knows the infant and can communicate most sensitively around that particular infant's various experiences of threat to novelty and other stressors.
- Regulation of the HPA axis in the infant by co-created emergent interactive patterns between infant and caregiver, which continue to evolve over development. These co-created patterns are a means by which the infant has a sense of predictable influence on the caregiver's behavior through shared patterns of communication.
- Because of the primacy of communication in the regulation of fear in human development, maternal separation is not an inclusive-enough paradigm for understanding the development and regulation of the infant attachment system.
- The ongoing regulation of fear-related behavior within a hierarchy of attachment relationships over time (hierarchy based on close reading of the infant's fear-related communications, not biological relatedness) needs to be understood.

For further discussion, see Hennighausen and Lyons-Ruth (this volume).

ISSUES OF CONTINUITY AND CHANGE, INCLUDING PSYCHOPATHOLOGY

Stability of Early Attachment Classification

The quality of attachment, as reflected in the traditional classification system, appears moderately stable in some samples (Vondra et al. 2001) and unstable in others (Belsky et al. 1996), even during early childhood. Of the samples studied, some of that stability can be attributed to stable living conditions; those which included more change exhibited lower stability estimates.

After infancy, stability estimates range from no significant relationship (Bar Haim et al. 2000) to impressive stability (Grossmann and Grossmann 1991). One methodological issue here is the change of measurement instruments, which have to be age appropriate. Thus, we have to compare behaviors directly aimed at maintaining proximity in the presence of a stranger to coherence in a discourse about relationships with parents many years ago. In between are other instruments, including projective tests. Diverse instrumentation increases the probability of underestimating true continuity. In meta-analyses, a moderate degree of stability is found at least into adolescence. Several authors have pointed to the importance of explaining continuity and discontinuity rather than just rejecting or confirming the stability hypothesis (e.g., Bar Haim et al. 2000).

Beyond the early continuity in the phenomenon, there have been numerous efforts to determine whether continuity in attachment covaries with developmental outcomes in other domains. For example, it has been reported that, on the whole, securely attached children appear to be more advanced in achievement motivation (Matas et al. 1978) and social competence (Suess et al. 1992; Easterbrooks and Goldberg 1990). In at least one at-risk-sample, lower rates of psychopathology and problem behavior were reported (Sroufe 1983). Securely attached children were also shown to have more advanced theory of mind abilities (Meins 1997). This latter relationship may be spurious since the mothers of secure infants in Meins's study also included more mental references in their communication with their infants during the first year, which could account for the difference in a more direct way. Additionally, language differences were reported in favor of securely attached children (van IJzendoorn et al. 1995). Stability of psychological features may in itself be a trait-like phenomenon (e.g., some children may reorganize more easily than others and thus display less continuity over time).

For all of these reasons, the expectation of predictability of general psychopathology or specific disorders on the basis of the quality of the attachment relationship within the A, B, and C classifications appears to be unrealistic. Indeed, Belsky (this volume) concludes that attachment security exhibits modest but significant stability from infancy to adulthood. There are reasons to expect, however, that attachments will be stable over time for some, but not all, individuals. Several studies indicate that a high proportion of children are consistent in remaining secure or insecure for many years whereas others show that infants and young children change dramatically in the security of attachment over a matter of months (e.g., Thompson 2000, 2006). Under what conditions is attachment security likely to remain stable or change?

Evidence suggests two provisional conclusions (Thompson 2006). First, children with secure attachments and those with the disorganized classification are more likely to remain consistent in their attachment status over time than are children with the two insecure classifications (avoidant and resistant). This is likely to be true for different reasons: secure relationships are stable because they are mutually rewarding; disorganized relationships are stable because their atypical nature becomes self-perpetuating in the responses children and their caregivers elicit and provoke. Second, children and parents living in more stable circumstances are likely to enjoy more stable relationships, whereas those who experience disruptive family events are more likely to change because of the impact of those events on their relationship. It remains for researchers to identify clearly the kinds of events that are likely to provoke change in attachment security over time, and in which individuals (Thompson 2000, 2006; Thompson, pers. comm.).

Differential Susceptibility to Rearing Experience

Evidence is increasingly emerging that infants who display higher levels of negative emotionality during their first 18 or so months of life (or even later) may be more strongly affected by rearing experiences than other children. Consistent with this observation is evidence which van IJzendoorn left out of his attachment intervention meta-analysis, because the effect on sensitivity and attachment was so great that the study was considered an anomaly (Bakermans-Kranenburg et al. 2003; van IJzendoorn et al. 1995). Of notable interest is the intervention study by van den Boom (1994), which explicitly targeted mother–infant dyads in which infants were twice measured during the neonatal period and found to have very high levels of negativity.

This is not the only experimental study which suggests that highly negative infants may be more susceptible to rearing experience. Blair (2002) recently reanalyzed data from the multisite "Infant Health and Development Project," a home- and center-based early intervention project for premature infants. Although effects were found for the experimental treatment compared to a randomly assigned control condition, Blair observed, with respect to both cognitive and problem-behavior outcomes, that infants who scored higher on negative emotionality were disproportionately likely to benefit from the intervention. These data are also in accord with monkey data (Suomi and Ripp 1983), which shows that good and bad rearing had disproportionate (positive and negative, respectively) effects on the "up-tight" and thus highly anxious and negatively prone infants than the "laid back" ones.

Beyond the Mother–Infant and Family Relationship

Although family experiences are likely to be most influential, events outside the family might also affect the security of parent–child attachments if they impose stress on either or both partners. Conversely, extra-familial sources of social support might buffer difficulties in the parent–child relationships and can thus provide avenues to the development of greater security. The alternatives are that the parent–child/family interaction promotes child adaptation and the expression of developmental capacity; the interaction allows the child to develop; or the interaction interferes with "what could have been" for the child.

One concept views the mother–infant relationship as needing to be "just good enough"; that is, there is a minimum standard where the child is adequately cared for in the attachment and bonding relationship. Beyond that, it is up to the offspring (Winnicott 1965a, b).

Another takes the mother–infant relationship as deflecting the long-term abilities of the child to behave in one way or another. That this is true is established at this point, but the eventual "impact" or societal value deserves some consideration. One must ask why the maternal care patterns of being "withdrawn," "dismissive," or "coercive" — each carries a negative connotation and is thought to be related to a form of insecure attachment style, or to the "disorganized" classification — continue to exist. More specifically, how can maternal care styles propagate down through generations if the offspring, which is a product of that style, is maladapted and perhaps less fit as a result of it?

One answer is that insecure or even (more controversially) disorganized attachment patterns in early life are associated with adult behavioral styles that are "adaptive" and successful in some contexts. Thus, if a particular maternal rearing style (e.g., coercive) is associated with offspring that are unduly impulsive, aggressive, or unable to maintain sustained attention, then this may be maladaptive in a sedate classroom. In a "street" or "juvenile gang" environment, however, such attributes will be highly adaptive, even though the group itself may be maladaptive when viewed from a larger social context.

Indeed, among our nomadic foraging ancestors living in the Pleistocene, infants whose mothers were less than fully committed, detached, avoidant, or neglectful were unlikely to survive, yet presumably some did. Almost by definition, these would be youngsters born to mothers without a lot of kin support, a lack of which would be reflected in the child's IWM of relationships (Hrdy 1999). The most adaptive developmental trajectory for such a child (requiring considerable phenotypic flexibility) might be quite different than for an infant securely attached to a responsive and committed mother surrounded by kin and supportive group members (Belsky et al. 1991; Chisholm 1999). Although empathetic feelings for others along with a willingness to share and cooperate are normative in most foraging societies, and would be highly adaptive traits for children surrounded by supportive kin, this might not be the case for such a "wretch"(i.e., a lonely, exiled person, lacking kin). No one would likely share with such a person nor help in an emergency, or even in such ordinary life tasks as finding a mate (Sarah Hrdy, pers. comm.).

In some cases, the mother withdraws and does not provide for the infant's wants. The infant responds by becoming more assertive and demanding, and "takes over" dominance in the relationship. This situation normally would be defined as maladaptive. By focusing solely on the mother–child interaction, one can lose sight of other people who are in the larger social field in which the dyad is embedded. For example, a mother may persist in a withdrawal mode because she is aware that there are other available caretakers. Her "strategy," not necessarily consciously expressed, would thus draw out solicitous behavior from some other caretaker whom she deems to be eligible. When data on such disorganized attachments are collected, one could also collect information on such things as the number and kind of other people in the household. Note, however, that a mother must cooperate in letting a child take over the relationship. She could assert herself even in a negative way and abuse or kill the child, but by remaining in the attachment dyad she leaves open the relationship while signaling to others that her performance is inadequate.

Attachments to Peers

One contention, present in the literature, is that distinctions in early attachment of the A, B, and C groups are relatively insignificant when one considers the social environmental influences exerted by peers (Harris 2000a, b; Plomin 1989). At base, about 50% of the variation in personality differences or traits (e.g., extraversion vs. introversion, risk-taking vs. conservative, inhibited vs. uninhibited) can be accounted for by genetic factors. Although the rest of the variation is presumably due to environmental factors, variation in early attachment to parents accounts for very little of it. If securely attached children have attentive, compassionate, and understanding parents, and insecurely attached or disorganized attached children have parents who are neglectful yet demanding, aggressive, dismissive, and so on, genetic loading has to be considered (Scarr and McCartney 1993). Harris (2000a) proposes that socialization is context specific and that outside-the-home socialization takes place in the peer groups of childhood and adolescence. Intra- and inter-group processes, not dyadic relationships, are responsible for the transmission of culture and for environmental modification of children's personality characteristics. Presently, however, there is not enough empirical data to support or reject this hypothesis.

Attachment to Adults Other than Parents

Bowlby was explicit in relating early separation and deprivation to the risk for and vulnerability to social stressors later in life, as well as to inadequacy in the rearing of subsequent offspring, i.e., transgenerational effects (Bowlby 1982, p. 37). The risk was expressed in the form of conflicting working models that ultimately leave the mature individual unable to manage disruptions of the social environment cognitively. Indeed, Bowlby asserted that having multiple caretakers early in development was a risk factor for later problems. This was because the child would have multiple and potentially conflicting IWMs of the "caretaker role." This construct also tells us that children reared in poor social environments are not likely to do well later in life because the cognitive foundations of how they understand social affiliation and confront social and affective problems is jumbled and dysfunctional.

It seems, however, that some children grow up in terrible environments and do well later, while others grow up in optimal environments and do not fare well. These exceptions to the social developmental "rules" have often suggested that some organismic and possibly genetic characteristic of the individual must be responsible for the exhibition of psychopathology in "good" environments and for exhibition of health and well-being in "bad" environments.

A proportion of social-developmental exceptions can be accounted for by the child's social environment outside of the caretaker–infant dyad. Werner's (1989a, b) report of a longitudinal study conducted on Kauai illustrates this point. Of 698 infants born in 1955, 30% ($n = 201$) were identified as being "at risk" for mental illness or criminal delinquency on the basis of factors that included perinatal stress, chronic poverty, low socio-economic status and education of parents, parental discord, divorce, alcoholism, or parental mental illness. Of this population, 64% ($n = 129$) conformed to expectations and had mental health or delinquency records by age 18. The remainder, 36% (n = 72), "grew into competent young adults who loved well, worked well, and played well" (Werner 1989a, p. 109).

Among the "survivors," Werner asserts that constitutional factors (including a fairly high activity level, low degree of excitability and distress, and a high degree of sociability) combined with "the opportunity to establish a close bond with at least one caretaker from whom they received positive attention during the first years of life" (Werner 1989a, p. 109) were major protective factors that distinguished these children from those who did not do well. In addition, as survivors developed, they demonstrated an adequate ability to concentrate, they had average or above problem-solving and reading skills, and seemed to find a great deal of emotional support outside of their immediate family. This analysis does not rule out genetic resilience among the survivors. Indeed, the factors having to do with excitability, concentration, problem-solving, and reading skills begs the question. Werner's analysis does indicate, however, that such resilience is expressed in relation to the development of social attachment and not some vague organismic resource that manifests itself in any environment.

At this stage we are left with the conclusion that attachments change for some children and remain consistent for others (Thompson 2000). Developmental formulations that assume long-term influences from early attachment relationships must accommodate the fact that attachment relationships themselves often change over time, and thus the consequences of early attachment may also be malleable (see, e.g., the evolutionary formulation by Belsky et al. 1991). Moreover, such a conclusion underscores the dynamic nature of parent–child–sibling–peer relations, which is consistent with the cascade of developmental changes occurring in the child, the changing parent, and family ecology, which constitutes the child's home, and social surround.

Attachment and Performance in Diverse Domains of Human Endeavor

Attachment theory predicts that early secure parent–child relationships will yield beneficial consequences later in life and that early insecure attachment sends children on developmental pathways that are likely to be less successful. Attachment researchers have explored the relations between attachment security and a wide variety of expected outcomes in consequent or contemporaneous relations to the security of attachment. Predicted outcomes have included teacher–child relationships, cognitive and language development, frustration tolerance, self-recognition, behavior problems, relations with peers, friends, and siblings, interactions with unfamiliar adults, exploration and play, competence in preschool and kindergarten, curiosity, psychopathology, ego resiliency, and math achievement (Thompson, pers. comm.).

Researchers in this field disagree over the scope of the theoretically predicted sequels of attachment security. Attachment theory is not especially clear about the range of social consequences that could reasonably be anticipated from early security. Greater theoretical clarity is thus needed to inform hypotheses and the design and interpretation of findings. How can the claims of attachment theory be properly evaluated if researchers are unclear about its central hypotheses concerning the consequences of early attachment? Nevertheless, sifting through a large body of empirical literature that examine the contemporaneous and predictive correlates of attachment security in infancy and early childhood yields several conclusions (Thompson 1999, 2006).

Secure attachment seems to be associated with greater competence and success in close relationships. Most notably, a harmonious parent–child relationship heightens the child's receptiveness to the parent's socialization incentives and fosters mutual cooperation and responsiveness (Waters et al. 1991). Securely attached children are more successful in other close relationships, such as with friends, teachers, and counselors. It is unclear whether this is due to social skills, social expectations (such as IWMs of relationships), maternal support, or other reasons. There is also evidence that securely attached young children have different ways of thinking about the social world. This is reflected in a more acute understanding of emotions, more positive friendship conceptions, and advances in conscience development. These conclusions can be challenged in relation to probable confounds.

There is little systematic evidence that attachment security is associated with personality characteristics, such as ego resiliency, or with behavioral problems and other potential precursors of clinical difficulties (although research indicates that the disorganized classification may be a risk factor for later clinical problems). Attachment security is not strongly associated with a child's interactions with unfamiliar partners.

Overall, the strongest evidence for the broader influences of a secure or insecure attachment arises from contemporaneous assessments of attachment and other behaviors. The studies do not permit, however, unequivocal causal conclusions. In predictive studies, short-term associations between attachment and outcomes are stronger than longer-term predictive associations. At best, the strength of the relation between attachment security and its psychological correlates is modest. There are many reasons for this (Thompson 1999). The sequels with which attachment security is associated are themselves multi-determined and are likely to be affected by a variety of influences in addition to the parent–child relationship. Moreover, children typically experience multiple attachment relationships that may have complementary or conflicting influences on aspects of the child's later psychological growth. Parent–child relationships also change over time, as noted earlier, such that later relational experience at home may confirm the influences of early attachment security, or may alter earlier developmental influences. Taken together, the security of attachment has an important but modest influence on children's subsequent relational experience, but its broader effects have yet to be systematically established.

A model compatible with this pattern of stability and change is one where experience shapes and adjusts the underlying physiological system in a process over time. The resulting reactivity and regulatory capacities of that particular individual are then the basis for the transformation of new experiences into meaning. Relevant aspects of the physiological system include autonomic reactivity, hormones, and neurotransmitters. The mutual adjustment of the physiological system and the behavioral organization continue over the lifespan; however, animal models and human data suggest that early experiences (extending up to pre-adolescence) may be of relatively greater importance than later experiences.

By contrast, the dimension of disorganization, as is observable in Strange Situation tests, seems to index an increased risk of psychopathology. Stronger concordance, however, exists in the presence of stable risk factors, which in themselves may be predictive of psychopathological disorders.

PSYCHOBIOLOGICAL ATTACHMENT AND PSYCHOPATHOLOGY

Psychobiological attachment theory differs from Bowlby's theory by suggesting that variation in social development is synonymous with variation in biological development. The phenotype of the optimum social genome usually conforms to the social environment in which it develops. As individuals deviate from this optimum they will be more or less "in tune," matched or mismatched, stressed, survivable, and challenged or accepted in some social environments but not in others. Substantial neurobiological differences in human populations are likely to be attributable as much to variations in social development as they are to genetic variation.

Consistent with Hofer's concept of hidden regulators, the primary caregiving relationship appears to have multiple biological effects on the infant, and multiple biological systems may contribute to the infant's seeking of the caregiver. From an evolutionary perspective, why is the infant so dependent on the mother for regulation? Much of what we claim to know at this level is derived from research on animals, as were Hofer's seminal contributions.

One characteristic feature of many vertebrate species is that individual members of the species are able to adapt behaviorally and physiologically to different environments and/or changing conditions within a given environment. Plasticity in behavioral mechanisms is clearly exhibited in mammalian mother–young interactions; however, it is also exhibited across species and in a number of developmental contexts (e.g., song learning, food caching, food preference development, imprinting, and mate selection. This suggests that the mechanisms of neurobiological plasticity, which must underpin behavioral plasticity, have deep evolutionary roots.

What might be the adaptive and hence selective value of plasticity and dependence on learning, rather than "hard-wiring" of innate behavioral control mechanisms for mother–infant recognition, attachment, and caregiving? Plasticity permits a certain latitude or flexibility in the relevant features that enable offspring to identify the mother and for the mother to identify her offspring. On one hand, olfactory cues and other characteristics of the mother may vary depending on her sources of food and dietary regimen. These resources vary geographically, and over time, and are thus not likely to be the same for all offspring. Hence, the offspring's expression of attachment behaviors cannot be locked into a predetermined, invariant set of salient maternal characteristics, or preset to narrowly defined environmental conditions.

From the maternal viewpoint, a mother must be able to tolerate differences in offspring, which may occur over successive births. Variation in maternal diet and environmental effects on maternal pre-parturitional physiology may affect infant odors, body size and conformation, and neonatal behavior. Successive offspring may differ in paternal genotype as well as phenotype. If the expression of maternal behaviors were narrowly locked into invariant neonatal characteristics, then the diversity of offspring nurtured and thus surviving would also be narrow. Thus, plasticity in mammalian mother–infant behavior allows for offspring to be nurtured in widely varying environments and circumstances, and provides for preservation of genetic/behavioral diversity in those offspring. In addition, by using conditioning mechanisms, a complex multimodal stimulus (e.g., of an infant with a characteristic odor, cry, or visual appearance) comes to be easily located and identified based on any one of these cues. This is important when not all cues are present (e.g., when the infant is concealed within a nest or strays away from the nest or mother).

Finally, plasticity in the maternal brain increases reproductive fitness by allowing experience with one infant to modify care of subsequent offspring in the changing environment in which the mother lives. Among many primate species, mothers of first infants are considerably less competent and motivated than are mothers of subsequent offspring. The experiences of the multiparous female are not limited to interactions with offspring. They include somatic and physiological experiences associated with pregnancy and parturition, as well as exposure to infants, peers, and the larger environment and society. This effect of parity and the associated experiences usually insures that young of experienced (multiparous) mothers have an advantage over the firstborns of primiparous mothers. They are more likely to be cared for during adversity, and they receive more abundant nutrition, attention, and social stimulation provided by an older, more mature, less timid, and better-socialized mother.

The mother and her young usually constitute for one another the earliest and most pervasive stimulus set present in the postpartum environment. To the degree that the nervous system of the infant is dependent on an extended series of interactions with a mother for its development, deprivation of those interactions might have proportional adverse effects. Plastic brain mechanisms take time to adapt, and their development can be adversely affected if they are not exposed to the expected or common set of species-specific experiences.

Maladaptation in Relation to Gene and Environment Interaction

Mother–infant attachment is the major intersection between what the infant brings to the world and the society it is about to enter. Gene–environment interactions are most likely subject to selection. Biological "code" exists to insure variability in the production of different outcomes in diverse environments. Perhaps this needs to be emphasized. Genes are not selected independently of how what they interact with a cellular, organismic, and environmental surround. Genetic endowment varies across individuals. Variability in the control of genetic expression is built-in and is known to be responsive to a number of different factors: pre- and postnatal exposure to chemicals, hormones, changes in temperature, nutritional quantity and quality, con-specific social environmental conditions (including the behavior of peers). However, just because an individual carries a particular aspect of genetic code does not mean that it will be expressed.

The expression of the genetic code in the infant and child clearly impacts the interaction with the mother and others. Genes do not determine behavior, rather the resources that an environment affords, life experiences, as well as past and ongoing behavior determine how the available genes are expressed in an individual. What is expressed constitutes the capabilities of the organism. One suggestion is that individual variances in the genetic code are set to produce different outcomes depending on what environmental factors have an impact on the individual at various stages of development. Ultimately expression of the "code" translates to differences in the expression of brain neurotransmitter mechanisms, synthetic mechanisms, and so on. How the code is expressed, and in response to what, is the key (Keverne, this volume). By implication, expression of a particular "genetic package" might be quite adaptive in one environment, but not in another (or in the same environment, in one individual with a particular role, function, and status, but not another with different obligations and relationships).

One example of the interaction between the genetic code and the environment is the different physiological and behavioral consequences of the early rearing environment on subsequent stress and drug abuse. Changes in central serotonin (5-hydroxytryptamine, 5-HT) neurotransmitter system function have been linked to several forms of psychopathology in humans, especially depression (Tamminga et al. 2002). Synaptic transmission of signals in the 5-HT system depends both on neuronal release of 5-HT and reuptake of the released 5-HT into the presynaptic terminal. Reuptake of 5-HT is mediated by the serotonin transporter (5-HTT). This is a presynaptic membrane-bound protein ultimately produced by the transcription of code in a specific 5-HTT gene. The gene itself comes in two versions, long and short (i.e., the gene is polymorphic). These genes differ only in the length of the promoter region preceding the code for the amino acid sequence of the transporter protein. One effect of long versus short promoter regions is variation in the efficiency with which the gene can be transcribed into RNA and then into protein. Individuals can be homozygous, i.e., have two short (S/S) or long alleles (L/L), or heterozygous, i.e., have a short and a long allele (S/L).

In rhesus macaques separated from their mothers and reared in peer groups, distribution of 5-HTT polymorphism interacts with early experience to affect the long-term impact of the early experience on brain neurochemistry (Bennett et al. 2002). These genetic interaction effects are not observed at the same magnitude in mother-reared monkeys. For example, overall brain 5-HT system activity can be assessed by measuring the concentration of the major metabolite of 5-HT, 5-hydroxyindoleacetic acid (5-HIAA), in cerebrospinal fluid (CSF). Monkeys with peer-only early rearing experiences, bearing at least one copy of the short allele (S/S or S/L), have lower levels of CSF 5-HIAA when compared to (a) peer-only reared monkeys that are homozygous for the long allele (L/L) and (b) mother-reared monkeys, regardless of genotype (Bennett et al. 2002). Moreover, in rhesus macaques separated from their mothers and reared in peer-only groups but not in mother-reared animals, 5-HTT polymorphism distribution predicted adult alcohol consumption (Barr et al. 2003). Hence, behavioral outcome (alcohol intake) of subjects with the short variant (S/L and S/S) depends on the rearing environment (mother/peer). One could imagine that this effect is perhaps adaptive from an evolutionary perspective for a species, but pathological for an individual.

Thus, there can be a gene–environment interaction such that the genetic endowment leaves an individual more, or less, affected by environmental contingencies, if such occur, than if there was no endowment. The report by Bennett et al. (2002) illustrates the point: Monkeys bearing one version of the serotonin transporter gene are likely to be significantly affected by maternal deprivation and peer-only rearing. Monkeys not having that version of the gene are less affected. Among the monkeys that are maternally reared, the gene polymorphism has little bearing on their development. The "gene" effect surfaces most predominantly under certain environmental circumstances and adversity, and perhaps not otherwise.

Findings such as these may help to explain why stressful experiences lead to depression in some humans and not in others. If genes are not transmitted in a dominant way, a particularly high-risk genotype might only be phenotypically expressed every other or third generation and therefore would be conserved. Recently it has been reported that individuals with one or two copies of the short allele of the 5-HTT promoter polymorphism (S/L or S/S) exhibited more depressive symptoms, diagnosable depression, and suicidality in relation to stressful life events than individuals homozygous for the long allele (Caspi et al. 2003). This provides a clinically relevant example of how an individual's response to the environment might be influenced by their genetic code. Hence, adaptive or maladaptive individual development depends in part on the interaction between the experiences and the genetic makeup of the individual. The next section introduces another distinction.

Attachment and Infant Biological Systems

There is an extensive literature on the mechanisms regulating maternal recognition and care of offspring among animals. Less is known about the neurobiological basis of infant recognition of and attachment to the mother in animals, and comparatively little is known about the neurobiology of attachment mechanisms in human mothers or infants through direct study.

Much of what are inferred to be active biological systems in human or animal infant attachment are derived from studies of what goes wrong if the infant's attachment to a caregiver is disrupted. By reasoning backwards, we find biological differences between individuals with secure attachment and those in which attachment has been disrupted; we infer that the differences between the two result from or reside in changes in neurobiological "attachment mechanisms." This approach contains multiple pitfalls, not the least of which is that animals separated from their mothers grow up in quite different environments than those that have mothers. Hence, environmental demands and opportunities are quite different. Nevertheless, some biological influences that we have evidence for in other species can be cited.

Long-term Broad Spectrum Effects of Maternal Deprivation and/or Social Isolation in Rhesus Monkeys

In rhesus monkeys, a brief list of reported effects of being reared in a nursery (as opposed to by a rhesus mother) includes altered temperature regulation, immune system function, body weight regulation, eating patterns (polydipsia and hyperphagia); exhibition of self-injurious behavior, motor stereotypies, hyper- or hypo-emotionality and aggressiveness; failure to be able to use facial expression as a discriminative stimulus in learning tasks, failure to inhibit well learned responses, "unusual" performance on cognitive learning tasks (better at some, worse at others, impulsivity and attention seem to be factors) (Kraemer and Bachevalier 1998); and disrupted sexual and maternal behavior (Kraemer 1992b; Lubach et al. 1995; Lubach et al. 1992). In sum, maternal privation affects almost every aspect of what it means to be a social monkey. If the monkeys also do not have peers to interact with and duration of social privation extends over the first six to nine months of postnatal life, the majority of effects listed above persist into adulthood (Harlow et al. 1971; Kraemer 1992a; Suomi and Ripp 1983). These effects are also associated with altered responsiveness to pharmacological agents (primarily drugs of abuse such as alcohol, amphetamine, and cocaine (Kraemer et al. 1984; Kraemer and McKinney 1985).

Sympathetic Nervous System

The emergence of concordance between patients and therapists in galvanic skin response and heart rate (using time-series analysis) is correlated with rated empathy of the therapist for the patient. This suggests that there may be an entrainment of physiology in a sensitive and responsive relationship. This is one potential mechanism in which the infant and the mother mutually regulate each other, but it has yet to be examined in parent–infant dyads (Marci and Orr 2003).

Neurohormonal Influences

Regulation of HPA axis responses, cortisol, and corticotropin-releasing hormone (CRH), in relation to attachment formation and disrupted attachment, are considered by Fleming and Gunnar (both this volume). One unifying finding cited here is that early separation/isolation from the mother appears to produce a blunted HPA axis response to stressors. In rhesus monkeys this occurs even though the behavioral response (distress, agitation) may be exaggerated (Clarke 1993; Clarke et al. 1994). Other effects on HPA axis function are cited below in relation to neurotransmitter systems.

Neurotransmitter Function

A number of psychobiological studies in rhesus monkeys have focused on the development of the brain biogenic amine neurotransmitter systems and the HPA axis. "Biogenic amine systems" in this context refers collectively to the brain norepinephrine (NE), dopamine (DA), and 5-HT systems. These neurotransmitter and neuroendocrine systems are thought to play a role in brain mechanisms regulating reward (NE, DA), information gating and impulse control (5-HT), as well as response and adaptation to stress (HPA axis) (Kraemer 1992a). It has also been suggested that malfunction of the NE, DA, and 5-HT systems may be causal factors in some human psychiatric disorders. Thus, affective disorders may be caused by aberrations in NE and/or 5-HT system function, schizophrenia by aberrations in DA system function, and impulsive violence and suicide may be related to aberrations in 5-HT system function (see Higley et al. 1991, 1992; Kraemer 1992a, b; Kraemer et al. 1989). The development of these systems is affected by social rearing conditions, attachment, and mothering.

Peer-reared monkeys have been found to differ from mother-reared monkeys in measures of levels of activity in all of the above-mentioned neurochemical- and neuroendocrine-dependent measures (Kraemer 1997). A unifying theme across the studies is that peer-reared monkeys are biologically different from mother-reared monkeys; magnitude and even direction of difference in dependent measures may vary over development and in relation to prior or ongoing environmental circumstances (Higley et al. 1991, 1992; Kraemer 1997). For example, juvenile peer-reared monkeys housed in stable social groups generally maintain lower baseline levels of cerebrospinal fluid (CSF), NE, and the DA metabolite homovanillic acid (HVA) by comparison to juvenile mother-reared monkeys housed in stable social groups (Kraemer and Clarke 1996). When challenged, however, the behavioral response of peer-reared monkeys to social stressors or drugs that activate NE and DA neurotransmitter systems is exaggerated and inordinate by comparison to mother-reared monkeys.

Juvenile peer-reared monkeys housed in stable social groups also maintain lower baseline levels of adrenocorticotropic hormone (ACTH) and cortisol than mother-reared monkeys, but have a blunted HPA axis response (little increase in ACTH and/or cortisol) to psychosocial stressors, such as separation from cage mates (Clarke 1993). Thus, the exaggerated behavioral response to stressors in peer-reared monkeys, perhaps mediated in part by hypersensitive brain NE and/or DA systems, is not paralleled by comparably enhanced or even normal neuroendocrine responses. Overall, altered responsiveness is the feature of peer-reared monkeys that characterizes them across ages and environments.

Disorganized Attachment and Neurotransmitter System Relationships

It appears that the development and actions of the brain 5-HT, NE, and DA systems are usually interrelated. Part of the evidence for this is that the levels of these biogenic amines and/or their metabolites in CSF are usually correlated (Higley et al. 1992; Kraemer et al. 1989). Mother-reared offspring tracked from birth to pre-adolescence exhibit significant and substantial intercorrelations among NE, 5HIAA, and HVA beginning within two months after birth (Kraemer et al. 1989). Thus, 5HIAA levels usually covary with measures of other biogenic amine systems. Also, measures of NE and/or DA system activity covary with exhibition of social behavior, social development, and the exhibition of behavioral responses to stressors, such as separation from companions (Kraemer et al. 1989, 1991). Many of the interrelationships cited above as developing soon after birth do not materialize in peer-reared rhesus infants (Kraemer et al. 1989). This suggests that important aspects of neurobiological organization are attributable to infant–mother attachment and do not occur if the infant monkey has peer companionship but no mother (Kraemer et al. 1991).

MECHANISMS THAT PROMOTE OR FACILITATE SELF-REPAIR

When thinking about continuity and discontinuity, it is important to focus on the construct of the attachment system, namely the IWM and what might influence changes to it. Developmental research has shown that once a set of affect-laden experiences and interactions form a set of representations of self and other, those representations are resistant to change. However, Bowlby maintained that IWMs can be and are constantly updated, thus retaining the potential for change across the lifespan (Bowlby 1982, pp. 126–136).

Looking at changes to attachment representations among children who suffered maltreatment and were subsequently placed in permanent adoptive homes could be especially revealing. Steele et al. (2003) demonstrated that even children who bring a set of negative representations of caregivers and themselves to new attachment relationships are influenced by new interactions in a rather immediate way. That is, over the course of a two-year period, a decrease in negative representations and an increase in positive representations on measures derived from story telling can be observed. Children begin to depict attachment figures as being capable of providing care, protection, and acknowledgement of distress in the child and show a decrease in representations of the adult as unable to deliver care (i.e., depictions of adults as injured or dead). The children with the least chance for change are those that have been placed with mothers rated as "Unresolved" on the Adult Attachment Interview (AAI). Here, children show a propensity for aggressive themes in their stories. Interestingly, even when there are changes in the ratio of positive themes across the sample, what remains are themes of disorganized representations such as bizarre and atypical depictions.

Intervention and How Change Transpires

Daniel Stern (1995) has reviewed a variety of parent–infant psychotherapy paradigms ranging from those that focus on maternal behavior and parenting style to those that focus on the mother's representations of attachment from her own childhood history. Stern postulates that it may be the case that where one intervenes in the cycle of maternal attachment representations → maternal sensitivity → infant responsiveness → infant attachment sequence may not matter, as each junction impacts the system and can create change in it.

Hypervigilance

One of the interesting features that we sometimes see in the interactions between previously maltreated children and their attachment figures is that of a hypervigilant state or tendency. For these children, the need to be hypervigilant makes sense in terms of their survival in highly charged, often inconsistent, unpredictable, and dangerous contexts. For these children, to be ultrasensitive to the contents of the caregiver's mind may represent a highly adaptive strategy. However, if these children are set in the context of a caregiving environment, where the caregiver is also hypervigilant to the nuances of the child's state of mind and behavioral expressions, then a less than optimal situation may result (e.g., a child who cowers as if ready to be physically stuck in response to a parent reaching for the salt across the dinner table). For the parent who may themselves be unresolved with regard to past losses or trauma, there may be a tendency to interpret the child's behavior in the context of their own mental state ruminations rather than being able to reflect upon the behavior from the child's perspective. Based on the data of Steele et al. (2003), the perseverance of the hypervigilant state in the child can be ameliorated by the careful, sensitive, and reflective interactions initiated by the mother or in response to interactions initiated by the child. In this way, a new narrative can build in the child's mind, with the affective and cognitive features of a more secure type of narrative.

Attachment and Other Motivational Systems, as Related to the Therapeutic Context: Adults

Attachment dynamics have been extensively studied in relation to a few other motivational systems, as personality development unfolds. We know much concerning the complex dialectics between attachment and exploration, both in "attachments for care" and in "attachments for companionship as shared exploration and play" (Grossmann and Grossmann, and C. Trevarthen, both in this volume). We also know much concerning the relation between attachment in infancy and parental caregiving in adulthood, as it has been studied within the paradigm of intergenerational attachment.

Attachment disorganization suggests that we pay attention to other, less familiar reciprocal influences between attachment and different motivational systems. For instance, in disorganized infants the care-seeking and the defense system are activated simultaneously toward the same person (Liotti 2000). Later on, when disorganized infants grow up to become controlling children, it seems that the care-seeking and the caregiving systems may work together in controlling caregiving strategies, or that the care-seeking and competitive ranking (i.e., dominance-submission) systems may be simultaneously active in controlling-punitive strategies. Perhaps much of psychopathological development could be studied and understood in terms of abnormal dialectics between attachment and other motivations (examples of abnormal dialectics being provided by attachment disorganization).

How do mental states and IWMs of attachment change during the psychotherapy of adult patients with borderline personality disorder (BPD) and dissociative identity disorders (DID)? There is an ongoing study of the psycho-therapy process with BPD/DID patients, based on M. Linehan's Manual of Dialectic Behavior Therapy (DBT). Two therapists, strictly collaborating but operant in independent settings (usually but not always individual and group setting), are involved in the treatment of each patient.

An analysis of the transcripts of therapeutic sessions allows for the assessment of patients' metacognitive capacity at the beginning of treatment and in its later phases. The assessment procedures have been derived from the AAI and Fonagy's Reflective Self-Scale (RSS). They allow for separate evaluations of components of metacognition; that is, the ability to identify mental states, the ability to discriminate between mental states (e.g., of shame and of guilt), and the ability to provide one's narratives with coherence. Preliminary data from this study could contribute to the clarification of how adult IWMs may change in therapy (R. Framba, pers. comm.; E. Prunetti, pers. comm.):

1. An immediate increase in the ratings of a patient's metacognition have been observed in a session of individual therapy following the engagement of the second therapist (E. Prunetti, pers. comm.) — in sporadic cases when the second therapist was available only a few months after the beginning of the first individual therapy (because of difficulties with the availability of therapeutic resources).
2. At the beginning of treatment, following the therapist's (manualized) interventions aimed at "validating" the patient's emotions, there is, usually, a within-session *increase* in the patient's ability to identify/discriminate mental states, and a concurrent *decrease* in the coherence of narrative.
3. Later during the course of treatment, these two components of metacognition usually come into alignment, with both being fostered in response to "validating" interventions.

According to attachment theory, a plausible interpretation of these data is that:

1. BPD/DID patients often come from a dramatic history of disorganized attachment that brings with it three related consequences: (a) expressions of multiple, dramatically unintegrated IWMs, which become active whenever the patient's attachment wishes/needs are evoked by mental pain, separations, etc.; (b) easily evoked fear of being abandoned (a central diagnostic features of BPD); (c) context-dependent deficits of metacognition. These deficits are contingent on activation of the attachment system and the dramatic split/multiple representations of self-with-other composing the IWM of disorganized attachment (Liotti 2000).

   The engagement of the second therapist reduces the fear of being abandoned: "two secure bases are better than only one" (Liotti 2000). This is accompanied by less frequent activation of the attachment system within the first therapeutic relationship. Consequently, an exercise of metacognition closer to the optimum becomes (transiently) possible.

2. The experience of having one's emotions "validated" by an empathic (i.e., caregiving) therapist fosters a feeling of security in the patient, and this becomes the basis for exploring his/her inner world more freely. This shows up as increased capacity to identify mental states. However, the unintegrated IWMs of self-with-other are also activated concurrently with an activation of the patient's attachment system. The activation of an unintegrated self-representation hampers the integrative functions of consciousness; this accounts for the observed *decrease in coherence* of within-session narratives.

3. As favorable attachment interactions (with both therapists) accumulate over time, a patient's IWM changes. It is not clear whether it changes through the construction of a new, more unitary/coherent IWM, which temporarily "displaces" the old IWM, or through integration of the previously split/dissociated representations of self-with-other composing the old IWM. This change, however, is heralded by the fact that the two components of metacognition, identifying mental states and coherence of narrative, come into alignment in showing a simultaneous increase as a response to "validating" interventions.

IMPLICATIONS FOR ADVANCES IN TREATMENT AND CLINICAL INTERVENTION

Our final topic concerns the relational and communication processes that mediate behavior and physiological regulation. A recent meta-analysis examined the effects of a variety of random assignment interventions aimed at promoting maternal sensitivity and or attachment security (Bakermans-Kranenburg et al. 2003). Results revealed that the most effective interventions were not large scale or extremely ambitious in terms of targeting multiple foci (e.g., provide social support, enhance maternal IWM, focus upon parenting skill), but rather ones that took a narrow, parenting-skill development approach and which were of short rather than long duration. It appeared like the more that an intervention tried to do and the longer it lasted, the less likely it was to either enhance maternal sensitivity or foster attachment security. Moreover, in the few studies that focused upon sensitivity and attachment security as outcomes of intervention, evidence emerged that the effect of the intervention on attachment security was via its effect on maternal sensitivity. The latter finding is consistent with an earlier meta-analysis by van IJzendoorn et al. (1995), which showed that sensitivity, however operationalized, was predictive of security (to a modest, but significant extent). However, very different conclusions emerged from a recent meta-analysis of intervention studies attempting to reduce the incidence of disorganized forms of attachment (Juffer et al. 2005).

Knowledge about attachment and bonding is of relevance for intervention in individuals with attachment disorders or disorganized attachment patterns.

Moreover, it has important implications for the diagnostic process, prevention, and treatment of a great variety of other mental disorders and even physical illnesses. Some important points concerning intervention with disorganized/controlling families are outlined below. Implications for the diagnostic procedure as well as the integration of psychological and biological information are highlighted. The interdependence between attachment research and intervention from a more general point of view is discussed. Finally, an example designed to illustrate how attachment research and treatment strategies could be mutually stimulating in the future is provided.

Intervening with Disorganized/Controlling Families

Intervention programs designed to modify disorganized attachment strategies have generally focused on the parent–infant relationship. Treatment goals have usually included building a warm therapeutic relationship to provide a corrective emotional experience for the parent, helping the parent to understand the effects of prior relationships on current feelings and interactions, coaching the parent on sensitive, age-appropriate responses to the child's signals, and connecting the family to additional resources. These interventions are based on attachment literature, which show that developing a relationship can serve as a regulatory function and has the potential to increase security. The goal is to change regulatory processes so that the parent responds to challenge or surprise in an organized way.

Therapeutic results in disorganized/controlling families have been mixed. Comparisons among existing studies are complicated by variable sample characteristics, design and length of treatments, as well as type and timing of outcome measures. Interventions that have successfully prevented or changed disorganized attachment classifications in infancy have involved more clinically impaired populations and have been characterized by frequent home visits with parent and infant over longer periods of time: 42 visits over 12 months (Heinicke et al. 1999) and 47 visits over 18 months (Lyons-Ruth et al. 1990). Less successful interventions have typically been shorter and conducted with lower risk families: 3 visits (van den Boom 1994; 4 visits (Bakermans-Kranenburg et al. 2003). To date the evidence suggests that longer and more intensive interventions may be necessary to modify deeply entrenched disorganized attachment representations and behaviors.

Outside the attachment tradition, an array of early intervention models for stressed low-income parents have now shown positive long-term effects on child and adolescent life outcomes and decreased aggression (Lyons-Ruth et al. 2005; Hennighausen and Lyons-Ruth, this volume). Thoughtful clinical models and additional well-designed controlled treatment trials are now needed to evaluate which service designs best meet the needs of children with disorganized attachment patterns and their parents. Randomized intervention trials constitute one of the strongest methodologies for assessing basic causal mechanisms involved in the development and maintenance of disorganized/controlling attachment strategies.

Intervention strategies are complicated by indications that the disorganized attachment spectrum encompasses dramatically different subgroups (Hennighausen and Lyons-Ruth, this volume). This increased variability complicates assessment and makes it unlikely that a single treatment approach will be effective for all families. Therefore, interventions around parenting will need to be flexible and responsive to these wide individual differences in the maladaptive behaviors displayed. Taken together, effective intervention programs to modify disorganized attachment strategies are characterized by a moderate duration and by targeting specific foci.

Diagnostic/Assessment Procedures

Because of the attachment focus, diagnostic procedures need to focus more on the past and present relational context, as well as the function of the symptomatic behavior in its ecological context. From an attachment perspective we would also assess IWMs or the appraisal processes by which the individual assesses his/her experiences within its ecological context. It is difficult to specify what biological systems might be of special relevance to assess changes in attachment on a physiological basis. Within the outcome measures that have some research validation, cortisol reactivity shows the strongest correlations with the attachment system. In addition, the dopamine D4 receptor gene (DRD4) has been linked to attachment disorganization (Lakatos et al. 2000). Based on animal models, it is likely that a number of neurochemical systems are involved in and affected by the attachment relationship. There is a strong need to develop further measurement techniques (e.g., oxytocin) that can be used in children to establish their relationship to attachment. In summary, implementing aspects from attachment theory adds several important foci to the diagnostic process.

Attachment Research and Intervention

When looking at research on attachment and bonding from a clinical perspective, it is important to consider how study results can be applied to intervention. We see attachment as a process that becomes not only relevant after stress or threat, but as a phenomenon that enables the individual to regulate her/himself in contact with significant others. Therefore, attachment theory should be applied not only for secondary (identify and treat asymptomatic subjects with risk factors or preclinical disease) and tertiary prevention measures (therapy of disease), but also for primary prevention measures (prevention of the onset of a targeted condition) (see U.S. Preventative Services Task Force 1996).

Attachment theory can help develop preventive measures that are applicable for single individuals (children, adolescents, adults, elderly persons), but also for dyads, families, or groups. As the formation of bonds is strongly influenced by cultural and societal traditions and regulations, even action on the level of the society can be informed by results from the field of attachment theory (see Pedersen et al., this volume).

As described by Leckman et al. (this volume), research in the field of attachment and bonding includes studies on different animal species (especially mammals) as well as humans from behavioral and physiological perspectives. Therefore, interventions derived from attachment research can target physiological, mental, or behavioral processes or a combination thereof, by intervening on a biological (e.g., medication), psychological (e.g., psychotherapy, counseling), or societal level (e.g., policy making). As these levels are cross-linked, intervention on one will usually lead to changes on different levels: the administration of drugs (e.g., selective serotonin reuptake inhibitors) will not only change brain physiology, but also behavior; moreover, psychotherapy, which aims to improve interpersonal functioning (Klerman 1984), alleviates depressive symptoms and also leads to changes in neurotransmitter activity (e.g., Brody et al. 2001).

Over the last decades, attachment theory and intervention have been brought together in different ways, and can be summarized in three categories:

1. "Bringing forward": Several attachment researchers have discussed the relevance of their findings for clinical interventions (e.g., Bowlby 1978).
2. "Taking backward": There have been several attempts to interpret and better understand the effects of interventions (e.g., psychotherapy) with the help of attachment theory (Lewis 2000).
3. "Translating": Several groups have developed and successfully applied intervention strategies that are based on attachment theory, e.g., "interpersonal psychotherapy" (Klerman 1984) which focuses on relations of the patient with significant others and has been found to be effective for depression and several other forms of psychopathology (Perry et al. 1999; Thase et al. 1997), or the attachment theory informed model of "preschooler–parent psychotherapy" (Toth et al. 2002).

From our point of view, all three approaches can be very beneficial in integrating attachment theory into clinical use. We even believe that they are most effective when brought together. "Bringing forward" helps clinicians or clinical researchers invent new forms or refine interventions. Researchers who keep "bringing forward" in mind might also design their studies in such a way that they become more relevant for intervention. "Taking backwards" helps clinicians to increase the theoretical and empirical basis of their activities. Moreover, it can point out the weaknesses and needs for further research activities. Both can lead to a "translation" of attachment theory into interventions that then should be refined and assessed for their effectiveness and efficacy.

We want to illustrate these processes with the following example, which demonstrates how research results from a psychological and physiological level can be brought together for the development of clinical interventions:

It has been shown that a weekly supportive group therapy in patients with metastatic breast cancer augments the time of survival from 18.9 to 36.6 months (Spiegel and Sephton 2001). Taking these results backwards, we can hypothesize that the supportive group therapy allows the patients to create new bonds which help them regulate physiologic reactions to stressors. From animal studies on the biological basis of attachment, we know that oxytocin is a key player in the regulation of bonds (Young et al. 2001). Moreover oxytocin dampens the HPA axis responses to stress (Neumann et al. 2000). Bringing the results forward, it has been suggested that oxytocin is the physiological link between positive social interactions and suppression of the HPA axis (DeVries et al. 2003). Relatively high cortisol can negatively influence natural killer cell activity that is important in the defense against tumors (Spiegel and Sephton 2001). Greater quality of social support is associated with lower cortisol concentrations in women with metastatic breast cancer (Turner-Cobb et al. 2000). Based on the "bringing forward" and "taking backward" approaches, future research could focus on such questions as: How can group therapy be improved to strengthen the creation of new bonds and relationships of the patients? What characteristics of these bonds and relationships are relevant to increase the dampening effects of oxytocin on the HPA axis, and how can bonds with these characteristics be fostered in the patients? Answers to these questions will help improve the intervention for patients with metastatic breast cancer. Taken together, we hope that researchers from the field of attachment and bonding and clinicians will interact more to foster the translation of psychological and biological research results into interventions.

CONCLUSIONS AND COMMENTS

The central issue for Bowlby and for this Dahlem Workshop has not yet been resolved: How do we translate theory and scientific findings into clinical practice? For this to happen, there needs to be a better bridge between theories and systems in psychology and neuroscience. There are at least four broad (psychological) models of the influence of early experiences on long-term development (O'Connor 2003; Thompson 2001):

1. "Programming" model: Early experiences exert a lasting effect because of the early malleability of biological (or personality or conceptual) systems that become subsequently less plastic. Evidence for this model often derives from studies of animals or human infants exposed to antenatal or early postnatal stressors (e.g., Barker 1998; O'Connor et al. 2003).

2. "Developmental sensitivity" model: Effects of particular events or experiences depend on the developmental period in which they occur. Contrary to the programming model, early experiences are not necessarily formative. Experiences occurring at later ages (such as giving birth) can have an equal developmental influence.

3. "Cumulative experience" model: Both early and later influences are important. Early experiences have an enduring effect when they are maintained or supported by subsequent experiences. Conversely, early adversity does not necessarily impair healthy development if it is corrected and replaced by supportive care (Clarke and Clarke 2000).

4. "Cognitive/affective processing" model: The effect of early experiences on long-term development depends on how these events are interpreted and/or internalized by the individual. Like the cumulative experience model, the relationship between early influences and later development are probabilistic rather than deterministic.

Psychological and psychobiological theories need to be brought into closer alignment or amalgamated. Presently, it is not possible to assess whether or how interactions among early attachment experiences and neurobiological predisposing factors might promote and sustain maladaptive behavior. For example, if an infant arrives with what now would be considered a subtle neurobiological problem, and if there is no means to assess that, then preventative measures cannot be implemented when they might be most effective and, failing that, subsequent developmental difficulties may be assigned to other causes.

The practical approaches to promoting and limiting neurobiological plasticity need to be better understood. Contemporary studies on multiple neurotransmitter, neuromodulator, and neuroendocrine systems indicate that the neurobiological substrates of attachment mechanisms can be identified. It is also clear that biologically active chemicals (drugs) can alter behaviors associated with attachment, separation, and loss (i.e., protest, despair, and detachment), or early social isolation, neglect, and perhaps abuse. We have much to do before we fully understand the psychopharmacology of attachment mechanisms. Pragmatic, moral, and ethical applications of any new found knowledge in this domain to clinical issues will depend on improved assessment. One should have a neurobiological problem before a neurobiological fix is implemented.

An objective for the future is to develop and encourage a cross-disciplinary approach to research on attachment and psychosocial development spanning biological and social-cultural levels of analysis. One major impediment to this is that different constructs and concepts related to "attachment" are used by investigators in different disciplines. In some cases there is also a lack of clarity and rigor in definition and use of constructs within a discipline. Therefore, clarifying concepts and improving communication may be the first step in promoting interdisciplinary research.

REFERENCES

Ainsworth, M.D.S., M.C. Blehar, E. Waters, and S. Wall. 1978. Patterns of Attachment: A Psychological Study of the Strange Situation. Hillsdale, NJ: Erlbaum.

Astington, J.W., and J.M. Jenkins. 1999. A longitudinal study of the relation between language and theory-of-mind development. *Dev. Psychol.* **35**:1311–1320.

Bakermans-Kranenburg, M.J., M.H. van IJzendoorn, and F. Juffer. 2003. Less is more: Meta-analyses of sensitivity and attachment interventions in early childhood. *Psychol. Bull.* **129**:195–215.

Bar Haim, Y., D.B. Sutton, N.A. Fox, and R.S. Marvin. 2000. Stability and change of attachment at 14, 24, and 58 months of age: Behavior, representation, and life events. *J. Child Psychol. Psych. Allied Disc.* **41**:381–388.

Barker, D.J. 1998. *In utero* programming of chronic disease. *Clin. Sci.* **95**:115–128.

Barr, C.S., T.K. Newman, M.L. Becker et al. 2003. Serotonin transporter gene variation is associated with alcohol sensitivity in rhesus macaques exposed to early-life stress. *Alcohol. Clin. Exp. Res.* **27**:812–817.

Belsky, J., S.B. Campbell, J.F. Cohn, and G. Moore. 1996. Instability of infant–parent attachment security. *Dev. Psychol.* **32**:921–924.

Belsky, J., L. Steinberg, and P. Draper. 1991. Childhood experience, interpersonal development and reproductive strategy: An evolutionary theory of socialization. *Child Dev.* **62**:647–670.

Bennett, A.J., K.P. Lesch, A. Heils et al. 2002. Early experience and serotonin transporter gene variation interact to influence primate CNS function. *Molec. Psychiatry* **7**:118–122.

Bernstein, I.S., and C. Ehardt. 1986. The influence of kinship and socialization on aggressive behaviour in rhesus monkeys (*Macaca mulatta*). *Anim. Behav.* **34**:739–747.

Blair, C. 2002. Early intervention for low birth weight preterm infants: The role of negative emotionality in the specification of effects. *Dev. Psychopathol.* **14**:311–332.

Bowlby, J. 1951. Maternal Care and Mental Health. New York: Columbia Univ. Press. Abridged version: Child Care and the Growth of Love. Harmondsworth: Penguin, 2nd ed., 1965.

Bowlby, J. 1969. Attachment. Attachment and Loss, vol. 1. New York: Basic.

Bowlby, J. 1978. Attachment theory and its therapeutic implications. *Adolesc. Psychiatry* **6**:5–33.

Bowlby, J. 1982. Attachment and loss: Retrospect and prospect. *Am. J. Orthopsychiatry* **52**:664–678.

Bowlby, J. 1988. A Secure Base: Parent–Child Attachment and Healthy Human Development. New York: Basic.

Brody, A.L., S. Saxena et al. 2001. Brain metabolic changes associated with symptom factor improvement in major depressive disorder. *Biol. Psychiatry* **50**:171–178.

Bruner, J.S. 1990. Acts of Meaning. Cambridge, MA: Harvard Univ. Press.

Caspi, A., K. Sugden, T.E. Moffitt et al. 2003. Influence of life stress on depression: Moderation by a polymorphism in the 5-HTT gene. *Science* **301**:386–389.

Cheney, D., R. Seyfarth, and B. Smuts. 1986. Social relationships and social cognition in nonhuman primates. *Science* **234**:1361–1366.

Chisholm, J. 1999. Death, Hope, and Sex: Steps to an Evolutionary Ecology of the Mind and Morality. New York: Cambridge Univ. Press.

Clarke, A.M., and A.D.B. Clarke. 2000. Early Experience and the Life Path. London: Kingsley.

Clarke, A.S. 1993. Social rearing effects on HPA axis activity over early development and in response to stress in young rhesus monkeys. *Dev. Psychobiol.* **26**:433–447.

Clarke, A.S., D.J. Wittwer, D.H. Abbott, and M.L. Schneider. 1994. Long-term effects of prenatal stress on HPA axis activity in juvenile rhesus monkeys. *Dev. Psychobiol.* **27**:257–270.

Damasio, A.R. 1999. The Feeling of What Happens: Body, Emotion and the Making of Consciousness. London: Heinemann.

DeVries, A.C., E.R. Glasper, and C.E. Detillion. 2003. Social modulation of stress responses. *Physiol. Behav.* **79**:399–407.

Donald, M. 2001. A Mind So Rare: The Evolution of Human Consciousness. New York: Norton.

Easterbrooks, M.A., and W.A. Goldberg. 1990. Security of toddler–parent attachment: Relation to children's sociopersonality functioning during kindergarten. In: Attachment in the Preschool Years: Theory, Research, and Intervention, ed. M.T. Greenberg and D. Cicchetti, pp. 221–244. Chicago: Univ. of Chicago Press.

Edelman, G.M. 1989. Topobiology. *Sci Am.* **260**:76–89.

Freeman, W. 1999. How Brains Make up Their Minds. London: Weidenfeld & Nicolson.

Frodi, A., L. Bridges, and W. Grolnick. 1985. Correlates of mastery-related behavior: A short-term longitudinal study of infants in their second year. *Child Dev.* **56**:1291–1298.

Grossmann, K.E., and K. Grossmann. 1991. Attachment quality as an organizer of emotional and behavioral responses in a longitudinal perspective. In: Attachment across the Life Cycle, ed. C.M. Parkes and J. Stevenson-Hinde, pp. 93–114. New York: Tavistock/Routledge.

Harlow, H.F., M.K. Harlow, and S.J. Suomi. 1971. From thought to therapy: Lessons from a primate laboratory. *Am. Sci.* **59**:538–549.

Harris, J.R. 2000a. The outcome of parenting: What do we really know? *J. Pers.* **68**: 625–637.

Harris, J.R. 2000b. Socialization, personality development, and the child's environments: Comment on Vandell. *Dev. Psychol.* **36**:711–723.

Harris, P.L. 1998. Fictional absorption: Emotional responses to make-believe. In: Intersubjective Communication and Emotion in Early Ontogeny, ed. S. Bråten, pp. 336–353. Cambridge: Cambridge Univ. Press.

Heinicke, C.M., N.R. Fineman, G. Ruth et al. 1999. Relationship-based intervention with at-risk mothers: Outcome in the first year of life. *Infant Mental Hlth. J.* **20**:349–374.

Higley, J.D., S.J. Suomi, and M. Linnoila. 1991. CSF monoamine metabolite concentrations vary according to age, rearing, and sex, and are influenced by the stressor of social separation in rhesus monkeys. *Psychopharm.* **103**:551–556.

Higley, J.D., S.J. Suomi, and M. Linnoila. 1992. A longitudinal study of CSF monoamine metabolite and plasma cortisol concentrations in young rhesus monkeys: Effects of early experience, age, sex, and stress on continuity of individual differences. *Biol. Psychiatry* **32**:127–145.

Hobson, P. 2002. The Cradle of Thought: Exploring the Origins of Thinking. London: Macmillan.

Hofer, M.A. 1987. Early social relationships: A psychobiologist's view. *Child Dev.* **58**: 633–647.

Holstege, G., R. Bandler, and C.B. Saper, eds. 1996. The Emotional Motor System, vol. 107. Amsterdam: Elsevier.

Hrdy, S.B. 1999. Mother Nature: A History of Mothers, Infants and Natural Selection. New York: Pantheon.

Juffer, F., M.H. van IJzendoorn, and M.J. Bakermans-Kranenburg. 2005. Enhancing children's socio-emotional development: A review of intervention studies. In Handbook of Research Methods in Developmental Science, ed. D.M. Teti, pp. 213–232. Oxford: Blackwell.

Klerman, G.L. 1984. Interpersonal Psychotherapy of Depression. New York: Basic.

Kraemer, G.W. 1992a. Psychobiological Attachment Theory (PAT) and psychopathology. Behav. Brain Sci. 15:525–534.

Kraemer, G.W. 1992b. A psychobiological theory of attachment. Behav. Brain Sci. 15:493–511.

Kraemer, G.W. 1997. Psychobiology of early social attachment in rhesus monkeys: Clinical implications. Ann. NY Acad. Sci. 807:401–418.

Kraemer, G., and J. Bachevalier. 1998. Cognitive changes associated with persisting behavioral effects of early psychosocial stress in rhesus monkeys: A view from psychobiology. In: Adversity, Stress, and Psychopathology, ed. B. Dohrenwend, pp. 438–462. Oxford: Oxford Univ. Press.

Kraemer, G.W., and A.S. Clarke. 1996. Social attachment, brain function, and aggression. Ann. NY Acad. Sci. 794:121–135.

Kraemer, G.W., M.H. Ebert, C.R. Lake, and W.T. McKinney. 1984. Hypersensitivity to d-amphetamine several years after early social deprivation in rhesus monkeys. Psychopharm. 82:266–271.

Kraemer, G.W., M.H. Ebert, D.E. Schmidt, and W.T. McKinney. 1989. A longitudinal study of the effects of different rearing environments on cerebrospinal fluid norepinephrine and biogenic amine metabolites in rhesus monkeys. Neuropsychopharm. 2:175–189.

Kraemer, G.W., M.H. Ebert, D.E. Schmidt, and W.T. McKinney. 1991. Strangers in a Strange Land: A psychobiological study of mother–infant separation in rhesus monkeys. Child Dev. 62:548–566.

Kraemer, G.W., and W.T. McKinney. 1985. Social separation increases alcohol consumption in rhesus monkeys. Psychopharm. 86:182–189.

Lakatos, K., Z. Nemoda, I. Toth et al. 2000. Dopamine D4 receptor (DRD4) gene polymorphism as associated with attachment disorganization in infants. Molec. Psychiatry 5:633–637.

Leckman, J.F., and L.C. Mayes. 1998. Understanding developmental psychopathology: How useful are evolutionary perspectives? J. Am. Acad. Child Adoles. Psychiatry 37:1011–1021.

Lewis, J.M. 2000. Repairing the bond in important relationships: A dynamic for personality maturation. Am. J. Psych. 157:1375–1378.

Lewis, M. 1990. Challenges to the study of developmental psychopathology. In: Handbook of Developmental Psychopathology, ed. M. Lewis and S.M. Miller, pp. 29–40. New York: Plenum.

Liotti, G. 2000. Disorganized attachment, models of borderline states and evolutionary psychotherapy. In: Genes on the Couch: Explorations in Evolutionary Psychotherapy, ed. P. Gilbert and K.G. Bailey, pp. 232–256. London: Brunner-Routledge.

Locke, J. 1993. Child's Path to Spoken Language. Cambridge, MA: Harvard Univ. Press.

Lubach, G.R., C.L. Coe, and W. Ershler. 1995. Effects of early rearing environment on immune responses of infant rhesus monkeys. Brain Behav. Immun. 9:31–46.

Lubach, G.R., E.M.W. Kittrell, and C.L. Coe. 1992. Maternal influences on body temperature in the primate infant. Physiol. Behav. 51:987–994.

Lyons-Ruth, K., D.B. Connell, H.U. Grunebaum, and S. Botein. 1990. Infants at social risk: Maternal depression and family support services as mediators of infant development and security of attachment. *Child Dev.* 61:85–98.

Lyons-Ruth, K., C. Yellin, S. Melnick, and G. Atwood. 2005. Expanding the concept of unresolved mental states: Hostile/helpless states of mind on the Adult Attachment Interview are associated with disrupted mother–infant communication and infant disorganization. *Dev. Psychopath.*, in press.

Main, M. 1983. Exploration, play, and cognitive functioning related to infant-mother attachment. *Infant Behav. Dev.* 6:167–174.

Main, M., and J. Solomon. 1990. Procedures for identifying infants as disorganized/disoriented during the Ainsworth Strange Situation. In: Attachment in the Preschool Years: Theory, Research, and Intervention, ed. M. Greenberg, D. Cicchetti, and E.M. Cummings, pp. 121–160. Chicago: Univ. of Chicago Press.

Malloch, S. 1999. Mother and infants and communicative musicality. In: Rhythms, Musical Narrative, and the Origins of Human Communication: Musicae Scientiae, spec. iss. 1999–2000, ed. I. Deliège, pp. 29–57. Liège, Belgium: European Society for the Cognitive Sciences of Music.

Marci, C.D., and S.P. Orr. 2003. Psychophysiologic Correlates of Empathy. Psychiatry Research Conference. Cambridge, MA: Harvard Medical School.

Maslin-Cole, C., and S.J. Spieker. 1990. Attachment as a basis for independent motivation. In: Attachment in the Preschool Years: Theory, Research, and Intervention, ed. M.T. Greenberg, D. Cicchetti, and E.M. Cummings, pp. 245–272. Chicago: Univ. of Chicago Press.

Matas, L., R.A. Arend, and L.A. Sroufe. 1978. Continuity of adaptation in the second year: The relationship between quality of attachment and later competence. *Child Dev.* 49:547–556.

McElwain, N.L., M.J. Cox, M.R. Burchinal, and J. Macfie. 2003. Differentiating among insecure mother-infant attachment classifications: A Focus on child-friend interaction and exploration during solitary play at 36 months. *Attach. Hum. Dev.* 5:136–164.

Meins, E. 1997. Security of Attachment and the Social Development of Cognition. London: Psychology Press.

Murray, L., C. Kempton, M. Woolgar, and R. Hooper. 1993. Depressed mothers' speech to their infants and its relation to infant gender and cognitive development. *J. Child Psychol. Psychiat.* 34:1083–1101.

Murray, L., and C. Trevarthen. 1985. Emotional regulation of interactions between two-month-olds and their mothers. In: Social Perception in Infants, ed. T.M. Field and N.A. Fox, pp. 177–119. Norwood, NJ: Ablex.

Murray, L., M. Woolgar, S. Briers, and A. Hipwell. 1999. Children's social representations in dolls' house play and theory of mind tasks, and their relation to family adversity and child disturbance. *Soc. Dev.* 8:179–200.

Nadel, J., I. Carchon, C. Kervella, D. Marcelli, and D. Réserbat-Plantey. 1999. Expectancies for social contingency in 2-month-olds. *Dev. Sci.* 2:164–173.

Neumann, I.D., S.A. Kromer, N. Toschi, and K. Ebner. 2000. Brain oxytocin inhibits the (re)activity of the hypothalamo-pituitary-adrenal axis in male rats: Involvement of hypothalamic and limbic brain regions. *Regul. Pept.* 96:31–38.

O'Connor, T.G. 2003. Early experiences and psychological development: Conceptual questions, empirical illustrations and implications for intervention. *Dev. Psychopathol.* 15:671–690.

O'Connor, T.G., R.S. Marvin, M. Rutter et al. 2003. Child-parent attachment following early institutional deprivation. *Dev. Psychopathol.* 15:19–38.

Perry, J.C., E. Banon, and F. Ianni. 1999. Effectiveness of psychotherapy for personality disorders. *Am. J. Psych.* **156**:1312–1321.

Plomin, R. 1989. Environment and genes: Determinants of behavior. *Am. Psychol.* **44**:105–111.

Porges, S.W. 1997. Emotion: An evolutionary by-product of the neural regulation of the autonomic nervous system. In: The Integrative Neurobiology of Affiliation, ed. C.S. Carter, B. Kirkpatrick, and I.I. Lederhendler, vol. 807, pp. 62–78. New York: New York Academy of Sciences.

Reddy, V. 2001. Mind knowledge in infancy: Understanding attention and intention in the first year. In: Blackwell Handbook of Infancy Research, ed. G.J. Bremner and A. Fogel, pp. 241–264. New York: Blackwell.

Reddy, V. 2003. On being the object of attention: Implications for self–other consciousness. *Trends Cogn. Sci.* **7**:397–402.

Rogoff, B. 2003. The Cultural Nature of Human Development. Oxford: Oxford Univ. Press.

Sapolsky, R.M. 1990. Stress in the wild. *Sci. Am.* **262**:116–123.

Scarr, S., and K. McCartney. 1993. How people make their own environments: A theory of genotype-environment effects. *Child Dev.* **54**:424–435.

Schölmerich, A., and A. Lengning. 2005. Neugier, Exploration und Bindungsentwicklung. In: Ursprünge und Frühentwicklungen von Bindungsbeziehungen: Ein Lehrbuch, ed. L. Ahnert. Munich: Reinhard.

Schore, A.N. 1994. Affect Regulation and the Origin of the Self: The Neurobiology of Emotional Development. Hillsdale, NJ: Erlbaum.

Schore, A.N. 2003a. Affect Dysregulation and Disorders of the Self. New York: Norton.

Schore, A.N. 2003b. Affect Regulation and the Repair of the Self. New York: Norton.

Selby, J.M., and B.S. Bradley. 2003. Infants in groups: A paradigm for study of early social experience. *Hum. Dev.* **46**:197–221.

Spiegel, D., and S.E. Sephton. 2001. Psychoneuroimmune and endocrine pathways in cancer: Effects of stress and support. *Sem. Clin. Neuropsychiatry* **6**:252–265.

Sroufe, L.A. 1983. Infant-caregiver attachment and patterns of adaptation in preschool: The roots of maladaptation and competence. In: The Minnesota Symposium on Child Psychology, ed. M. Perlmutter, vol. 16, pp. 41–83. Hillsdale, NJ: Erlbaum.

Sroufe, L.A. 1986. Bowlby's contribution to psychoanalytic theory and developmental psychology. *J. Child Psychol. Psychiat.* **27**:841–849.

Steele, M., J. Hodges, J. Kaniuk, S. Hillman, and K. Henderson. 2003. Attachment representations in newly adopted maltreated children and their adoptive parents: Implications for placement and support. *J. Child Psychother.* **29**:187–205.

Stern, D.N. 1995. The motherhood constellation: A unified view of parent–infant psychotherapy. New York: Basic.

Stern, D.N. 1999. Behavioural and neural bases: The temporal contour of feelings as a basic unit for constructing the infant's social experience. In: Early Social Cognition: Understanding Others in the First Months of Life, ed. P. Rochat, pp. 67–90. Mahwah, NJ: Erlbaum.

Stern, D.N. 2000. The Interpersonal World of the Infant: A View from Psychoanalysis and Development Psychology, 2nd ed. New York: Basic.

Stone, E., K. Bonnet, and M.A. Hofer. 1976. Survival and development of maternally deprived rats: Role of body temperature. *Psychosom. Med.* **39**:242–249.

Suess, G. J., K.E. Grossmann, and L.A. Sroufe. 1992. Effects of infant attachment to mother and father on quality of adaptation in preschool: From dyadic to individual organisation to self. *Intl J. Behav. Dev.* **15**:43–62.

Suomi, S.J., and C. Ripp. 1983. A history of motherless monkey mothering at the University of Wisconsin Primate Laboratory. In: Child Abuse: The Non-human Primate Data, ed. M. Reite and N. Caine, pp. 49–78. New York: A.R. Liss.

Tamminga, C.A., C.B. Nemeroff, R.D. Blakely et al. 2002. Developing novel treatments for mood disorders: Accelerating discovery. *Biol. Psychiatry* **52**:589–609.

Taylor, M., and S.M. Carlson. 1997. The relation between individual differences in fantasy and theory of mind. *Child Dev.* **68**:436–455.

Thase, M.E., J.B. Greenhouse, E. Frank et al. 1997. Treatment of major depression with psychotherapy or psychotherapy-pharmacotherapy combinations. *Arch. Gen. Psychiatry* **54**:1009–1015.

Thompson, R.A. 1998. Early sociopersonality development. In: Handbook of Child Psychology, 5th ed.,vol. 3., Social, Emotional, and Personality Development, ed. W. Damon, pp. 25–104. New York: Wiley.

Thompson, R.A. 1999. Early attachment and later development. In: Handbook of Attachment, ed. J. Cassidy and P.R. Shaver, pp. 265–286. New York: Guilford.

Thompson, R.A. 2000. The legacy of early attachments. *Child Dev.* **71**:145–152.

Thompson, R.A. 2001. Sensitive periods in attachment? In: Critical Thinking about Critical Periods, ed. D.B. Bailey, J.T. Bruer, F.J. Symons, and J.W. Lichtman, pp. 83–106. Baltimore: Brookes.

Tomasello, M. 1988. The role of joint attentional processes in early language development. *Lang. Sci.* **10**:69–88.

Toth, S.L., A. Maughan, J.T. Manly, M. Spagnola, and D. Cicchetti. 2002. The relative efficacy of two interventions in altering maltreated preschool children's representational models: Implications for attachment theory. *Dev. Psychopathol.* **14**:877–908.

Trevarthen, C.I. 1979. Communication and cooperation in early infancy: A description of primary intersubjectivity. In: Before Speech: The Beginning of Human Communication, ed. M. Bullowa, pp. 321–347. London: Cambridge Univ. Press.

Trevarthen, C. 2001a. Intrinsic motives for companionship in understanding: Their origin, development and significance for infant mental health. *Infant Mental Hlth. J.* **221**:95–131.

Trevarthen, C.I. 2001b. Neurobiology of early communication. In: Handbook on Brain and Behavior in Human Development, ed. A. Kalverboer and A. Gramsbergen, pp. 841–882. Dordrecht: Kluwer.

Trevarthen, C., and K.J. Aitken. 1994. Brain development, infant communication, and empathy disorders: Intrinsic factors in child mental health. *Dev. Psychopathol.* **6**:599–635.

Trevarthen, C., and K.J. Aitken. 2001. Infant intersubjectivity: Research, theory, and clinical applications: Annual Research Review. *J. Child Psychol. Psychiat. Allied Disc.* **42**:13–48.

Trevarthen, C., and K.J. Aitken. 2003. Regulation of brain development and age-related changes in infants' motives. In: Regression Periods in Human Infancy, ed. M. Heimann and F. Plooij, pp. 107–184. Mahwah, NJ: Erlbaum.

Trevarthen, C., and P. Hubley. 1978. Secondary intersubjectivity confidence, confiding and acts of meaning in the first year. In: Action, Gesture and Symbol: The Emergence of Language, ed. A. Lock, pp. 183–229. London: Academic.

Tronick, E.Z., H. Als, L. Adamson, S. Wise, and T.B. Brazelton. 1978. The infant's response to entrapment between contradictory messages in face-to-face interaction. *J. Am. Acad. Child Psychiatry* **17**:12–13.

Turner-Cobb, J.M., S.E. Sephton, C. Koopman, J. Blake-Mortimer, and D. Spiegel. 2000. Social support and salivary cortisol in women with metastatic breast cancer. *Psychosom. Med.* **62**:337–345.

Tzourio-Mazoyer, N., S. De Schonen, F. Crivello, and B. Reutter. 2002. Neural correlates of woman face processing by 2-month-old infants. *NeuroImage* **15**:454–461.

U.S. Preventative Services Task Force. 1996. Guide to Clinical Preventative Services. Baltimore: Williams and Wilkins.

van den Boom, D.C. 1994. The influence of temperament and mothering on attachment and exploration: An experimental manipulation of sensitive responsiveness among lower-class mothers with irritable infants. *Child Dev.* **65**:1457–1477.

van IJzendoorn, M.H., F. Juffer, and M. Duyvesteyn. 1995. Breaking the intergenerational cycle of insecure attachment: A review of the effects of attachment-based interventions on maternal sensitivity and infant security. *J. Child Psychol. Psychiat.* **36**: 225–248.

Vondra, J.I., D.S. Shaw, L. Swearingen, M. Cohen, and E.B. Owens. 2001. Attachment stability and emotional and behavioral regulation from infancy to preschool age. *Dev. Psychopathol.* **13**:13–33.

Vygotsky, L.S. 1987. Problems of general psychology. In: The Collected Works of L.S. Vygotsky, vol. 1, ed. R.W. Rieber and A.S. Carton. New York: Plenum.

Waters, E., K. Kondo-Ikemura, G. Posada, and J. Richters. 1991. Learning to love: Mechanisms and milestones. In: Self Processes and Development, ed. M.R. Gunnar and L.A. Sroufe, pp. 217–255. Minnesota Symp. on Child Psychology 23. Hillsdale, NJ: Erlbaum.

Werner, E.E. 1989a. Children of the garden island. *Sci. Am.* **260**:106–111.

Werner, E.E. 1989b. High risk children in young adulthood: A longitudinal study from birth to 32 years. *Am. J. Orthopsychiatry* **59**:72–81.

Winnicott, D.W. 1965a/1962. Ego Integration and Child Development. New York: Intl. Univ. Press.

Winnicott, D.W. 1965b/1952. Psychoses and Child Care. New York: Intl. Univ. Press.

Young, L.J., M.M. Lim, B. Gingrich, and T.R. Insel. 2001. Cellular mechanisms of social attachment. *Horm. Behav.* **40**:133–138.

Name Index

Subject Index

Printed in the United States
by Baker & Taylor Publisher Services